Analgesics

From Chemistry and Pharmacology to Clinical Application

Edited by
Helmut Buschmann, Thomas Christoph, Elmar Friderichs,
Corinna Maul, Bernd Sundermann

Further titles of interest

McGuire, John L. (Ed.)
Pharmaceuticals
Classes, Therapeutic Agents, Areas of Application
4 Volumes
2000, ISBN 3-527-29874-6

Molema, Grietje / Meijer, Dirk K. F. (Eds.)
Drug Targeting
Organ-Specific Strategies
2001, ISBN 3-527-29989-0

Negwer, Martin, Scharnow, H.-G.
Organic-Chemical Drugs and Their Synonyms
5 Volumes
2001, ISBN 3-527-30247-6

Smith, Dennis A. / van de Waterbeemd, Han / Walker, Don K.
Pharmacokinetics and Metabolism in Drug Design
2001, ISBN 3-527-30197-6

Analgesics

From Chemistry and Pharmacology to
Clinical Application

Edited by
Helmut Buschmann, Thomas Christoph,
Elmar Friderichs, Corinna Maul,
Bernd Sundermann

with contributions by
Gregor Bahrenberg, Johannes Bartholomäus, Petra Bloms-Funke,
Helmut Buschmann, Thomas Christoph, Werner Englberger,
Robert Frank, Elmar Friderichs, Clemens Gillen,
Hagen-Heinrich Hennies, Ulrich Jahnel, Corinna Maul,
Michael Przewosny, Claudia Pütz, Klaus Schiene, Wolfgang Schröder,
Bernd Sundermann, Thomas Tzschentke

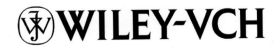

Dr. Gregor Bahrenberg
Dr. Johannes Bartholomäus
Dr. Petra Bloms-Funke
Dr. Helmut Buschmann
Dr. Thomas Christoph
Dr. Werner Englberger
Dr. Robert Frank
Dr. Elmar Friderichs
Dr. Clemens Gillen
Dr. Hagen-Heinrich Hennies
Dr. Ulrich Jahnel
Dr. Corinna Maul
Dr. Michael Przewosny
Dr. Claudia Pütz

Dr. Klaus Schiene
Dr. Wolfgang Schröder
Dr. Bernd Sundermann
Dr. Thomas Tzschentke

Grünenthal GmbH
Center of Research
P.O. Box 50 04 44
52088 Aachen
Germany

Cover picture after an original illustration by René Descartes (17th century)

Library of Congress Card No. applied for.
British Library Cataloguing-in-Publication Data: A catalogue record for this book is available from the British Library.
Die Deutsche Bibliothek - CIP Cataloguing-in-Publication-Data
A catalogue record for this publication is available from Die Deutsche Bibliothek

Preface

Pain has been a human problem since the beginning of time but the last decade has seen an explosion of information about the transmitters, receptors and channels involved in the transmission and modulation of noxious messages generated in peripheral tissues. This has lead to the identification of a number of potential new targets for analgesic therapy. We now have more experimental drugs available, which allows us to study the roles of transmitters and receptors in physiological events. There are now numerous animal models for clinical pain states such as inflammation and neuropathies, and these models have shown that several transmitter systems which have minor actions in acute pains can play important roles in more persistent pains.

This ability to test drugs in contexts other than acute pain models has arisen from good communication between bench scientists, clinicians and industry. Until recently investigations into the mechanisms of clinical pain syndromes all relied on animal studies using acute stimuli. The symptoms of pain arising from nerve injury, neuropathic pain, such as allodynia, spontaneous pain, hyperalgesia, sensory deficits and in some cases a sympathetic component are simply not seen in the older acute models. There are now several animal models which mimic peripheral and central neuropathic states. The same is true for inflammation.

A number of major discoveries over the last thirty years, such as the opioid receptors and the endogenous opioids, the spinal, supraspinal and peripheral sites of action of opioids, the key role of glutamate in signalling in the nervous system, the important actions of peptides such as substance P, the ability of descending controls, both noradrenergic and serotoninergic, to influence pain transmission may not yet have yielded many new drugs but has enormously aided the conceptual basis for understanding pain and analgesia. The Gate Theory of Pain, published in 1965, was the first study to make us think about the ways in which transmission of pain could alter yet the pharmacological details have only recently been eluidated. Plasticity, the capacity of the pain signalling and modulating systems to alter in different circumstances, has changed our ways of thinking about pain control. Signalling events are not fixed, not the same in all pain conditions, but subject to alteration. Types of pain, symptoms of pain, the intensity and area are all factors that alter the pharmacology.

High throughput screening should expedite the identification of useful agents, which, combined with improved combinatorial chemistry, should lead to fast and efficient production of novel agents with good affinity for particular targets. Genomics can be used to identify targets related to specific disease, and, in the field of pain and analgesia, to identify targets associated with particular pathological processes within this area. Here again, the validity of the models will be critical in screening molecules. Realistically many discoveries are still serendipitous, but with a better understanding of the neurobiology of pain their effects can be better verified. Molecular and genetic approaches have recently allowed the identification of channels or receptors that has lead to a far better understanding of the peripheral processes that lead to pain from thermal, chemical and other stimuli. At the level of the peripheral nerve, the roles of particular sodium channels in the generation of activity after tissue damage may provide local-anaesthetic-like drugs that target only pain-related activity. Agents acting on calcium channels that control both neuronal activity and transmitter release also have potential.

Within the last 10, years several new compounds were launched in the field of non-steroidal antiinflammatory drugs (NSAIDs) with a clear focus on cyclooxygenase type 2 selective compounds. In the field of opioids on the other hand no new drugs have passed phase III clinical trials. In this field innovation has been achieved through new pharmaceutical formulations of known drugs such as transdermal systems, e.g. buprenorphine patch, transmucosal systems, e.g. fentanyl lollipop, or rectal delivery systems containing e.g. morphine. These were developed in order to reduce opioid side effects, but also to overcome pharmacokinetical limitations, in particular to prolong compliance and duration of action.

This book deals with established analgesics as well as with new chemical entities for established and new targets. Compounds are classified with respect to their physiological target. In every case the structural formula is given as well as further information e.g. on the pharmacological profile, synthetic routes or major metabolites if important. In addition, structure-activity relationships are discussed if available. Consequently following this scheme, a huge number of compounds is evaluated and a clear picture especially of pain research in the industrial setting is constructed.

Based on the snapshot-like collection of information in this book the cyclooxygenase and the opioid systems are still the most attractive targets and ligands acting on this system are still not surpassed by ligands of other targets. It is also clear, however, that we are at the beginning of an era of promising new approaches to pain therapy. The future will show which targets will survive the race for the best therapy.

The book presented here will be highly valuable for advanced students in pharmaceutical and medicinal chemistry as well as for scientists in the field of chemistry, biochemistry and pharmacology in industrial and academic research.

August 2002

Anthony Dickenson, London
Ulrike Holzgrabe, Würzburg

A View from Grünenthal

Pain research is a traditional and well established field within the pharmaceutical industry. Beginning with the isolation of morphine in a small pharmacy by Adam Sertürner (1806), the next major breakthrough in pain treatment was achieved by the synthesis of acetylsalicylic acid by Felix Hoffmann in the Bayer Laboratories in Wuppertal (1897). Further outstanding contributions by the pharmaceutical industry were the first fully synthetic opioids pethidine (1939) and methadone (1946). Continued efforts up to now have resulted in many potent and clinically accepted analgesics with reasonable side effects and covering nearly all facets of pain treatment. However, pain treatment is far from being satisfactory in respect to more complex pain states, e.g. neuropathy, visceral pain or migraine.

Grünenthal's interest in pain research started in 1962, when Kurt Flick designed a simple molecule containing the essential structural elements of morphine to be a potent analgesic. This prediction was clinically confirmed and today this compound – tramadol – is one of the leading centrally acting analgesics.

Forty years after the discovery of tramadol, research at Grünenthal is still focused on the search for even better analgesics. Due to the intense accumulation of knowledge about pain the idea was born to collect this in a comprehensive overview with the intention to stimulate further scientific efforts in this area. It is our hope that this book will be a useful reference meeting the challenge to improve pain therapy.

Klaus-Dieter Langner and Eric-Paul Pâques

Aachen, August 2002

Contents

Part I

Introduction

1   What is Pain?

Helmut Buschmann

Introduction

Pain is the most common symptomatic reason for seeking a medical consultation.

Everyone is affected by pain at some point in their lives, whether it is from headaches, cuts and bruises or more severe pain resulting from surgery, which would be pre-controlled in anticipation of the event.

Although chronic types of pain may generally appear to have no purpose, acute pain acts as an important warning mechanism to the person by instructing the brain to remove the individual from that particular pain stimulus. If for example a person lifts a hot object, pain signals to the brain to put the object down to avoid severe burns.

The treatment of pain, a major problem in medicine, is complicated by many factors. Pain is not a uniform sensation, as illustrated by its many common descriptions, e.g. sharp, dull, aching, burning, shooting, cramping, stabbing and throbbing. There are several ways to classify pain, but the first distinction usually made is that between acute and chronic pain. Pain is a subjective sensation which cannot be measured objectively, and its intensity is not always a direct reflection of the nociceptive inputs provoking it. Nociceptive inputs which are easily ignored by an individual in one situation may be unbearable in another.

Definition of Pain

Various definitions of pain have been proposed but the most widely accepted is that of the International Association for the Study of Pain (IASP):

Pain - a common phenomenon

Acute pain as a warning mechanism

The treatment of pain, a major problem in medicine

A definition of pain (IASP)

Pain is an unpleasant sensory and emotional experience associated with actual or potential tissue damage, or described in terms of such damage. Pain is always subjective. Each individual learns the application of the word through experiences related to injury in early life. It is unquestionably a sensation in part of the body, but it is also unpleasant and therefore also an emotional experience. Many people report pain in the absence of tissue damage or any likely pathophysiological state; usually this happens for psychological reasons. There is no way to distinguish their experience from that due to tissue damage, if we take this subjective report. If they regard their experience as pain and if they report it in the same way as pain caused by tissue damage, it should be accepted as pain (Merksey, 1979).

Before the 1960s, pain was considered an inevitable sensory response to tissue damage, but since that time the definition has broadened to encompass the affective dimension of pain with greater consideration of the effects of genetic differences, past experience, anxiety and expectation.

...pain remains grossly undertreated and is frequently mistreated...

Research in understanding the underlying mechanisms behind people's pain has progressed rapidly, but despite these critical advances pain remains grossly undertreated and is frequently mistreated. In the words of Jean-Marie Besson, President of the IASP at the 9th IASP Congress in Vienna, Austria, in August 1999: '*Some pain states can now be controlled, yet there are still others which are far from being treatable.*'

Side-effects of analgesics

Pain, as a whole, is currently a very active area for pharmaceutical R&D, largely because of its undertreatment and frequent mistreatment, but also because the older and still widely-used compounds can cause unacceptable side-effects.

Side-effects of NSAIDs

This is especially true for the traditional non-steroidal anti-inflammatory drugs (NSAIDs) which are associated with serious gastrointestinal complications such as bleeding, lesions and ulcers.

Side-effects of central acting analgesics

Conversely, the perceived dangerous side-effects and fears of addiction and tolerance associated with potent opioid analgesics (e.g. morphine) has led to restrictions and controversy regarding their use. Clinical studies, however, have demonstrated that these risks are low and potent opioid analgesics today are more widely accepted for treating severe cancer pain, but experts are still calling for broader use of opioids in non-malignant chronic pain.

Class	2000 sales ($ billion)	% of global sales	% growth (vs. 1999)
Anti-ulcer	17.4	5.5	+ 13
Cholesterol & triglyceride reducers	15.9	5.0	+ 21
Antidepressants	13.4	4.2	+ 18
Calcium antagonists (plain)	9.8	3.1	+ 2
NSAIDs	9.5	3.0	+ 26
ACE inhibitors	7.3	2.3	+ 3
Cephalosporins & combinations	6.9	2.2	- 5
Antipsychotics	6.0	1.9	+ 22
Non-narcotic analgesics	6.0	1.9	+ 3
Oral antidiabetics	5.9	1.9	+ 26

Table 1: Global pharma sales - the leading therapeutic classes.

Source: IMS Health Word Reviews 2001, SCRIP No. 2630, March 30th 2001, p. 18.

Physiology and Pathophysiology of Pain

The physiological aspects of lasting pain become apparent when a mechanical, thermal, chemical or electrical stimulus strong enough to damage tissue or affect cellular metabolism stimulates the nociceptive free nerve endings of C-fibers, which are found all over the surface of the body and its organs. Several subtypes of A-fibers also carry afferent nociceptive impulses. The damaged tissue sends out nerve impulses through nerve tracts in the spinal cord to the brain (cerebral cortex) where the stimulus translates to a conscious pain sensation.

Pain transmission

In addition to nervous pain impulses, injured tissues produce inflammatory pain-producing substances, including bradykinin and other kinins, serotonin, histamine, acetylcholine, excesses of potassium ions, proteolytic enzymes and prostaglandins, which can act in synergy to increase pain levels. Many of these substances, especially the proteolytic enzymes, can cause direct damage to the pain nerve endings, but others, such as bradykinin and prostaglandins, can cause extreme direct stimulation of pain nerve fibers without actually damaging them. Local changes accompanying the injury, such as muscular spasm, ischeamia and inflammation, can also contribute to the intensity and character of the pain.

Contribution of endogenous inflammatory and/or pain-producing substances

Severe and sustained pain can cause long-lasting reflexes in the spinal cord and sympathetic nervous system that can lead to changes in the secretion of hormones and other substances and to a chronic state of increased pain sensitivity known as hyperalgesia. This, in turn, can give rise to pain sensations even in response to non-noxious stimuli that can be difficult to treat. Hyperalgesia characteristically develops during inflammation and research has shown that prostaglandins are the main inflammatory mediators responsible for the development of hyperalgesia. Futhermore, both prostaglandins and leukotrienes play a key role in the sensitization of pain mediating receptors. In fact, the basis for the analgesic actions of non-steroidal anti-inflammatory drugs (NSAIDs) is their ability to prevent the production of prostaglandins.

Peripheral pain mechanisms

Pain receptors in the skin (cutaneous) and other tissues (non-cutaneous) are all free nerve endings. They are widespread in the superficial layers of the skin and in certain internal tissues such as the arterial walls and joints. Most other deep tissues contain few free nerve endings and so tissue damage there is more likely to cause a slow, chronic, dull ache rather than acute pain in these areas.

Different groups of nerve endings

Different groups of nerve endings in the skin relay messages about four basic sensations:

- **Warmth:** very sensitive non-myelinated fibers
- **Cold:** thinly myelinated A-fibers
- **Touch:** mechano-receptive afferent fibers
- **Pain:** nociceptive fibers

Nociceptors

Nociceptors, or nociceptive fibers, are peripheral nerve endings. They are mostly found in the skin but can also be of non-cutaneous origin. Nociception itself is a response to the excitation of these nociceptors, which will only occur after a strong stimulus such as a pinch or knock that may hurt briefly or a more severe injury causing bruising and/or broken skin. The signals transmitted from the nociceptors following this stimulus reach the brain and are interpreted as pain. Although nociception may give rise to the experience of pain, pain may also arise in the absence of nociception. Conversely, nociception may also occur in the absence of pain. The complex relationship between pain and injury is highlighted by the fact that analgesics such as morphine cannot abolish pain due to nerve injury (neuropathic pain) as efficiently as they abolish pain due to tissue damage (nociceptive pain). Furthermore, the intensity of chronic pain frequently bears little relation to the extent of tissue damage, making the perception of pain itself an important issue.

The central nervous system (CNS) - the brain and spinal cord - is involved in the reception and interpretation of peripheral afferent nociceptive impulses. Reflexes mediated by spinal interneurons and the gating functions of the dorsal horn of the spinal cord are particularly crucial. However, our knowledge of brain mechanisms is still limited.

Central pain mechanisms

If a spinal cord is cross-sectioned, the gray matter appears as a roughly H-shaped area in its middle which is, divided into dorsal (posterior), lateral, and ventral (anterior) horns. The horns are interconnected by a crossbar, the gray commissure. The rest of the spinal cord is the white matter, made up largely of tracts of myelinated nerve fibers (axons). Ascending tracts carry afferent sensory impulses towards the brain, descending tracts transmit motor impulses from the brain to the motor neurons in the ventral or lateral horns of the gray matter.

The spinal cord

Neurons in different regions of the gray matter can connect with each other, forming spinal reflex arcs between sensory nerves bringing together noxious stimuli and motor nerves controlling avoidance responses. The behavioral consequences of such spinal reflexes are familiar in everyday life: the eye blinks as an object approaches, the hand is withdrawn from a hot plate, both without conscious control.

... spinal reflexes

The dorsal horn of the spinal cord houses a type of pain-inhibitory complex where the pain signals can be blocked before they are relayed to the brain. The dorsal horn itself contains axons from sensory spinal neurons that pass into the dorsal ascending tracts and to higher levels of the spinal cord and the brain. The neurons in the dorsal horn are immediately involved in the processing of pain signals and the control of pain. Mechanisms by which they modulate pain messages transferred to the brain are referred to as segmental and supraspinal. Nerve tracts ascend from the dorsal horn to parts of the brain, including the periaqueductal gray matter, and on to the cerebral cortex, where the pain is localized to a particular body region. Conscious appreciation of pain occurs in the frontal lobes of the brain.

... the dorsal horn

The dorsal horn of the spinal cord contains many transmitters and receptors. Some of these include: peptides, e.g. substance P, somatostatin and neuropeptide Y; excitatory amino acids, e.g. glutamate and aspartate; inhibitory amino acids, e.g. γ-aminobutyric acid (GABA); nitric oxide; endogenous opioids; adenosine; and the monoamines, e.g. serotonin and noradrenaline. There is, therefore, diverse therapeutic potential for pharmacological control of the transmission of nociceptive information to the brain.

... dorsal horn neurons

Available evidence suggests that the neurons of the dorsal horn do not have fixed functions, that their functional characteristics are modifiable, and that pathological processes can have a potent influence on them. Wall (1989) summarizes three main processes that can affect the functioning of dorsal horn cells and thus, by implication, the experience of pain: gate control, sensitivity control and connectivity control.

... gate control

The widely accepted theory of gate control was put forward by Melzack and Wall (1965). Wall (1978) later restricted the term to describe the immediate reception and control of sensory inputs that lead to effector triggering and sensation. Descending impulses from the raphe nuclei, reticular formation and other regions of the brain affect - and, in particular, inhibit - the activity of neurons in the dorsal horn, where gating functions are thought to be localized. Only when the gate is open does pain information pass to the brain.

... sensitization

Unlike most receptors, nociceptors can become increasingly sensitive after injury (i.e. when the stimulus is very strong) or when the stimulus is continuing or repeated. This sensitization means that there can be a reduction in the threshold for activation (i.e. pain signals will be transmitted in response to even gentle stimuli), an increase in the response to a given stimulus, or even the appearance of spontaneous activity.

Sensitization results from the actions of second messenger systems activated by the release of inflammatory mediators such as the prostaglandins described above. These effects cause some of the features of hyperalgesia produced by pathological processes as opposed to physiological pain that occurs in response to a noxious stimulus. Much of the peripheral sensitization of nociceptors is caused by primary hyperalgesia occurring at the site of the damaged tissue, although some sensitization appears to be due to central mechanisms of hyperexcitability (Besson, 1999).

Pathological pain involves:

- **Allodynia**: a lowered pain threshold
- **Hyperalgesia**: increased responsiveness
- **Hyperpathia**: prolonged pain sensations after the initial stimulus

Psychology of Pain

Organic factors alone cannot explain why different patients report different levels of pain. There is an important psychological reaction to pain that must be assessed and physicians must adopt a comprehensive approach, encompassing psychosocial and behavioral factors as well as organic ones. Melzack and Wall's (1965) gate control theory explains this as the suppression of nociceptive afferent peripheral impulses in the dorsal horn by descending central messages relating to the individual's emotional, cognitive and attention state.

Everyday evidence exists to support the notion that physical pain is closely associated with emotion, cognition and attention. For example, people who have injured themselves whilst participating in a sporting event may not fully realize the extent of their injuries until they stop and their concentration is focused on the injury rather than the game.

Even the placebo effect goes some way towards demonstrating that if patients believe that they are taking a strong drug this will improve their condition and they will start to feel better even if the drug is really an inactive imitation. Similarly, if during an examination patients are advised that nothing is wrong with their health, their mind's logic may be strong enough to convince them that the pain has no pathological cause and therefore does not really exist. The placebo response is of vital importance in pain management and pain research. In the clinical setting, one may seek to optimize the placebo response to achieve a greater success rate during treatment, but in research one aims to rule out the placebo response.

Placebo effect

Although in the majority of cases, a physician would find an underlying pathological cause to explain a patient's physical pain, it is possible for pain to be brought on by emotional disturbances such as a reaction to grief, anxiety (panic disorder), depression or anger (Ray and Yoham 1992). These emotions themselves can be consequences of pain, perhaps even reinforcing each other, or lead to pain. Painful conditions can be mimicked by neuroendocrine and autonomic changes brought on by emotional distress. Furthermore, a great problem for terminally-ill patients is the resulting distress or suffering from the belief that their pain cannot be cured or pain relief improved. This creates a negative outlook leaving the patient with feelings of despair, hopelessness, helplessness and pessimism.

The role of emotions

On the other hand the body can also control pain by producing its own analgesic molecules (endorphins).

Individual perception and tolerance

The way a person relates to pain is in the domain of cognitive psychology. How sufferers cope depends on their own cognitive evaluation of the situation, and if their treatment or prognosis is incorrect the patient will respond inappropriately by over- or under-reacting to it.

Pharmaceutical Pain Management

Analgesics and anesthetics adequately cover pain management and are sometimes used with adjuvant therapies such as sedatives, antidepressants and anxiolytics. In the following sections, and for convenience, general pain therapy will refer to opioid and non-opioid analgesics that normally are given orally (or transdermally). Non-general pain therapy will refer to peripheral localized analgesia and anesthesia, such as that provided by topically applied agents and regional or central blockade methods (nerve blocks, spinal and epidural anesthesia/analgesia).

Principal treatment of pain
- NSAIDs (non-opioid analgesics)
- Opioids
- Adjuvants

At present, the principal treatment for pain are non-steroidal anti-inflammatory drugs (NSAIDs) and opioids, but both of these classes suffer from drawbacks in clinical use. The third group of drugs which is currently used for the treatment of pain is represented by analgesic adjuvants, a class of compounds that include antidepressants and local anesthetics that are used empirically to treat chronic pain states. Some of the NSAIDs are associated with gastric damage as well as kidney and liver toxicity and an increase in blood clotting time, while the opioids can produce tolerance and dependence, along with constipation, nausea, respiratory depression and sedation. In certain pain states, both NSAID and opioid use are ineffective.

Non-opioid analgesics (NSAIDs)

Almost all non-opioid analgesics are non-steroidal anti-inflammatory drugs (NSAIDs) and have varying degrees of analgesic, anti-inflammatory and antipyretic activity. Acetylsalicylic acid (Aspirin®), used to relieve mild to moderate pain and certain types of severe pain, is the archetypal NSAID and is probably the best known and most used therapeutic drug worldwide.

The basis for the analgesic action of NSAIDs is their ability to prevent the production of prostaglandins. Prostaglandins are derived from the arachidonic acid cascade and are implicated in the production of inflammatory pain and in sensitizing nociceptors to the actions of other mediators.

Their antipyretic action means that NSAIDs do not reduce normal body temperature or elevated temperatures in heat stroke, which is due to hypothalamic malfunction. During fever, interleukin-1 (IL-1) is released and acts directly on the thermoregulatory centre in the hypothalamus to increase body temperature. This is associated with an increase in brain prostaglandins. Aspirin prevents the temperature-raising effects ol IL-1 and the rise in brain prostaglandin levels.

Older and still widely-used analgesic compounds can cause unacceptable side-effects. This is especially the case for the traditional non-steroidal anti-inflammatory drugs (NSAIDs) which are associated with serious gastrointestinal complications such as bleeding, lesions and ulcers. Every year it is estimated that 16,500 NSAID-related deaths occur in the US alone, with 75,000 patients hospitalized.

COX-2 selective inhibitors

The main advantage of the highly selective COX-2 inhibitors may be a significant improvement in the unacceptable gastrointestinal side-effects commonly caused by NSAIDs in patients with chronic pain of an inflammatory origin. Other adverse events of conventional NSAIDs include: nephrotoxicity, since prolonged analgesic use over several years is associated with papillary necrosis and chronic renal failure; bronchospasm; skin rash and other allergies.

Opioid analgesics

Opioid analgesics, some of which are the most powerful analgesics (narcotics) are used to relieve moderate to severe pain and can also be used as adjuncts to anesthesia.

Many myths surround the stronger opioids and their use can become restricted when the definitions of addiction, tolerance and physical dependence are confused. Some opioids, e.g. codeine, are less potent and are readily available in OTC products.

Morphine is the gold standard opioid against which all others are compared (McQuay, 1999) and it is the analgesic of choice for terminal pain.

Local legislation limits the availability and choice of opioids in many countries, but there can also be a reluctance to prescribe opioids for non-cancer pain due to the assumption that susceptible individuals may become addicted to these potent drugs through abuse. However, if opioids are prescribed on an individual basis with adequate support and education for the patients as well as their familes or carers, a great deal of unnecessary chronic pain and suffering can be prevented. But today there are still several unresolved clinical issues surrounding opioid use for which there is no data to construct a suitable policy.

Adjuvants are agents other than the primary opioid analgesics, which can be used to assist total pain management. They can directly diminish pain, counteract opioid side-effects, or help manage concurrent psychiatric symptoms. Adjuvants include agents such as non-opioid analgesics (e.g. NSAIDs), corticosteroids, anticonvulsants, antidepressants and muscle relaxants that can decrease pain directly. In addition, antinauseants, laxatives and psychostimulants can also be administered alongside opioids to help counteract the three most common problems of opioid therapy - nausea, constipation and sedation. This ensures that patients can tolerate higher doses of opioids if their pain so dictates. Furthermore, pain can be aggravated by feelings of depression and anxiety, so various antidepressants and anxiolytics can also be given.

Outlook

Continuing advances in understanding the pharmacology of pain and analgesia that have resulted from the application of molecular biology techniques and the development of selective ligands for the various receptor classes involved in nociceptive transmission, have established that pain is an extremely complex and dynamic process involving multiple, interrelated neurotransmitter/neuromodulator systems in the spinal cord, in ascending and decending spinal pathways, and at supraspinal sites.

The identification of novel compounds which more effectively treat both acute and chronic pain states, and which lack side-effects associated with current therapies, remains a major challenge in biomedical and pharma-ceutical research. Over the last two decades analgesia research has focused largely on identifying safer NSAIDs resulting in the current COX-2 inhibitors and safer opioids.

This situation was commented on in a review article as follows (Williams et al., 1999):

'Despite an intensive research effort over the past two decades involving many innovative approaches in the global academic community and by the pharmaceutical industry, the latter representing an aggregate investment in excess of $ 2.5 billion, the only new opioid-based pain medications either in clinical development or on the market are alternative dosage forms of the classical opioids, morphine, loperamide, and fentanyl, or compounds such as tramadol.'

| Loperamide | Fentanyl | Tramadol | Morphine |

References

Besson, J. M.: *The neurobiology of pain*, Lancet **1999**, *353*, 1610-1614.

McQuay, H.: *Opioids in pain mangement*, Lancet **1999**, *353*, 2229-2232.

Melzack, R., Wall, P.D.: *Pain mechanisms: a new theory*, Science Wash CD **1965**, *150*, 971-979.

Merksey, H.: *Pain terms: a list with definitions and notes on usage; recommended by the IASP subcommittee on taxonomy*, Pain **1979**, *6*, 249-252.

Ray, A. L., Yoham, M.: *Emotional pain*, in Pain-Clinical Aspects and Therapeutic Issues, Part I, edited by K. Linz. Edition Selva Verlag **1992**.

Wall, P. D.: *The gate control theory of pain mechanisms. A re-examination and restatement*, Brain **1978**, *191*, 1-18.

Wall, P. D.: *The dorsal horn*, in Textbook of Pain, edited by P.D. Wall and R. Melzack. Churchill Livingstone, Edinburgh, **1989**, 102-111.

Williams, M., Kowaluk, E. A., Arneric, S. P.: *Emerging molecular approaches to pain therapy*, J. Med. Chem. **1999**, *42*, 1481-1500.

Part II

Pain Therapy Today

2   Cyclooxygenase Inhibiton: From NSAIDs to Selective COX-2 Inhibitors

Thomas Christoph and Helmut Buschmann

History of NSAIDs

For many decades the pain relieving properties of willow bark extracts have been used in folk medicine (Fig.1). Glycoside cleavage and oxidation is necessary for the biosynthesis of salicylic acid from the plant precursor β-D-glucopyranoside, the so-called saligenins.

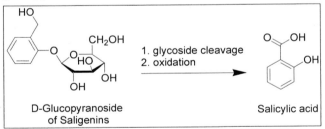

D-Glucopyranoside of Saligenins → Salicylic acid

Scheme 1: Biosynthesis of salicylic acid.

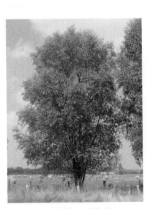

Figure 1: Willow (*Salix alba*).

The active principle was shown to be salicin by Buchner in 1828 but the bitter taste and damage to the gastric mucosa limited its use. Piria isolated salicylic acid from salicin in 1838. In 1859, Kolbe discovered the structure and synthesis of salicylic acid and in 1897 acetylsalicylic acid was synthesized by Hoffmann. Two years later, in 1899, acetylsalecylic acid, the first nonsteroidal anti-inflammatory drug was registered under the name Aspirin (Fig. 2).

More than 100 years later, acetylsalicylic acid is still the best-known nonsteroidal anti-inflammatory drug and is used in almost every household for the treatment of mild to moderate pain states and fever. Despite the fact that there had already been a long period from the initial use of aspirin to ist introduction as a registered drug, it took

NSAIDs in Plants?

Salicylic acid and related molecules are involved in endogenous defence mechanisms (Dong, 2001). Infection with tabac mosaic virus leads to an induction of salicylic acid in the infected leafs of a tabac plant (Hennig et al., 1993).

another 70 years until the mechanism of action of acetylsalicylic acid could be elucidated. In 1971, it was shown that the analgesic action of nonsteroidal anti-inflammatory drugs is due to the inhibition of the enzymatic production of prostaglandins (Vane, 1971).

Cyclooxygenase (COX), one of the two activities of prostaglandin endoperoxide synthase (PGHS), is the key enzyme in the conversion of arachidonic acid derived from lipids of the cell membrane to prostaglandins and other eicosanoids (Fig. 3).

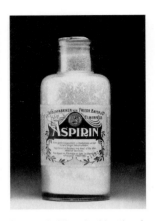

Figure 2: Historical bottle of Aspirin.

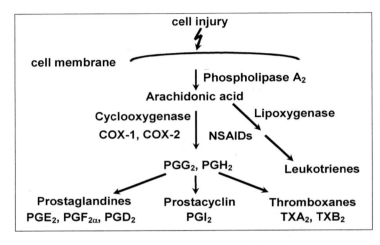

Figure 3: Simple schema of the biosynthesis of prostaglandins (PG), thromboxanes (TX), and leukotrienes from arachidonic acid consequent to cell injury (modified after Bonica, 1990).

Prostaglandin Receptors and Pain

EP1 receptor knock-out mice show reduced pain sensitivity, suggesting an important role for this receptor subtype in pain perception (Stock et al., 2001). Furthermore these mice show a significant reduction in systolic blood pressure and an increased renin angiotensin activity, suggesting a role also in cardiovascular homeostasis.

The eicosanoids (Fig. 4) are important mediators in pain and inflammation leading to hyperalgesia by sensitization of nerve fibers and fever. Furthermore they fulfill important roles in the protection of the gastric mucosa, in platelet aggregation and maintenance of normal kidney function (Vane et al., 1998). The diversity of physiological functions of the eicosanoids is reflected by a variety of different receptors. Five main receptor types have been described, designated DP, FP, IP, TP, and EP which show the greatest apparent affinity for PGD, PGF, PGI_2, TXA_2, and PGE, respectively (Pierce et al., 1995). PGE_2, the eicosanoid which plays a key role in pain perception, exerts this and other functions via the four subtypes of the EP receptors, EP1 to 4.

Isoforms of Cyclooxygenase

Two different isoforms, COX-1 and COX-2, encoded by two genes have been cloned and sequenced (Table 1; Funk et al., 1991; Kujubu et al., 1991; Hla and Neilson, 1992; O'Banion et al., 1992). The cloning of the two isoforms led to further characterization of the enzymes by means of a whole range of molecular biology tools from experiments using knock-out mice (Dinchuk et al., 1995; Langenbach et al., 1995; Morham et al., 1995) to protein structure determination (Picot et al., 1994; Kiefer et al., 2000).

COX-1 is constitutively expressed in many cells of the body and responsible mainly for the production of eicosanoids serving normal physiological functions. One important physiological role is the protection of the gastric mucosa. Inhibition of COX-1 therefore often brings pain relief together with gastrointestinal side-effects.

Arachidonic Acid Metabolism via Cyclooxygenase Enzyme

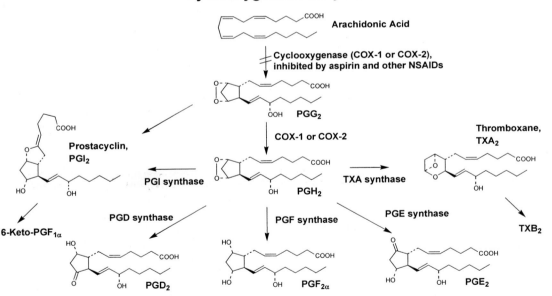

Figure 4: Chemical structure of eicosanoids.

COX-2 expression is induced during inflammation and is thought to be responsible for the production of eicosanoids in inflammatory conditions related to fever and pain. Furthermore, COX-2 is expressed in the central nervous system and might play a more direct role in central pain processing.

The characteristic differences in expression of the two COX isoforms suggest a potential for new drugs addressing inflammatory and painful conditions specifically via inhibition of COX-2. This analgesic and anti-inflammatory potential should come without the well-known gastrointestinal side-effects of classical NSAIDs which target COX-1 in combination with COX-2 or alone. As usual, nature is not that simple. COX-1 expression is also subject to regulatory processes and can be increased in inflammatory conditions (Crofford et al., 1994). COX-2 expression on the other hand is increased in the gastric mucosa by inflammatory stimuli and *Helicobacter pylori* infection (Sawaoka et al., 1998, McCarthy et al., 1999). Finally, analysis of COX-1 and COX-2 knock-out mice indicate that both isoforms can contribute to an inflammatory response and have significant roles in the maintenance of physiological homeostasis and in carcinogenesis (Langenbach et al., 1999). These data suggest that the initial roles attributed to COX-1 and COX-2 under normal and inflammatory conditions, respectively, should be re-assessed.

Ultimately, comparison of clinical data from the COX-2 selective drugs with those of the classical NSAIDs will answer the question of whether or not COX-2-inhibitors will take a leading position within the NSAIDs.

Table 1: Comparison of COX-1 and COX-2 (Dannhardt and Laufer, 2000).

Parameter	COX-1	COX-2
Sequence identity	60 %	
Gene size	22 kb	8.3 kb
Exons	11	10
Molecular weight	67,000 Da	72,000 Da
Chromosome	9q32-q33,3	1q25,2-q25,3
MRNA	2.8 kb	4,1 kb
mRNA regulation	Constitutive	Inducible (>50 fold)
Inducers	-	Cytokine, LPS, Phorbolester
Amino acids	599	604
Localization	Nuclear membrane, ER	Nuclear membrane, ER

Table 1: continued

Parameter	COX-1	COX-2
Co-factors	1 Mol Heme	1 Mol Heme
Glycosylation	-N, 3 site	-N, 3 or 4 site
Acetylsalicylic acid (ASS)-acetylation site	Ser 529	Ser 516
Substrate specificity	Arachidonic acid (AA) γ-linolenic acid	Arachidonic acid (AA) γ- linolenic acid, eicosapentenoic acid
Activity	23 mmol AA/mg/min	11 mmol AA/mg/min
Role of COX-1 and COX-2	Homeostatic functions • Protection of normal gastric mucosa • Platelet function • Renal	Pathological functions a) Inflammation, pain, fever b) Dysregulated proliferation Physiological functions 1. Tissue repair 2. Vasculature 3. Reproduction 4. Renal 5. Bone 6. Islet cells 7. Lung 8. Brain

AA, arachidonic acid; LPS, endotoxin lipopolysaccharide; ER, endoplasmic reticulum.

Classification of NSAIDs According to their Chemical Structure

Many nonsteroidal anti-inflammatory drugs of different chemical structures (Fig. 5) have been introduced for the treatment of inflammatory and painful conditions. Many years of clinical experience with these drugs have shown that there is no induction of tolerance or dependence and no respiratory depression as seen with opioids. The major side-effects of these compounds with COX-1 selectivity or balanced COX-1 and COX-2 inhibition are damage to the gastric mucosa, prolongation of bleeding time and renal failure.

According to their chemical structure the following classification of the classical NSAIDs can be made:

- Salicylates
- Anthranilates
- Arylacetic acids
- Arylpropionic acids

Christoph and Buschmann

- Pyrazolinone derivatives
- Para-aminophenol derivatives
- Acidic enolic compounds (pyrazolidine-3,5-diones, oxicams)

Salicylates

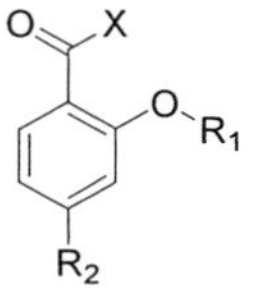

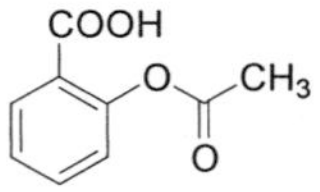

Acetylsalicylic acid

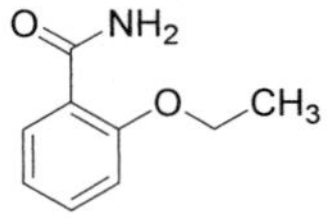

Ethenzamide

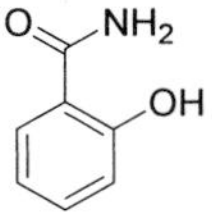

Salicylamide

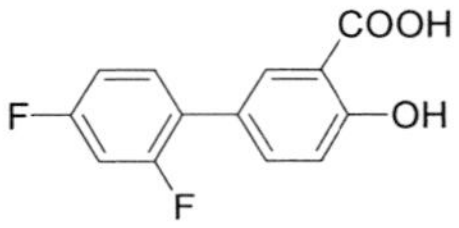

Diflunisal

Anthranilates

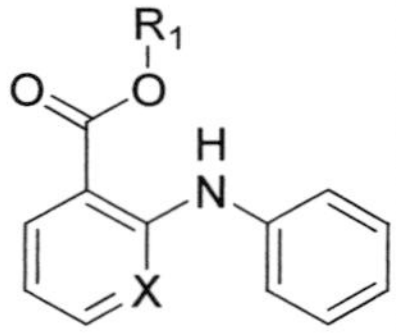

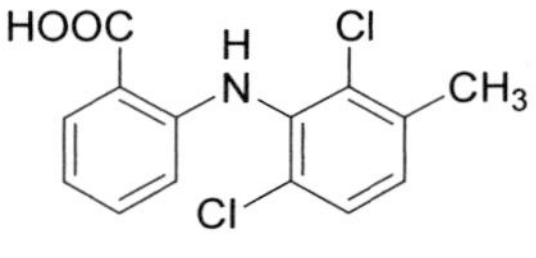

Meclofenamic acid

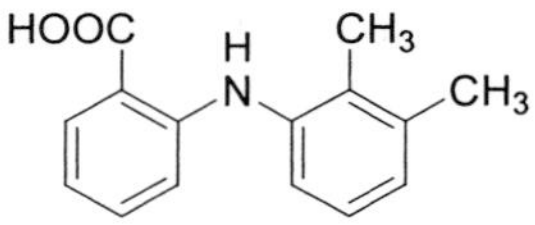

Mefenamic acid

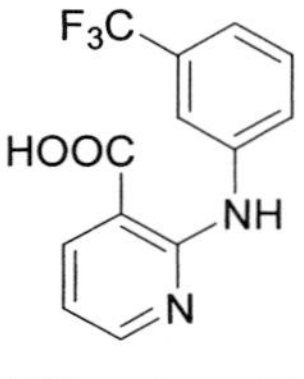

Niflumic acid

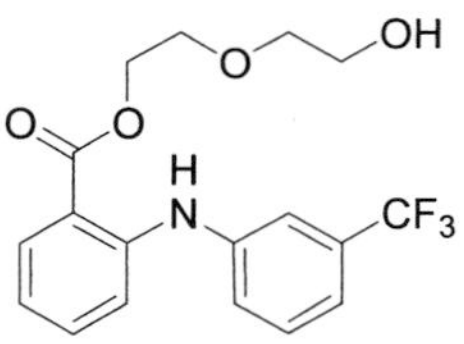

Etofenamate

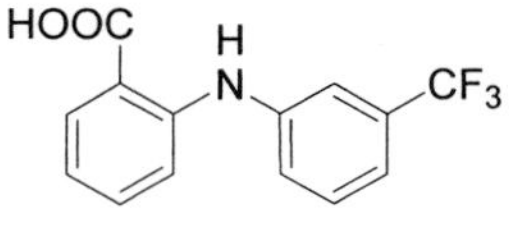

Flufenamic acid

Arylacetic Acids

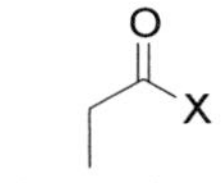

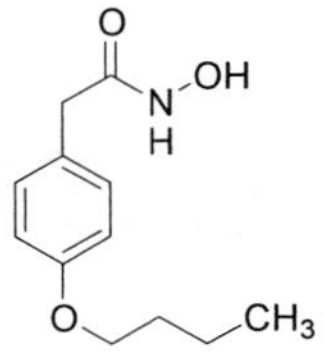

Bufexamac

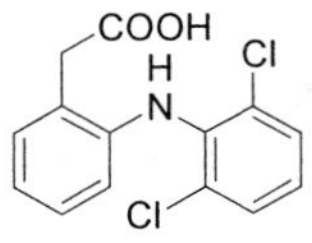

Diclofenac

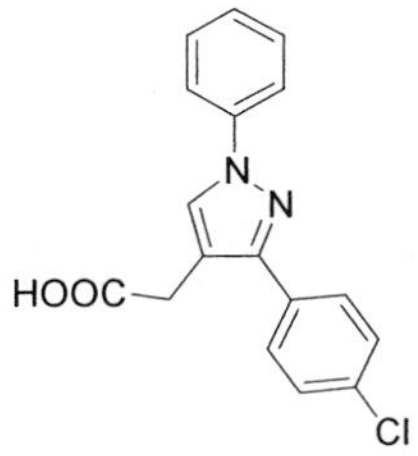

Lonazolac

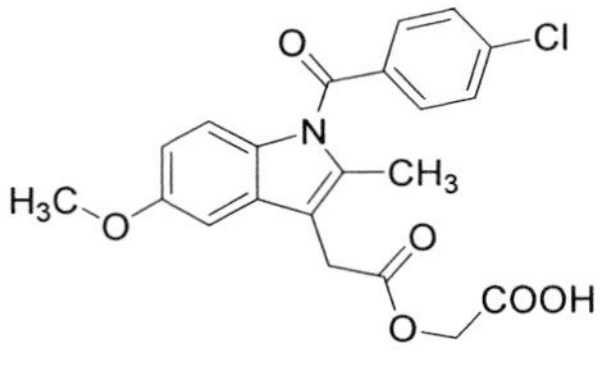

Acemetacin

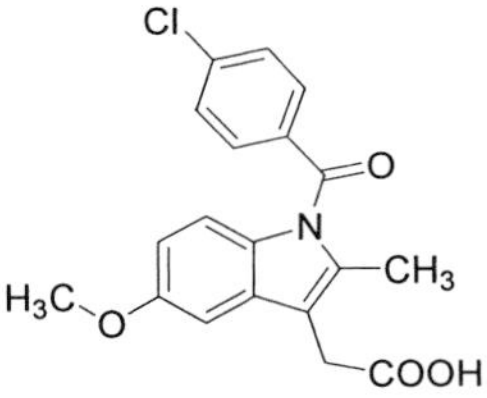

Indomethacin

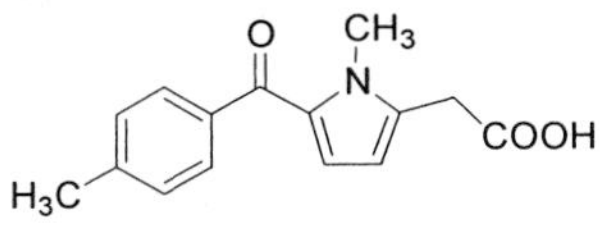

Tolmetin

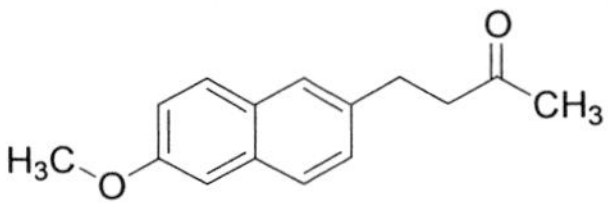

Nabumetone

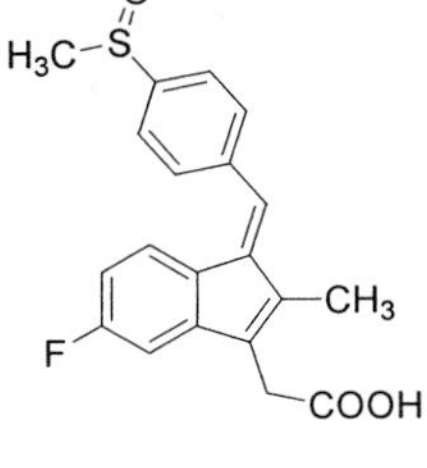

Sulindac

Arylpropionic Acids

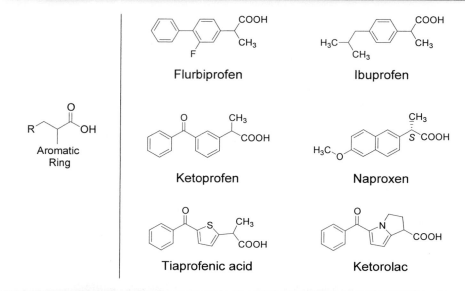

Flurbiprofen

Ibuprofen

Ketoprofen

Naproxen

Tiaprofenic acid

Ketorolac

Pyrazolinone Derivatives

Metamizol

Propyphenazone

Para-Aminophenol Derivatives

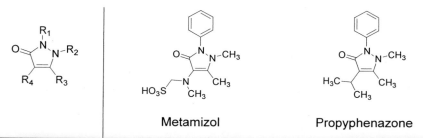

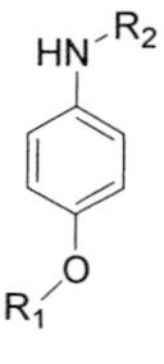

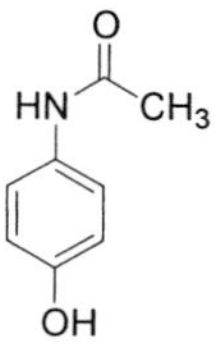

Paracetamol

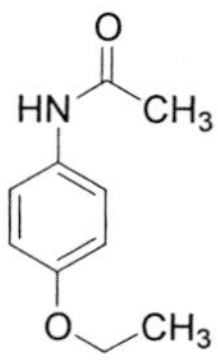

Phenidine

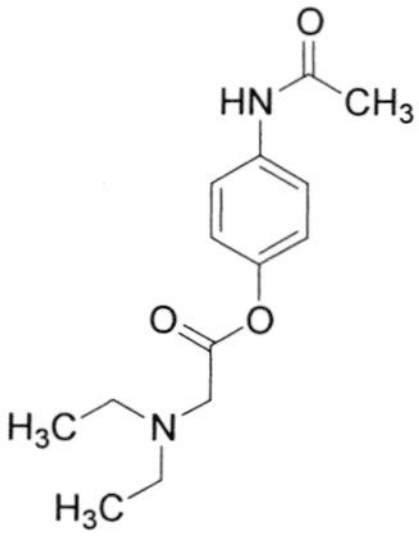

Propacetamol

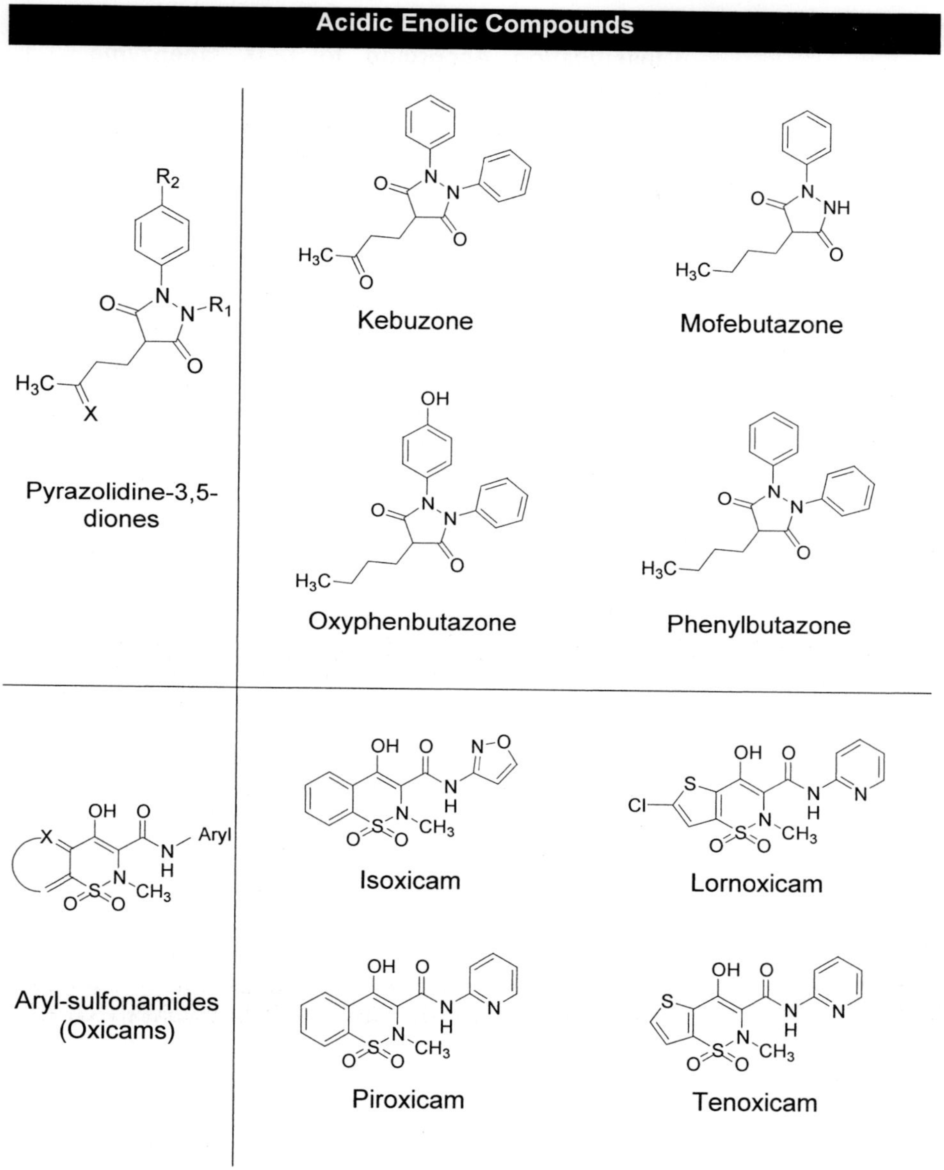

Acidic Enolic Compounds

Kebuzone

Mofebutazone

Pyrazolidine-3,5-diones

Oxyphenbutazone

Phenylbutazone

Isoxicam

Lornoxicam

Aryl-sulfonamides (Oxicams)

Piroxicam

Tenoxicam

Figure 5: Chemical diversity of NSAIDs.

The Development of COX-2 Selective Inhibitors

Classification According to COX Isoenzyme Selectivity

The discovery of the inducible isoform led to the identification of drugs that show a stronger inhibition of COX-2 compared to COX-1 (Table 2).

Table 2: COX-2 selective inhibitors.

Group	Compound	COX-2 Selectivity (enzyme)	COX-2 Selectivity (whole blood)
first generation	etodolac	n.d.	10 [1]
	meloxicam	75 [2]	11.2 [1]
	nimesulide	n.d.	18 [1]
second generation	celecoxib	375 [3]	7.6 [4]
	rofecoxib	76 [5]	75 [6]
third generation	etoricoxib	>20 [4]	105 [4]
	valdecoxib	28000 [6]	30 [4]
	parecoxib	valdecoxib prodrug	valdecoxib prodrug

Selectivity of inhibition of COX-2 vs. COX-1 based on enzyme assays and whole blood cellular assays (IC50 COX-1/IC50 COX-2)

(1) Patrignani et al. (1997)
(2) Churchill et al. (1996)
(3) Penning et al. (1997)
(4) Riendeau et al. (2001)
(5) Chan et al. (1999)
(6) Warner et al. (1999)
(7) Talley et al. (2000a)

COX Inhibition Assays

Inhibition of COX can be quantified in recombinant or natural enzyme preparations, cellular systems, isolated human cell populations such as platelets (COX-1) and white blood cells (COX-2), or in *ex vivo* stimulated whole blood samples The closer the experimental system is to the physiological state, the lower the selectivity for most COX-2-inhibitors. The standard test for comparison is considered to be a whole blood assay which mimics *in vivo* conditions like plasma binding (e.g. Patrignani et al., 1996). It is commonly accepted that reasonable variations occur between different laboratories (see data for Piroxicam). Therefore, whenever possible, data of several compounds generated with a given test system should be compared with each other.

Table 2 shows the classification of COX-2 selective inhibitors based mainly on their historical development. The first generation of COX-2 inhibitors such as meloxicam still shows inhibition of COX-1 in physiological plasma concentrations and hence, still generate the same gastrointestinal side-effects as COX-1 inhibitors although to a lower degree. These compounds were developed before the discovery of the inducible isoform of COX. The second generation COX-2 inhibitors, which have been identified by screening their inhibitory potentials on both COX isoforms, reached the market in 1999 with celecoxib and rofecoxib and shows a clear selectivity for COX-2 compared to COX-1 in enzyme preparations and whole blood assays. The gastrointestinal side-effects of these drugs seem to be clearly lower than those of classical NSAIDs such as naproxen. Nevertheless, the FDA has so far rejected claims of reduced side-effect profile of celecoxib. The third generation of COX-2 inhibitors is under development showing an even greater selectivity for COX-2.

The fastest-growing product in 2000 was Pharmacia/Pfizer's COX-2 inhibitor, Celebrex (Celecoxib), for osteoarthritis, which was launched in early 1999.

Celecoxib generated $ 2.4 billion in sales, up by 65 % from previous year (Table 3).

Table 3: The top ten selling drugs in 2000.

Product	2000 sales ($ billion)	% of global sales	% growth (vs. 1999)
Losec / Prilosec	6.1	1.9	+ 9
Lipitor	5.4	1.7	+ 44
Zocor	4.4	1.4	+ 15
Norvasc	3.3	1.1	+ 15
Orgastro / Prevacid	3.1	1.0	+ 33
Prozac	2.9	0.9	- 1
Seroxat / Paxil	2.4	0.8	+ 20
Zyprexa	2.4	0.8	+ 30
Celebrex	**2.4**	**0.7**	**+ 65**
Zoloft	2.2	0.7	+ 12

Source: IMS Health Word Reviews 2001, SCRIP No 2630 March 30th 2001 p. 18

Including the classical NSAIDs in a classification based on isoenzyme selectivity, it turns out that beside low dose aspirin there is no COX-1 selective inhibitor on the market. Instead, most of the classical NSAIDs belong to the group of nonselective COX inhibitors.

- **Selective COX-1 inhibitors** (low dose aspirin)
- **Nonselective COX inhibitors** (e.g. high dose aspirin, indomethacin)
- **Preferential COX-2 inhibitors** (e.g. meloxicam)
- **Highly selective COX-2 inhibitors** (e.g. celecoxib, second and third generation of COX-2 inhibitors, sometimes called coxibs)

Classification According to Drug-Protein Interactions

Another classification is based on the mode of interaction between drug and enzyme (Kurumbail et al., 1996).

APHS (2-**a**cetoxy-**p**henyl-
hept-2-ynyl **s**ulfide)

- **Irreversible inhibitors of COX-1** (aspirin) **or COX-2** (2-acetoxyphenylhept-2-ynyl sulfide, APHS; Kalgutkar et al., 1998). Aspirin and APHS acetylate the amino acid serine so that endogenic arachidonic acid is prevented from reaching the catalytic center of the enzymes.

- **Reversible, competitive inhibitors of COX-1 and COX-2.** Inhibitors such as ibuprofen, piroxicam or mefenamic acid compete against arachidonic acid to bind at the catalytic center.

- **Slow, time-dependent, reversible inhibitors of COX-1 and COX-2.** E.g. indomethacin and flurbiprofen seem to act by ionic interactions between their carboxylic acid function and the arginine residue of the enzyme. This effect seems to influence the helix D of the protein followed by a significant loss of flexibility in the enzyme protein.

- **Slow, time-dependent irreversible inhibitors of COX-2** (e.g. celecoxib and rofecoxib) The last group shows a weak competitive inhibition of COX-1 which is of minor clinical relevance compared to the slow, time-dependent COX-2 inhibition.

Chemical Classification of Selective COX-2 Inhibitors

The large number of newly developed COX-2 inhibitors demonstrates how promising this field of anti-inflammatory agents is expected to be. More than 1000 COX-2 inhibitors have been described over the past few years (Prous database, March 2002). The chemical structures of COX-2 inhibitors are heterogenic. Contrary to the classical NSAIDs, this new class of enzyme inhibitors lacks a carboxylic acid group, thus effecting COX-2 affinity by a different orientation within the enzyme without formation of a salt bridge in the hydrophobic channel of the enzyme.

Most of the selective COX-2 inhibitors belong to one of the following different structural classes (Thalley et al., 1999; Dannhardt and Kiefer, 2001; Jiménez et al., 2000):

- **Diaryl- or aryl-heteroaryl ethers and thioethers** (sulfonanilide inhibitors) such as nimesulide or flosulide

- **Heterocycles or carbocycles with vicinal diaryl substitution**, e.g. celecoxib and rofecoxib

- **Modified, known NSAIDs to improve COX-2 selectivity**: L-748780, L-761066, meloxicam, etodolac

- **Antioxidative compounds**

- **1,2-Diarylethylene derivatives** (*cis*-stilbenes)

- **Miscellaneous structures**

Diaryl- and Aryl-Heteroaryl Ether and Thioether

Diaryl- and aryl-heteroaryl ether and thioether compounds belong to the first generation of selective COX-2 inhibitors (Fig. 6). One of the first COX-2 inhibitors was compound NS-398 wich has a completely different structure from classic NSAIDs.The compound showed inhibition of prostaglandin synthesis in inflammatory cells and was largely free of unwanted gastrointestinal effects in animal models. Moreover, NS-398 did not affect prostaglandin production in the stomach or kidney. On recognizing that NS-398 was a more or less preferential selective inhibitor of COX-2, new interest in this class of anti-inflammatory agents evolved. Nimesulide and flosulide are two other compounds with a diaryl ether and thioether structure, respectively, which bear a methansulfonanilide moiety. The sulfonamide structure with its NH-acidity in all these compounds seems to be obligatory.

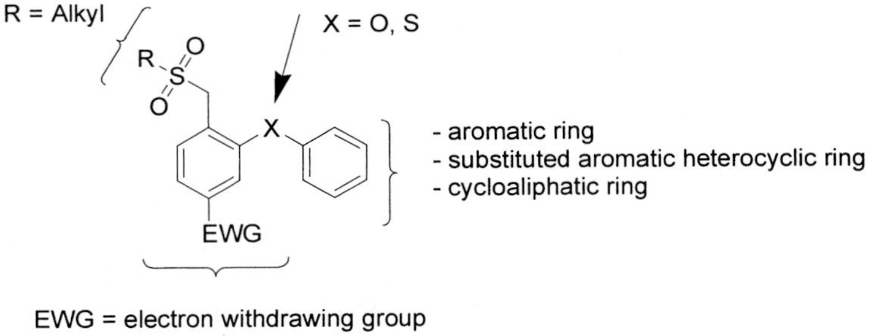

- aromatic ring
- substituted aromatic heterocyclic ring
- cycloaliphatic ring

EWG = electron withdrawing group

Scheme 2: General structure of a sulfonanilide COX-2 inhibitor (first generation scaffold).

Carbocycles and Heterocycles with Vicinal Aryl Substitution (Second Generation of COX-2 Inhibitors)

By far the greatest amount of research in the area of COX-2 inhibition has been carried out in the preparation and evaluation of this class of compounds. The compounds are characterized by a central carboxylic or heterocyclic ring system bearing two vicinal aryl moieties. These compounds represent the most important group of COX-2 inhibitors. During the last few years a large number of compounds has been developed as potential candidates.

Celecoxib, rofecoxib, valdecoxib, parecoxib sodium, and etoricoxib all belong to this chemical class.

The diaryl heterocycles described in the last 2 years can be classified into the following subcategories according to the nature of their linkages (Fig. 7; Jiménez et al., 2000):

- Diaryl heterocyles linked via a 4-membered ring
- Diaryl heterocyles linked via a 5-membered ring
- Diaryl heterocyles linked via a 6-membered ring
- Diaryl heterocyles linked via a fused-ring system

It is assumed that the heterocyclic core structure is responsible for the appropriate orientation of the aromatic rings in space and finally for binding to the enzyme. A wide variety of heterocycles can serve as templates, i.e. pyrrole, thiazole, oxazole furane, furanone, imidazole, isoxazole, pyrimidine and thiophene, but at the moment pyrazole and cylopentenone seem to be the most appropriate for achieving COX-2 specificity. For optimal activity, one aromatic ring must be substituted with a methylsulfonyl or a sulfonamide substituent in the para position. Substitution at position 4 of one of the aromatic systems with a sulfonamide or a methylsulfonyl group is essential for COX inhibition. Replacement of the methylsulfonyl group by a sulfonamide group reduces COX-2 selectivity but improves oral bioavailability.

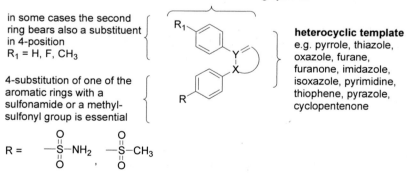

two vicinal aromatic ring systems

in some cases the second ring bears also a substituent in 4-position
R_1 = H, F, CH_3

4-substitution of one of the aromatic rings with a sulfonamide or a methyl-sulfonyl group is essential

R_1

heterocyclic template
e.g. pyrrole, thiazole, oxazole, furane, furanone, imidazole, isoxazole, pyrimidine, thiophene, pyrazole, cyclopentenone

R

R = —S(=O)(=O)—NH$_2$, —S(=O)(=O)—CH$_3$

Scheme 3: General structure of carbocycles and heterocycles with vicinal aryl substituents. The structural pre-requisites shown are obligatory for enhanced activity towards COX-2.

Diaryl- or aryl-heteroaryl-ethers and thioethers

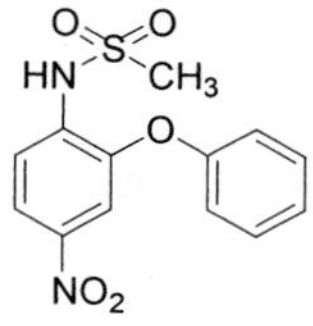

Nimesulid

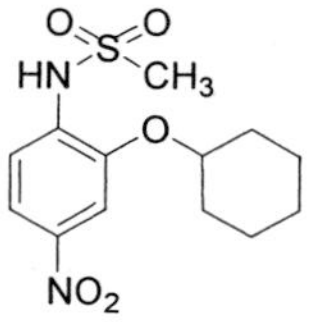

NS-398

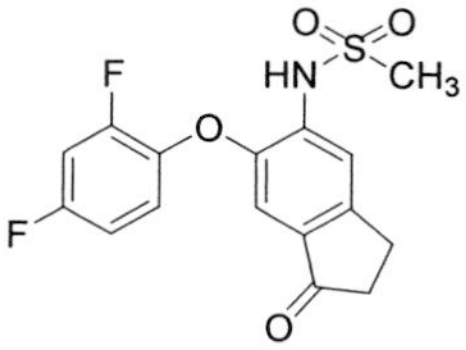

Flosulid

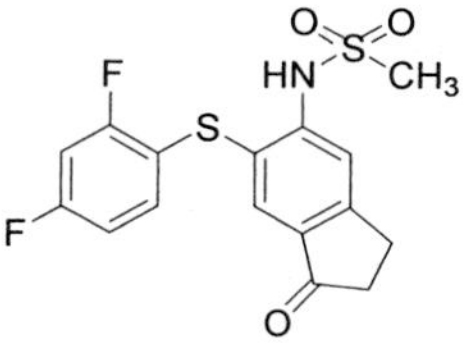

L-745337

COX-1: IC_{50} > 30 µM

COX-2: IC_{50} = 9.67 µM

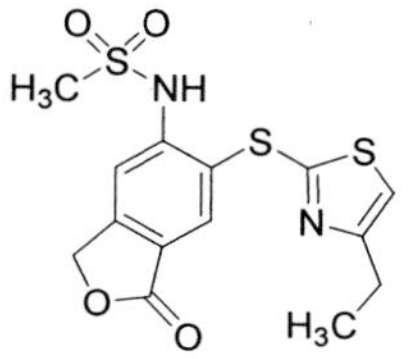

COX-2: IC_{50} = 0.005 µM

COX-1: IC_{50} > 100 µM

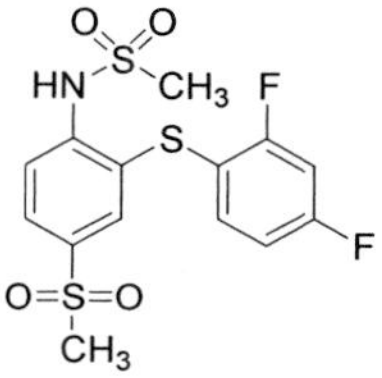

(Nycomed Austria)

Figure 6: Chemical structures of diaryl- or aryl-heteroaryl-ethers and thioethers

Carbocycles and heterocycles with vicinal diaryl substituents

• Diaryl heterocycles linked via a 4-membered ring

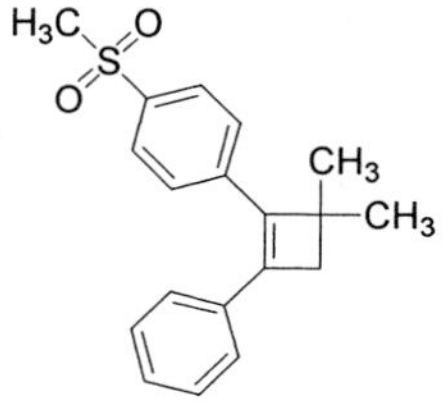

COX-1: IC_{50}=0.12 µM

COX-2: IC_{50} = 0.002 µM

COX-2/COX-1 = 0.017

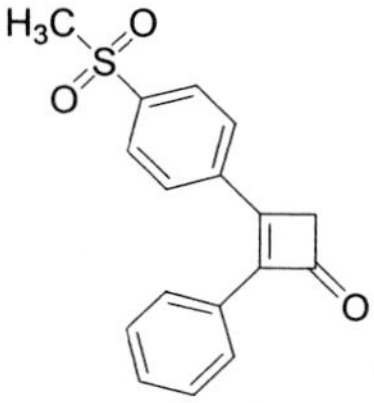

COX-1: IC_{50} > 5 µM

COX-2: IC_{50} = 0.11 µM

COX-2/COX-1 < 0.022

- Diaryl heterocycles linked via a 5-membered ring

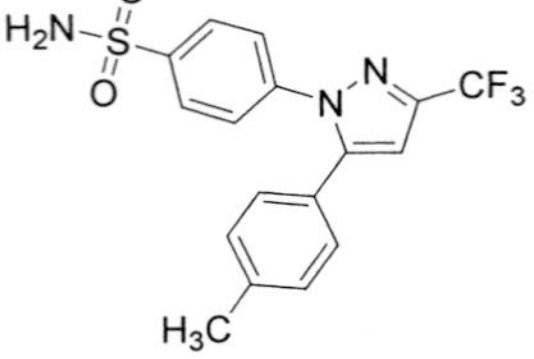

Celecoxib (Celebrex)

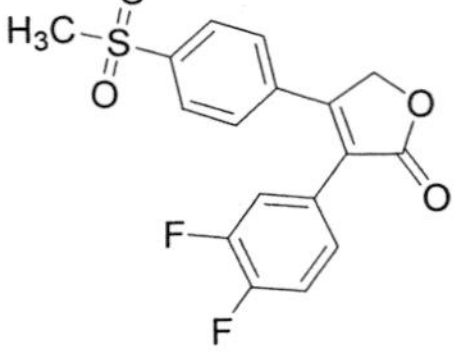

Rofecoxib (Vioxx)

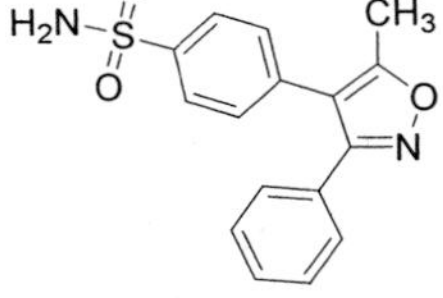

Valdecoxib

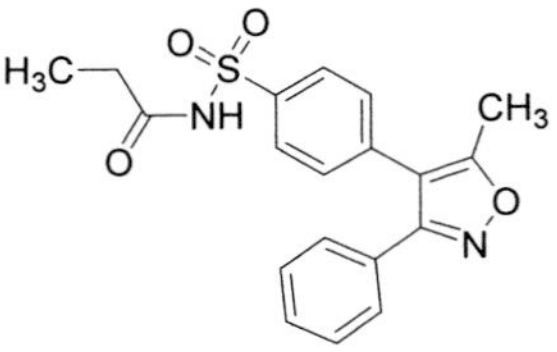

Parecoxib

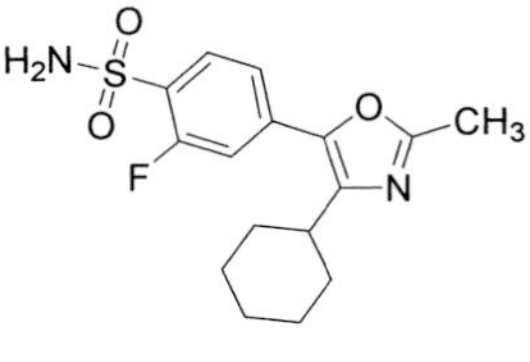

JTE-522

COX-2: IC_{50} = 0.085 µM

COX-1: IC_{50} = 0.64 µM

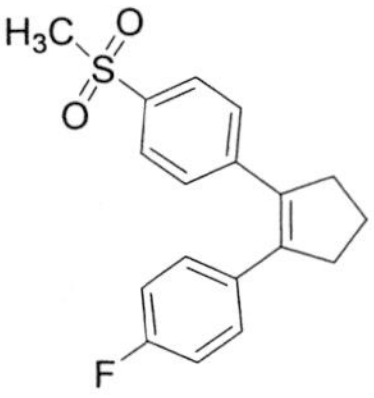

SC-57666

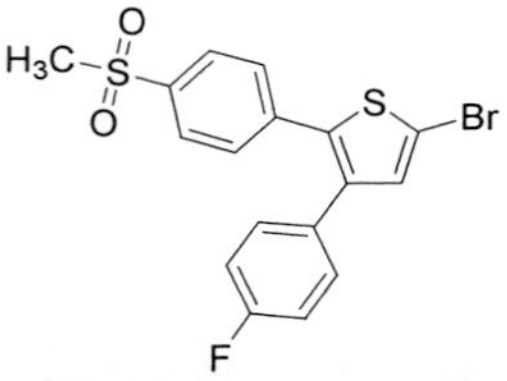

DuP-697

COX-1: IC_{50} = 1.18 µM

COX-2: IC_{50} = 0.06 µM

COX-2/COX-1 = 0.051

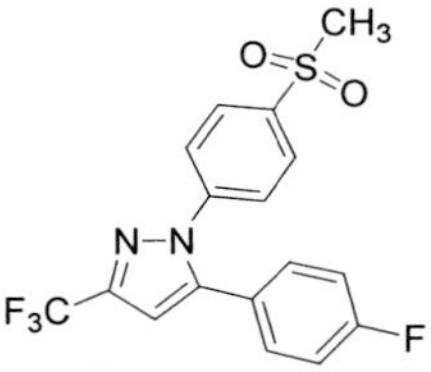

SC-5812 5

COX-1: IC_{50} > 30 µM

COX-2: IC_{50} = 2.25 µM

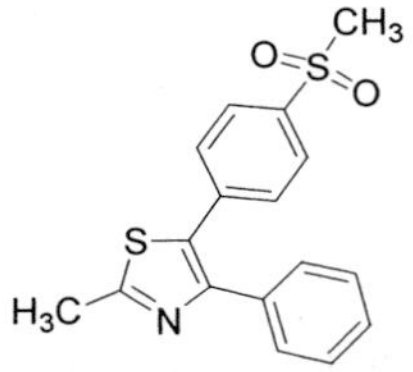

(GD Searle & Co)

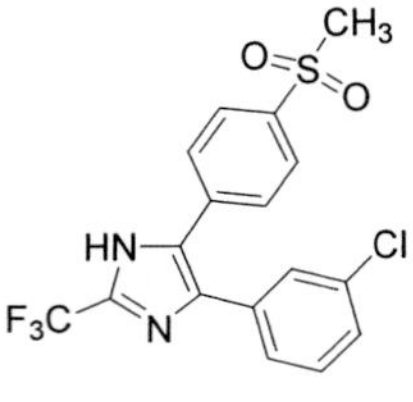

(GD Searle & Co)

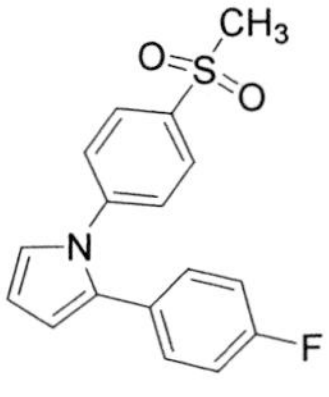

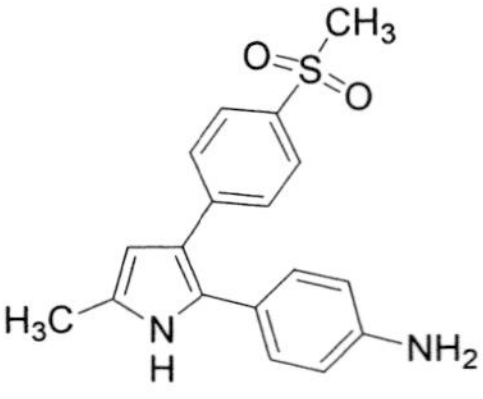

(GD Searle & Co)

(Nissin Foods Products)

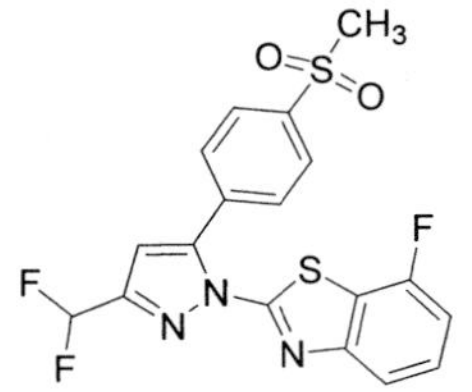

(Grelan Pharmaceutical)

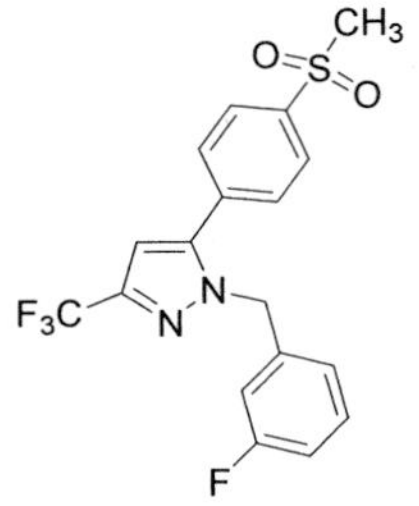

(Fujisawa Pharm.)

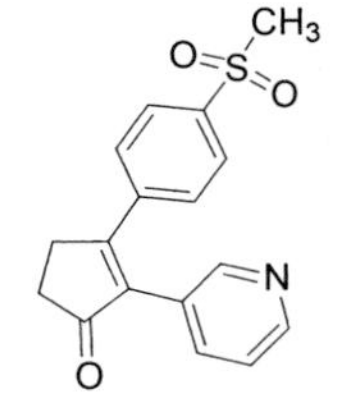

L-784506

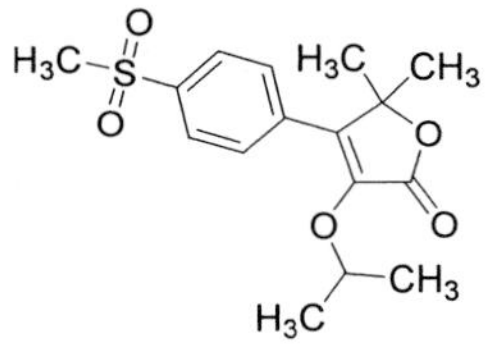

DFP

COX-2: IC_{50} = 0.3 μM

COX-1: IC_{50} = 3 μM

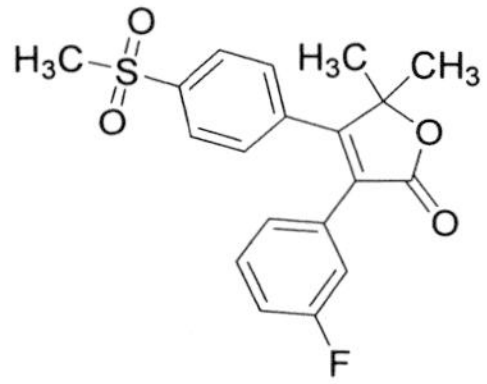

DFU

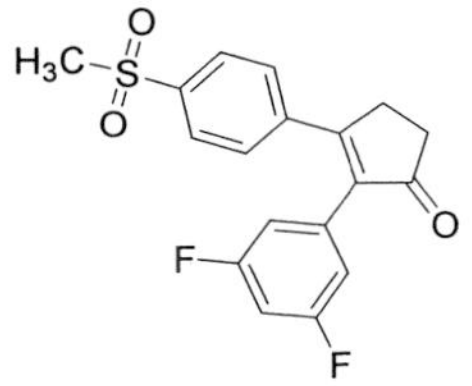

L-776967

COX-2: IC_{50} = 0.03 μM

COX-1: IC_{50} = 0.1 μM

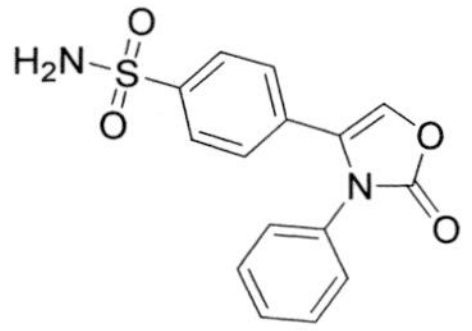

(Almirall Prodesfarma)

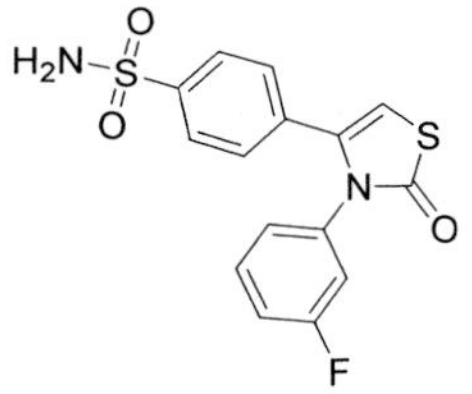

(Laboratoires UPSA)

COX-2: IC_{50} = 0.06 μM

COX-1: IC_{50} = 328 μM

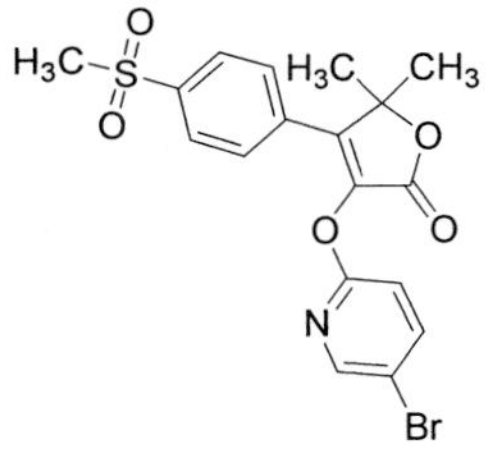

L-778736

- Diaryl heterocycles linked via a 6-membered ring

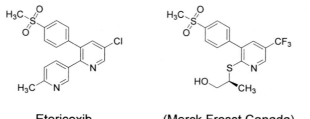

Etoricoxib (Merck Frosst Canada)

COX-1: IC$_{50}$ = 5.5 μM

COX-2: IC$_{50}$ = 0.002 μM

COX-2/COX-1 = 0.00036

L-804600

- Diaryl heterocycles linked via a fused ring system

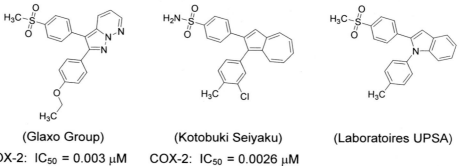

(Glaxo Group)   (Kotobuki Seiyaku)   (Laboratoires UPSA)

COX-2: IC$_{50}$ = 0.003 μM   COX-2: IC$_{50}$ = 0.0026 μM

COX-1: IC$_{50}$ = 90 μM   COX-1: IC$_{50}$ = 4.2 μM

Figure 7: Chemical structures of heterocycles or carbocycles with vicinal diaryl substitution.

Metabolism Considerations in the Discovery and Selection of COX-2 Inhibitors

Compound DuP-697 with a bromo-substituted thiophene ring is a typical representative which fulfills these pre-requisites. However, the clinical data obtained from DuP-697 showed a very long plasma half-life of 242 h in humans as a result of its enterohepatic recirculation and rendered in unacceptable for further evaluation. Today this compound serves as a pharmacological tool.

A continuous effort was made in chemical research to develop a second generation of COX-2 inhibitors, structurally different from existing ones, that would show very high COX-2 selectivity, a suitable pharmacokinetic profile and *in vivo* efficacy in animal models. Based on these properties, DFP (5,5-dimethyl-3-(2-isopropyl)-4-(4-methanesulfonyl-phenyl)-2-(5*H*)-furanone and DFU (5,5-dimethyl-3-(3-fluorophenyl)-4-(4-methylsulfonyl)phenyl-2(5*H*)-furanone) were selected for human clinical trials (Chauret et al., 2001). However, during phase I clinical studies, both of these compounds showed poor pharmacokinetic characteristics in humans: DFP had a very long half-life (64 h) while DFU exhibited pharmacokinetics that varied significantly from individual to individual (12.2 h to > 72 h). In addition, pharmacokinetic studies in rats showed that the clearance of DFP was significantly increased upon multiple dosing. The basis of these pharmacokinetic behaviors was investigated through *in vitro* metabolic studies. It was found that DFP was poorly metabolized in human microsomes and hepatocytes, and a low rate of metabolism *in vivo* probably accounts for the very long half-life. *In vivo* studies in hepatocytes indicated that DFP induces its own metabolism in the rat, probably through the induction of CYP3A, and this phenomenon was related to the faster clearance of DFP upon multiple dosing. Regarding the metabolism of DFU, it was discovered that the compopund was metabolized by a single, polymorphic cytochrome P450 (CYP2C19), which explains the variable pharmacokinetics obtained *in vivo*.

In light of these observations, it was considered critical that the metabolic fate of any potential second generation COX-2 inhibitor should be carefully examined as early as possible.

Modification of Known NSAIDs and Compounds Without Common Structural Features

Modifying well-known NSAIDs into more selective COX-2 inhibitors represents an interesting strategy (Dannhardt and Laufer, 2000). However, the methodology utilized in NSAID modification does not follow a general scheme.

Modification of indomethacin

Indomethacin

COX-2: IC$_{50}$ = 0.96 µM (human)

COX-1: IC$_{50}$ = 0.08 µM (human)

Classic NSAIDs such as indomethacin possess both COX-1 and COX-2 inhibiting affinity. Various attempts have been made to shift the enzyme selectivity of indomethacin from COX-1 to COX-2 while keeping the potency at the same level and reducing the unwanted side-effects at the same time. In principle, the strategy consisted of introducing larger substituents to fit the active site volume of COX-2 resulting in compounds like L-748780. Introducing a larger trichlorobenzoyl analog instead of the chlorobenzoyl analog optimized COX-2 selectivity. Altering the side chain by introducing a beta-branched butyric acid and replacing the benzoyl group of indomethacin with a 4-bromo benzyl-substituent finally produced compound L-761066 which has a high potency and remarkable selectivity (Black et al., 1996; Leblanc et al., 1996) Transformation of the aryl acetic acid moiety of indomethacin to esters or amides produces molecules capable of binding tightly to COX-2 but not COX-1 (Kalgutkar, 2000a).

Abbott (Brooks et al. (Abbott), 1998a; Woods et al. (Abbott), 1998) published two patent applications in which the carboxyl moiety of indomethacin was substituted with an iminooxy or substituted thiazole. On the other hand, Kotobuki Seiyaku (Tomiyama et al. (Kotobuki Seiaku Co. LTD), 1998) used a novel approach, exchanging the indole nucleus for an azulene (Jiménez et al., 2000).

Conversion of indomethacin to selective COX-2 inhibitors

Some of the most potent and selective indomethacin derivatives are shown

L-748780

COX-2: IC$_{50}$ = 0.06 µM

COX-1: IC$_{50}$ > 10 µM

L-761066

COX-2: 0.04 µM (human)

COX-1: 66 µM (bovine)

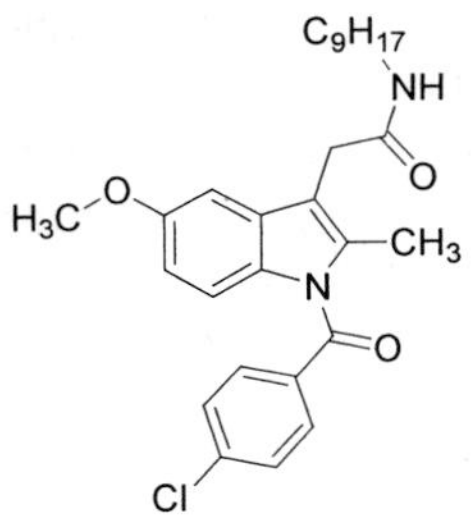

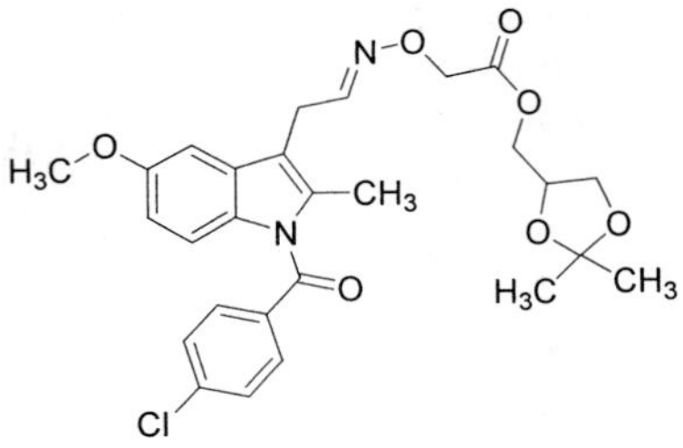

(Abbott Laboratories)

COX-2: IC_{50} = 0.0003 μM

COX-1: IC_{50} > 100 μM

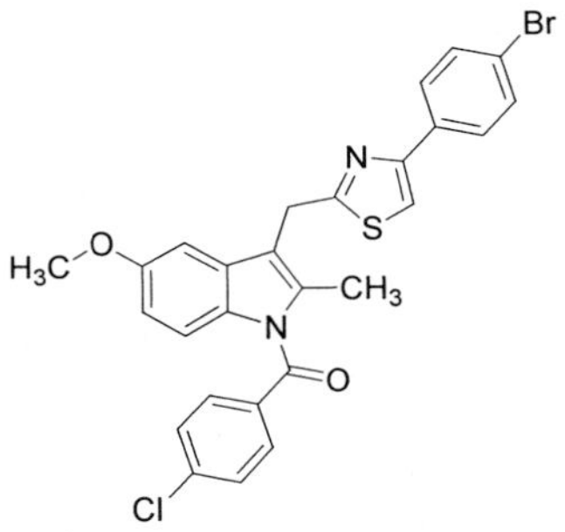

(Abbott Laboratories)

COX-2: IC_{50} = 0.003 μM

COX-1: IC_{50} = 0.09 μM

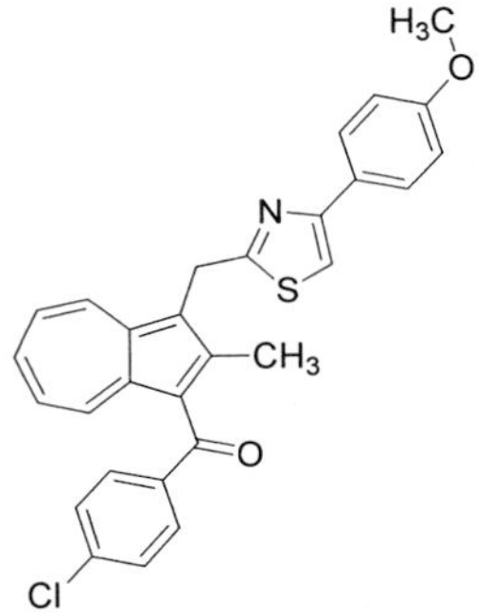

(Kotobuki Seiyaku)

COX-2: IC_{50} = 0.0008 μM

COX-1: IC_{50} > 100 μM

Figure 8: Modification of known NSAIDs.

A similar strategy was used for the modification of zomepirac, basically a COX-1 selective drug. The desired COX-2 selectivity was achieved by replacing the acetic acid group by other moieties such as a pyridazinone ring or an N-acyl aminosulfonyl phenyl group to yield RS-57067 and RS-1048934, respectively (Barnett et al., 2000)

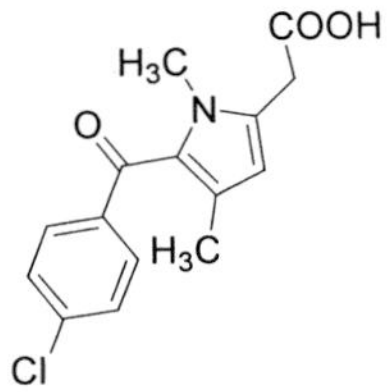

Modification of zomepirac

zomepirac

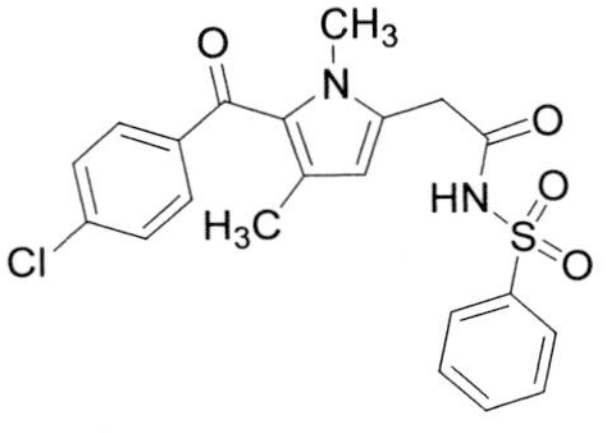

RS-1048934 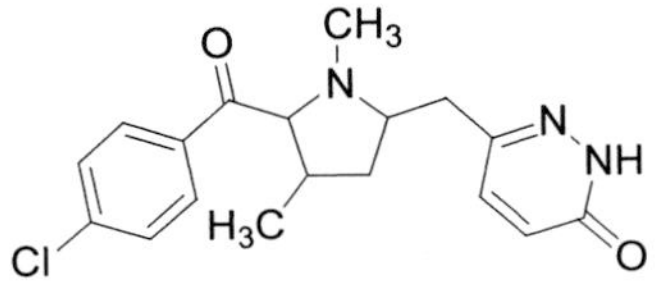   RS-57067

Figure 9: Modification of zomepirac.

Modification of sulindac

American Home Products (Failli et al. (American Home Products), 1998a; 1999) has described analogs of sulindac that act as selective COX-2 inhibitors, where a tetronic acid moiety is used as an isosteric replacement for the carboxylic acid group (Jiménez et al., 2000).

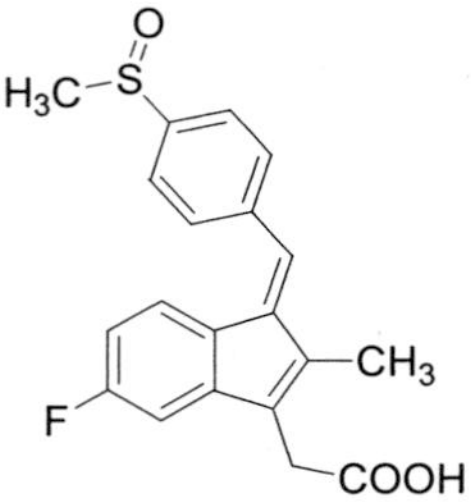

Sulindac

COX-2: IC_{50} = 10.43 μM

COX-1: IC_{50} = 1.02 μM

(sulfide derivative, active metabolite)

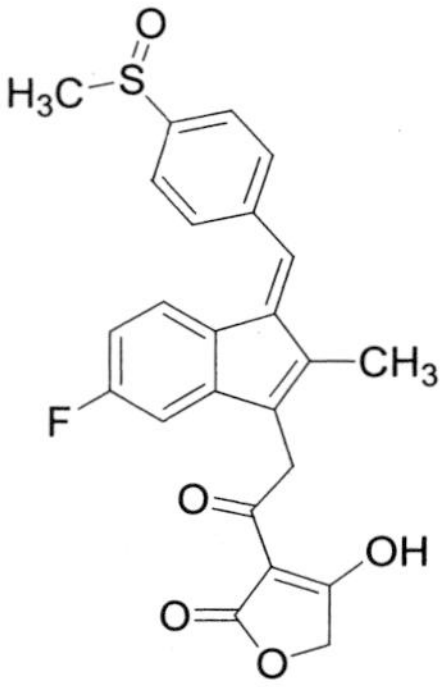

(American Home Products)

COX-2: IC_{50} = 0.027 μM

COX-1: IC_{50} = 10 μM

Figure 10: Modification of sulindac.

Modification of diclofenac

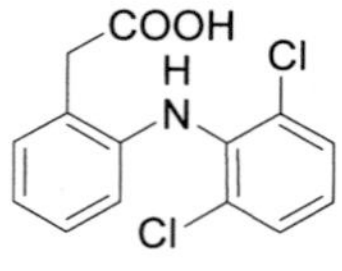

diclofenac

COX-2: IC_{50} = 0.05 μM

COX-1: IC_{50} = 0.14 μM

Two different strategies have been used in the modification of diclofenac. First Novartis (Fujimoto et al. (Novartis), 1999) described the substitution of ring A of diclofenac with an alkyl group resulting in a compound, which has very good COX-2 potency and selectivity, while Abbott Laboratories (Brooks et al. (Abbott), 1998b; 1999), using a modification of the acidic moiety, obtained moderately selective inhibitors (Jiménez et al., 2000).

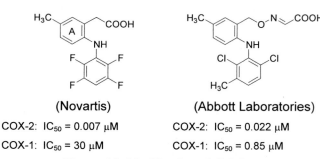

(Novartis)

COX-2: IC_{50} = 0.007 μM

COX-1: IC_{50} = 30 μM

(Abbott Laboratories)

COX-2: IC_{50} = 0.022 μM

COX-1: IC_{50} = 0.85 μM

Figure 11: Modification of diclofenac.

In 1995, etodolac (American Home Products) was shown to be a selective COX-2 inhibitor (Glaser et al., 1995). An increase in selectivity was achieved by replacing the oxygen with a methylene group at the 4-position of the pyran ring, by transformation of the ketone into an oxime or by complete reduction of the pyran ring (Failli et al. (American Home Products), 1998b; Kreft et al. (American Home Products), 1998a; 1998b; Jiménez et al., 2000).

Modification of etodolac

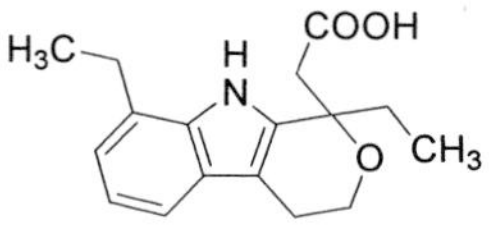

etodolac

COX-2: IC_{50} = 0.041 μM

COX-1: IC_{50} = ~50 μM

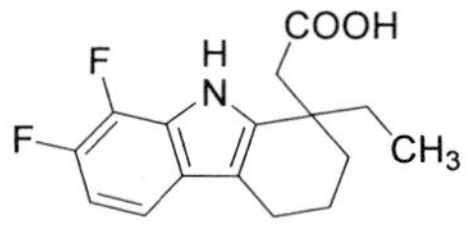

(American Home Products)

COX-2: IC_{50} = 0.7 μM

COX-1: IC_{50} = 23 μM

Figure 12: Modification of etodolac.

Flurbiprofen has been successfully modified by Merck Frosst using comparative computer modeling studies of the X-ray crystal structures of COX-1 and COX-2 (Bayly et al., 1999, (Merck Frosst), 1999). Optimal selectivity was conferred by a 3-atom lipophilic substitution at the 3′ position of the unsubstituted phenyl ring. The most effective analog was obtained by introducing two ethoxy groups at the 3′ and 5′ position of flurbiprofen, yielding a compound, which has 77-fold greater selectivity than the parent compound (Jiménez et al., 2000).

Modification of flurbiprofen

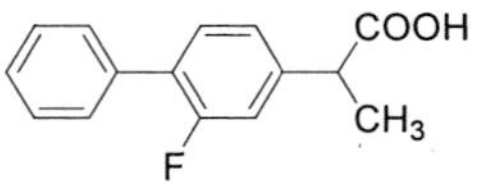

Flurbiprofen

COX-2: IC_{50} = 6.42 μM

COX-1: IC_{50} = 0.41 μM

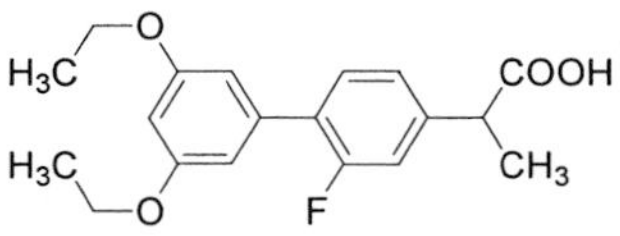

(Merck Frosst)

(S)-Flurbiprofen (Dannhardt and Kiefer, 2001)

COX-2: IC_{50} = 2.56 μM

COX-1: IC_{50} = 0.29 μM

Figure 13: Modification of flurbiprofen.

Meloxicam was discovered to be an anti-inflammatory agent with relatively few gastrointestinal side-effects, when compared with other NSAIDs (Ogino et al., 1997). New attempts to modify the modestly selective COX-2 inhibitor led to a new series of isoquinoline-1,3-diones, which are orally active COX-2-selective inhibitors (Lazer et al. (Boehringer Ingelheim), 1997; 1998). The most

Modification of meloxicam

representative example of this series is BIRL-790 (Boehringer Ingelheim).

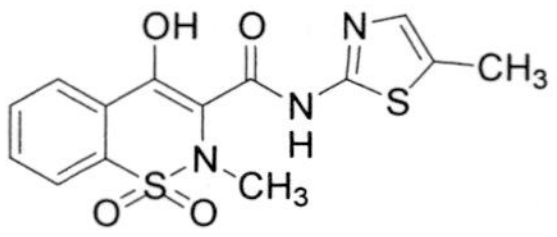

melioxicam 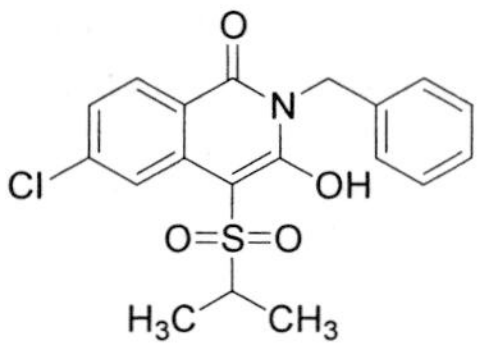   BIRL-790

COX-2: IC_{50} = 0.06 μM

COX-1: IC_{50} = 1.44 μM

Figure 14: Modification of melioxicam.

Aspirin is the only known NSAID that covalently bonds to serine and inhibits COX-1 more significantly than COX-2. Many systematic structural modifications have been carried out resulting in the development of APHS characterized by a 60-fold increase in activity and a 100-fold increase in selectivity for COX-2 than aspirin. Inhibition of COX-2 also occurs by acetylation of the same serine residue that is acetylated by aspirin, indicating that the mechanism of APHS inhibition is not identical to that of other selective COX-2 inhibitors (Kalgutkar et al., 1998a; 1998b).

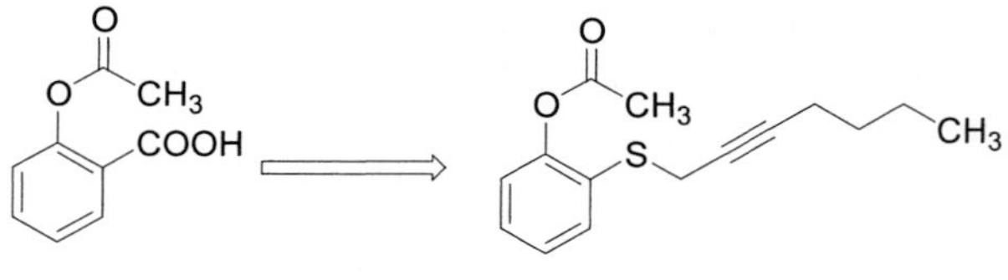

aspirin   APHS
                                  (Vanderbilt University)

COX-2: IC_{50} = 0.8 μM

COX-1: IC_{50} = 17 μM

Figure 15: Modification of aspirin.

Compounds with Antioxidative Moieties

The mode of action of these compounds, which are under investigation, is via an antioxidative mechanism. Since COX enzyme catalysis involves radical intermediates, a radical scavenging moiety such as a di-*tert*-butylphenol interferes with the cyclooxygenase reaction. Linkage of phenolic substructure with a thiazolone, oxazolone, thiadiazole or oxadiazole derivative produces non-ulcerogenic, orally active anti-inflammatory agents as a novel class of COX-2 inhibitors. The most potent and COX-2 selective compound of this class was the thiadiazole derivative (Song et al., 1999).

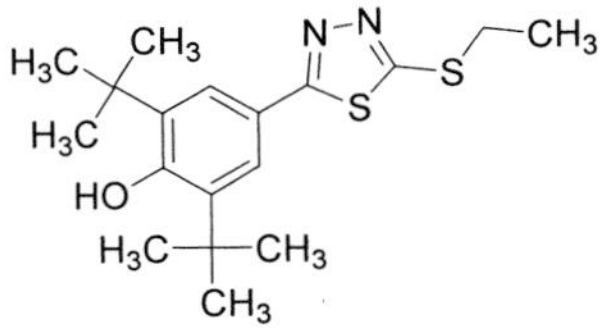

COX-1: IC_{50} > 100 μM

COX-2: IC_{50} = 0.14 μM

(purified enzymes)

Figure 16: COX-2 inhibitor with an antioxidative moiety.

Dual COX-2 and 5-LO Inhibitors

A new class of compounds is reported to have dual inhibitory properties. They have a γ-sultam skeleton and show potent inhibitory effects towards both COX-2 and 5-lipoxygenase as well as production of IL-1 in *in vitro* assays. These compounds have also proved to be effective in several animal arthritic models without any ulcerogenic activity. Among these compounds S-2474 ((*E*)-(5)-(3,5-di-*tert.*-butyl-4-hydroxy-benzylidene)-2-ethyl-1,2-isothiazolidine-1,1-dioxide) was selected as an anti-arthritic drug candidate and is now under clinical investigations (Inagaki et al., 2000).

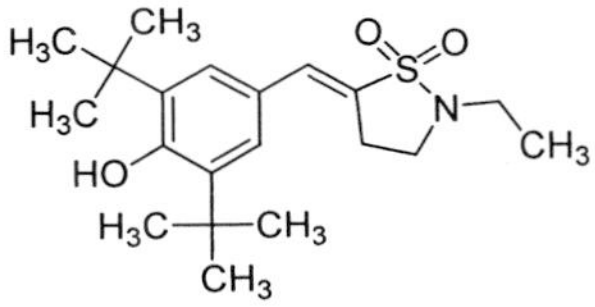

ML-3000 ((2,2-dimethyl-6-(4-chlorophenyl)-7-phenyl-2,3-dihydro-1H-pyrrolizine-5-yl)-acetic acid) is a non-antioxidant dual inhibitor of both cyclooxygenase and 5-lipoxygenase. ML-3000 has been compared to indomethacin in a number of experimental models of inflammation. The analgesic effects of ML-3000 have also been assessed in a number of animal models. Phase II studies have shown a wide range of activities, including anti-inflammatory, analgesic, antiplatelet and anti-asthmatic properties (Laufer et al., 1994; Chin and Wallace, 1999).

S-2474

Non-antioxidant dual COX-2 and 5-LO inhibitors

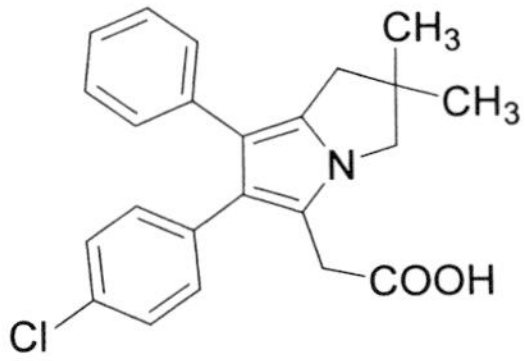

ML-3000

COX: IC_{50} = 0.21 μM

5-LO: IC_{50} = 0.18 mM

Diarylethylene Derivatives (*cis*-Stilbene Compounds)

Reduction of the furanone ring led to active inhibitors with an open-ring diol structure. Ring opening and elimination of the heteroatom led to *cis*-stilbene derivatives which still contain the prerequisites for COX-2 inhibition: vicinal orientation of two aromatic rings, substitution pattern at the aryl moiety as seen in potent COX-2 inhibitors, i.e. a methylsulfonyl moiety in combination with a halogen. This group of compounds is presently undergoing biological testing (Dannhardt and Kiefer, 2001).

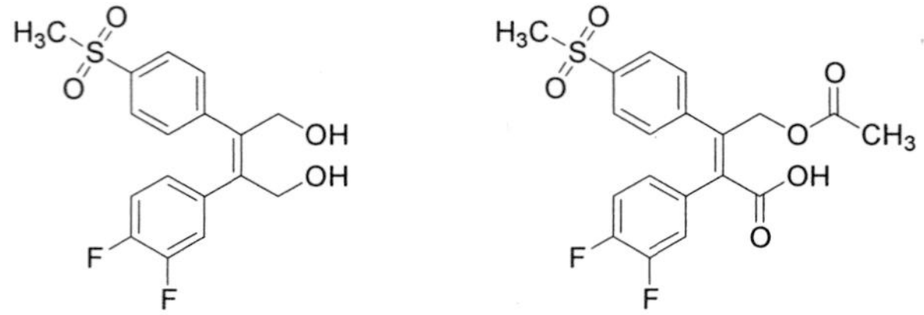

Figure 17: COX-2 inhibitors with a diarylethylene moiety.

Miscellaneous Structures

Novel structural series that do not fit the above-mentioned categories have been included in the miscellaneous group. Hoffmann-La Roche (Rotstein and Sjorgen (Hoffmann-La Roche), 1998) has described aroylnaphthalene derivatives, which exhibit good *in vitro* activity and selectivity. Searle (Carter, 1998) has also disclosed a series of chromenes with good COX-2 selectivity and remarkable oral activity (57 % inhibition of paw edema at 30 mg/kg p.o.). Chugai Seiyaku claimed a series of indoles and diazaindoles, as well as substituted indenes. Interestingly, these compounds lack the alkanoic acid side chain typical of COX inhibitors (Matsuoka et al. (Chugai Seiyku Kabushiki Kaisha), 1998; 1999). Pfizer (Nakao et al. (Pfizer), 1999; Okumura et al. (Pfizer), 1999) has also reported indole derivatives as selective COX-2 inhibitors. Additionally, Pfizer modified the indole framework, yielding benzimidazole derivatives (Stevens et al. (Pfizer), 1999; Jiménez et al., 2000).

Computational and combinatorial chemistry methodology helped to create a highly selective phenothiazine derivative which can serve as a novel lead compound for further development in the field of COX-2 inhibitors (Dannhardt and Kiefer, 2001).

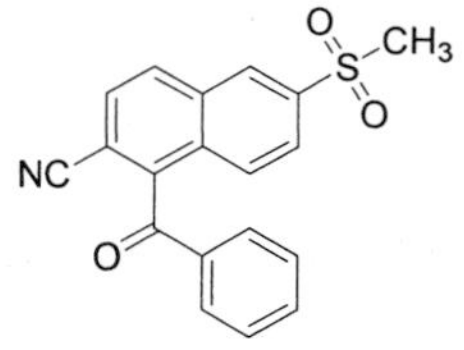

(Hoffmann La Roche) 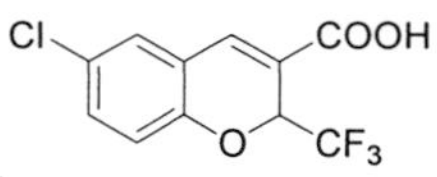   (GD Searle & Co)

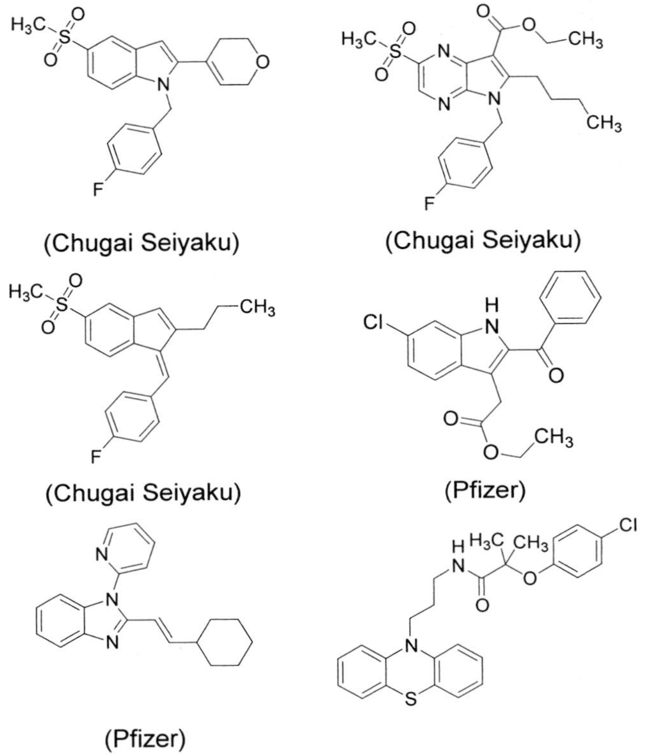

(Chugai Seiyaku)   (Chugai Seiyaku)

(Chugai Seiyaku)   (Pfizer)

(Pfizer)

Figure 18: Miscellaneous structures.

Clinical Experiences with COX-2 Inhibitors

A variety of clinical studies have shown the efficacy of the new COX-2 inhibitors in several indications of pain and inflammation. Two large clinical studies have been performed in order to assess clinical efficacy and side-effects of rofecoxib (VIGOR trial) and celecoxib (CLASS trial), respectively (Fitzgerald and Patrono, 2001). Both studies show an increased gastrointestinal safety profile compared to the standard medication, although only rofecoxib shows a statistically significant improvement. In terms of cardioprotection, naproxen had a better outcome compared to rofecoxib. This may represent the negative aspects of the COX-1-sparing novel COX-2 inhibitors, since they do not inhibit platelet-derived thromboxanes, which are important in indications such as myocardial infarction. Likewise, the influence of COX-2 inhibition on renal function and hypertension has to be addressed in future studies, since COX-2 expression is essential for kidney development and function (Dinchuk et al., 1995; Komhoff et al., 2000).

Gastro-intestinal safety

The Vioxx Gastrointestinal Outcomes Research (VIGOR) trial (Bombardier et al., 2000) and the Celecoxib Long-Term Arthritis Safety Study (CLASS) trial (Silver-stein et al., 2000) were designed to assess both efficacy and gastrointestinal side-effects. The VIGOR trial included 8076 patients with rheumatoid arthritis receiving either rofecoxib or naproxen. The CLASS trial comprises of a total of 8059 patients with rheumatoid arthritis or osteoarthritis in two studies, comparing cele-coxib to diclofenac and ibuprofen, respectively.

Colon cancer

Celecoxib leads to a significant reduction in the number of colorectal polyps in patients with familial adenomatous polyposis in a 6-months study (Steinbach et al., 2000).

Alzheimer's disease

A prospective, population-based cohort study of 6989 patients aged 55 years or older, who were free of dementia at baseline, showed a beneficial effect of long-term treatment with NSAIDs (in't Veld et al., 2001).

NSAIDs and COX-2 inhibitors show good potencies and efficacies in mild to moderate pain conditions and in inflammation. Many combinations of NSAIDs with other principles are on the market or under development. Misoprostol (on the market) and NO donors (under development) reduce the side-effects of NSAIDs on the gastric mucosa and opioid analgesics (standard WHO ladder of pain treatment) add to the analgesic potency of NSAIDs.

In addition to the treatment of pain and inflammation, COX-2 inhibitors might be of benefit in other indications. Expression of COX-2 in colon cancer, intestinal adenomas, and other cancer cells as well as clinical studies with COX-2 inhibitors, suggest the use of COX-2 inhibitors in cancer (Masferrer et al., 1999). Expression of COX-2 in angiogenesis follows the same route since angiogenesis is important for blood supply and hence the growth of many tumors.

COX-2 expression was also found in brain areas related to memory (hippocampus, cortex) in patients with Alzheimer's disease (Ho et al., 1999, Yasojima et al., 1999). These findings together with clinical data suggest new options for the use of COX-2 inhibitors in this indication.

Aspirin has gained additional importance in the last few years due to its inhibition of platelet aggregation. Low dose treatment with aspirin leads to irreversible acetylation of COX-1 in platelets and is used in the acute treatment and chronic prevention of myocardial infarction and stroke (Higgs et al., 1987).

Additional Effects of COX-inhibitors

Some NSAIDs show anti-inflammatory and anti-proliferative effects independent of their COX activity. Modulation of intracellular signalling pathways might contribute to these activities (Tegeder et al., 2001). A key question with respect to those additional activities is whether or not concentrations of the respective compound at the presumed sites of actions is sufficient in order to add to the main mode of action, COX inhibition.

NSAIDs as Transcriptional Modulating Drugs

In addition to bioactive eicosanoids, the inflammatory response involves the sequential activation of various signaling pathways, including reactive oxygen intermediates, cytokines, growth factors, enzymes, receptors, and adhesion molecules. Increased expression of most of these proteins is the result of enhanced gene transcription. Changes in gene transcription of proteins involved in inflammation are usually regulated by transcription factors such as modulators of activated T cells (NF-AT), nuclear factors (NF-κB), and activated protein (AP-1).

Therefore, drugs able to inhibit transcription of genes involved in the inflammatory process could be potent anti-inflammatory agents. Thus among the most effective anti-inflammatory drugs are the glucocorticoids, whose actions occur by inhibition of the transcription of several genes which are responsible for the induction of cytokines, chemokines and COX-2 in response to inflammation. Inhibition of pro-inflammatory transcription factors such as AP-1, NF-AT or NF-κB is thought to be the major action of glucocorticoids

The role of glucocorticoids

Another class of transcription-modulating drugs is the immunosuppressants such as cyclosporin A (CsA), which inhibit T cell activation and proliferation, events playing a central role in the immune response and therefore in the inflammatory process. CsA blocks transcriptional induction of cytokines by inhibiting the phosphatase calcineurin, and by the subsequent inhibition of the activation of NF-AT and NF-AT-dependent activation genes.

The role of other immunosuppressants such as cyclosporin A (CsA)

Several studies have demonstrated that certain NSAIDs have anti-inflammatory and anti-proliferative effects that seem to be mediated through mechanisms independent of cyclooxygenase activity and prostaglandin production. These effects are generally mediated through inhibition of several transcription factors such NF-AT, NF-kB, or AP-1. It may be these properties of NSAIDs that add to the therapeutic benefits of these drugs in diseases such carcinogenesis and Alzheimer´s disease. In most cases, the doses required to ameliorate chronic inflammatory diseases and tumor progression are much higher than those doses required to inhibit prostaglandin synthesis. In addition, NSAIDs which are poor inhibitors of COX-2 are able to reduce inflammation and hyperalgesia. The ani-tumor activity of NSAIDs such as inhibition of cell cycle progression, induction of apoptosis and inhibition of angiogenesis has become apparent at high concentrations of the drugs. This suggests that the effects of high doses of certain NSAIDs are mediated by cyclooxygenase-independent mechanisms. Some of these mechanisms decribed for NSAIDs are summarized below. The enzymatic inhibition of NSAIDs as well as the transcriptional regulation is shown in Fig. 19.

Cyclooxygenase-independent mechanisms of NSAIDs

Christoph and Buschmann

Summary of mechanisms of actions of NSAIDs as transcriptional regulators on the functional and molecular level

Functional level

- Inhibition of immune cell activation
- Inhibition of cytokine production
- Induction of apoptosis

Molecular level

- Inhibition of transcription factors NF-κB, NF-AT, and AP-1
- Alteration of MAP kinases cascade
- Modulation of the activity of nuclear receptors (PPARs)
- Induction of transcription factors and genes (STAG, NAG, NFGI-B)

PPAR (Peroxisome Proliferator-Activated Receptor)

PPAR is a nuclear receptor-transcription factor and is ligand-dependent and expressed in several tissues. It is initially involved in adipocyte differentiation and fatty acid synthesis. Fatty acid and eicosanoids bind to PPAR and regulate transcription. PPAR activation inhibits monocyte differentiation and expression of several pro-inflammatory genes such as iNOS, TNF, etc. PPAR activation inhibits tumor cell proliferation (epithelial, colon, prostate). PPAR is involved in angiogenesis.

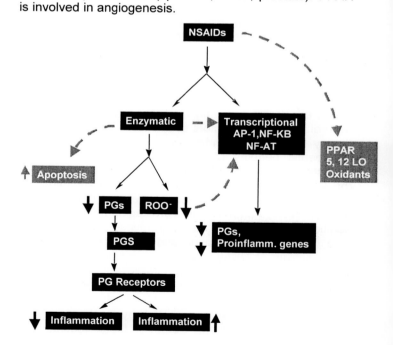

Figure 19: Mechanism of action of NSAIDs as enzyme inhibitors and/or transcriptional regulators.

COX-1 and COX-2 Inhibitors in Clinical Use

Acemetacin

Synthesis (Boltze and Kreisfeld, 1977; Kleemann et al., 1999):

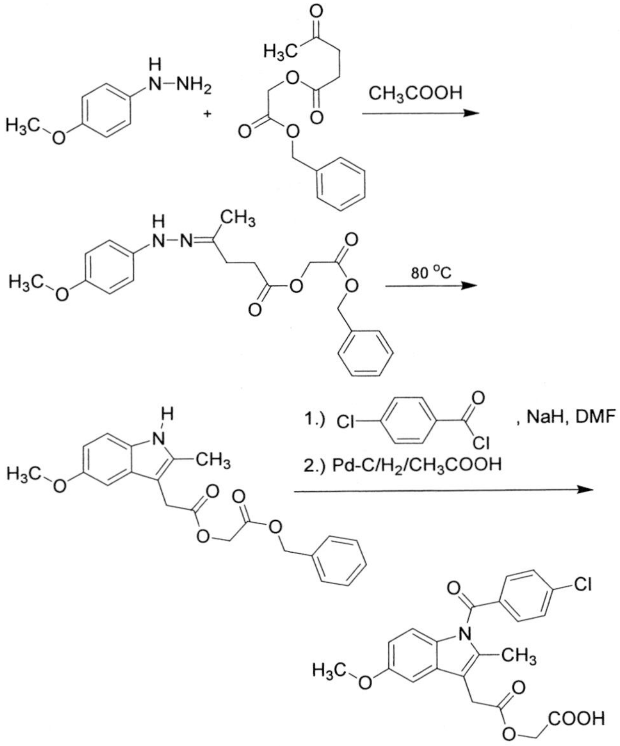

Acemetacin

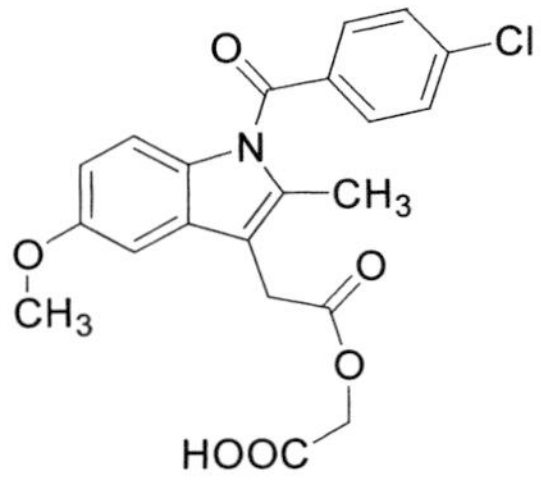

[53164-05-9], [1-(4-Chloro-benzoyl)-5-methoxy-2-methyl-1*H*-indol-3-yl]-acetic acid carboxymethyl ester, $C_{21}H_{18}ClNO_6$, M_r 415,82, *mp* 150-153 °C (fine pale yellow crystals)

Scheme 4: Synthesis of acemetacin.

The reaction product of indomethacin (see below) with benzyl bromo acetate can also be hydrogenated to Acemetacin.

Clinical use: Acemetacin (Jacobi and Dell, 1980) is a nonsteroidal anti-inflammatory drug which acts directly via its major metabolite indomethacin. Acemetacin is used in chronic joint pain as well as in postoperative pain. The recommendation for oral dosing is between 120 and 360 mg daily.

Trade name: Rantudil (Ger), Emflex (UK)

Acetylsalicylic Acid

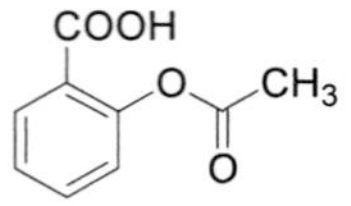

COOH

[structure of acetylsalicylic acid]

[50-78-2], 2-Acetoxy-
benzoic acid, $C_9H_8O_4$, M_r
180.04, *mp* 135 °C

Acetylsalicylic Acid

Synthesis (Kleemann et al., 1999; Kuhnert, 1999):

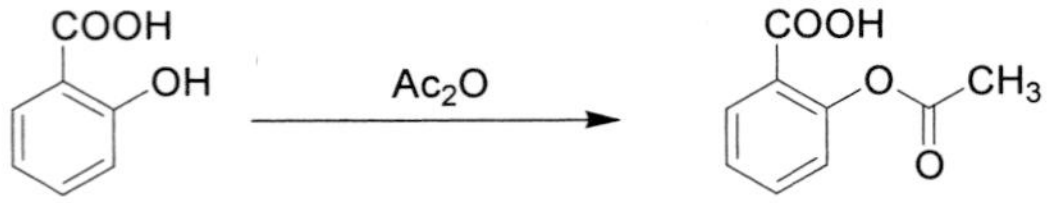

COOH Ac_2O COOH

Scheme 5: Synthesis of acetylsalicylic acid.

Clinical use: Acetylsalicylic acid is the prototype of a nonsteroidal anti-inflammatory drug and is used in a large number of inflammatory and pain indications including musculoskeletal, soft tissue and joint disorders, headache, dysmenorrhoea and fever (Symposium on new perspectives on aspirin therapy 1983, various authors). Furthermore, acetylsalicylic acid is used as an antiplatelet drug in the acute treatment of myocardial infarction in combination with thrombolytics and for the prevention of myocardial infarction and stroke (Patrono, 1994).

Depending on the assay system, acetylsalicylic acid shows a balanced inhibition of COX-1 and COX-2 or a selectivity towards COX-1. When used in low doses as antiplatelet drug, the main target is COX-1. In addition to a COX inhibition, acetylsalicylic acid modulates the activities of several cellular kinases which may contribute to its anti-inflammatory effects (Tegeder et al., 2001).

COX selectivity

IC50 [µM]	COX-1	COX-2	ratio
cell culture (1)	9.6	16.0	0.6
cell culture (2)	0.3	50	0.006
whole blood (3)	4.4	13.9	0.3

(1) Berg et al. (1997)

(2) Mitchell et al. (1993)

(3) Cryer and Feldman (1998)

The inhibition of COX-1 and COX-2 does not follow a competitive mechanism like other nonsteroidal anti-inflammatory drugs but rather is due to a covalent enzyme inhibition via acetylation. After absorption, acetylsalicylic acid is hydrolyzed to salicylate which itself still shows some COX inhibition. Both compounds are bound (80-90%) to plasma proteins. The plasma elimination half-life is about 15 min for acetylsalicylic acid and between 3 and 22 h for salicylate depending on the dose (Needs and Brooks, 1985).

The metabolic pathway of acetylsalicylic acid is shown in scheme 6.

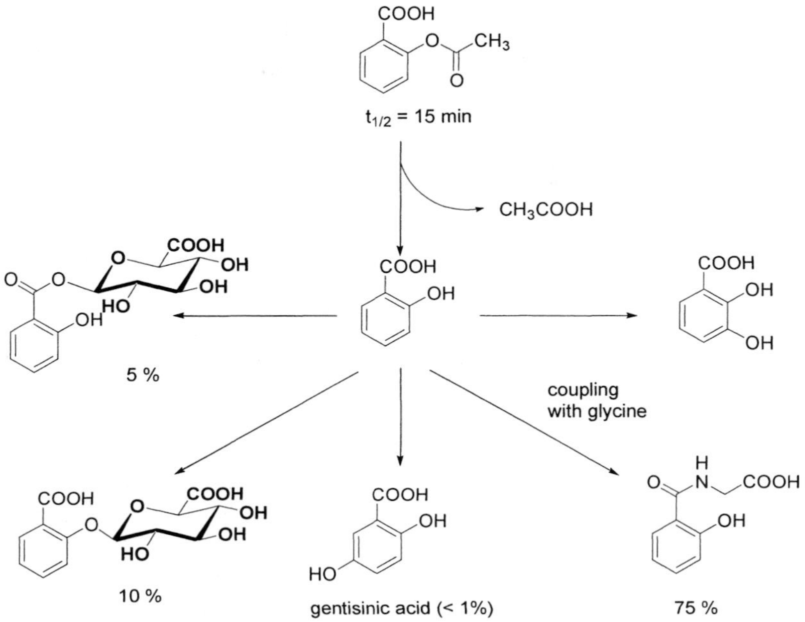

Scheme 6: Metabolic pathway of acetylsalicylic acid

Acetylsalicylic acid is usually given by oral administration (0.5-8 g/day) for pain and inflammation and for antiplatelet therapy (75-100 mg/day). It is also available in rectal and topical formulations and as a soluble lysine derivative for intravenous or intramuscular application. Acetylsalicylic acid is often used in multi-drug preparations. The main side-effects are gastrointestinal disorders. Use in children is limited due to the risk of Reye's syndrome (Waldmann et al., 1982). The lithium, magnesium, calcium, and aluminium salts of acetylsalicylic acid are used in some special preparations.

Trade name: Aspirine (F), Aspirin, Aspisol (Ger), Aspro (UK), Alka Seltzer (US)

Bufexamac

Synthesis (Buu-Hoi, 1965; Kleemann et al., 1999):

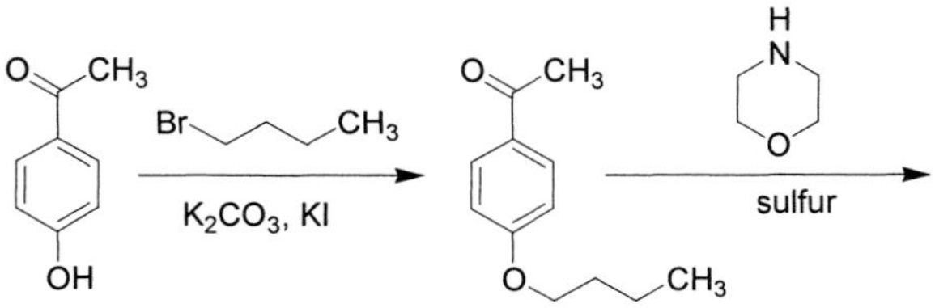

Bufexamac

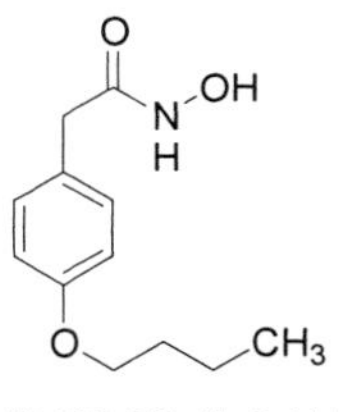

[2438-72-4], 2-(4-Butoxy-phenyl)-N-hydroxy-acetamide, $C_{12}H_{17}NO_3$, M_r 223.12, *mp* 153-155 °C

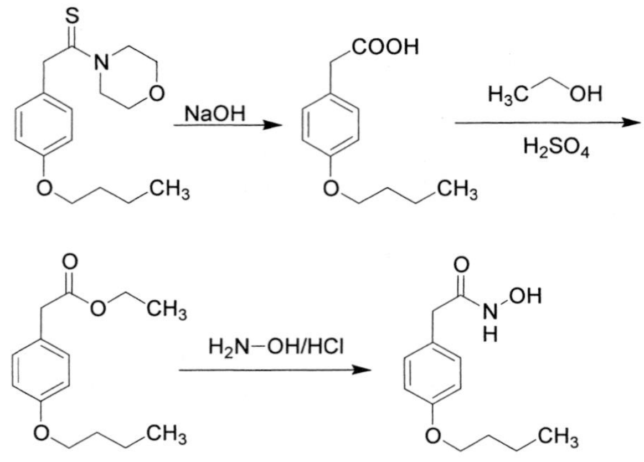

Scheme 7: Synthesis of bufexamac.

Trade name: Duradermal
(Ger), Parfenac (France,
Ger)

Clinical use: Bufexamac (Brogden et al., 1975) is a nonsteroidal anti-inflammatory drug used in topical formulations for mild skin disorders and as suppositories (250-500 mg/day) for haemorrhoids.

Celecoxib

Celecoxib

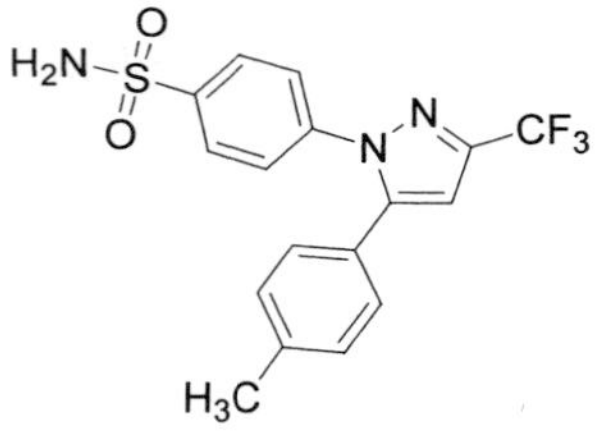

[169590-42-5], 4-(5-p-Tolyl-3-trifluoromethyl-pyrazol-1-yl)-benzenesulfonamide, $C_{17}H_{14}F_3N_3O_2S$, M_r 381.37; *mp* 157-159 °C (pale yellow solid)

Synthesis: The condensation of 4-methylacetophenone with ethyl acetate by means of NaOMe in refluxing methanol gives 4,4,4-trifluoro-1-(4-methylphenyl)butane-1,3-dione, which cyclized with 4-hydrazinophenyl-sulfonamide in refluxing ethanol (Graul et al., 1977; Talley et al. (Searle & Co.), 1995.

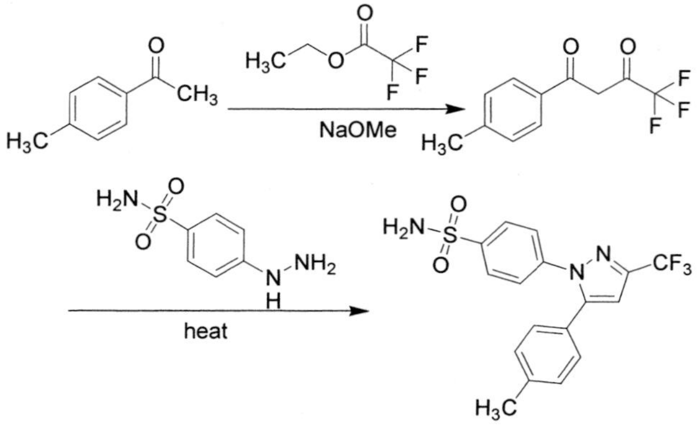

Scheme 8: Synthesis of celecoxib.

Clinical use: Celecoxib (Graul et al., 1997; Wallace and Chin, 1999) is a second generation selective COX-2 inhibitor and the first drug of this group which reached the market. Its selectivity for COX-2 compared to COX-1 is about 375-fold greater in human recombinant enzyme preparations and about 8-fold in a whole blood assay. Celecoxib has been approved for rheumatoid arthritis, osteoarthritis, acute pain and primary dysmenorrhoea in the US and has been launched in an increasing number of countries since 1999.

Plasma peak concentrations are achieved within 2 h and the elimination half-life is about 12 h. Within the clinical dose range, there is high plasma protein binding (~97%). Celecoxib is metabolized primarily via cytochrome P450 2C9 to three inactive main metabolites. It is excreted in faeces (~57%) and urine (~27%) as determined by administration of a single oral dose of radiolabeled drug. Celecoxib is given orally (200-400 mg/day).

COX selectivity

IC50 [µM]	COX-1	COX-2	ratio
recomb. enzyme (1)	15.0	0.040	375
whole blood (2)	6.7	0.87	7.6

(1) Penning et al. (1997)

(2) Riendeau et al. (2001)

Proposed metabolic pathway for celecoxib in humans (Paulson et al., 1999, 2000)

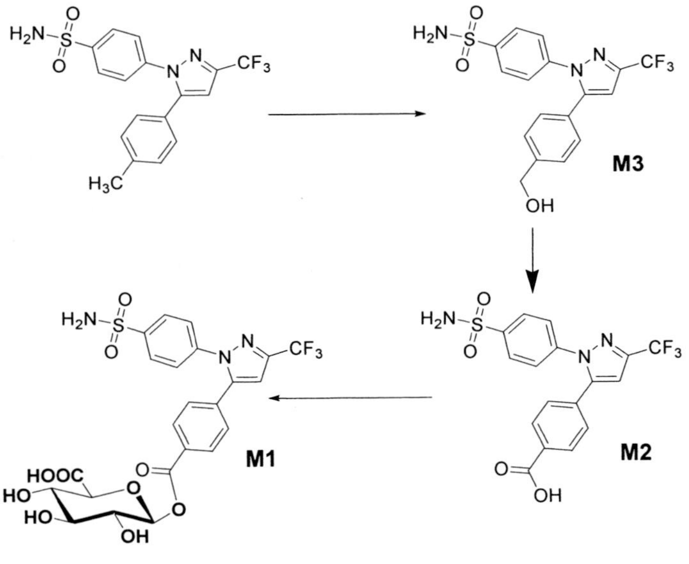

Scheme 9: Metabolic pathway of celecoxib.

Use of celecoxib is associated with a reduced incidence of gastroduodenal ulcers in comparison to naproxen (Goldstein et al., 2001) ibuprofen, or diclofenac (Silverstein et al., 2000) in patients with arthritis.

Celecoxib is approved for the use in familial adenomatous polyposis in the US and leads to a reduction in the number of colorectal polyps in these patients (Steinbach et al., 2000).

Trade name: Celebrex (US, EC)

Diclofenac

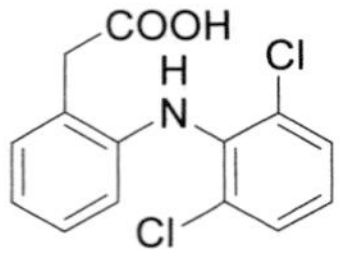

[*15307-86-5*], [2-(2,6-
Dichloro-phenylamino)-
phenyl]-acetic acid,
$C_{14}H_{11}Cl_2NO_2$, M_r 296.15,
mp 156-158 °C; sodium salt
[*15307-79-6*],
$C_{14}H_{10}Cl_2NNaO_2$, M_r
318.13, *mp* 283-285 °C

Diclofenac

Synthesis (Moser et al., 1990): acylation of *N*-phenyl-2,6-dichloroaniline with chloroacetyl chloride gives the corresponding chloroacetanilide, which is fused with aluminum chloride to give 1-(2,6-dichlorophenyl)-2-indolinone. Hydrolysis of the indolinone with dilute aqueous-alcoholic sodium hydroxide affords the desired sodium salt directly.

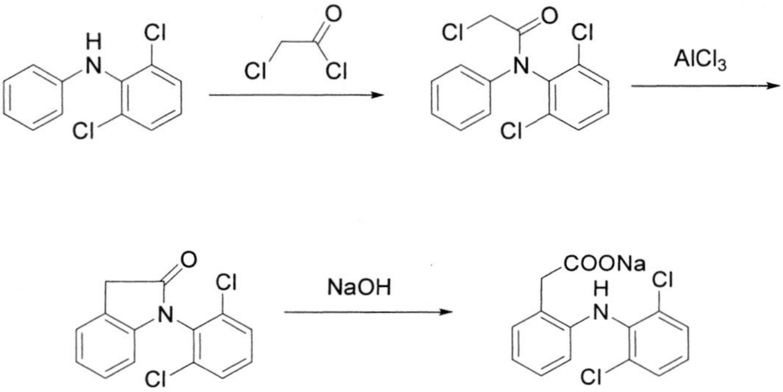

Scheme 10: Synthesis of diclofenac.

Another synthesis using 2-chloro benzoic acid as starting material is shown below.:

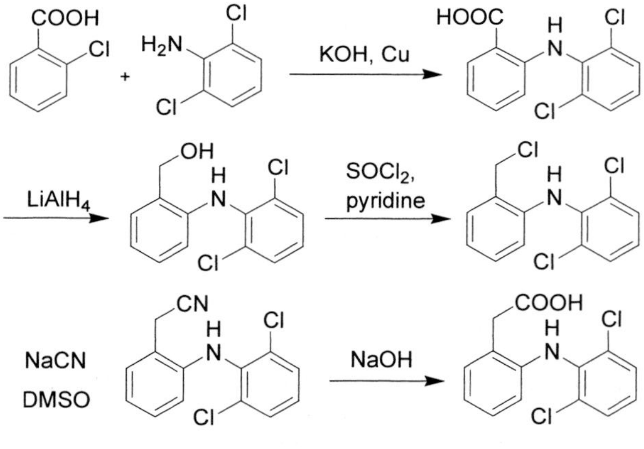

Scheme 11: Synthesis of diclofenac.

Clinical use: Diclofenac (Todd and Sorkin, 1988) is a nonsteroidal anti-inflammatory drug with balanced COX-1 and COX-2 inhibition. It is commonly used for a variety of inflammatory and pain conditions such as musculoskeletal and joint disorders, periarticular disorders, soft tissue disorders, renal colic, acute gout, dysmenorrhoea as well as postoperative pain.

The plasma protein binding of diclofenac is greater than 99.5 % and the plasma elimination half-life is between 1 and 2 h. The metabolites of diclofenac, 4'-hydroxy-diclofenac, 5-hydroxydiclofenac, 3'-hydroxy-diclofenac, and 4',5-dihydroxydiclofenac are excreted as glucuronide and sulphate conjugates in the urine (~65%) and in the bile (~35%).

COX selectivity

IC50 [µM]	COX-1	COX-2	ratio
recomb. Enzyme (1)	0.059	0.031	1.9
cell culture (2)	0.5	0.35	1.4
whole blood (3)	0.14	0.05	2.8

(1) Churchill et al. (1996)
(2) Mitchell et al. (1993)
(3) Brideau et al. (1996)

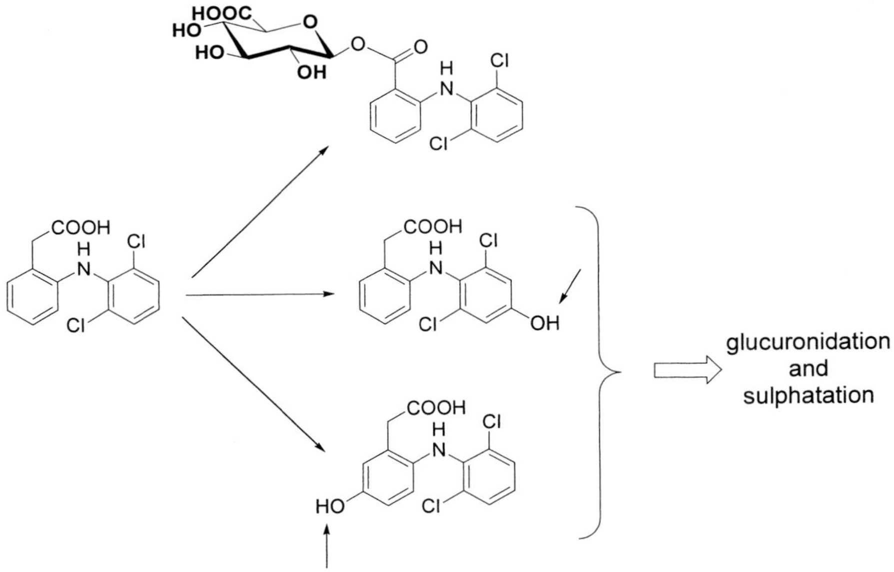

Scheme 12: Metabolic pathway of diclofenac.

Diclofenac is used mainly as the sodium salt orally or parenterally (75-150 mg/day) and as an ophthalmic solution. Topical formulations may contain the diethylammonium or epolamine salt. Diclofenac is combined with misoprostol to reduce gastrointestinal effects, which are the main side-effects.

Trade name: Voltaren (Ger, US), Voltarène (France), Voltarol (UK)

Diflunisal

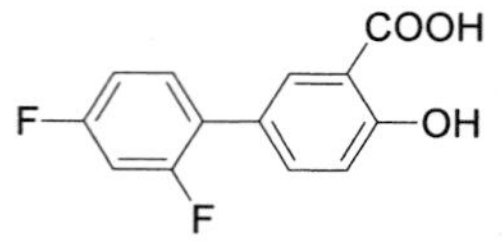

[*22494-42-4*], 2'4'-Difluoro-4-hydroxy-biphenyl-3-carboxylic acid, $C_{13}H_8F_2O_3$, M_r 250.20, *mp* 210-211 °C (also reported as 212-213 °C)

Diflunisal

Synthesis (Arrigoni-Martelli, 1978a; Hannah et al., 1978; Jones and Hauser (Merck & Co.), 1980; Kleemann et al., 1999): The diazotation of 2,4-difluoroanaline with isoamyl nitrite and condensation with anisole gives 4-(2,4-difluorophenyl)anisole, which is hydrolyzed with HI in refluxing acetic acid yielding 4-(2,4-difluorophenyl)phenol. Finally this compound is carbonated with K_2CO_3 and CO_2 at 175 °C and 90 bar.

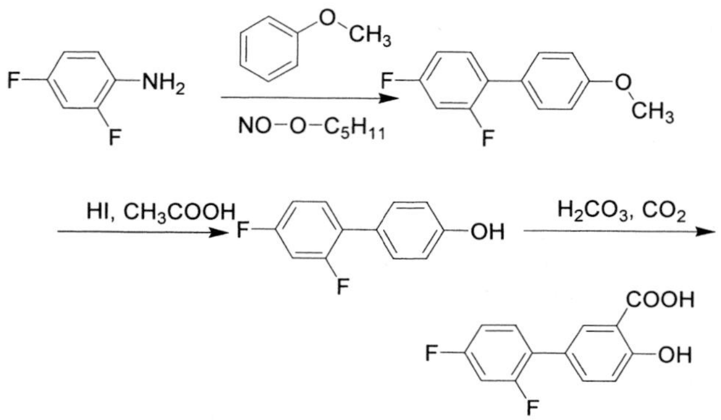

Scheme 13: Synthesis of diflunisal.

Clinical use: Diflunisal (Brogden et al., 1980) is a nonsteroidal anti-inflammatory drug used in the treatment of mild to moderate pain including osteoarthritis, rheumatoid arthritis and primary dysmenorrhoea. It is used as base or lysine- or arginine-salt for oral or parenteral application.

Diflunisal shows weak inhibition of both, COX-1 and COX-2 in a whole blood assay.

Peak plasma concentrations are reached within 2 to 3 h after oral dosing. Diflunisal is heavily bound to plasma protein (>99 %), has a long elimination half-life (8-12 h) and non-linear kinetics. Hence, it is used with an initial loading dose (1000 mg) and a lower maintenance dose (500-1000 mg/day). Diflusinal is excreted as glucuronide in the urine.

The main side-effects are gastrointestinal disturbances, headache and rash.

COX selectivity

IC50 [µM]	COX-1	COX-2	ratio
whole blood (1)	232	52	4.5

(1) Young et al. (1996)

Trade names: Dolobis (France), Dolobid (UK, USA)

Ethenzamide

Synthesis: Salicylamide (see below) is ethylated with diethyl sulfate (Lundbeck, 1948; Kleemann et al., 1999).

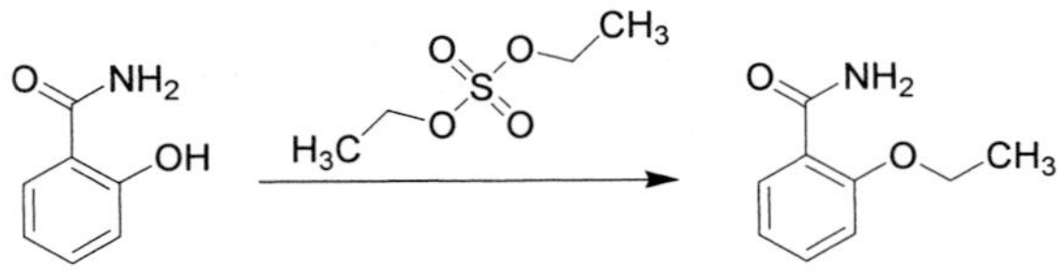

Scheme 14: Synthesis of ethenzamide.

Clinical use: Ethenzamide is a nonsteroidal anti-inflammatory drug used mainly in combination with other ingredients for the treatment of mild to moderate pain including musculoskeletal and joint disorders.

Etodolac

Synthesis (Demerson et al. (American Home Products), 1974; Demerson et al., 1975; 1976; Castaner and Arrigoni-Martelli, 1977a):

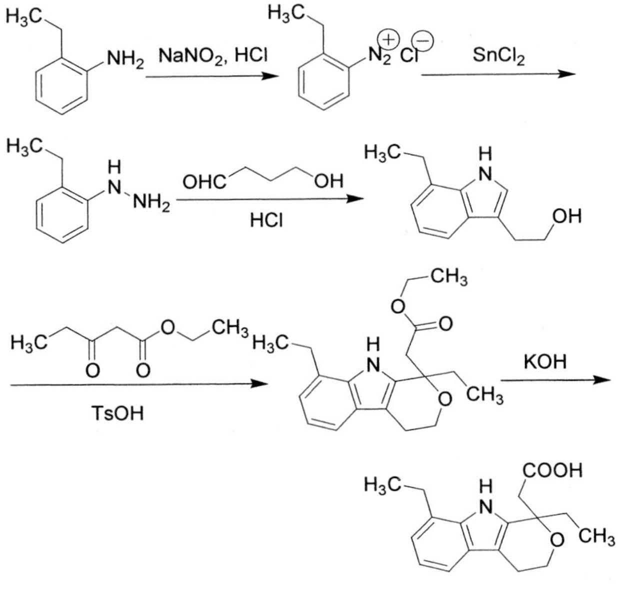

Scheme 15: Synthesis of etodolac.

Ethenzamide

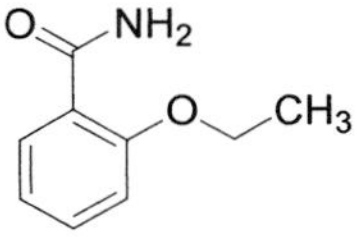

[*938-73-8*], 2-Ethoxy-benzamide, $C_9H_{11}NO_2$, M_r 165.19, *mp* 132-134 °C

Trade name: Trancalgyl (France), Kolton, Antiföhnon-N (Ger)

Etodolac

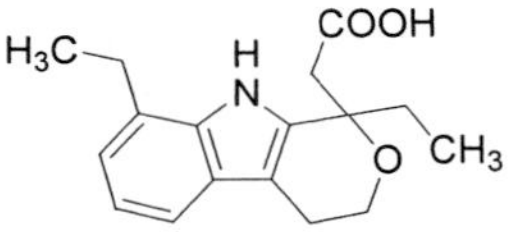

[*41340-25-4*], (1,8-Diethyl-1,3,4,9-tetrahydro-pyrano[3,4-*b*]indol-1-yl)-acetic acid, $C_{17}H_{21}NO_3$, M_r 287.35, *mp* 145-148 °C

COX selectivity

IC50 [µM]	COX-1	COX-2	ratio
cell culture (1)	~50	0.041	~1000
whole blood (2)	34	3.4	10

(1) Riendeau et al. (1997)

(2) Patrignani et al. (1997)

Trade name: Lodine (USA, UK, France)

Etofenamate

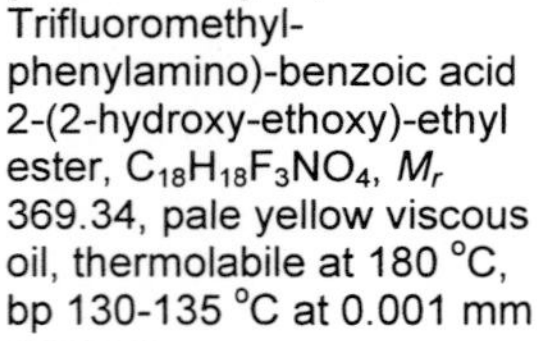

[*30544-47-9*], 2-(3-Trifluoromethyl-phenylamino)-benzoic acid 2-(2-hydroxy-ethoxy)-ethyl ester, $C_{18}H_{18}F_3NO_4$, M_r 369.34, pale yellow viscous oil, thermolabile at 180 °C, bp 130-135 °C at 0.001 mm pressure

Trade name: Rheumon (Austria, Ger, Switz.)

Clinical use: Etodolac (Bellamy, 1997) is a drug, invented before the discovery of the COX isoenzymes. Thus, there was clinical experience with the drug, before it was shown, that etodolac has a 10-fold selectivity for COX-2 compared to COX-1 in human whole blood. Etodolac belongs to the first generation of COX-2 inhibitors (Vane et al., 1998). Clinical data indicate fewer gastrointestinal side-effects in comparison to naproxen (Taha et al., 1989; Bianchi Porro et al., 1991). Etodolac is a racemate with an active (S)-enantiomer and an inactive (R)-enantiomer.

Etodolac shows efficacy in a wide variety of diverse pain states. It is used for the treatment of mild to moderate acute and chronic pain including rheumatoid arthritis and osteoarthritis. Etodolac is administered orally (400-1200 mg/day).

Peak plasma concentrations are reached within 2 h. Etodolac shows 99 % binding to plasma protein and an elimination half-life of about 7 h (Brooks and Jamali, 1994). Etodolac is metabolized almost completely to the main metabolites 6- or 7-hydroxy-etodolac, acyl-glucuronide, 8-(1'-hydroxyethyl)-etodolac and 4-ureido-etodolac. The metabolites and a small quantity of etodolac are excreted in the urine. A small amount of conjugated etodolac is excreted through the biliary tract.

Etofenamate

Synthesis: The esterification of the potassium salt of flufenamic acid (see below) with 2-(2-chloroethoxy)ethanol in dimethyl formamide as solvent yields Etofenamate (Boltze and Kreisfeld, 1977; Kleemann et al., 1999).

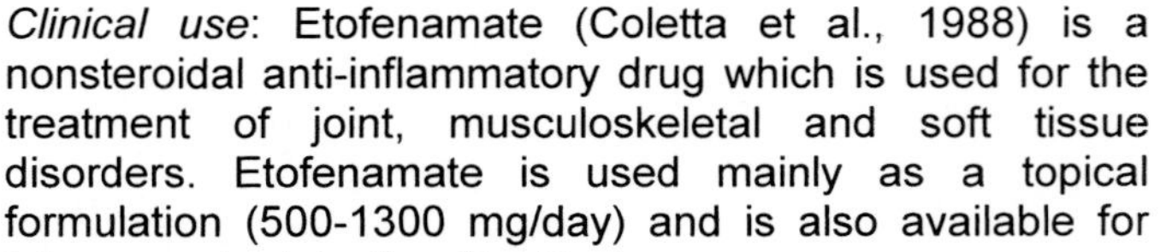

Scheme 16: Synthesis of etofenamate.

Clinical use: Etofenamate (Coletta et al., 1988) is a nonsteroidal anti-inflammatory drug which is used for the treatment of joint, musculoskeletal and soft tissue disorders. Etofenamate is used mainly as a topical formulation (500-1300 mg/day) and is also available for intramuscular injection (1 g/day).

Etoricoxib

Synthesis: A number of synthetic strategies to the COX-2 specific inhibitor etoricoxib have been described (Dube et al. (Merck Frosst), 1998; Davies et al., 2000; Sobera et al., 2001a). In schemes 17-20 the two major routes via a dichloropyridine derivative or a ketosulfone, respectively, as the key intermediates are discussed.

The bromination of 5-chloro-2-hydroxypyridine with bromine gives 3-bromo-5-chloro-2-hydroxypyridine, which is treated with benzyl bromide and silver carbonate yielding the benzyl ether-protected derivative (**i**). Condensation of (**i**) with 4-(methylsulfanyl)phenylboronic acid by means of Pd(PPh$_3$)$_4$ in refluxing ethanol(benzene affords 2-(benzyloxy)-5-chloro-3-(4-(methylsulfanyl) phenyl)pyridine (**ii**), which is treated with osmium tetroxide and sodium sulfite to furnish sulfone (**iii**). Treatment of the sulfone (**iii**) with TFA provides the 2-hydroxypyridine derivative, which is reacted with POCl$_3$ to yield the key intermediate 2,5-dichloro-3-(4-(methylsulfonyl)phenyl) pyridine (**iv**). An alternative pathway to (**vi**) starts with the bromination of 2-chloropyridine with bromine in acetic acid to yield 2-amino-3-bromo-5-chloropyridine, which is coupled with (methylsulfanyl)phenylboronic acid by means of Pd(PPh$_3$)$_4$ and sodium carbonate in refluxing ethanol/benzene to give 5-chloro-3-(4-methanesulfonyl-phenyl)-pyridin-2-ylamine (**v**). The subsequent oxidation of (**v**) with osmium tetroxide as before yield compound (**vi**), which is converted to the key intermediate (**iv**) by treatment first with NaNO$_2$ and HCl and then chlorination with POCl$_3$.

Etoricoxib

[*202409-33-4*], [*202409-40-3*] (mono HCl) , 5-Chloro-3-(4-(methyl-sulfonyl)phenyl)-2-(6-methylpyridin-3-yl)pyridine; 5-chloro-6′-methyl-3-(4-(methylsulfonyl)phenyl)-2,3′-bipyridine C$_{18}$H$_{15}$ClN$_2$O$_2$S, 358.848; crystals mp 271.5-138.1 °C (136.7 °C DSC onset)

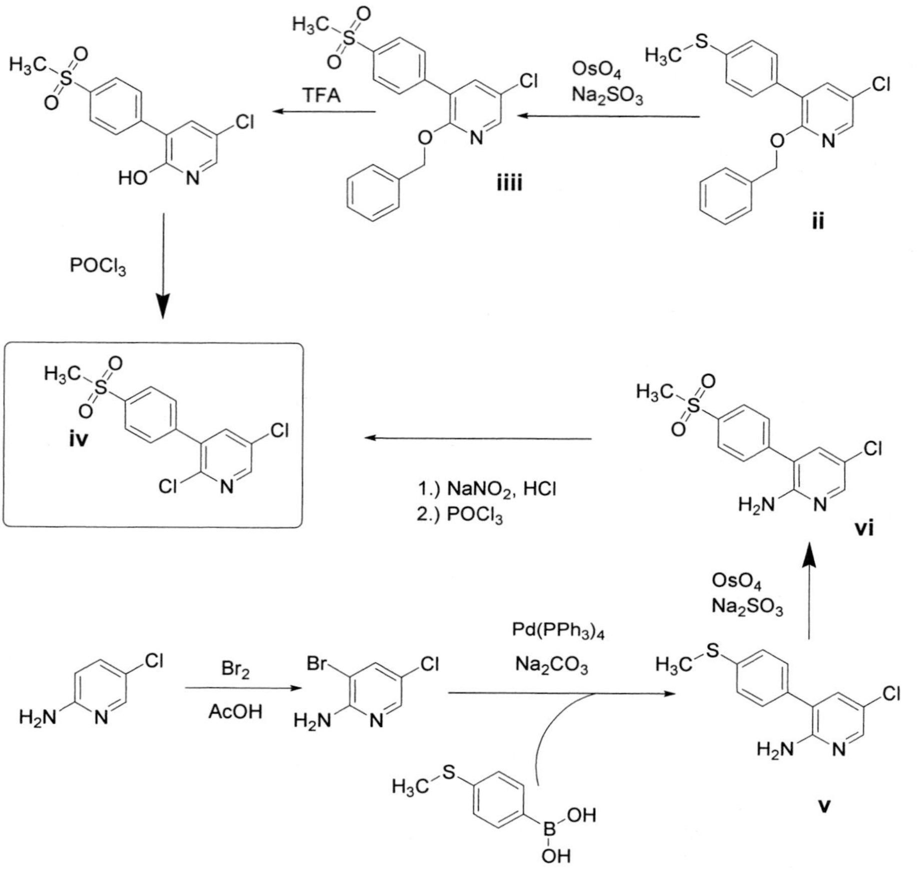

Scheme 17: Synthetic pathways to the key intermediate 2,5-dichloro-3-(4-
(methylsulfonyl)phenyl) pyridine (**iv**).

Finally, compound (**iv**) is condensed with either
trimethyl(6-methyl-3-pyridyl)tin or the boronate ester by
means of Pd(PPh$_3$)$_4$ to afford etoricoxib. The metallated
pyridine (**vii**) is obtained by esterification of 3-hydroxy-2-
methylpyridine with triflic anhydride to give the
corresponding triflate, which is treated with a tin reagent to
yield the target tin intermediate. The boron lithium salt
(**viii**) is prepared by treatment of 5-bromo-2-methylpyridine
with butyllithium followed by addition of triisopropyl borate.

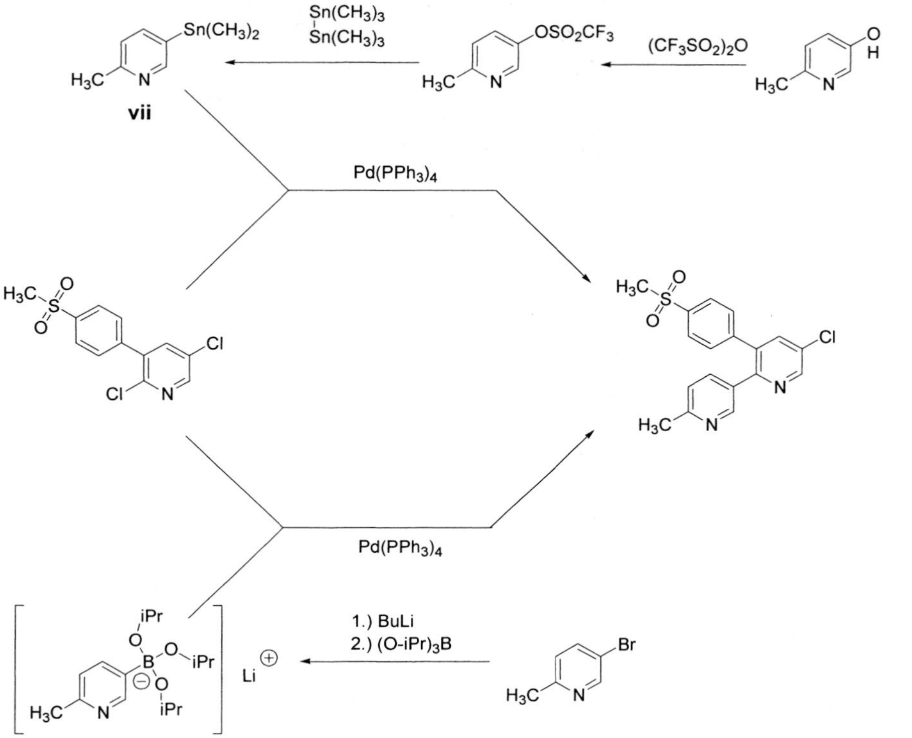

Scheme 18: Condensation pathways from the key intermediate 2,5-dichloro-3-(4-(methylsulfonyl)phenyl) pyridine (**iv**) with the tin or boronate derivative, respectively, to afford etoricoxib.

The reaction of 6-methylpyridine-3-carboxylic acid methyl ester with N,O-dimethylhydroxylamine and isopropyl-magnesium chloride in toluene gives the N-methoxyamide derivative (**x**), which is reduced with diisobutyl aluminium hydride (DIBAL) to afford 6-methylpyridine-3-carbaldehyde (**xi**). The reaction of the aldehyde (**xi**) with a phosphite provides the diphenyl phosphonate derivative, which is condensed with 4-(methylsulfonyl)benzaldehyde in the presence of potassium *tert*-butoxide in HF to yield the enimine (**xii**). Finally, this compound is hydrolyzed with HCl to yield the ketosulfone (**ix**).

Another synthetic route starts with the condensation of N-methoxyamide (**x**) with 4-(methylsulfanyl) benzyl-magnesium bromide to give 1-(6-methylpyridin-3-yl)-2-(4-(methylsulfanyl)phenyl)ethanone (**xiii**), which is finally oxidized with the wolframate to ketosulfone (**ix**).

Alternatively the oxidation of 4´-(methylsulfonyl) acetophenone with S_8 and morpholine produces the 2-(4-(methylsulfonyl)phenyl)acetic acid ethyl ester (**xiv**), which is condensed with 2-methylpyridine-3-carboxylic acid methyl ester by means of *tert*-butyl magnesium chloride in hot tetrahydrofurane to give the ketosulfone (**ix**).

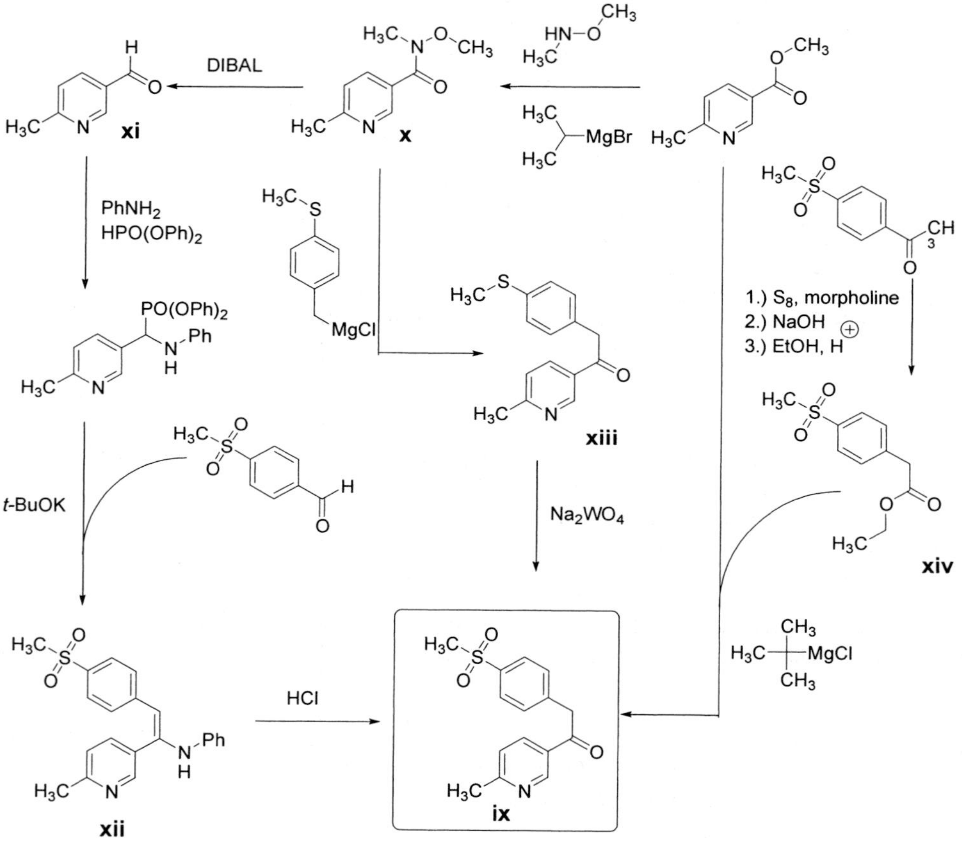

Scheme 19: Synthetic pathways to the ketosulfone (**ix**) as the key intermediate for the etoricoxib synthesis.

Finally etoricoxib can be obtained by several related cylization reactions:

- Cyclization of the ketosulfone (**ix**) with 2-chloro-3-hydroxy-propenal (**xv**) in the absence of ammonium acetate

- Cyclization with the aniline derivative (**xvi**) in the absence of ammonium acetate

- Cyclization with aminoacrolein (**xvii**), which is prepared by treatment of with 2-chloro-3-hydroxy-propenal (**xv**) with isopropanol, yielding the ether derivative and followed by reaction with ammonium hydroxide

- Cyclization of the lithium enolate of the ketosulfone (**iv**) with 2,3-dichloroacrolein (**xviii**), obtained by treatment of 2-chloro-3-hydroxy-propenal (**xv**) with oxalyl chloride and DMF in toluene, followed by reaction with ammonium acetate or anhydrous ammonia

- Reaction of the ketosulfone (**ix**) with 2-chloro-1,3-bis(dimethylamino)trimethinium salt (**xix**) in the presence of an equimolar amount of *tert*-BuOK followed by treatment with acetic acid and TFA and reflux with an excess of ammonium hydroxide. 2-Chloro-1,3-bis(dimethylamino)trimethinium hexafluoro-phosphat (**xix**) is obtained by reaction of chloroacetic acid with hot dimethylformamide and $POCl_3$. Finally the reaction mixture is treated with NaOH and hexafluorophosphoric acid in water.

Clinical use: Etoricoxib (Sorbera et al., 2001a) is a third generation COX-2 inhibitor in clinical development. It shows a 100-fold selectivity for COX-2 in a whole blood assay. Classical recombinant enzyme preparations of COX-1 could not be blocked by etoricoxib. When lowering the substrate concentration (0.1µM arachidonic acid) in a microsomal enzyme preparation, thus generating an assay of high sensitivity, etoricoxib showed 6- and 240-fold lower IC_{50} values for COX-1 compared to rofecoxib and celecoxib, respectively (Riendeau et al., 2001). Etoricoxib shows efficacy in a variety of animal models of inflammation without affecting gastrointestinal permeability even at high doses (Riendeau et al., 2001).

Plasma peak concentrations are achieved within 1.0 to 1.5 h after administration in healthy volunteers and the elimination half-life is about 15 h. Etoricoxib is 60% metabolized via members of the cytochrome P450 3A family (Kassahun et al., 2001). *In vitro* studies provide no evidence for active metabolites with respect to COX-1 and COX-2 (Chauret et al., 2001).

COX selectivity

IC50 [µM]	COX-1	COX-2	ratio
recomb. enzyme (1)	>100	5.0	>20
cellular assay (1)	>50	0.079	>633
whole blood (1)	116	1.1	105

(1) Riendeau et al. (2001)

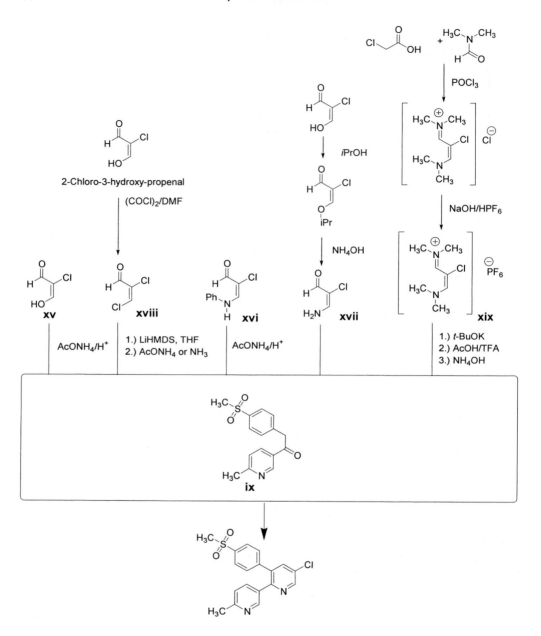

Scheme 20: Different cyclization pathways of of the ketosulfone to etoricoxib.

The metabolic profile of etoricoxib is shown below (Chauret et al., 2001):

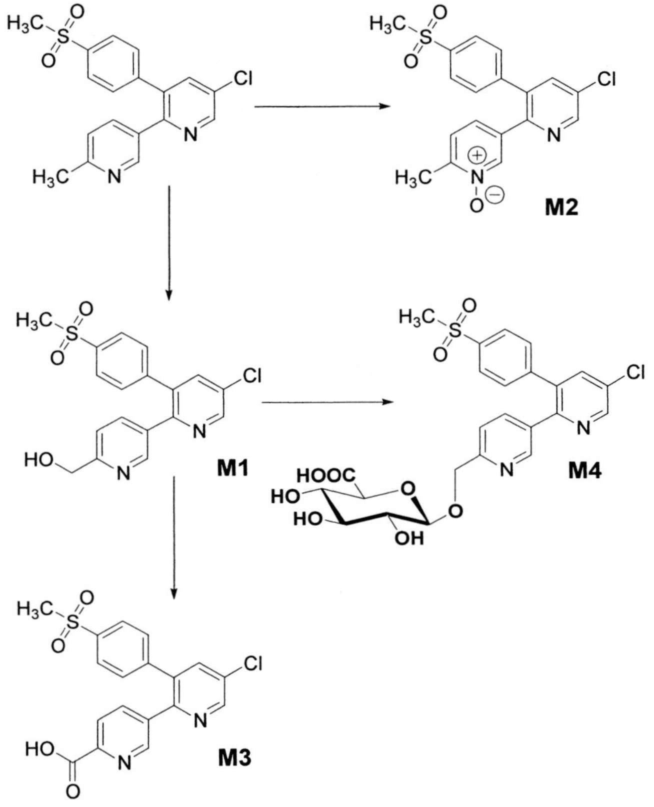

Scheme 21: *In vitro* metabolic pathways of etoricoxib.

Trade name: Arcoxia (US)

Fenbufen

Synthesis: Fenbufen is prepared by the Friedel-Crafts (aluminum chloride-nitrobenzene) acylation of biphenyl with succinic anhydride (Tomcufcik et al. (American Cyanamid Co.), 1972).

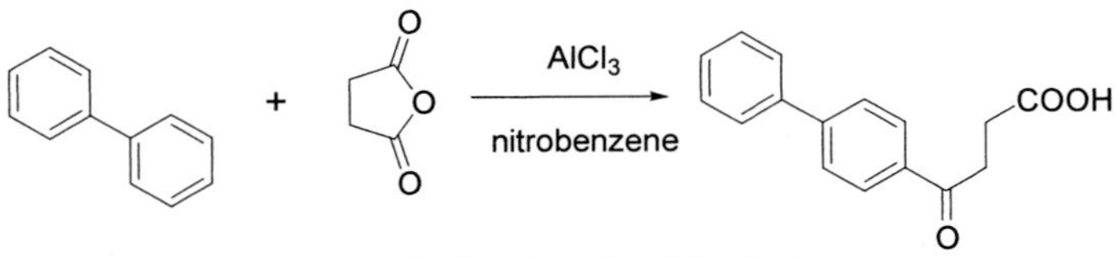

Scheme 22: Synthesis of fenbufen.

Fenbufen

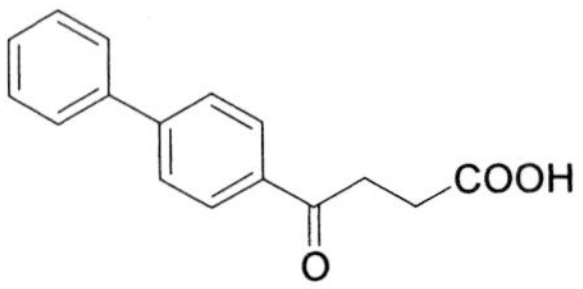

[*36330-85-5*], γ-oxo(1,1'biphenyl)- 4-butanoic acid, 4-Biphenyl-4-yl-4-oxo-butyric acid, $C_{16}H_{14}O_3$, M_r 354.29 , *mp* 185–187 °C

Clinical use: Fenbufen (Brogden et al., 1981a) has been found to be an effective, well-tolerated drug for the treatment of rheumatoid arthritis, osteoarthritis, and ankylosing spondylitis. The compound is metabolized in humans first to 4-hydroxy-4-biphenylbutyric acid (t_{max} 2.5 h) then to 4-biphenyl acetic acid (t_{max} 7.5 h). Both metabolites are more active than fenbufen itself (Kerwar, 1983) and circulate for several hours ($t_{1/2}$ 10 h). This slow conversion of fenbufen to active metabolites having relatively long plasma half-lives allows for once a day dosing (900 mg) with this agent.

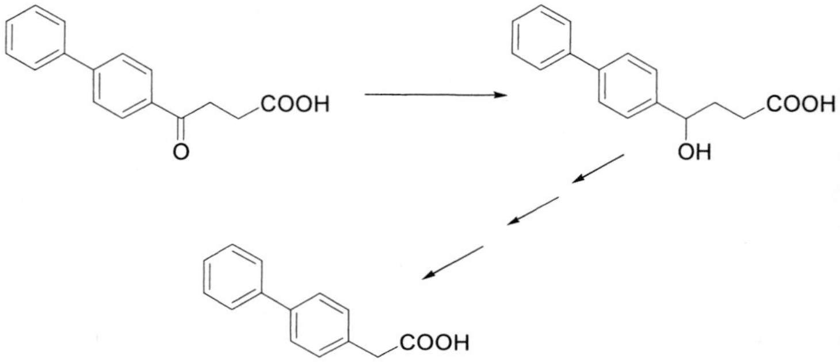

Trade names: Clincopal (Spain), Lederfen (UK), Napanol (Japan)

biphenyl acetic acid
(felbinac)

Scheme 23: Metabolic pathway of fenbufen.

Fenoprofen

Fenoprofen

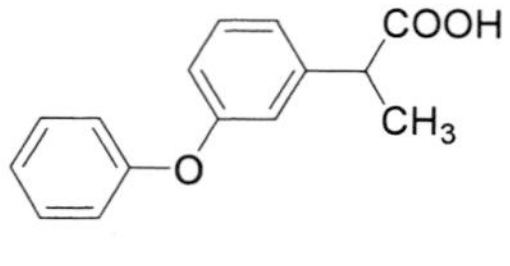

[*31879-05-7*], α-methyl-3-phenoxybenzeneacetic acid, 2-(3-Phenoxy-phenyl)-propionic acid, $C_{15}H_{14}O_3$, M_r 242.28, bp 168-171 °C (0.015 kPa)

Synthesis (Marshall (Eli Lilly & Co.), 1971): Sodium borohydride reduction of 3-phenoxyacetophenone followed by bromination of the resulting alcohol with PBr_3 gives α-methyl-3-phenoxybenzyl bromide. Reaction of this bromide with sodium cyanide in dimethyl sulfoxide gives the corresponding nitrile, which is hydrolyzed using sodium hydroxide. Acidification affords fenoprofen.

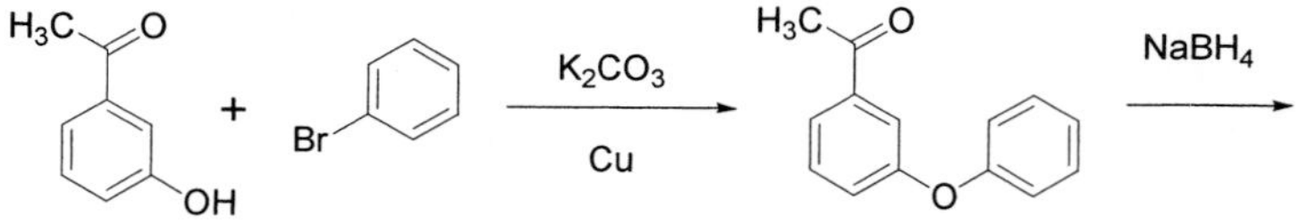

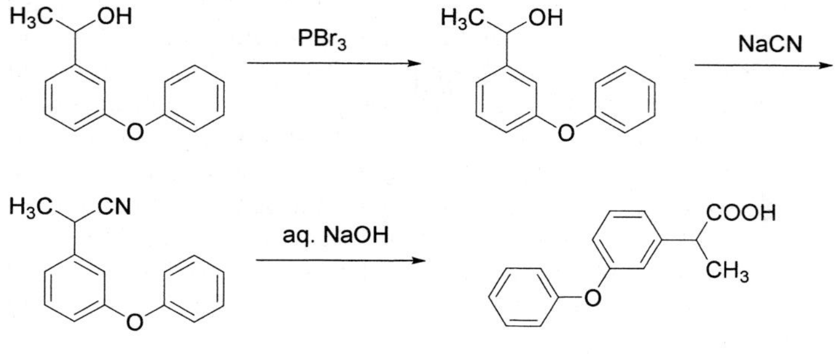

Scheme 24: Synthesis of fenoprofen.

Sonawane et al. (Sonawane et al., 1994) described a practical and efficient synthesis of fenoprofen using commercially available *m*-phenoxybenzaldehyde as the starting material. The key step in the synthesis is the transformation of the α-hydroxyacetal (**i**) into its chlorosulfonyl ester *in situ* and its concomitant rearrangement to the methyl ester (**ii**) in high yields. The required α-hydroxyacetal (**i**) can be readily prepared from *m*-methoxybenzaldehyde by the routine sequence of reactions: Grignard reaction with ethyl bromide or chloride, oxidation and finally α-chlorination with CuCl$_2$-LiCl/DMF.

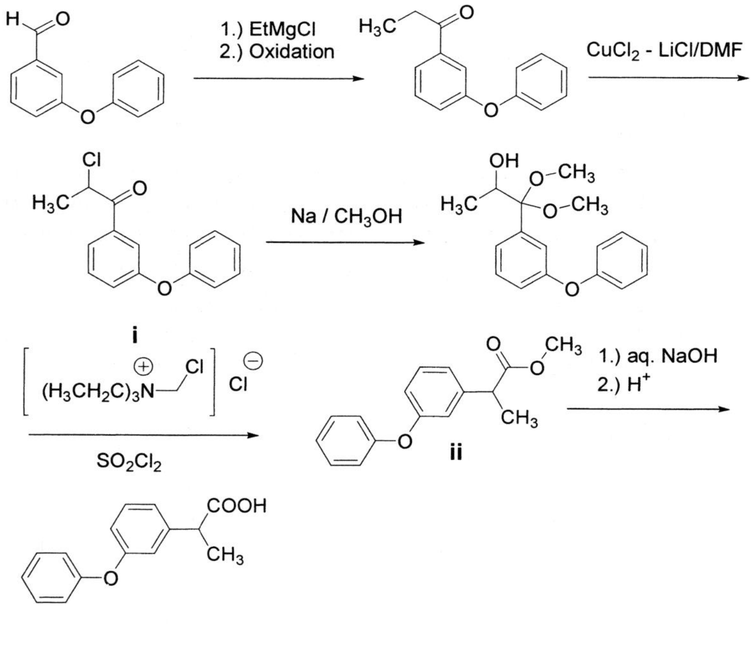

Scheme 25: Synthesis of fenoprofen.

Christoph and Buschmann

Trade names: Fenopron
(South Africa, UK), Fepron
(Italy), Nalfon (US, Austria,
Canada), Nalgesic (France),
Progesic (UK)

Clinical use: Fenoprofen (Gruber, 1976; Brogden et al.,
1977) is used as its calcium salt dihydrate in the treatment
of rheumatoid arthritis and osteoarthritis at a daily dose of
1.2-3.0 g. The drug is rapidly absorbed and excreted with
a plasma half-life of about 3 h despite being extensively
bound (99%) to plasma protein. Fenoprofen is well
tolerated, with dyspepsia being the main adverse effect.

Feprazone

Feprazone

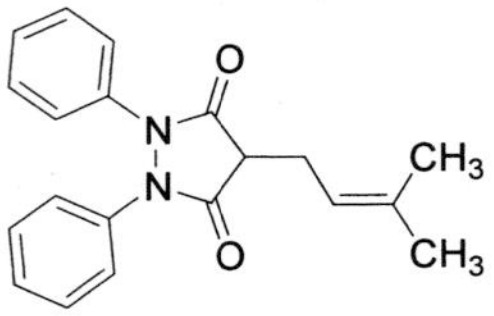

Synthesis: Feprazone is prepared by the condensation of
acetic acid 3-methyl-but-2-enyl ester with the lithium salt of
1,2-diphenyl-pyrazolidine-3,5-dione in the presence of
tetrakis(triphenylphosphin)palladium in anhydrous tetrahydrofuran.

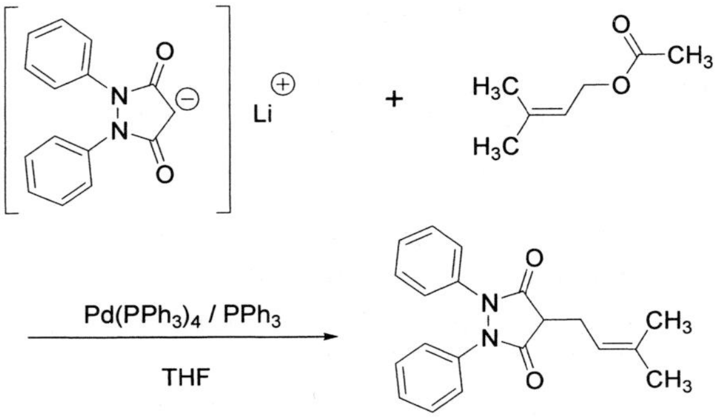

4-(3-Methyl-but-2-enyl)-1,2-
diphenyl-pyrazolidine-3,5-
dione

Scheme 26: Synthesis of feprazone.

Trade names: Zepelin
(Austria, Italy), Brotazona
(Spain)

Clinical use: Feprazone (Fletcher et al., 1975) is used in
conditions of mild to moderate pain associated with
musculoskeletal and joint disorders in daily oral doses of
400-600 mg. Peak plasma concentrations are seen 4-6 h
after oral administration. The plasma half-life is in the
range of 24 h.

Flobufen

Flobufen

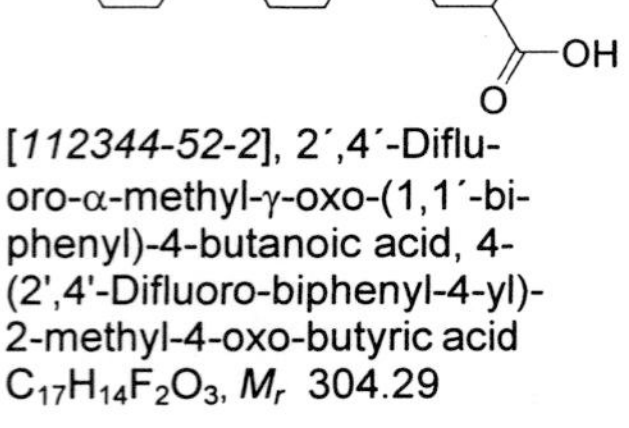

[112344-52-2], 2´,4´-Diflu-
oro-α-methyl-γ-oxo-(1,1´-bi-
phenyl)-4-butanoic acid, 4-
(2',4'-Difluoro-biphenyl-4-yl)-
2-methyl-4-oxo-butyric acid
$C_{17}H_{14}F_2O_3$, M_r 304.29

Synthesis (Rejholec, 1989; Fujimoto, 1999): Flobufen is
prepared by Friedel-Crafts acylation of 2,4-difluoro-
biphenyl with methylsuccinic anhydride. The biphenyl is
prepared by the Gomberg reaction of benzene with the
diazonium salt derived from 2,4-difluoroaniline.
Methylsuccinic anhydride is prepared by condensation of
ethyl 2-bromopropionate with ethyl cyanoacetate followed
by hydrolysis of the nitrile, decarboxylation of the resultant
β-ketoacid, and dehydration.

Clinical use: Flobufen (Fujimoto, 1999) an inhibitor of both,
cyclooxygenase and lipoxygenase, is in late clinical

development for the treatment of symptoms associated with rheumatoid arthritis and osteoarthritis.

Flufenamic Acid

Synthesis: 2-Chlorobenzoic acid is reacted with 3-trifluoromethylaniline in the presence of copper and potassium carbonate (Moffett and Aspergen, 1960; Parke Davis, 1961; Kleemann et al., 1999).

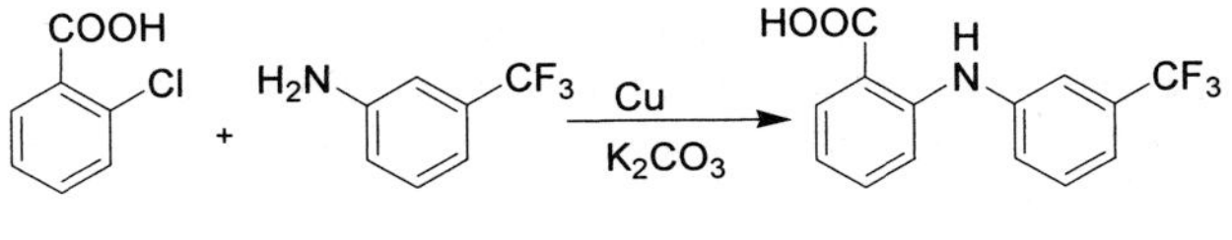

Flufenamic Acid

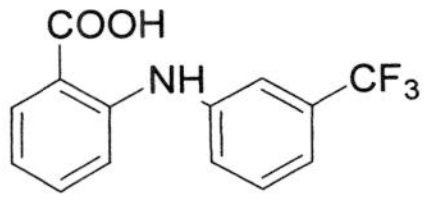

[*530-78-9*], 2-(3-Trifluoromethyl-phenylamino)-benzoic acid, $C_{14}H_{10}F_3NO_2$, M_r 281.23, mp 124-125 °C (also reported as 134-136 °C); aluminium salt (3 : 1) [*16449-54-0*], $C_{42}H_{27}AlF_9N_3O_6$, M_r 867.66

Scheme 27: Synthesis of flufenamic acid.

Clinical use: Flufenamate is a nonsteroidal anti-inflammatory drug used for the treatment of mild to moderate pain of musculoskeletal, joint or soft tissue origin.

Flufenamate shows a preference for COX-1 in enzyme preparations of recombinant human enzymes.

It is marketed in a variety of topical formulations alone or in combination with other ingredients.

Flufenamate is not recommended in patients with acute porphyria and was associated with a case of acute proctocolitis (Ravi et al., 1986).

The elimination half-life of flufenamate is about 2 h.

In addition to its action on prostaglandin synthesis, fenamates have been shown to modify several ion channel functions, e.g. inhibition of non-selective cation conductance (Gögelein et al., 1990), calcium-activated chloride channels (White and Aylwin, 1990), voltage-gated calcium channels, voltage-gated and ATP-sensitive potassium channels (Grover et al., 1994; Lee and Wang, 1999), as well as blocking gap junctions (Harks et al., 2001). The clinical relevance of these activities for the analgesic and anti-inflammatory potential of flufenamate is unknown.

COX selectivity

IC50 [µM]	COX-1	COX-2	ratio
purified enzyme (1)	2	29.5	0.07
whole blood (2)	30.6	n.d.	n.d.

(1) Gierse et al. (1995)

(2) Young et al. (1996)

Trade name: Dignodolin (Ger)

Flurbiprofen

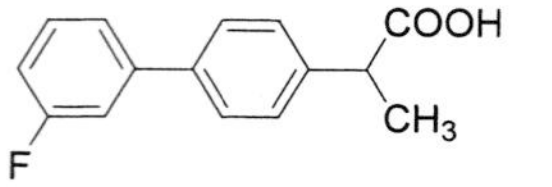

[5104-49-4], 2-(3'-Fluoro-
biphenyl-4-yl)-propionic
acid, 2-fluoro-a-methyl[1,1'-
biphenyl]-4-acetic acid,
$C_{15}H_{13}FO_2$, M_r 244.26, mp
110-111 °C; sodium salt
[56767-76-1], $C_{15}H_{12}FNaO_2$,
M_r 266.25

Flurbiprofen

Synthesis (Thiele and v. Bebenburg (Degussa), 1966;
1970; v. Bebenburg et al., 1979; 1981; 1983; Kleemann et
al., 1999):

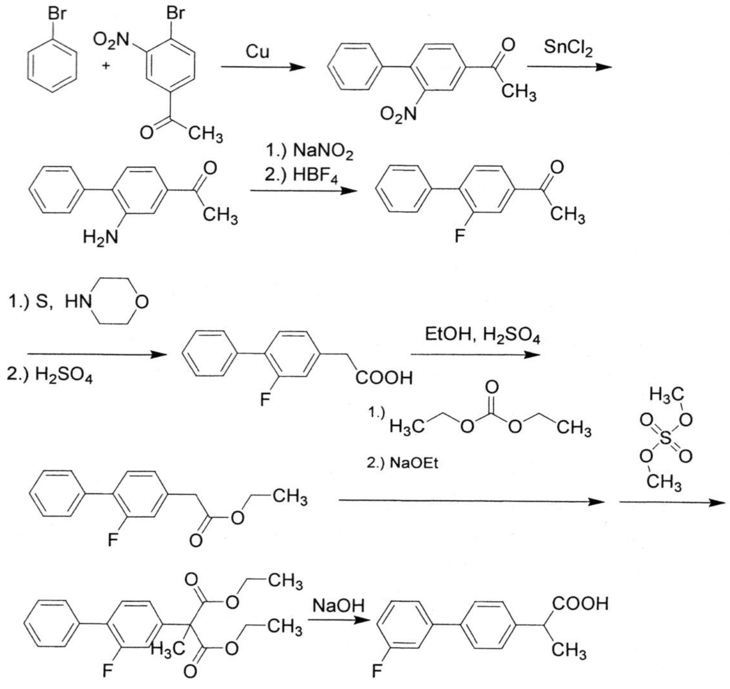

Scheme 28: Synthesis of flurbiprofen.

Clinical use: Flurbiprofen is a nonsteroidal anti-
inflammatory drug used for the treatment of pain and
inflammation associated with musculoskeletal and joint
disorders as well as neuralgias, dysmenorrhoea and
postoperative pain.

Flurbiprofen is a racemic mixture with the COX inhibitory
activity in the S-enantiomer. Flurbiprofen shows a
preference for COX-1 compared to COX-2.

Alternative synthesis:

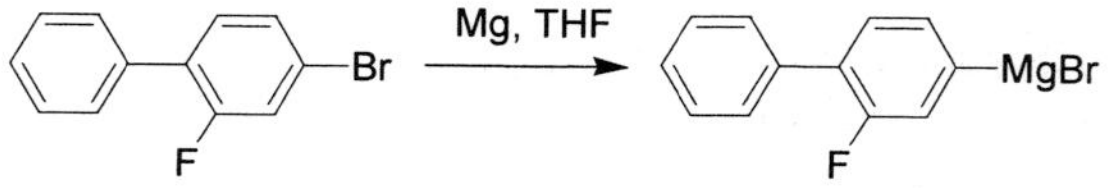

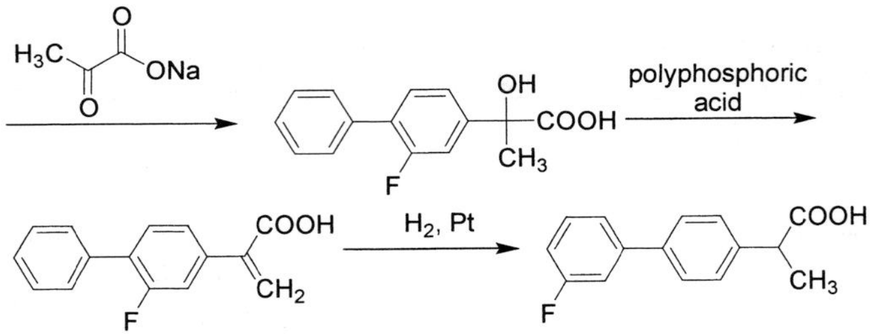

Scheme 29: Synthesis of flurbiprofen.

Flurbiprofen is given orally or rectally (150-200 mg/day, max. 300 mg/day) and as ophthalmic solutions. Peak plasma concentration appears 1 to 2 hours after oral administration. The plasma protein binding is about 99.5% and the elimination half-life is in the range of 3-5 h.

Flurbiprofen is metabolized mainly by hydroxylation and conjugation in the liver and excreted in the urine.

Flurbiprofen has been proposed as an anti-platelet agent following myocardial infarction (Brochier, 1993).

In addition to COX inhibition, flurbiprofen shows weak inhibition of the transcription factors NF-κB and AP-1. This activity resides in the R-enantiomer which has no COX-inhibiting properties (Tegeder et al., 2001). The clinical relevance of this activity is unknown. Furthermore, the anti-proliferative potential of R-flurbiprofen has been investigated in the treatment of cancer (Wechter et al., 2000).

COX selectivity

IC50 [µM]	COX-1	COX-2	ratio
Cell culture (1)	1.8	4.0	0.45
Whole blood (2)	0.44	6.42	0.07

(1) Riendeau et al. (1997)

(2) Brideau et al. (1996)

Trade name: Cebutid (France), Froben (Ger, UK), Ocufen (Ger, UK, US)

Ibuprofen

- 1960 patented by the Boots Pure Drugs Co.

- (*R*)- and (*S*)-isomers have similar *in vivo* potency

- Only the (*S*)-isomer inhibits prostaglandin synthetase *in vitro*

- Chiral inversion of the (*R*)-isomer to the active (*S*)-isomer occurs *in vivo*

- Production and sale of ibuprofen as a racemic mixture

- In 1985 the US patent on ibuprofen expired opening the generic prescription market.

- 1989 a US patent was filed: analgesia was more rapidly attained and enhanced in effect, when (*S*)- (+)-ibuprofen was used.

Ibuprofen

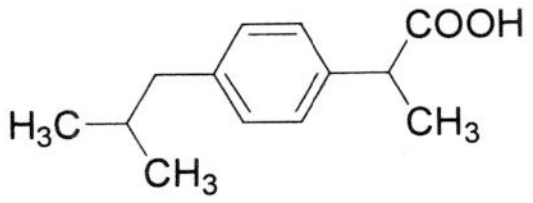

[*15687-27-1*], 2-(4-Isobutyl-phenyl)-propionic acid, $C_{18}H_{18}O_2$, M_r 206.28, *mp* 75-77 °C

Christoph and Buschmann

- The S(+)-enantiomer is available in some countries (dexibuprofen)

Synthesis (Mayer and Testa, 1997; Cleij et al., 1999; Kleemann et al., 1999): *a)* Treatment of ethyl 4-isobutylphenylacetate and diethyl carbonate with sodium ethoxide gives diethyl 4-isobutylphenylmalonate, which is methylated using methyl iodide and sodium ethoxide. Saponification followed by decarboxylation of the resulting malonic acid derivative affords ibuprofen.

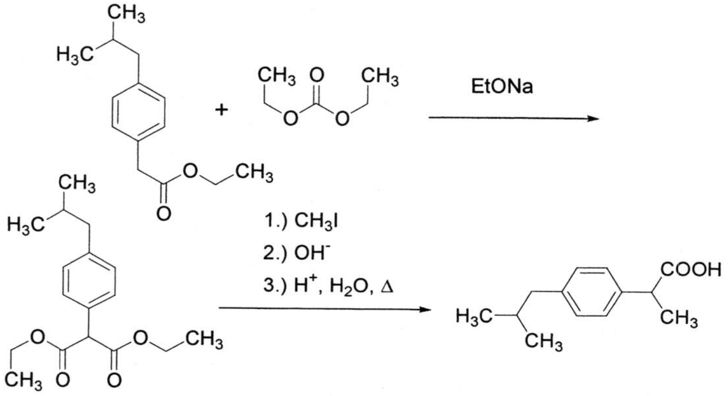

Scheme 30: Synthesis of ibuprofen.

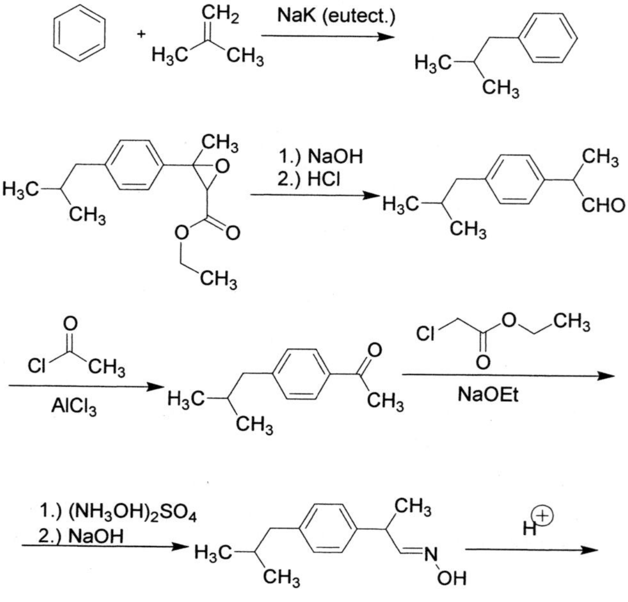

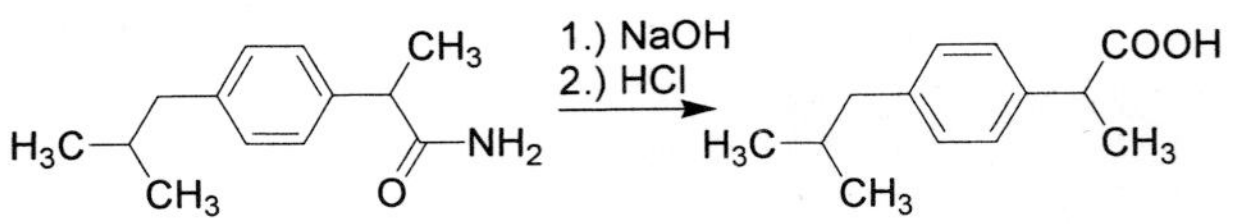

Scheme 31: Boots process (industrial process).

Boots-Hoechst-Celanese process: More recently, a shorter three-step catalytic route has been developed and is illustrated in the following scheme. Here, a Pd catalyzed carbonylation reaction is employed in the final step to introduce the carboxyl group.

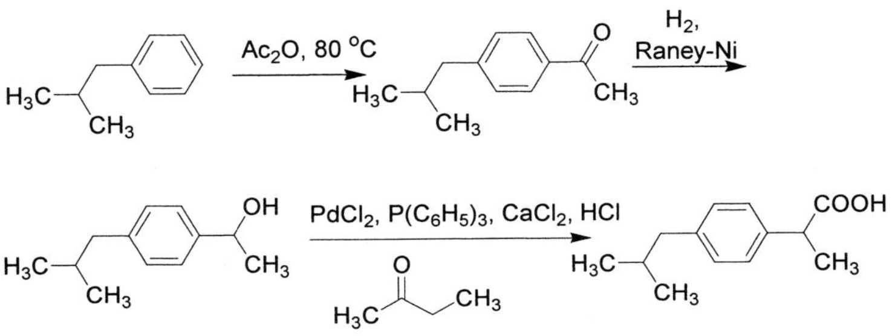

Scheme 32: Boots-Hoechst-Celanese process.

Several alternative processes are described in the literature.

For the preparation of the (*S*)-enantiomer an enzymatic racemic resolution process using *Aspergillus oryzae* protease was developed by Sepracor:

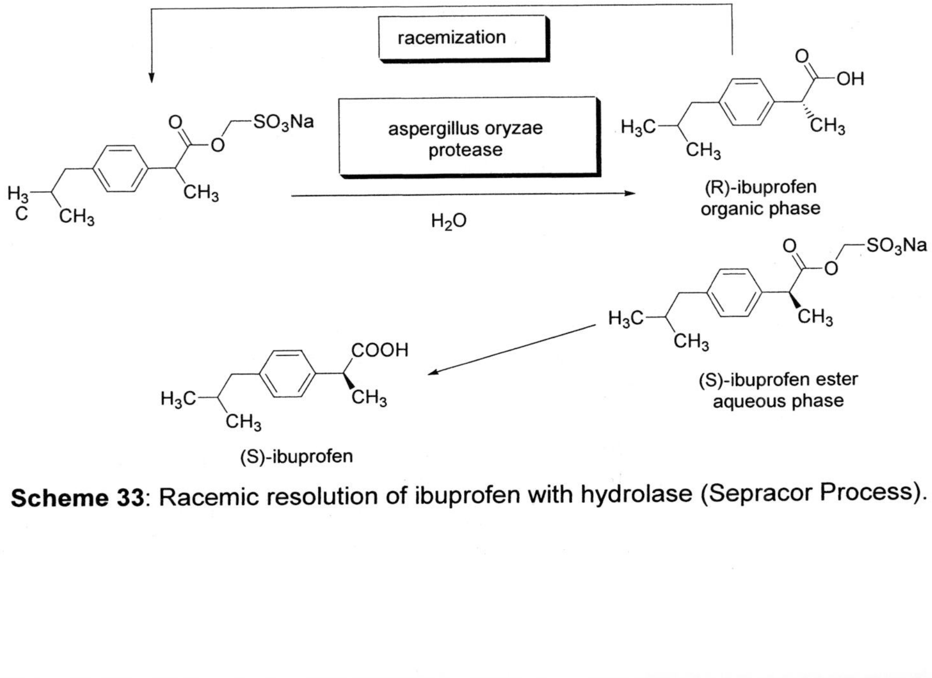

Scheme 33: Racemic resolution of ibuprofen with hydrolase (Sepracor Process).

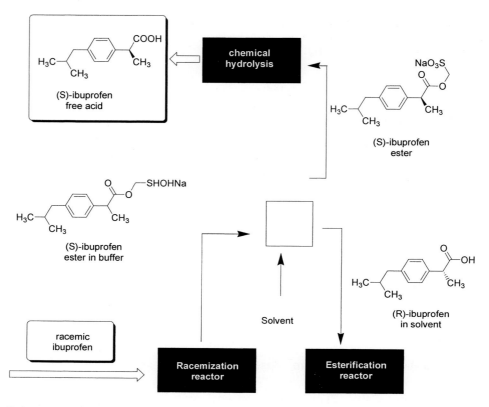

Scheme 34: Flow scheme for the enzymatic resolution process of ibuprofen.

COX selectivity

IC50 [μM]	COX-1	COX-2	ratio
purified enzyme (1)	1 μg/ml	46 μg/ml	0.02
cell culture (2)	1.07	1.12	0.95
whole blood (3)	4.75	>30	<0.1

(1) Mitchell et al. (1993)

(2) Berg et al. (1999)

(3) Brideau et al. (1996)

Clinical use: Ibuprofen (Busson, 1986) is a nonsteroidal anti-inflammatory drug, commonly used for the treatment of mild to moderate pain. It is used in conditions like rheumatoid arthritis, osteoarthritis, joint and soft tissue pain, dental pain, postoperative pain, dysmenorrhoea and headache, including acute migraine attacks.

Ibuprofen inhibits both COX-1 and COX-2 with some preference for COX-1, depending on the assay system.

Ibuprofen is given by oral, rectal or topical application (800-2400 mg/day) and in a lower dose (40 mg/kg day) for the treatment of fever in children. Ibuprofen is given as free base or a variety of salts, esters and other derivatives.

Peak plasma concentrations of ibuprofen occur 1 to 2 h after oral administration. It is heavily bound to plasma proteins (90-99%) and has a plasma half-life of 2 h. Ibuprofen is excreted as metabolites and conjugates in the urine (Davies, 1998a).

Ibuprofen is a racemate, the active enantiomer being the S(+)-enantiomer which is commercially available in some countries (dexibuprofen). (*R*)-ibuprofen is converted to the (*S*)-enantiomer via a metabolic chiral inversion process shown in Scheme 35.

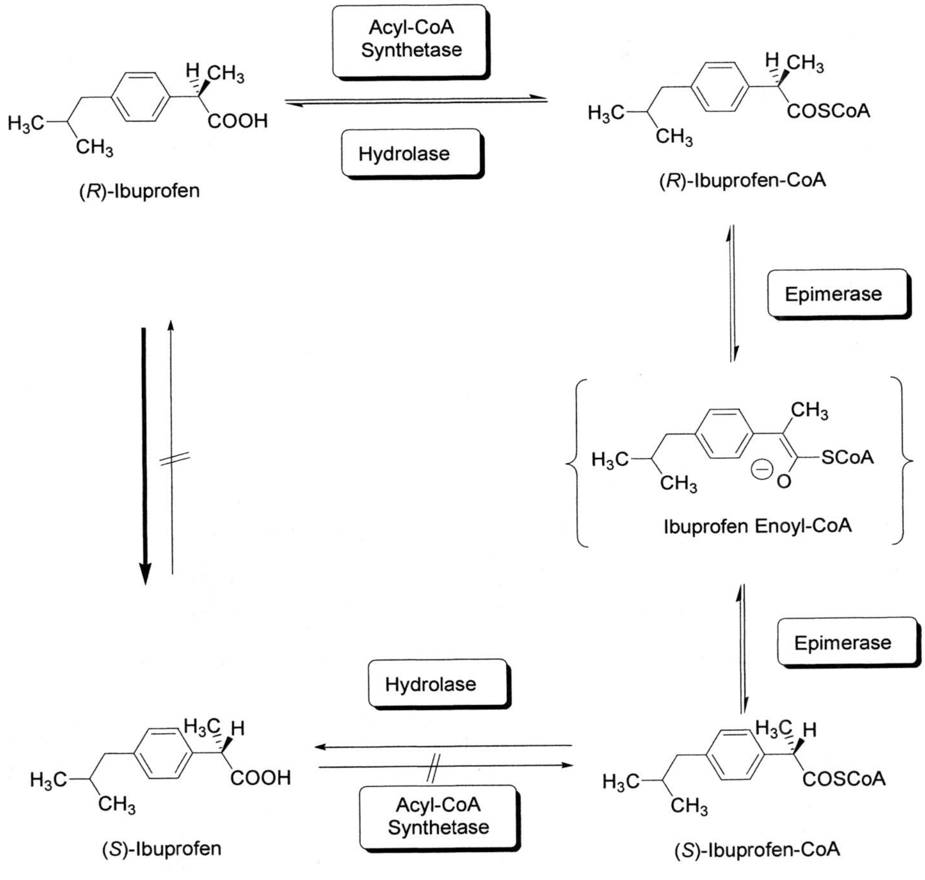

Scheme 35: Metabolic chiral inversion of (*R*)-ibuprofen to the (*S*)-enantiomer.

Ibuprofen shows the typical side-effects of nonsteroidal anti-inflammatory drugs but seems to be better tolerated than other such drugs. This may be due to its inhibition of COX-2.

Trade name: Anco (Ger), Imbim (Ger), Motrin (US)

Christoph and Buschmann

Indomethacin

Indomethacin

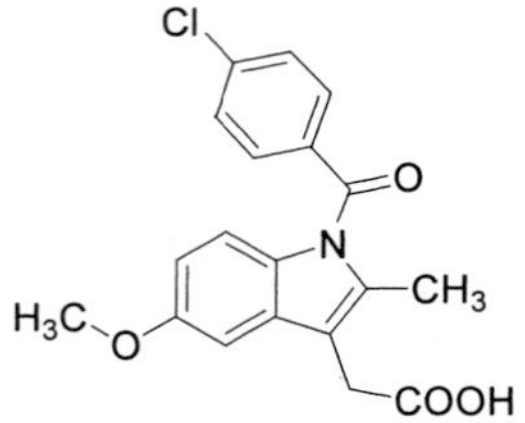

Synthesis (Shen et al., 1963; Kleemann et al., 1999):

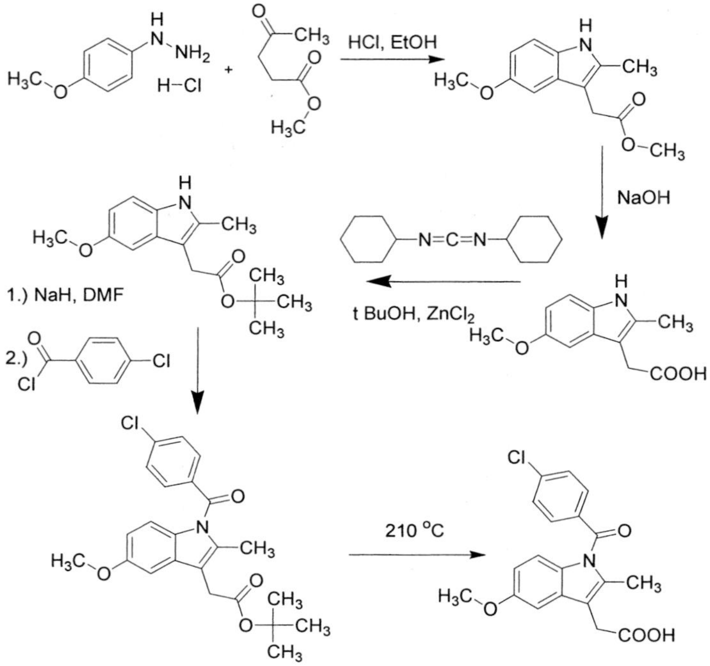

[*53-86-1*], [1-(4-Chloro-benzoyl)-5-methoxy-2-methyl-1*H*-indol-3-yl]-acetic acid, $C_{19}H_{16}ClNO_4$, M_r 357.79, *mp* 153-154 °C (crystals exhibiting polymorphism, *mp* for another form is 162 °C); sodium trihydrate [*74252-25-8*], $C_{19}H_{15}ClNNaO_4$. $3H_2O$, M_r 433.82, pale yellow crystaline powder

Scheme 36: Synthesis of indomethacin: Merck & Co. process (Shen (Merck & Co.), 1962; 1964).

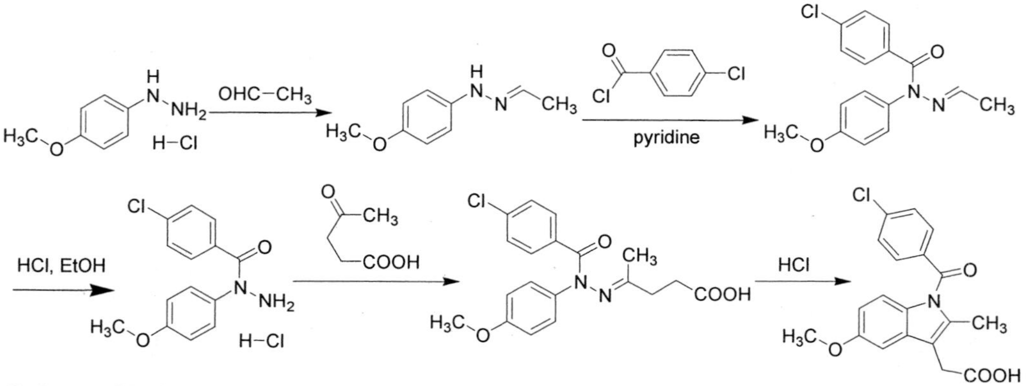

Scheme 37: Synthesis of indomethacin: Sumitomo process (Yamamoto et al., 1968).

Clinical use: Indomethacin is a nonsteroidal anti-inflammatory drug commonly used for the treatment of mild to moderate pain. It is also used in acute and chronic pain states such as rheumatoid arthritis, osteoarthritis, joint and soft tissue pain, dental pain, postoperative pain and dysmenorrhoea.

Indomethacin is a COX-1 selective inhibitor with up to 10-fold selectivity compared to COX-2 depending on the assay.

It is given by oral, rectal or topical administration (50-150 mg/day, maximal daily dose 200 mg) as well as an ophthalmic solution.

Indomethacin is absorbed after oral administration reaching peak plasma concentrations after 2 h. About 99% binds to plasma proteins and it has a variable terminal half-life from 2.6 to 11.2 h in adults and up to 30 h in neonates. The metabolites generated in the liver are desmethyl-indomethacin, desbenzoyl-indomethacin, desmethyl-desbenzoyl-indomethacin and glucuronides. Indomethacin and its conjugates undergo enterohepatic circulation and are excreted mainly in the urine.

The major side-effects of indomethacin are gastrointestinal and central nervous system disturbances such as depression, drowsiness, tinnitus and convulsions.

Indomethacin is available as the sodium, meglumine, or *L*-arginine salt or as the prodrug (proglumetacin maleate).

COX selectivity

IC50 [µM]	COX-1	COX-2	ratio
purified enzyme (1)	0.1	0.35	0.3
cell culture (2)	0.0045	0.045	0.1
whole blood (3)	0.16	0.46	0.3

(1) Churchill et al. (1996)

(2) Berg et al. (1999)

(3) Brideau et al. (1996)

Trade name: Indocid (F, UK), Amuno (Ger), Indocin (US), Protaxon (Proglumetacin, Ger)

Isoxicam

Synthesis (Lombardino and Wiseman, 1971; Zinnes et al. (Warner-Lambert), 1972; Zinnes et al., 1982; Kleemann et al., 1999):

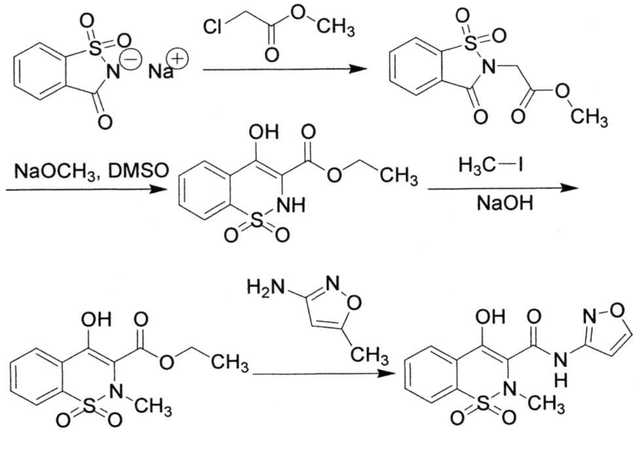

Isoxicam

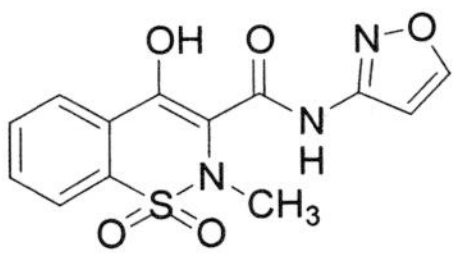

[*34552-84-6*], 4-Hydroxy-2-methyl-1,1dioxo-1,2-dihydro-$1\lambda^6$-benzo[*e*][1,2]thiazine-3-carboxylic acid isoxazo-3-ylamide, 4-hydroxy-2-methyl-*N*-(5-methyl-3-isoxazolyl)-2*H*-1,2-benzothiazine-3-carboxamide 1,1 dioxide, $C_{14}H_{13}N_3O_5S$, M_r 335.34, mp 265-271 °C (decomp.); sodium salt, $C_{14}H_{12}N_3NaO_5S$, M_r 343.29, mp 270-272 °C

Scheme 38: Synthesis of isoxicam.

Clinical use: Isoxicam (Downie et al., 1984) is a nonsteroidal anti-inflammatory drug withdrawn from the market following reports of fatal skin reaction.

Ketoprofen

Ketoprofen

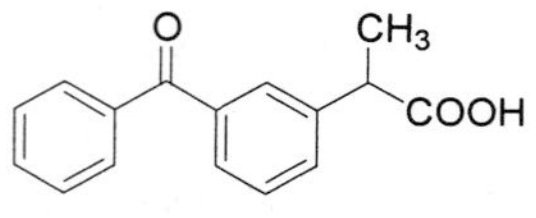

[22071-15-4], 2-(3-Benzoyl-phenyl)-propionic acid, 3-benzoyl-α-methylbenzene-acetic acid, $C_{16}H_{14}O_3$, M_r 254.28, mp 94 °C; lysine salt (1 : 1) [57469-78-0], $C_{16}H_{14}O_3 \cdot C_6H_{14}N_2O_2$, M_r 400.47; sodium salt [57495-14-4], $C_{16}H_{13}NaO_3$, M_r 276.27

Synthesis (Farge et al. (Rhône-Poulenc), 1972; Kleemann et al., 1999):

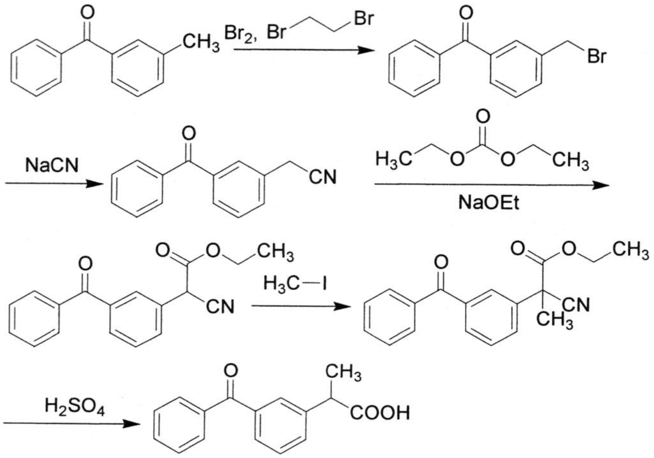

Scheme 39: Synthesis of ketoprofen.

Clinical use: Ketoprofen (Hommeril et al., 1994) is a nonsteroidal anti-inflammatory drug used for the treatment of a variety of acute and chronic pain and inflammatory conditions including rheumatoid arthritis, osteoarthritis, ankylosing spondylitis, postoperative pain and dysmenorrhoea. It is given by oral, rectal, topical or intramuscular application (100-200 mg/day, maximal dose 300 mg/day) as the sodium or lysine salt.

Ketoprofen is usually given as the racemate, the pharmacological action being mainly carried out by the S(+)-enantiomer. The active enantiomer is available in some countries since 1997 as the trometamol salt, which is said to be absorbed more quickly thus leading to an earlier onset of action.

Ketoprofen shows selectivity for COX-1 compared to COX-2.

COX selectivity

IC50 [µM]	COX-1	COX-2	ratio
cell culture (1)	0.0061	0.12	0.05
whole blood (2)	0.02	1.08	0.02
whole blood (3)	0.11	0.18	0.6

(1) Riendeau et al. (1997)

(2) Brideau et al. (1996)

(3) S-Ketoprofen, Patrignani et al. (1997)

Peak plasma concentration after oral application occurs within 2 h. Ketoprofen is bound to plasma protein up to 99% and shows a plasma elimination half-life of 1.5 to 4 h. It is metabolized mainly by glucuronidation and excreted mainly in the urine (Jamali and Brooks, 1990).

Trade name: Profénid (F), Orudis (Ger, UK, US), S(+)-Ketoprofen: Keral (UK)

Ketorolac

Synthesis: The benzoylation of 2-methylthiopyrrole with *N,N*-dimethylbenzamide by means of POCl₃ in refluxing CH₂Cl₂ gives 5-benzoyl-2-methylthiopyrrole, which is condensed with spiro[2,5]-5,7-dioxa-6,6-dimethyloctane-4,8-dione by means of NaH in DMF. The oxidation of this product with m-chloroperbenzoic acid in CH₂Cl₂ affords the sulfone, which is submitted to methanolysis with methanol and HCl giving 1-(3,3-dimethoxycarbonylpropyl)-2-me-thanesulfonyl-5-benzoylpyrrole. Cyclization with NaH in DMF yields dimethyl-5-benzoyl1,2-dihydro-3*H*-pyrrolo[1,2-a]pyrrole-1,1-dicarboxylate, which is finally hydrolyzed and decarboxylated with KOH in refluxing methanol (Franco et al., 1982; Synthex 1982; 1984; 1989); Arrigoni-Martelli, 1983; Muchowski et al., 1985; Guzman et al., 1986; Kleemann et al., 1999).

Ketorolac

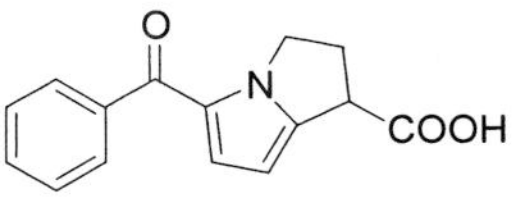

[*74103-06-3*], 5-Benzoyl-2,3-dihydro-1*H*-pyrrolizine-1-carboxylic acid, C₁₅H₁₃NO₃, *M*ᵣ 255.27, *mp* 160-161 °C; tromethamine salt (1 : 1) [*74103-07-4*], C₁₅H₁₃NO₃ · C₄H₁₁NO₃, *M*ᵣ 376.41, (+)-form *mp* 174 °C, [α]_D +173° (*c* = 1, CH₃OH), (-)-form *mp* 169-170 °C, [α]_D -176° (*c* = 1, CH₃OH); monosodium salt [*110618-38-7*], C₁₅H₁₂NNaO₃, *M*ᵣ 277.26

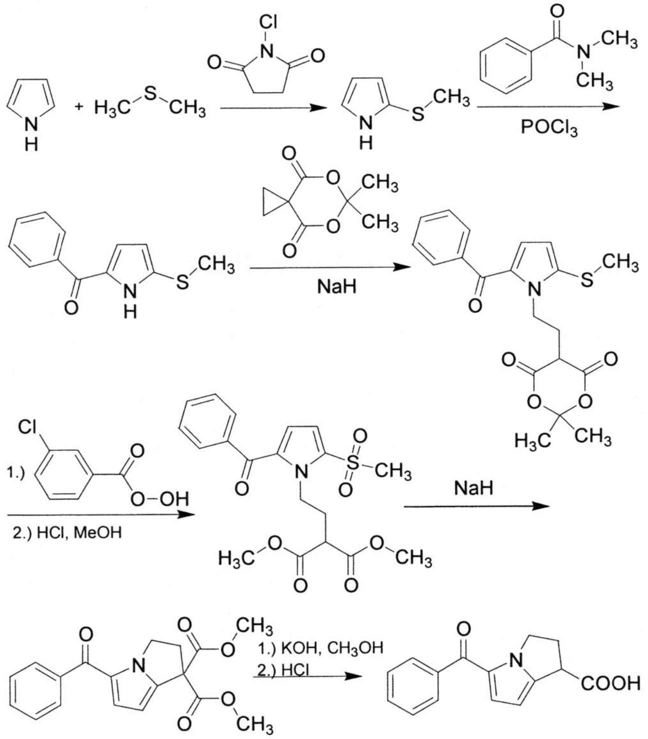

Scheme 40: Synthesis of ketorolac.

Clinical use: Ketorolac (Gillis and Brogden, 1997) is a nonsteroidal anti-inflammatory drug mainly used for the treatment of moderate to severe postoperative pain.

Ketorolac shows a balanced inhibition of both COX-isoenzymes in a variety of assay systems and is a racemate with an active (S)-enantiomer.

Ketorolac is given as the trometamol salt intramuscularly, intravenously, or orally. The maximal daily dose is 90 mg for the parenteral and the oral route. The duration of treatment is restricted due to side-effects. Ketorolac is also used as a 0.5% ophthalmic solution.

The peak plasma concentration of oral ketorolac is reached within 30 to 60 min and may be slower after intramuscular administration. It is bound to plasma proteins by more than 99%. The terminal plasma half-life is about 4 to 6 h and is prolonged in elderly and in patients with renal dysfunction. Ketorolac is metabolized mainly by glucuronidation and to a minor extent by para-hydroxylation and is excreted in the urine (~90%) and faeces (~10%) (Buckley and Brogden, 1990).

Due to a number of severe side-effects including gastrointestinal disturbances, liver function changes, renal failure, skin and other hypersensitivity reactions ketorolac has been withdrawn in many countries.

COX selectivity

IC50 [µM]	COX-1	COX-2	ratio
recomb. enzyme (1)	1.23	3.50	0.35
cell culture (2)	0.025	0.039	0.6
whole blood (3)	0.11	0.06	1.8

(1) Jett et al. (1999)

(2) Berg et al. (1999)

Trade name: Tora-Dol (F, I), Acular (Ger), Toradol (UK, US)

Lonazolac

Synthesis: The pyrazole-4-carbaldehyde synthesized according to Vilsmeier is reduced to the alcohol, which is chlorinated. The chloro derivative is reacted with sodium cyanide to give the nitrile, which is hydrolyzed to Lonazolac. The calcium salt, slightly soluble in water, is formed by adding calcium chloride to the free acid (Rainer et al., 1981; Unterhalt, 1982; Rainer et al. (Byk Gulden), 1969; 1982; Kleemann et al., 1999).

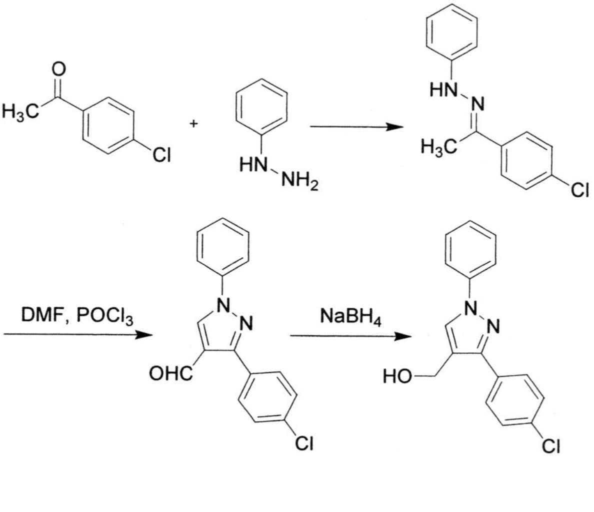

Lonazolac

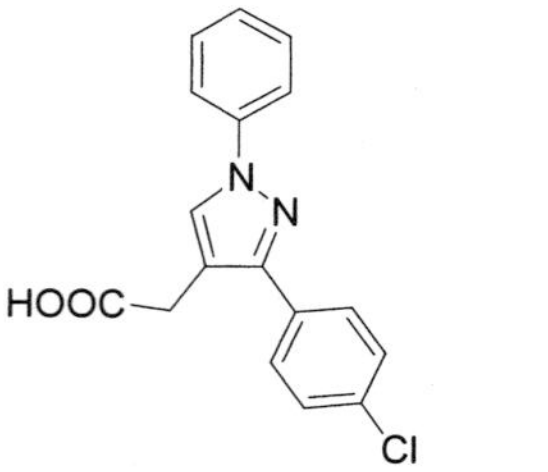

[53808-88-1], [3-(4-Chloro-phenyl-1H-pyrazol-4-yl]-acetic acid, $C_{17}H_{13}ClN_2O_2$, M_r 312.75, mp 150-151 °C; calcium salt (2 : 1) [75821-71-5], , $C_{34}H_{24}CaCl_2N_4O_4$, M_r 663.57, mp 270-290 °C (decomp.)

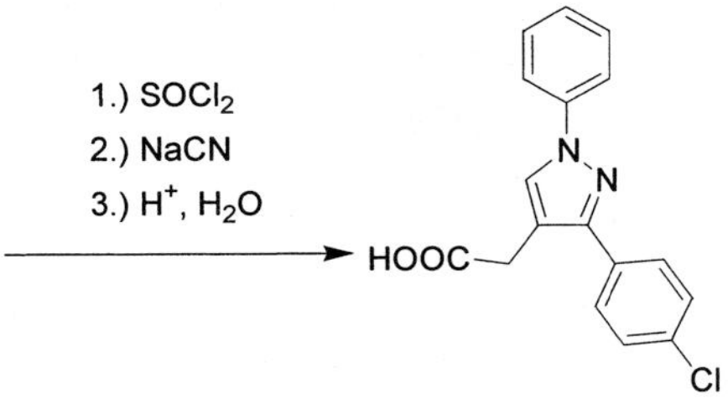

Scheme 41: Synthesis of lonazolac.

Clinical use: Lonazolac (Riedel et al., 1981) is a nonsteroidal anti-inflammatory drug used for the treatment of acute inflammatory pain conditions of joint and soft-tissue disorders as well as posttraumatic and postoperative pain. It is used as its calcium salt and is given by oral (600 mg/day, initial dose up to 900 mg/day) or rectal administration (800 mg/day).

Lonazolac has a terminal half-life of about 6 h in young volunteers. The terminal half-life is prolonged to about 12 h in elderly patients (Huber et al., 1990).

Trade name: Argun (Ger), Irritren (Austria, Belg., Switz.)

Lornoxicam

Synthesis: The sulfonation of 2,5-dichlorothiophen with $ClSO_3H/SOCl_2$ gives 2,5-dichlorothiophene-3-sulfonic acid chloride, which by reaction with methylamine in $CHCl_3$ yields the corresponding methylamide. Carboxylation with butyl lithium and CO_2 in ether affords 5-chloro-3-(N-methylsulfamoyl)thiophene-2-carboxylic acid, which is esterified with PCl_5 and methanol to the methyl ester. The condensation with methyl iodoacetate by means of NaH in DMF gives 5-chloro-3-[N-(methoxycarbonylmethyl)-N-methylsulfamoyl]thiophene-2-carboxylic acid methyl ester, which is cyclized with sodium methoxide in methanol yielding 6-chloro-4-hydroxy-2-methyl-2H-thieno[2,3-e]-1,2-thiazine-3-carboxylic acid methyl ester-1,1-dioxide. Finally this compound is treated with 2-aminopyridine in refluxing xylene (Drugs Fut., 1992).

Lornoxicam

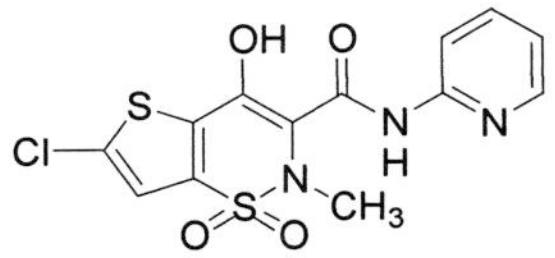

[*70374-39-9*], 6-Chloro-4-hydroxy-2-methyl-1,1-dioxo-1,2-dihydro-1l^6-thieno[2,3 e][1,2]thiazine-3-carboxylic acid pyridin-2-ylamide, 6-chloro-4-hydroxy-2-methyl-N-(2-pyridyl)-2H-thieno[2,3-e]-1,2-thiazine-3-carbox-amide-1,1-dioxide, $C_{13}H_{10}ClN_3O_4S_2$, M_r 371.81, mp 225-230 °C (decomp.)

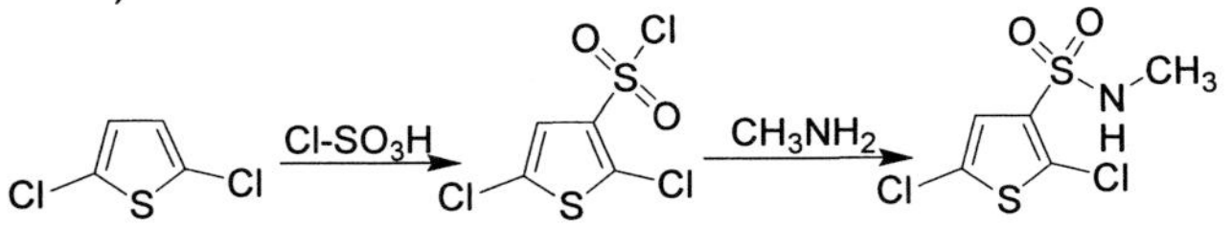

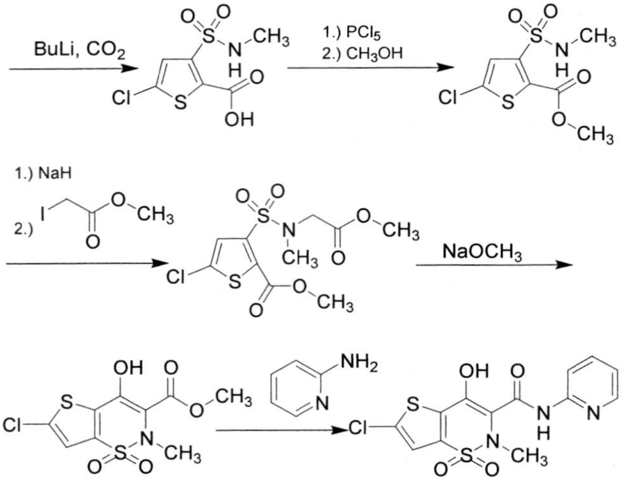

Scheme 42: Synthesis of lornoxicam.

COX selectivity

IC50 [µM]	COX-1	COX-2	ratio
cell culture (1)	0.003	0.008	0.4
whole blood (1)	0.13	0.13	1

(1) Berg et al. (1999)

Trade name: Xefo (Austria, I, D, Switz, UK)

Clinical use: Lornoxicam (Pruss et al., 1990) is a nonsteroidal anti-inflammatory drug with a strong and balanced inhibition of both COX isoenzymes.

It is used orally (8-24 mg/day) for the treatment of mild to moderate pain including postoperative pain, rheumatoid arthritis, osteoarthritis and ankylosing spondylitis (Balfour et al., 1996).

Lornoxicam reaches peak plasma concentrations within 2 to 6 h and shows high degree of binding to plasma protein (99.7%). In contrast to other oxicams, lornoxicam has a short plasma elimination half-life of about 4 h (Olkkola et al., 1994) and is metabolised mainly to the inactive compound 5'-hydroxy-lornoxicam (Dittrich et al., 1990) and excreted in the urine (~33%) and faeces (~66%) (Hitzenberger et al., 1990).

In addition to the inhibition of COX, lornoxicam shows weak inhibition of LPS-induced inducible nitric oxide synthase (iNOS; IC_{50} 65 µM) and LPS-induced interleukin-6 (IC_{50} 54 µM), both of which could contribute to its potent anti-inflammatory and analgesic action (Berg et al., 1999).

Meclofenamic Acid

Synthesis: By condensation of 2-bromobenzoic acid with 2,6-dichloro-3-methylaniline by means of CuBr$_2$ in diethyleneglycol dimethyl ether containing *N*-ethylmorpholine, and heating at 145-155 °C (Scherrer and Short (Parke Davis), 1961; 1967); Juby et al., 1968; Arrigoni-Martelli, 1978b; Kleemann et al., 1999).

Meclofenamic Acid

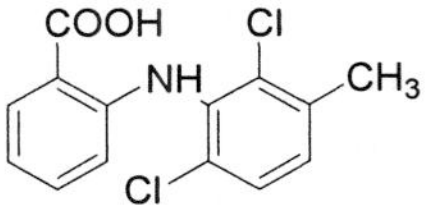

[*644-62-2*], 2-(2,6-Dichloro-3-methyl-phenylamino)-benzoic acid, $C_{14}H_{11}Cl_2NO_2$, M_r 296.15, *mp* 257-259 °C; monosodium salt monohydrate [*6385-02-0*], $C_{14}H_{10}Cl_2NNaO_2 \cdot H_2O$ M_r 336.15, *mp* 289-291 °C

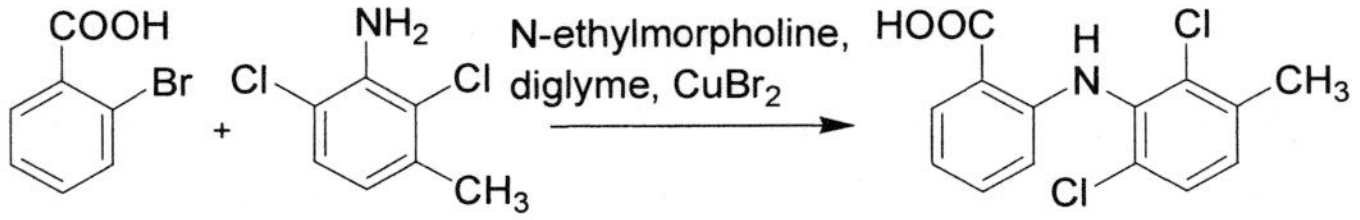

Scheme 43: Synthesis of meclofenamic acid.

Clinical use: Meclofenamate (McLean and Geuckman, 1983) is a nonsteroidal anti-inflammatory drug used for the treatment of mild to moderate pain, musculoskeletal and joint disorders such as rheumatoid arthritis and osteoarthritis as well as dysmenorrhoea.

Meclofenamate shows balanced inhibition of both COX-1 and COX-2 based on data with purified enzymes.

Meclofenamate is given by oral administration (300-400 mg/day).

Peak plasma concentration of meclofenamate occur 0.5 to 1 h after oral administration. The binding to plasma proteins is over 99% and the plasma elimination half-life is about 2 to 4 h. Meclofenamate is metabolized by oxidation, hydroxylation, dehalogenation, and glucuronidation. Metabolites are excreted mainly in the urine with about 20 to 30% being excreted in the faeces (Koup et al., 1990). A 3-hydroxymethyl metabolite of meclofenamate has been reported to be active.

In addition to its action on prostaglandin synthesis, fenamates have been shown to modify several ion channel functions, e.g. inhibition of non-selective cation conductance (Gögelein et al., 1990), calcium-activated chloride channels (White and Aylwin, 1990), voltage-gated calcium channels, voltage-gated and ATP-sensitive potassium channels (Grover et al., 1994; Lee and Wang, 1999), as well as blocking gap junctions (Harks et al., 2001). The clinical relevance of these activities for the analgesic and anti-inflammatory potential of meclo-fenamate is unknown.

COX selectivity

IC50 [µM]	COX-1	COX-2	ratio
purified enzyme (1)	0.040	0.050	0.8
whole blood (2)	2.3	n.d.	n.d.

(1) Kalgutkar et al. (2000a)

(2) Young et al. (1996)

Trade name: Meclomen (Austria, I, Spain, Switz., US)

Christoph and Buschmann

Mefenamic Acid

Mefenamic Acid

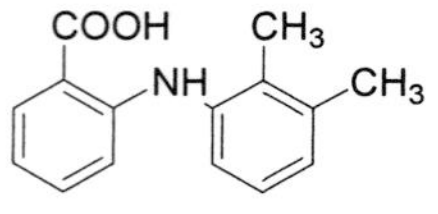

[*61-68-7*], 2-(2,3-Dimethyl-phenylamino)-benzoic acid, $C_{15}H_{15}NO_2$, M_r 241.29, *mp* 230-231 °C; monosodium salt $C_{15}H_{14}NNaO_2$, M_r 263.27

Mefenamic Acid

Synthesis (Scherrer (Parke Davis), 1961; 1967); Kleemann et al., 1999):

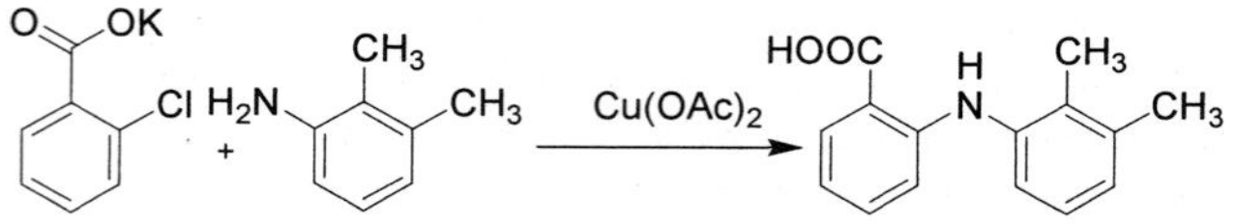

Scheme 44: Synthesis of mefenamic acid.

Clinical use: Mefenamic acid is a nonsteroidal anti-inflammatory drug which is used for the treatment of mild to moderate pain conditions, musculoskeletal and joint disorders such as rheumatoid arthritis and osteoarthritis, and dysmenorrhoea.

Mefenamate inhibits both COX isoforms with some preference for COX-2 in a whole blood assay and for COX-1 in an enzyme preparation of recombinant human enzymes and in a cellular assay. The COX-1 preference in the cellular assay shows a time dependency as pre-incubation of the cells decreases the ratio of COX isoform selectivity from 0.03 to 0.005 (Lora et al., 1998).

COX selectivity

IC50 [µM]	COX-1	COX-2	ratio
purified enzyme (1)	0.04	3	0.01
cell culture (2)	0.21	6.32	0.03
whole blood (3)	1.9	0.16	12

(1) Gierse et al. (1995)

(2) Lora et al. (1998)

(3) Cryer and Feldman (1998)

Mefenamic acid is given orally (1500 mg/day maximal dose).

After oral administration, mefenamic acid reaches peak plasma concentrations after 2 to 4 h. Mefenamic acid is heavily bound to plasma proteins and plasma elimination half-life is about 2 to 4 h.

The main side effects concern the gastrointestinal system and include diarrhea (Marks and Gleeson, 1975).

In addition to its action on prostaglandin synthesis, fenamates have been shown to modify several ion channel functions, e.g. inhibition of non-selective cation conductance (Gögelein et al., 1990), calcium-activated chloride channels (White and Aylwin, 1990), voltage-gated calcium channels, voltage-gated and ATP-sensitive potassium channels (Grover et al., 1994; Lee and Wang, 1999), as well as blocking gap junctions (Harks et al., 2001). The clinical relevance of these activities for the analgesic and anti-inflammatory potential of mefenamate is unknown.

Trade name: Ponstyl (F), Parkemed (Ger), Ponstan (UK), Ponstel (US)

Meloxicam

Synthesis: The reaction of benzothiazolo-3(2*H*)-one-1,1-dioxide with methyl chloroacetate gives the methyl 2(3*H*)-acetate derivative, which is isomerized with sodium methoxide in toluene/*tert*-butanol yielding methyl 4-hydroxy-2*H*-1,2-benzothiazine-3-carboxylate-1,1-dioxide. The subsequent methylation with methyl iodide in methanol yields the 2-methyl compound. Finally this compound is treated with 2-amino-5-methylthiazole in xylene (Trummlitz et al. (Thomae GmbH), 1979; Trummlitz et al., 1989; Kleemann et al., 1999).

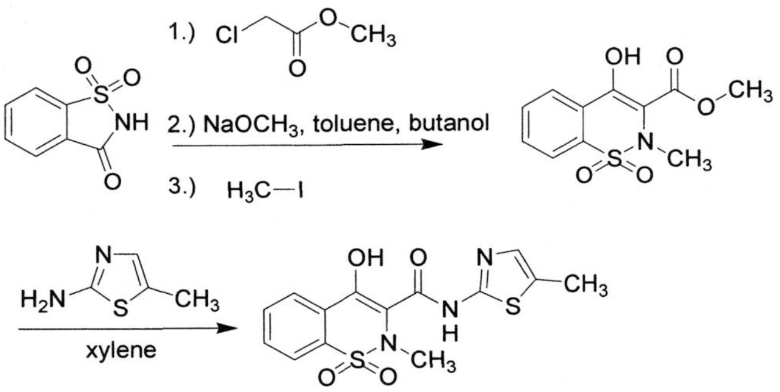

Meloxicam

[71125-38-7], 4-Hydroxy-2-methyl-1,1-dioxo-1,2-dihydro-1λ^6-benzo[e][1,2]thiazine-3-carboxylic acid (5-methyl-thiazol-2-yl)-amide, 4-hydroxy-2-methyl-*N*-(5-methyl-2-thiazoyl)-2*H*-1,2-benzothiazine-3-carboxamide-1,1-dioxide, $C_{14}H_{13}N_3O_4S_2$, M_r 351.40, mp 264 °C (decomp.)

Scheme 45: Synthesis of meloxicam.

Clinical use: Meloxicam (Engelhardt et al., 1995) is used for the acute and chronic treatment of mild to moderate pain including arthritis and ankylosing spondylitis.

Meloxicam is 10-times more selective for COX-2 compared to COX-1 in human whole blood and belongs to the first generation of COX-2 selective drugs (Vane et al., 1998).

Meloxicam is given by oral administration (7.5-15 mg/day).

Meloxicam reaches peak plasma concentrations about 8 h after oral dosing. More than 99.5% binds to plasma proteins and it has an elimination half-life of 20 h. Meloxicam is metabolized to four inactive metabolites and excreted in the urine and faeces.

Meloxicam shows central antinociceptive effects in rats which seem to be independent of the COX-inhibitory activity (Lopez-Garcia and Laird, 1998).

COX selectivity

IC50 [µM]	COX-1	COX-2	ratio
recomb. enzyme (1)	36.6	0.49	75
cell culture (2)	1.8	0.006	300
whole blood (3)	4.8	0.43	11.2

(1) Churchill et al. (1996)

(2) Riendeau et al. (1997)

(3) Patrignani et al. (1997)

Trade name: Mobic (US, EC, J)

Metamizol (Dipyrone)

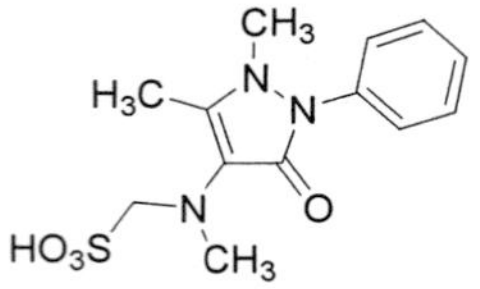

[*50567-35-6*] [(1,5-Dimethyl-3-oxo-2-phenyl-2,3-dihydro-1*H*-pyrazol-4-yl)-methyl-amino]-methanesulfonic acid, $C_{13}H_{17}N_3O_4S$, M_r 311.36; sodium salt [68-89-3], $C_{13}H_{16}N_3NaO_4S$, M_r 333.34; sodium salt monohydrate [*50567-35-6*], $C_{13}H_{16}N_3NaO_4S \cdot H_2O$, M_r 351.36

Metamizol (Dipyrone)

Synthesis (Boskmühl and Schwarz (I.G. Farben), 1922; Erhart and Ruschig, 1972; Kleemann et al., 1999):

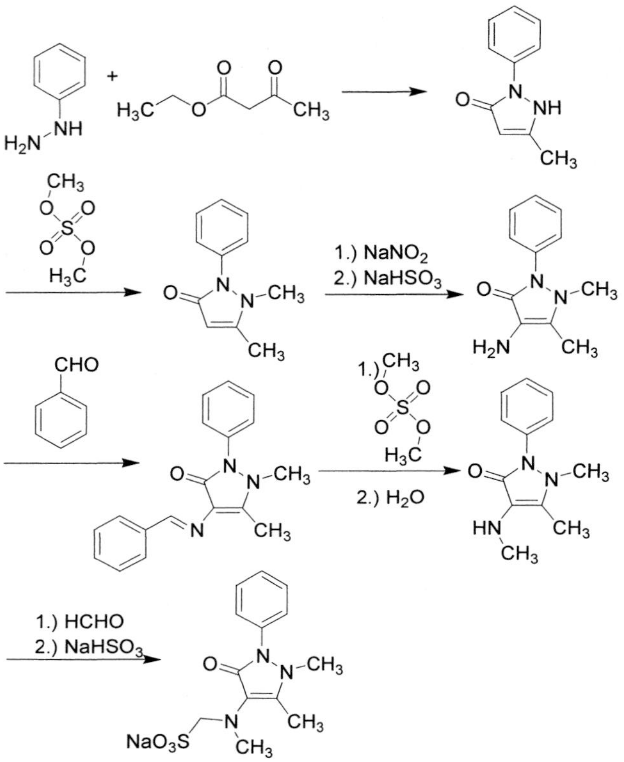

Scheme 46: Synthesis of metamizole.

COX selectivity

IC50 [µM]	COX-1	COX-2	ratio
purified enzyme (1)	420	420	1
whole blood (1)	4855	1364	3.6

(1) Campos et al. (1999)

Clinical use: Metamizol is the water-soluble sodium sulfonate of amidopyrine. After oral administration it is rapidly hydrolyzed to the active 4-methyl-amino-antipyrine and metabolized to various metabolites (Levy et al., 1995; scheme 47). Metamizol has strong analgesic, spasmolytic and antipyretic action, but no anti-inflammatory properties. The exact mechanism of action is unknown but may include inhibition of prostaglandin synthesis. Inhibition of both COX isoenzymes has been demonstrated, although only in extremely high concentrations, thus questioning the relevance of this activity.

Metamizol is used for the treatment of medium to severe pain, often in combination with opioids, for fever reduction and for the treatment of colic pain. It is given by mouth in doses of 500 mg up to 4 g daily, and by intravenous or rectal routes.

The active metabolite 4-methyl-amino-antipyrine reaches peak plasma concentrations 1.2 to 2 h after oral administration and is further metabolised with a mean elimination half-life of 2.6 to 3.5 h. Of the four main metabolites about 60% are excreted in the urine. Protein binding of these metabolites is less than 60% (Levy et al. 1995).

Metabolites of metamizol:

4-methyl-amino-antipyrine, 4-formyl-amino-antipyrine, 4-amino-antipyrine, 4-acetyl-amino-antipyrine

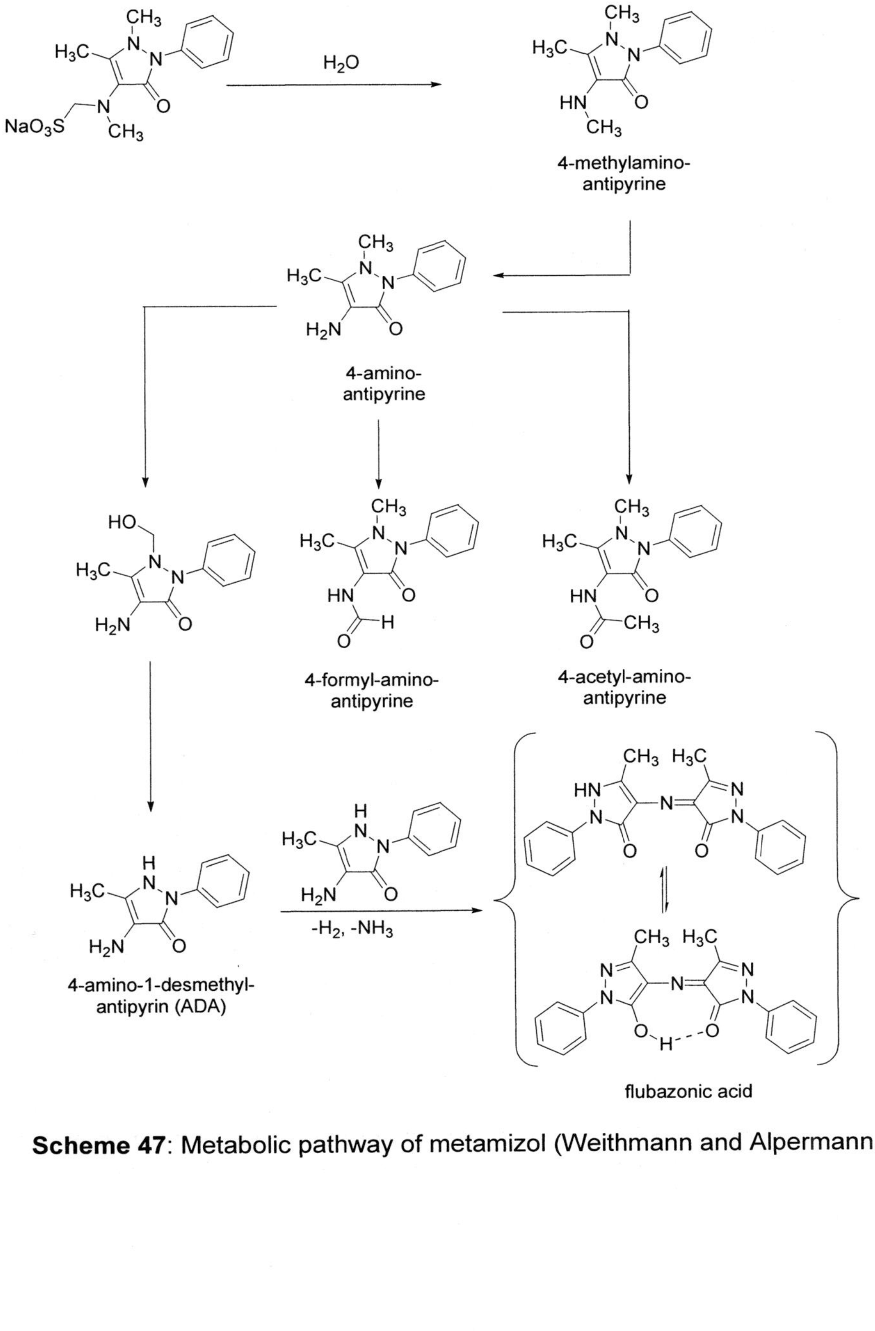

Scheme 47: Metabolic pathway of metamizol (Weithmann and Alpermann, 1983)

Trade name: Baralgin (Ger),
Novalgin (Ger)

Metamizol is relatively free of acute side-effects but in rare cases may induce severe and life-threatening allergic reactions such as agranulocytosis, allergic skin reactions and allergic shock. Therefore, the compound is not used in the UK, US or Scandinavian countries.

Mofebutazone

Mofebutazone

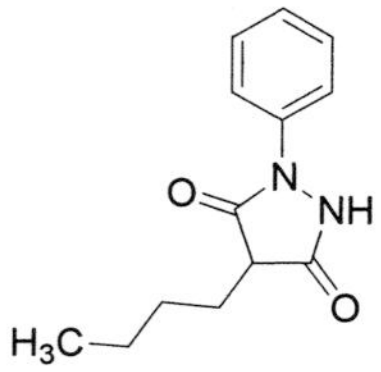

Synthesis (Büchi et al., 1953; Comm. Farmaceutica Milanese, 1957; Kleemann et al., 1999):

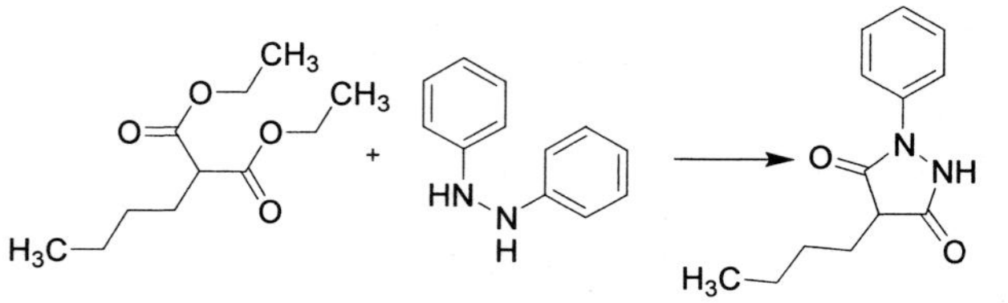

[*2210-63-1*], 4-Butyl-1-phenyl-pyrazolidine-3,5-dione, $C_{13}H_{16}N_2O_2$, M_r 232.28, *mp* 102-103 °C; sodium salt [*41468-34-2*], $C_{13}H_{15}N_2NaO_2$, M_r 254.27

Scheme 48: Synthesis of mofebutazone.

Clinical use: Mofebutazone is a nonsteroidal anti-inflammatory drug used for the treatment of mild to moderate pain including inflammatory and degenerative rheumatic disorders and musculoskeletal pain.

Mofebutazone is given as oral, rectal (900-1200 mg/day), or intramuscular preparations (650 mg/day).

Mofebutazone reaches peak plasma concentrations within 1.4 h and is extensively bound to plasma proteins (~99%). The plasma elimination half-life of mofebutazone is 1.9 h. Mofebutazone is excreted mainly as the glucuronides of its metabolites in the urine (Loew et al., 1985).

Trade name:Clinit (Austria),
Diadin, Mofesal (Ger)

Nabumetone

Nabumetone

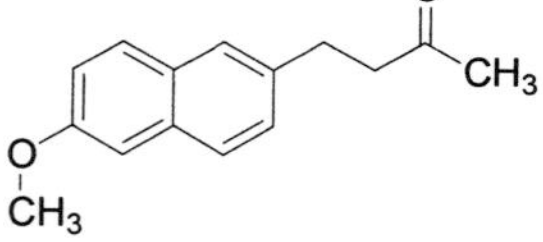

Synthesis: The condensation of 6-methoxy-2-naphthaldehyde with acetone by means of NaOH in water gives 4-(6-methoxy-2-naphthyl)-3-buten-2-one, which is reduced with H_2 over Pd-C in ethyl acetate (Goudie et al., 1978; Neumann, 1981; Lake and Rose (Beecham), 1974; 1983; Kleemann et al., 1999; Prabhakar et al., 1999).

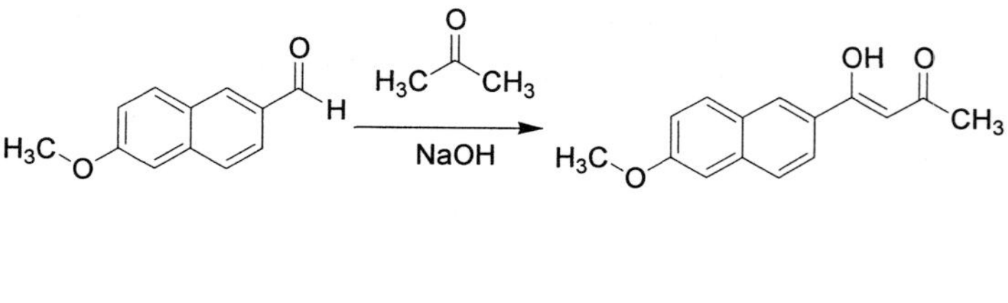

[*42924-53-8*], 4-(6-Methoxy-naphthalen-2-yl)-butan-2-one, $C_{15}H_{16}O_2$, M_r 228.29, *mp* 80 °C

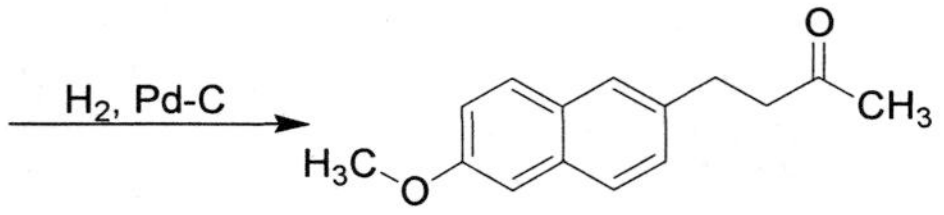

Scheme 49: Synthesis of nabumetone.

The following route starts with the bromination of β-naphthol, using molecular bromine and resulting in the formation of 2,5-dibromo-6-naphthol, which on monodebromination with tin metal affords the 6-bromo-2-naphthol in high yields. The bromophenol thus obtained is O-methylated using dimethyl sulfate to afford 2-bromonaroline in quantitative yields, which in turn is converted to 6-methoxy-2-naphthaldehyde via 6-methoxynaphthylmagnesium bromide using a Mg/DMF/THF protocol. The aldol condensation of the aldehyde with acetone resulted in the formation of the enone. The final reduction of the enone, using Pd/C or Raney-Ni, proceeded smoothly to produce nabumetone.

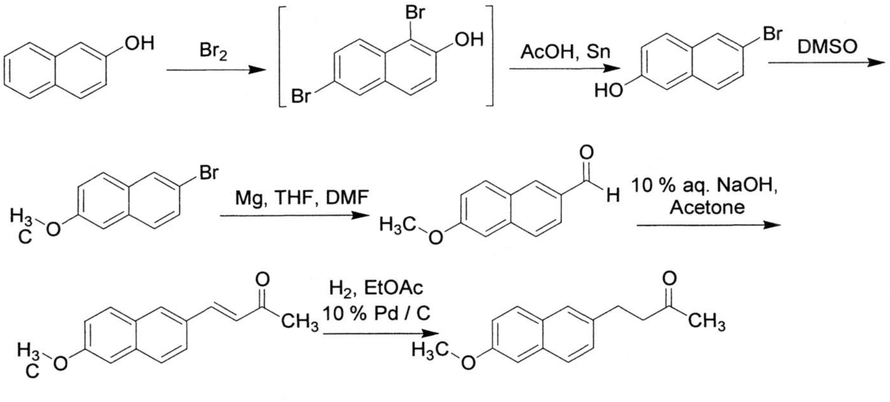

Scheme 50: Synthesis of nabumetone.

The reduction of methyl 6-methoxy-2-naphthyl acetate with lithium aluminium hydride in refluxing ether gives 2-(6-methoxy-2-naphthyl)ethanol, which by treatment with PBr$_3$ in refluxing benzene is converted into 2-(6-methoxy-2-naphthyl)ethyl bromide. Further reaction with KCN in refluxing ethanol-water affords 3-(6-methoxy-2-naphthyl) propionitrile, which is finally treated with methylmagnesium iodide in refluxing ethanol.

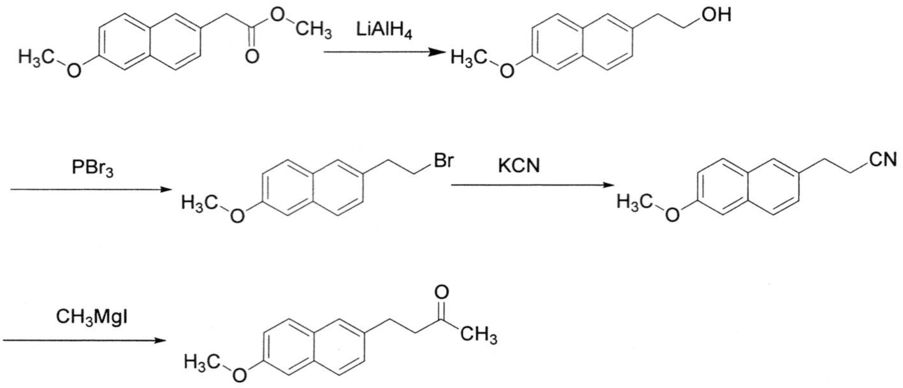

Scheme 51: Synthesis of nabumetone.

Several further synthetic methods have been described.

Clinical use: Nabumetone (Friedel et al., 1993) undergoes rapid first-pass metabolism to the active metabolite 6-MNA (6-methoxy-2-naphthyl acetic acid). 6-MNA shows balanced inhibition of both COX-1 and COX-2 in cell culture and a whole blood assay.

COX selectivity

IC50 [µM]	COX-1	COX-2	ratio
cell culture (1)	2.3	~5	~0.5
whole blood (2)	278	187	1.5

(1) Riendeau et al. (1997)

(2) Patrignani et al. (1997)

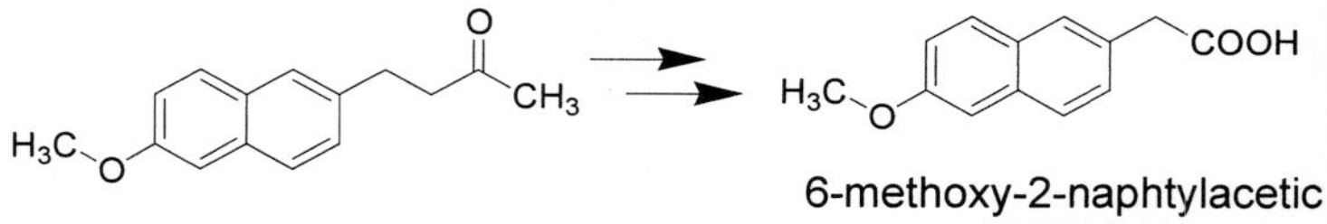

6-methoxy-2-naphtylacetic acid (6-MNA)

Scheme 52: 6-Methoxy-2-naphtylacetic acid (6-MNA), the active metabolite of nabumetone.

Nabumetone is used for the treatment of pain and inflammation associated with osteoarthritis and rheumatoid arthritis. The drug is is administered orally (500-2000 mg/day).

Trade name: Relafen (US), Relifex (UK)

Nabumetone is well absorbed from the gastrointestinal tract following oral administration and undergoes rapid and extensive first-pass metabolism in the liver to 6-MNA and other inactive metabolites. There is 99% binding of 6-MNA to plasma protein and it has an elimination half-life of up to 22 h with marked individual differences. 6-MNA is metabolized by O-methylation and conjugation and is excreted to about 80% in the urine as inactive or conjugated metabolites (Davies, 1997).

Naproxen

The 2-arylpropionic acid derivatives (profens) are important classes of NSAIDs that have been in clinical use for over 20 years. The profens have been used clinically as racemic agents with the exception of (S)-(+)-naproxen, which has been developed and used only as a single enantiomeric drug.

Naproxen

[22204-53-1], (+)-(S)-2-(6-Methoxy-naphthalen-2-yl)-propionic acid, $C_{14}H_{14}O_3$, M_r 230.26, mp 155.3 °C (also reported as 152-154 °C),), $[\alpha]_D$ +66° (c = 1, CHCl$_3$); sodium salt [26159-34-2], $C_{14}H_{13}NaO_3$, M_r 252.25, mp 244-246 °C, $[\alpha]_D$ -11° (c = 1, CHCl$_3$)

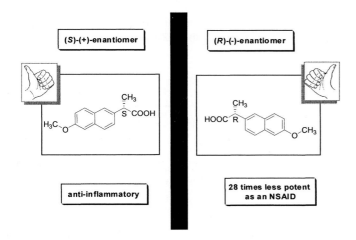

Figure 20: Enantiomers of naproxen.

- 1967 first publication (SYNTEX)
- 1972 intrudoction to the pharmaceutical market as an anti-inflammatory, analgesic and antipyretic drug in the form of the free acid, later as the sodium salt (naproxen sodium)
- 1988 expiry of the patent protection (development of the generic market in many countries)
- 1993 expiry of the patent protection in the US
- 2-Arylpropanoic acid derivative with one chiral center
- (S) enantiomer is 28 times more active as an anti-inflammatory agent than the (R) enantiomer
- Naproxen is the only NSAID drug currently on the market in an enantiomerically pure form
- Current production of naproxen and naproxen sodium: 1000 tons per annum
- Bulk price (1990) US $ 140-150 per kg.

Drug history

Synthesis (Shen, 1972; Dorfman, 1975; Sonawane et al., 1992; Kleemann et al., 1999)

Synthesis of racemic naproxene: Friedel-Crafts acylation (aluminum chloride - nitrobenzene) of β-naphthol methyl ether affords 2-acetyl-6-methoxy naphthalene, which, when treated with either dimethyl sulfonium or dimethylsulfoxonium methylide, gives 2-(6-methoxynaphthalen-2-yl)propylene oxide. Treatment of the latter with boron trifluoride etherate in tetrahydrofuran gives 2-(6-methoxynaphthalen-2-yl)propionaldehyde, which is oxidized using Jones reagent (4 M chromic acid) to yield the racemic 2-(6-methoxynaphthalen-2-yl)propionic acid.

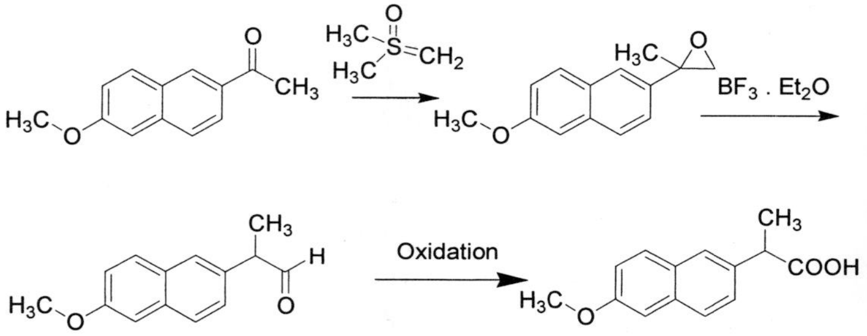

Scheme 53: Synthesis of racemic naproxen.

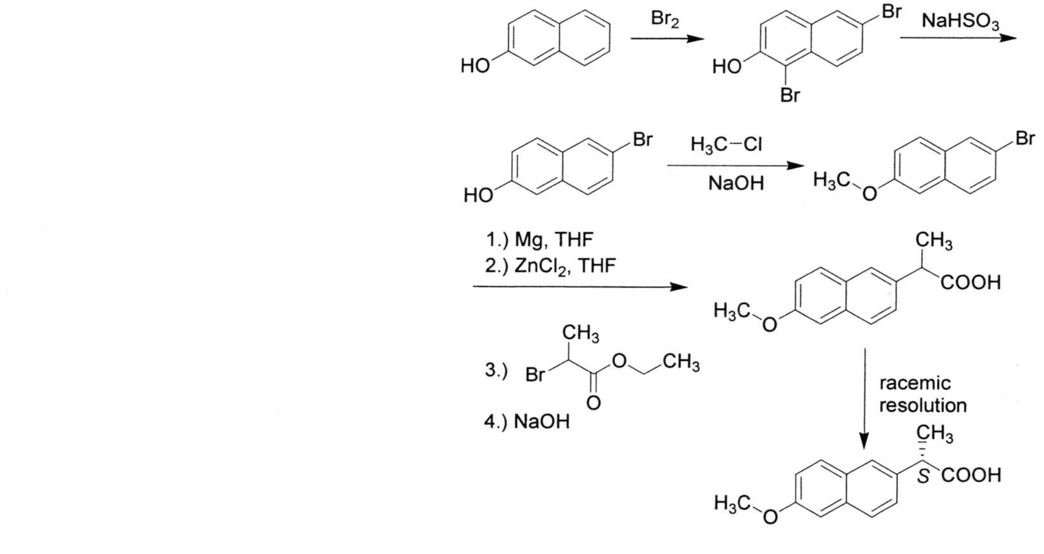

Scheme 54: First large-scale manufacturing process of Syntex (Alvarez, 1972):

For racemic resolution of naproxen the use of cinchonidine, *N*-alkyl-*D*-glucamine, dehydroabietylamine or (*S*)-α-phenylethylamine has been described.

For the enzymatic cleavage of esters of racemic naproxen, cloned esterases, which are cheap and easy to produce, have been developed (a 100 tons per annum process is planned).

Advantages of the enzymatic process

Cloned esterase (isolated from *Bacillus subtilis* and cloned in *E. coli*), cheap and easy to produce

Utilizes insoluble non-toxic ester, 150 g/l, conversion 39%

Very simple processing to recover product, 100 tons per annum (SHASUN Process)

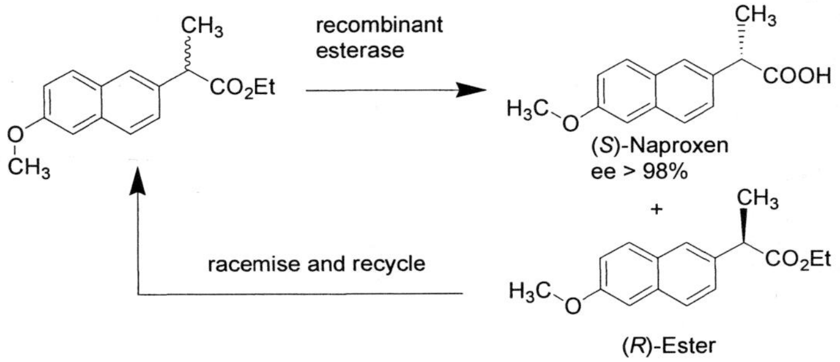

Scheme 55: Enzymatic cleavage of esters of racemic naproxen.

Other biocatalytic processes for (*S*)-naproxen production from the academic area are shown below:

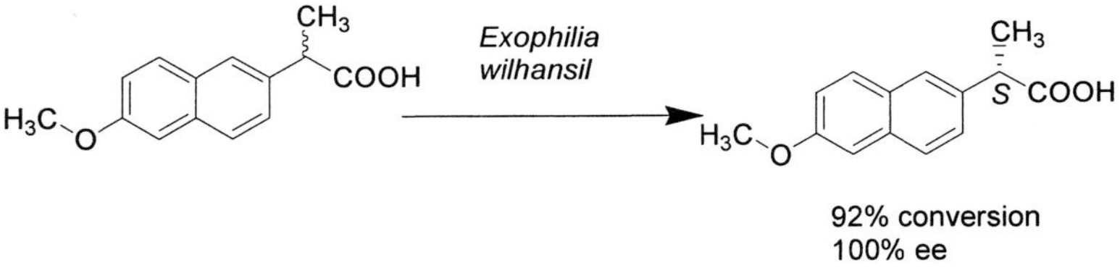

92% conversion
100% ee

Scheme 56: Direct isomerization of racemic naproxen using the biocatalyst *Exophialia wilhansil*.

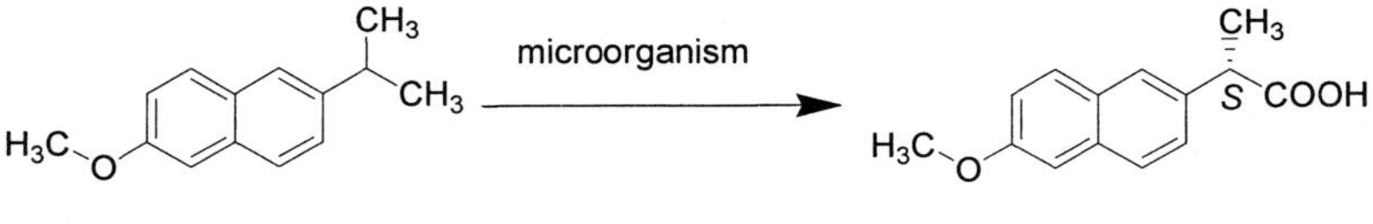

Scheme 57: One-step synthesis by microbial oxidation (IBIS).

Several other synthetic routes also exist. The stereospecific Syntex process is an example using chiral technology to produce enantiomerically pure naproxen:

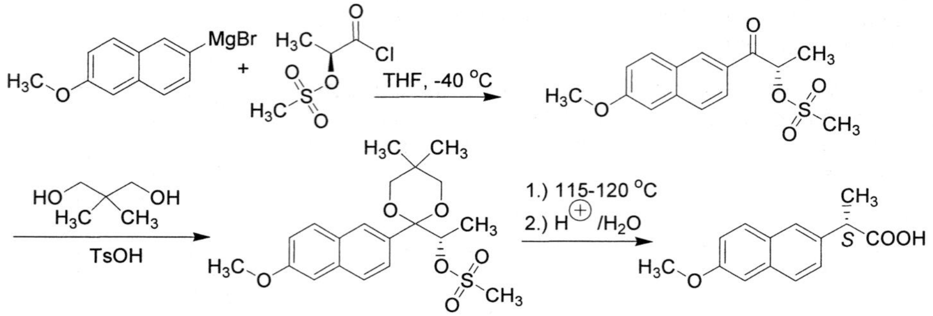

Scheme 58: Stereospecific Syntex process starting with ethyl-(S)-lactate (Schloemer (Syntex), 1986):

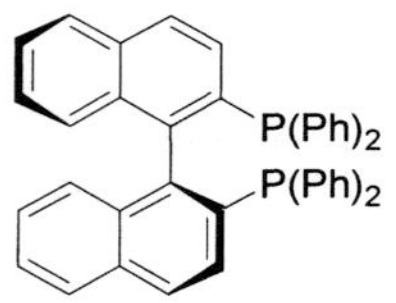

(S)-BINAP

The asymmetric hydrogenation of 2-(6-methoxy-2-naphthyl)acrylic acid using ruthenium-BINAP complexes also yields enantiomerically pure naproxen.

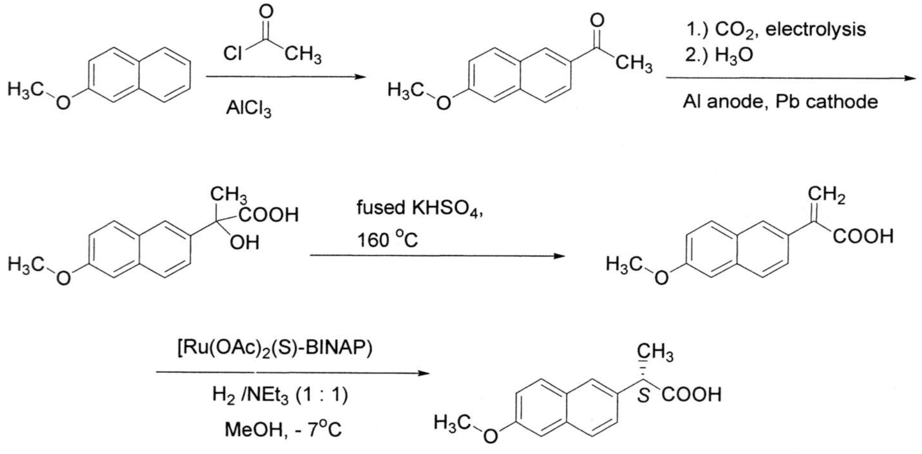

Scheme 59: Synthesis of naproxen by asymmetric hydrogenation.

Clinical use: Naproxen (Todd and Clissold, 1990) is a nonsteroidal anti-inflammatory drug used for the treatment of mild to moderate pain and inflammatory pain conditions such as rheumatoid arthritis, osteoarthritis, soft tissue disorders, postoperative pain and dysmenorrhoea. It is also used to treat migraine. Naproxen shows balanced inhibition of both COX isoenzymes in a cellular assay and a preference for COX-1 in a whole blood assay and in an enzyme assay using recombinant human enzymes.

Naproxen has fewer cardiovascular side-effects in comparison with the COX-2 selective inhibitor rofecoxib (Mukherjee et al., 2001).

Naproxen is the (+)-enantiomer. It is given orally or rectally with a common initial dose of 500 mg (up to 1250 mg/day). The major side-effects are gastrointestinal disturbances.

Naproxen is available as a free base, as sodium salt and in combination with misoprostol for the reduction of the gastrointestinal side-effects.

The plasma elimination half life of naproxen is about 13 h. Naproxen is heavily bound to plasma proteins (>99%) at therapeutic concentrations. Approximately 95% of the compound is excreted as naproxen and its 6-*O*-desmethyl metabolite (Davies and Andersson, 1997).

The synthesis and *in vitro* evaluation of novel morpholinyl- and methylpiperazinylacyloxyalkyl prodrugs of naproxen for topical drug delivery has been described recently (Rautio et al., 2000).

COX selectivity

IC50 [μM]	COX-1	COX-2	ratio
purified enzyme (1)	1.1	36	0.03
cell culture (2)	2.2	1.3	1.7
whole blood (3)	7.8	73.7	0.1

(1) Gierse et al. (1995)

(2) Mitchell et al. (1993)

(3) Brideau et al. (1996)

Trade name: Proxen (Ger), Apranax (F, Ger), Naprosyn (UK, US)

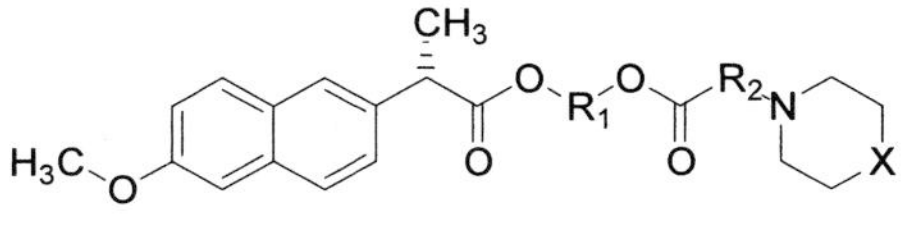

R$_1$ = (CH$_2$)$_2$, (CH$_2$)$_4$
R$_2$ = CH$_2$, (CH$_2$)$_2$
X = O, N-CH$_3$

Figure 21: Novel morpholinyl- and methylpiperazin-ylacyloxy alkyl prodrugs of naproxen for topical drug delivery.

Niflumic Acid

Synthesis: Condensation of 2-chloronicotinic acid with 3-trifluoromethylaniline or reaction of 2-aminonicotinic acid with 1-bromo-3-trifluoromethylbenzene yields niflumic acid (Sherlock and Sperber (Schering Corp.), 1967; Faure and Hoffman (Labs. U.P.S.A.), 1968; Kleemann et al., 1999).

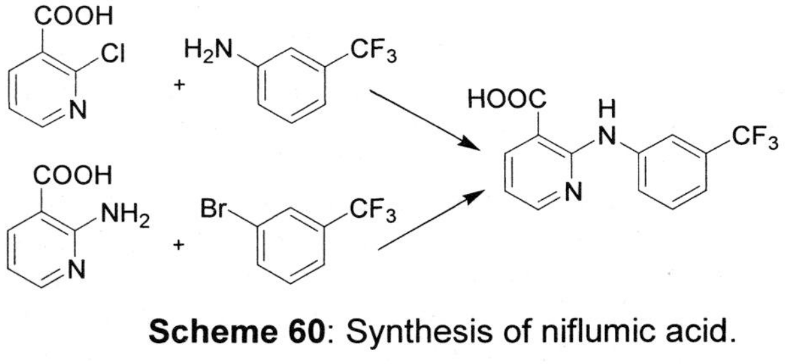

Niflumic Acid

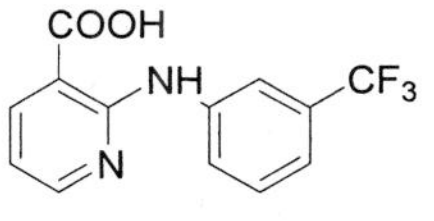

[*4394-00-7*], 2-(3-Trifluoromethyl-phenyl-amino)-nicotinic acid, 2-[[3-(trifluoromethyl)]amino]-3-pyrodinecarboxylic acid, C$_{13}$H$_9$F$_3$N$_2$O$_2$, *M$_r$* 282.22, *mp* 204 °C

Scheme 60: Synthesis of niflumic acid.

Clinical use: Niflumic acid (Auclair et al., 1989) is a nonsteroidal anti-inflammatory drug used for the treatment of inflammation and pain in musculoskeletal and joint disorders such as rheumatoid arthritis as well as traumatic and postoperative pain. Niflumic acid is used in oral, rectal or topical preparations (up to 750 mg/day).

The morpholinoethyl ester morniflumate, which is used in topical formulations was shown to inhibit both cyclooxygenase and 5-lipoxygenase, thus suggesting an additional potential in anti-inflammatory therapy (Civelli et al., 1991).

In addition to its action on prostaglandin synthesis, fenamates have been shown to modify several ion channel functions, e.g. inhibition of non-selective cation conductance (Gögelein et al., 1990), calcium-activated chloride channels (White and Aylwin, 1990), voltage-gated calcium channels, voltage-gated and ATP-sensitive potassium channels (Grover et al., 1994; Lee and Wang, 1999), as well as blocking gap junctions (Harks et al., 2001). The clinical relevance of these activities for the analgesic and anti-inflammatory potential of niflumic acid is unknown.

Trade name: Niflurid, Niflugel (B, F, Switz.), Actol (Austria, S)

Nimesulide

Nimesulide

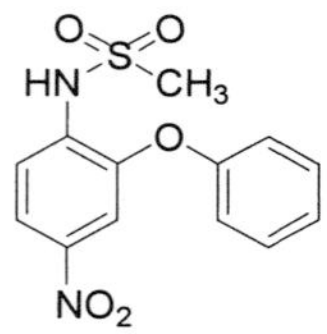

Synthesis (Riker, 1973; 1974; Kleemann et al., 1999):

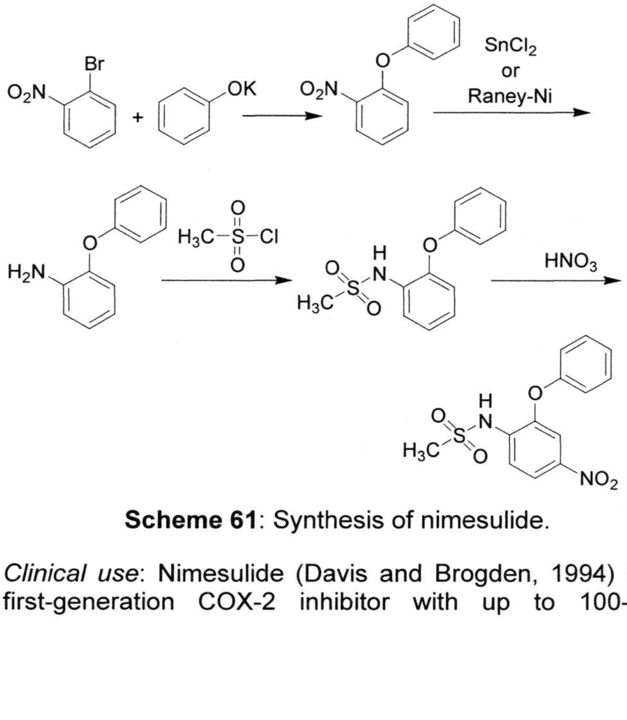

[51803-78-2], N-(4-Nitro-2-phenoxyphenyl)methanesulfonamide, $C_{13}H_{12}N_2O_5S$, M_r 308.05, *mp* 143-144.5 °C

Scheme 61: Synthesis of nimesulide.

Clinical use: Nimesulide (Davis and Brogden, 1994) is a first-generation COX-2 inhibitor with up to 100-fold selectivity for COX-2 compared to COX-1, depending on the assay system.

It is used for the short-term treatment of inflammatory conditions, fever and pain, including musculoskeletal and joint disorders. Nimesulide is used as an oral or rectal formulation (up to 400 mg/day).

Peak plasma concentrations are reached within about 2 to 3 h after oral administration. The terminal plasma elimination half-life is between 2 and 5 h. Nimesulide is subject to extensive metabolism. The principal active metabolite is 4-hydroxy-nimesulide. Nimesulide and its metabolites are excreted in the urine (~70%) and the faeces (~20%).

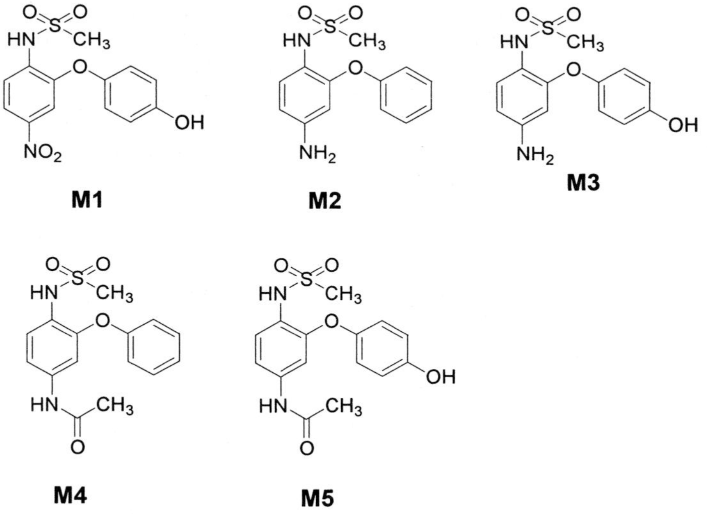

COX selectivity

IC50 [μM]	COX-1	COX-2	ratio
cell culture (1)	0.78	0.009	87
whole blood (2)	9.2	0.52	18

(1) Riendeau et al. (1997)

(2) Patrignani et al. (1997)

Figure 22: Urinary metabolites of nimesulide in man (Singla et al., 2000) including M1, 4-hydroxy-nimesulide, an active metabolite of nimesulide

Nimesulide has been reported to induce hepatic failure in some cases (McCormick et al., 1999; Ferreiro et al., 2000).

In addition to the inhibition of COX, nimesulide has been shown to inhibit the production of the pro-inflammatory cytokine TNF-α under inflammatory conditions (Azab et al., 1988).

Trade name: Nexen (France), Aulin (Italy, CH)

Oxaprozin

Oxaprozin

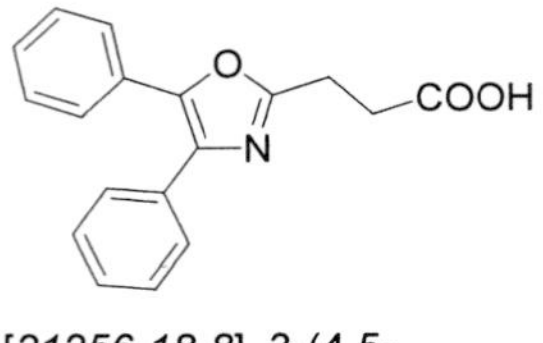

[*21256-18-8*], 3-(4,5-Diphenyl-oxazol-2-yl)-propionic acid, $C_{18}H_{15}NO_3$, M_r 293.32, *mp* 160.5-161.5 °C

Synthesis: Brown (Wyeth), 1971; Arrigoni-Martelli, 1978c; Kleemann et al., 1999):

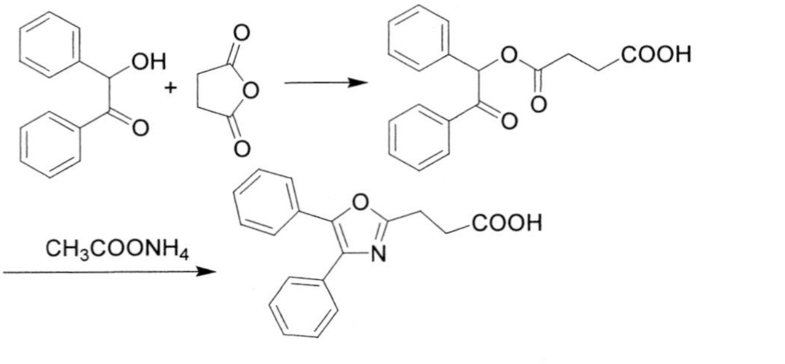

Scheme 62: Synthesis of oxaprozin.

Clinical use: Oxaprozin (Miller, 1992) is a nonsteroidal anti-inflammatory drug used for the treatment of mild to moderate pain including rheumatoid arthritis and osteoarthritis.

Oxaprozin shows selectivity for COX-1 in human cellular assays and a more balanced inhibition of both COX-1 and COX-2 in a whole blood assay. It is given orally (600-1200 mg/day, maximum dose 1800 mg/day).

Oxaprozin reaches peak plasma concentrations 2 to 6 h after oral administration (Davies, 1998b). It shows slow kinetics with an elimination half-life of about 24 h. Oxaprozin is metabolized and glucuronized and excreted in the urine and the bile. Two hydroxlated metabolites have been shown to have anti-inflammatory activity.

COX selectivity

IC50 [µM]	COX-1	COX-2	ratio
cell culture (1)	2.2	36	0.06
whole blood (2)	15	37	0.4

(1) Kawai et al. (1998)

(2) Cryer and Feldman (1998)

Trade names: Deflam (S. Afr.), Daypro (US)

Oxyphenbutazone

Oxyphenbutazone

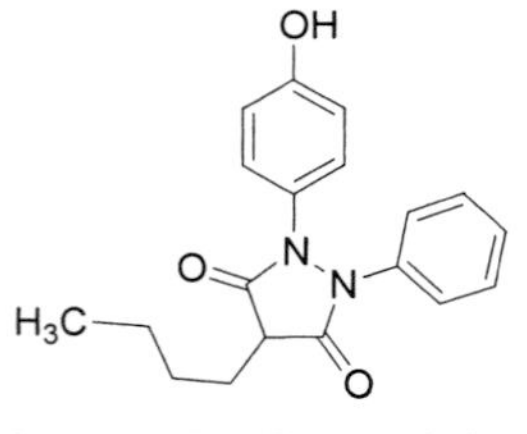

[*129-20-4*], 4-Butyl-1-(4-hydroxy-phenyl)-2-phenyl-pyrazolidine-3,5-dione, $C_{19}H_{20}N_2O_3$, M_r 324.37, *mp* 124-125 °C; monohydrate [*7081-38-1*], $C_{19}H_{20}N_2O_3 \cdot H_2O$, M_r 342.40, *mp* 96 °C

Synthesis (Häflinger (Geigy), 1956; Kleemann et al., 1999):

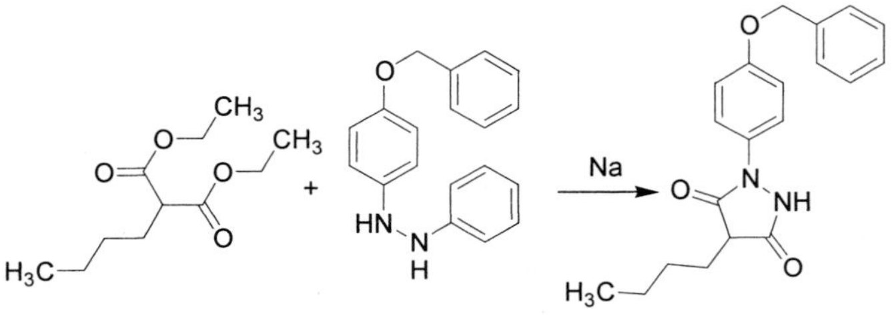

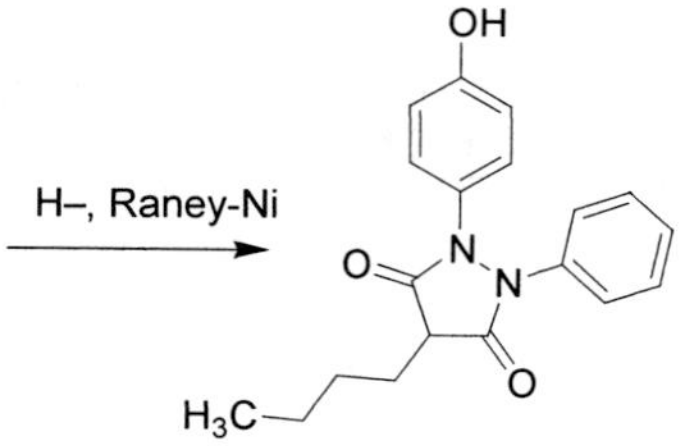

Scheme 63: Synthesis of oxyphenbutazone.

Clinical use: Oxyphenbutazone is a nonsteroidal anti-inflammatory drug used for the acute treatment of ankylosing spondylitis, chronic polyarthritis and gout. Oxyphenbutazone is a metabolite of phenylbutazone and is limited in use because of a high incidence of hematopoietic side-effects such as fatal agranulocytosis and aplastic anemia (Bottiger and Westerholm, 1973). Therefore, oxyphenbutazone should only be used if other nonsteroidal anti-inflammatory drugs do not show sufficient efficacy.

Oxyphenbutazone can be administered as oral, rectal or topical preparations (400-600 mg/day).

Trade name: Tanderil (Austria, Eire, Switz.), Phlogont (Ger)

Paracetamol (Acetaminophen)

Synthesis (Wilbert and DeAngelis (Warner-Lambert), 1961; Kleemann et al., 1999):

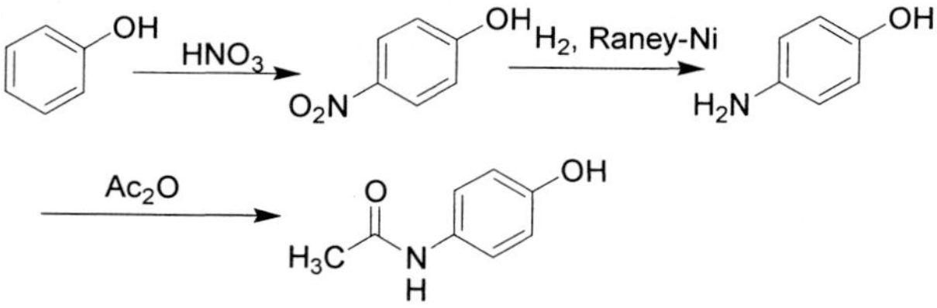

Paracetamol

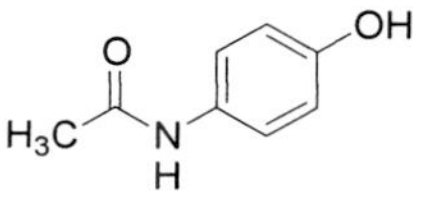

[103-90-2], N-(4-Hydroxy-phenyl)-acetamide, $C_8H_9NO_2$, M_r 151.16, *mp* 168-169 °C

Scheme 64: Synthesis of paracetamol, classical route.

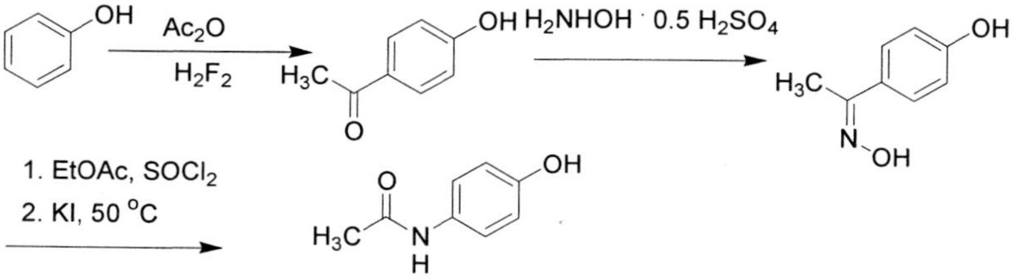

Scheme 65: Synthesis of paracetamol, Hoechst-Celanese process.

COX selectivity

IC50 [μM]	COX-1	COX-2	ratio
cellular assay (1)	2.7	20	0.1
whole blood (2)	>100	49	<2
whole blood (3)	42	11	4

(1) Mitchell et al. (1993)
(IC_{30} values are given, because 50% inhibition of COX-2 was not reached at concentrations up to 1 mg/kg)

(2) Warner et al. (1999)

(3) Cryer and Feldman (1998)

Clinical use: Paracetamol (Ameer and Greenblatt, 1977; Clissold, 1986) has analgesic and antipyretic properties, but no relevant anti-inflammatory action. It is used for the treatment of various mild to moderate pain conditions and to reduce fever. Paracetamol is one of the most popular analgesics as a single drug or in multi-ingredient preparations, often in combination with NSAIDs or weak opioids.

Despite its long clinical history after its discovery in 1893 (von Mering, 1893), the mechanism of action of paracetamol is not fully understood. It shows some weak inhibition of the COX isoenzymes and there is speculation on a third COX isoenzyme, COX-3, induced during the resolution phase of an inflammatory response, that might be specifically targeted by paracetamol (Willoughby et al., 2000). Furthermore, there is evidence for a possible central analgesic effect mediated indirectly by 5-HT (Courade et al., 2001).

Paracetamol is used orally or rectally as suppositories, the oral dose range is 500-1000 mg every 4-5 h up to 4 g daily.

Paracetamol reaches peak plasma concentrations within the first hour after oral administration and shows only a low tendency for plasma protein binding at therapeutic concentrations. The elimination half-life is between 1 and 3 h. Paracetamol is metabolized mainly in the liver and excreted in the urine as glucuronide and sulphate conjugates. The metabolic pathway of paracetamol is shown in Schemes 66 and 67:

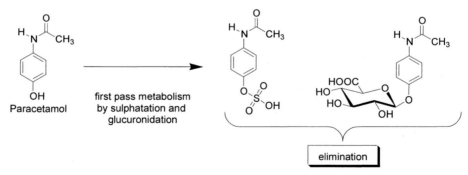

Scheme 66: Formation of the glucuronide and sulphate conjugates of paracetamol.

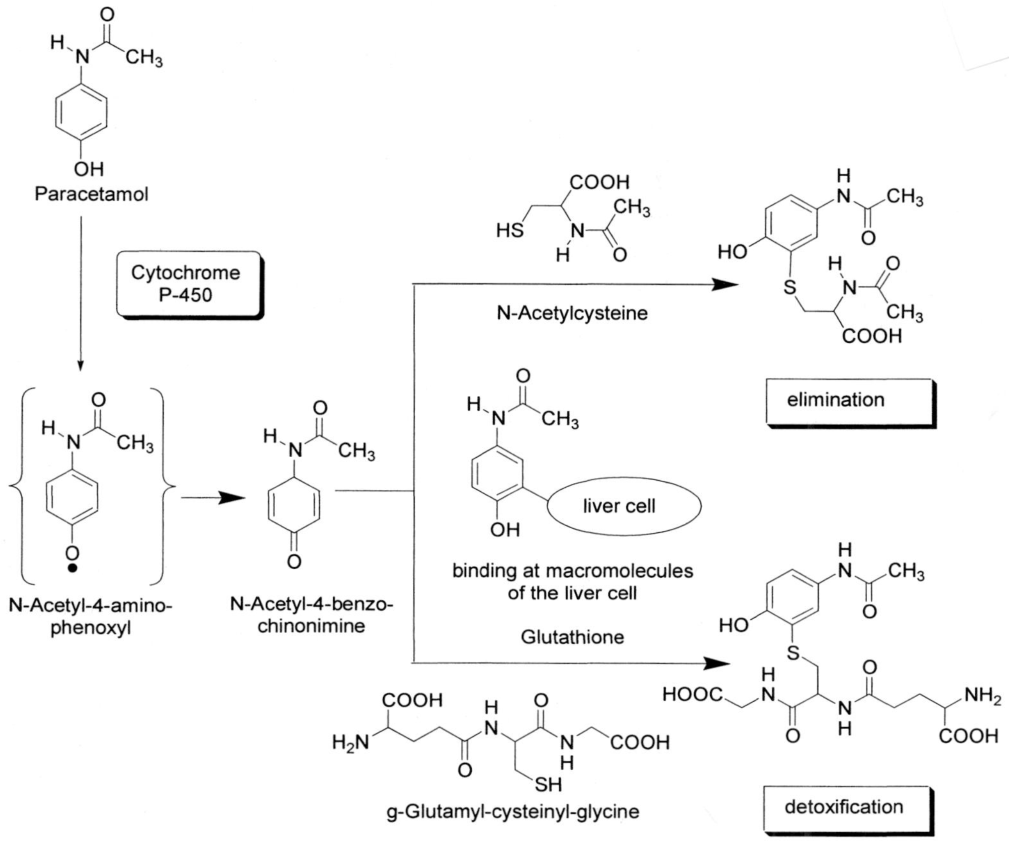

Scheme 67: Formation of the liver toxic metabolite *N*-acetyl-4-benzochinonimine and its elimination and detoxification with gluthathione or (*N*-acetyl)cysteine.

Side-effects are rare and may include hematological reactions, leucopenia, agranulocytosis and other hypersensitivity reactions. Paracetamol has a narrow therapeutic dose range and overdosage induces severe liver and renal damage (Lewis and Paloucek, 1991) via accumulation of a toxic metabolite, *N*-acetyl-benzoquinoneimine (NABQI). Acetylcysteine or methionine, which increase glutathione conjugation of the metabolite, are used as the antidote.

Paracetamol is not soluble in aqueous solutions and cannot be given parenterally. A soluble glycine prodrug derivative of paracetamol is on the market as parenteral form (propacetamol).

Trade name: Dafalgan (Fr), Benuron (Ger, Switz), Tylenol (Austr, Austral, Canad, US, Irl, Sp), Alvedon (Norw, Swed, UK)

Christoph and Buschmann

Parecoxib sodium

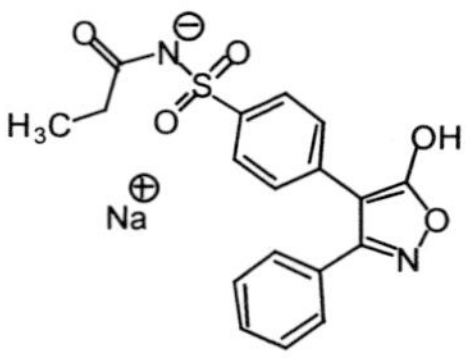

[198470-85-8],
[198470-84-7] (free acid) ,
N-(4-(5-methyl-3-
phenylisoxazol-4-yl)phen-
ylsulfonyl)propion-amide
sodium salt
$C_{19}H_{17}N_2O_4SNa$, 392.409;
crystals mp 271.5-272.7 °C

Parecoxib sodium

Synthesis: The acylation of 4-(5-methyl-3-phenylisoxazol-4-yl)benzenesulfonamide (valdecoxib), with propionic anhydride in a solution of TEA and DMAP in tetrahydrofurane gives N-(4-(5-methyl-3-phenylisoxazol-4-yl)phenylsulfonyl)propionamide, which is treated with NaOH in ethanol to give parecoxib sodium salt (Talley (Parmacia Corp.), 1996; 2000b; Sorbera, 2001b).

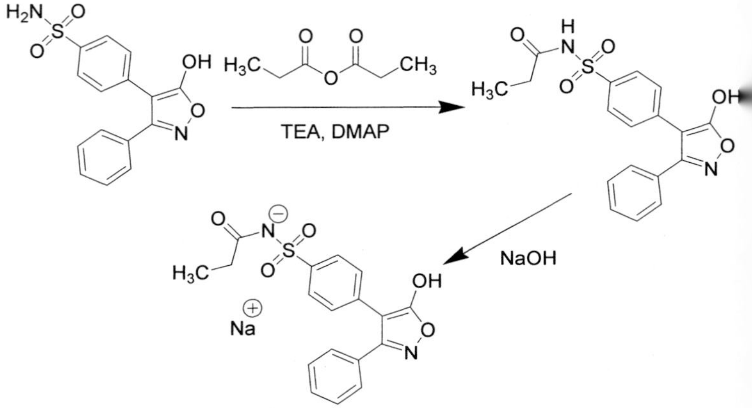

Scheme 68: Synthesis of parecoxib sodium.

Clinical use: Parecoxib (Cheer and Goa, 2001; Gotta, 2001; Sorbera et al., 2001b) is a third generation COX-2 inhibitor. Parecoxib is a prodrug of valdecoxib with aqueous solubility sufficient for the use of the substance in parenteral formulations. Valdecoxib shows about 30-fold selectivity for COX-2 in whole blood assays (see Valdecoxib; Talley et al., 2000a; Riendeau et al., 2001). Parecoxib shows efficacy in a variety of animal models of inflammation (Talley et al., 2000b).

Parecoxib is rapidly hydrolyzed by the liver to its active metabolite valdecoxib. Plasma peak concentrations for valdecoxib are achieved within 1.1 to 3.5 and 0.27 to 2 h after i.m. and i.v. administration, respectively, in healthy volunteers. The elimination half-life for parecoxib is 15 to 35 min and 5 min for i.m. and i.v. administration respectively, in healthy volunteers. Metabolism of parecoxib follows the metabolism of the active metabolite valdecoxib which is a substrate for cytochrome P450 3A4 and 2C9.

Trade name: Xapit,
Dynastat, Rayzon (EC)

Parecoxib is used in doses of 20 and 40 mg of its sodium salt for the short-term treatment of postoperative pain.

Phenidine (Phenacetin)

Synthesis (Kleemann et al., 1999):

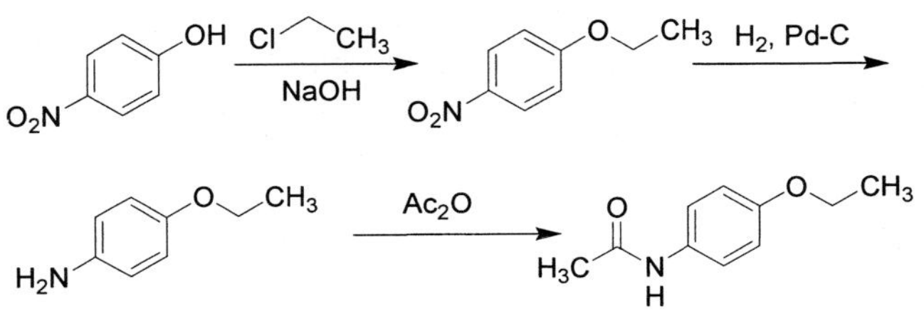

Phenidine

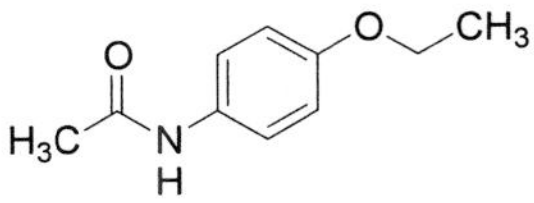

[62-44-2], *N*-(4-Ethoxy-phenyl)-acetamide, $C_{10}H_{13}NO_2$, M_r 179.22, *mp* 134-135 °C

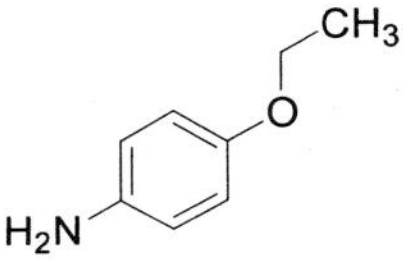

Scheme 69: Synthesis of phenidine

Clinical use: Phenidine (Clissold, 1986) is a weak analgesic and antipyretic compound without anti-inflammatory action. It has been used in combination with other compounds like aspirin, caffeine or codeine, but due to hematological and nephrotoxic side-effects (Dubach et al., 1983) has been withdrawn from many markets.

Phenidine is rapidly metabolized to a great extent to its metabolite paracetamol which seems to be responsible for the therapeutic action of phenidine. Another metabolite, *p*-phenetidine is responsible for the toxic side-effects.

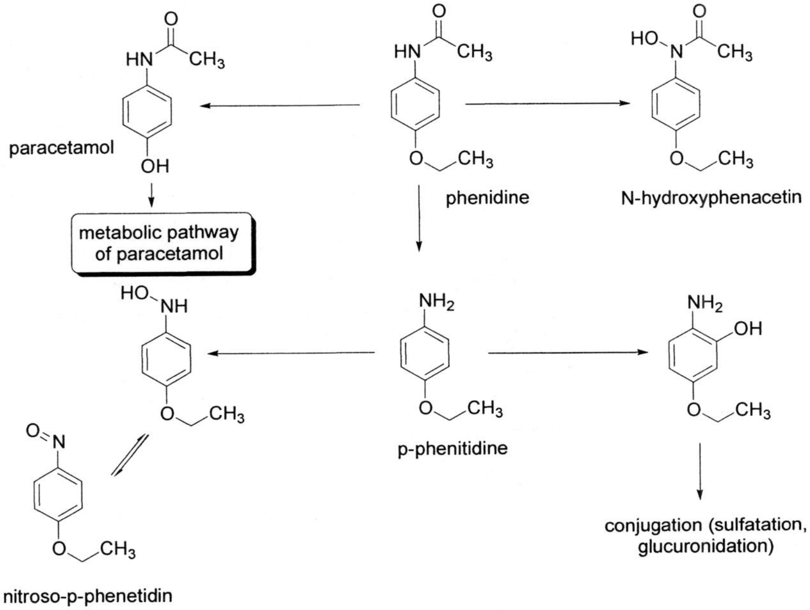

p-phenetidine, the toxic metabolite of phenidine

Trade name: Gripponyl (F), Cratodin (Spain)

Scheme 70: Metabolic pathway of phenidine with the formation of *p*-phenetidine, the toxic metabolite of phenidine.

Christoph and Buschmann

Phenylbutazone

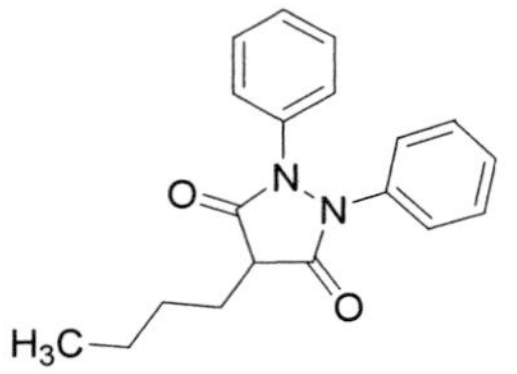

Phenylbutazone

Synthesis (Stenzl (Geigy), 1951; Kleemann et al., 1999):

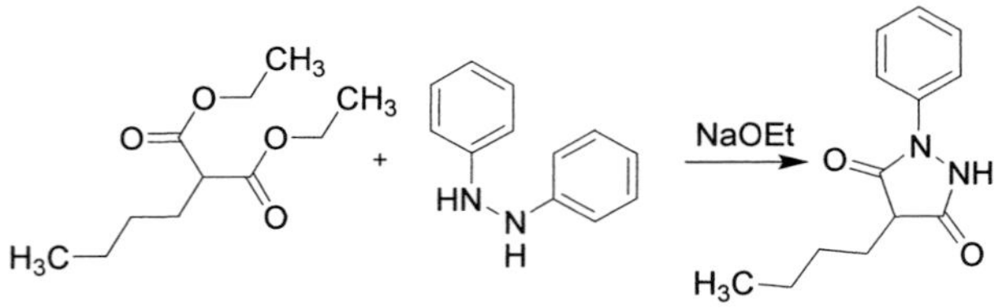

[*50-33-9*], 4-Butyl-1,2-diphenyl-pyrazolidine-3,5-dione, $C_{19}H_{20}N_2O_2$, M_r 308.37, *mp* 105 °C; sodium salt [*129-18-0*], , $C_{19}H_{19}N_2NaO_2$, M_r 331.36; calcium salt (2 : 1) [*36298-23-4*], , $C_{38}H_{36}CaN_4O_4$, M_r 656.83; piperazine salt (1 : 1) [*4985-25-5*], , $C_{19}H_{20}N_2O_2$. $C_4H_{10}N_2$, M_r 395.51, *mp* 140-141 °C

Scheme 71: Synthesis of phenylbutazone.

Clinical use: Phenylbutazone (Brogden, 1986) is a nonsteroidal anti-inflammatory drug used for the acute treatment of ankylosing spondylitis, chronic polyarthritis and gout. Phenylbutazone on its own shows only weak inhibition of COX-1 and COX-2 with IC50s >30 µM (Brideau et al., 1996) and active metabolites are mainly responsible for its actions.

Side-effects include disturbances of the hematopoietic system such as agranulocytosis and aplastic anaemia (Faich, 1987) and limit its use to the treatment of conditions in which other nonsteroidal anti-inflammatory drugs do not show sufficient efficacy.

Phenylbutazone is given as oral, rectal, intramuscular or topical formulation (up to 600 mg/day initial dose, up to 400 mg/day maintenance dose).

The peak plasma concentration is reached 2 h after oral administration. The degree of binding of phenylbutazone to plasma proteins is 98%. The long elimination half-life of phenylbutazone (mean ~70 h) exhibits large interindividual and intraindividual variation. It is metabolized in the liver by oxidation and glucuronidation and excreted in the urine and to a lower degree (~25%) in the faeces (Aarbakke, 1978). Oxyphenbutazone is an active metabolite of phenylbutazone. The metabolic pathway of phenyl-butazone is shown in Scheme 72.

Trade name: Butazolidin (F, Ger, UK, USA), Ambene (Ger)

Phenylbutazone is also used in veterinarian medicine in many species including camels (Wasfi et al., 1997).

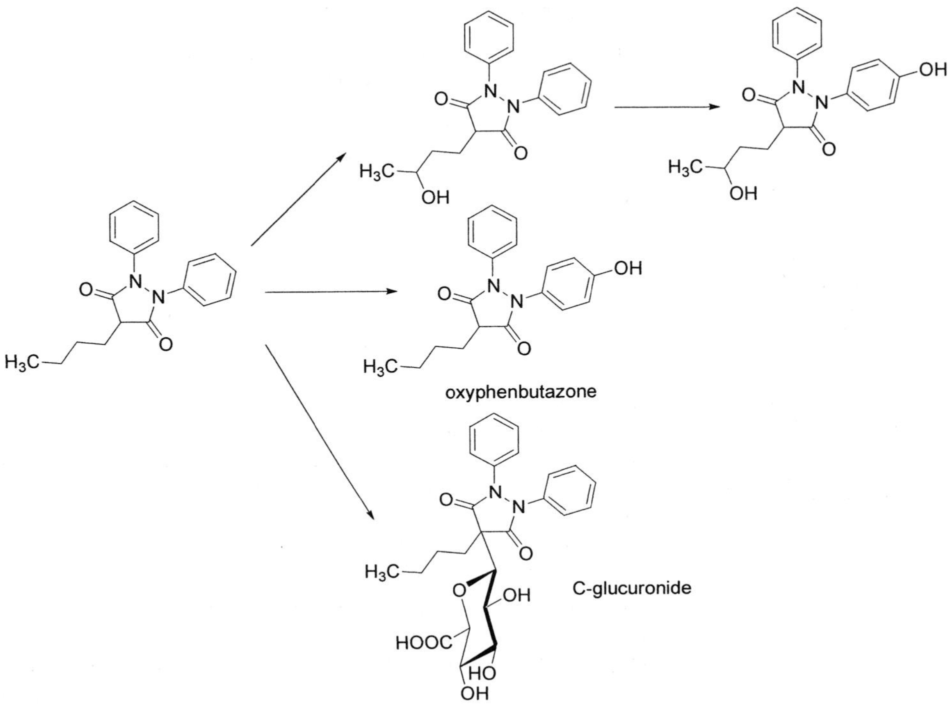

Scheme 72: Metabolic pathway of phenylbutazone.

Piroxicam

Synthesis (Lombardino (Pfizer), 1971; 1984); Lombardino et al., 1973; Hromatka et al. (Hoffmann-La Roche), 1975; Wiseman et al., 1976; Castaner and Arrigoni-Martelli, 1977b; Guzmann, 1986):

An improved procedure using 2-methoxyethyl 2-chloroacetate in place of methyl 2-chloroacetate for the alkylation of sodium saccharin has been described. The resulting 2-methoxyethyl saccharin-2-acetate is treated with sodium 2-methoxyethoxide in dimethyl sulfoxide, then acidified to give 2-methoxyethyl 4-hydroxy-2*H*-1,2-benzothiazine-3-carboxylate 1,1-dioxide, which is *N*-alkylated with methyl iodide in acetone-aqueous sodium hydroxide. The resulting 2-methoxyethyl 4-hydroxy-2-methyl-2*H*-1,2-benzothiazine-3-carboxylate 1,1-dioxide is heated with 2-aminopyridine in xylene to give piroxicam.

Piroxicam

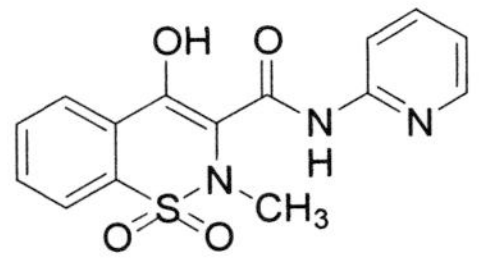

[*36322-90-4*], 4-Hydroxy-2-methyl-1,1-dioxo-1,2-dihydro-1λ^6-benzo[*e*][1,2] thiazine-3-carboxylic acid pyridin-2-ylamide, 4-hydroxy-2-methyl-*N*-2-pyridinyl-2*H*-1,2-benzothiazine-3-carboxamide-1,1-dioxide, $C_{15}H_{13}N_3O_4S$, M_r 331.35, *mp* 198-200 °C.

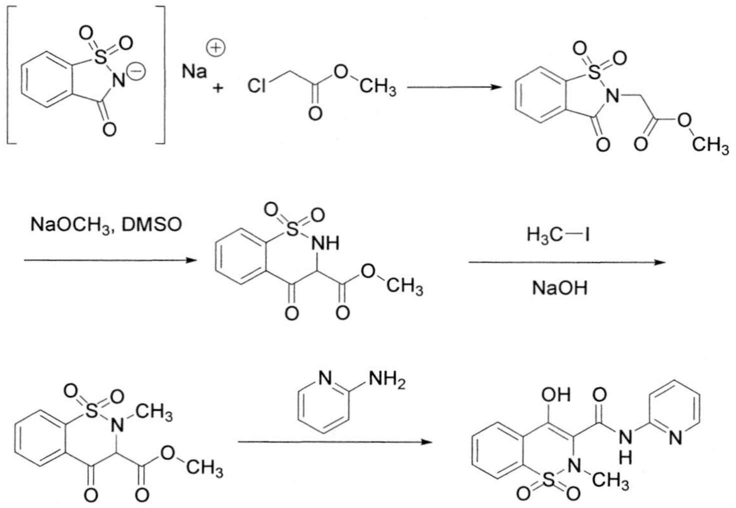

Scheme 73: Synthesis of piroxicam.

With a pK$_A$ of 5.5 piroxicam is a weak acidic enol. The resonance stabilization of the anionic form is shown below.

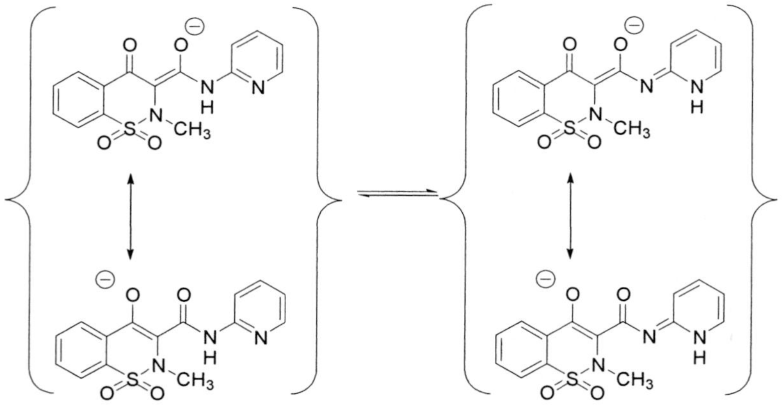

Scheme 74: Resonance stabilization of the anionic form of piroxicam.

Clinical use: Piroxicam (Brogden et al., 1981b) is a nonsteroidal anti-inflammatory drug used for the treatment of mild to moderate acute and chronic pain and inflammation including musculoskeletal, soft tissue and joint disorders such as ankylosing spondylitis, chronic polyarthritis and gout (Brogden et al., 1984).

Piroxicam shows up to 12-fold selectivity for COX-1 compared to COX-2 in several assay systems. The variations of the results in whole blood assays from different laboratories (see also Warner et al., 1999; ratio COX-1/COX-2: 0.3 and Young et al., 1996; ratio COX-1/COX-2: 0.4) stress the importance of careful interpretation of COX selectivity ratios.

Piroxicam is given by oral, rectal, intramuscular or topical administration (10-30 mg/day, maximal initial dose 40 mg/day) as the free base, as a complex with beta-cyclodextrin and as the cinnamate or pivalate.

After oral administration, piroxicam reaches peak plasma concentration after 3 to 5 h, shows 99% binding to plasma protein and a long half-life of about 50 h. Piroxicam is metabolized in the liver by hydroxylation and glucuronidation and excreted mainly in the urine.

The metabolic pathway of piroxicam is shown in Scheme 75.

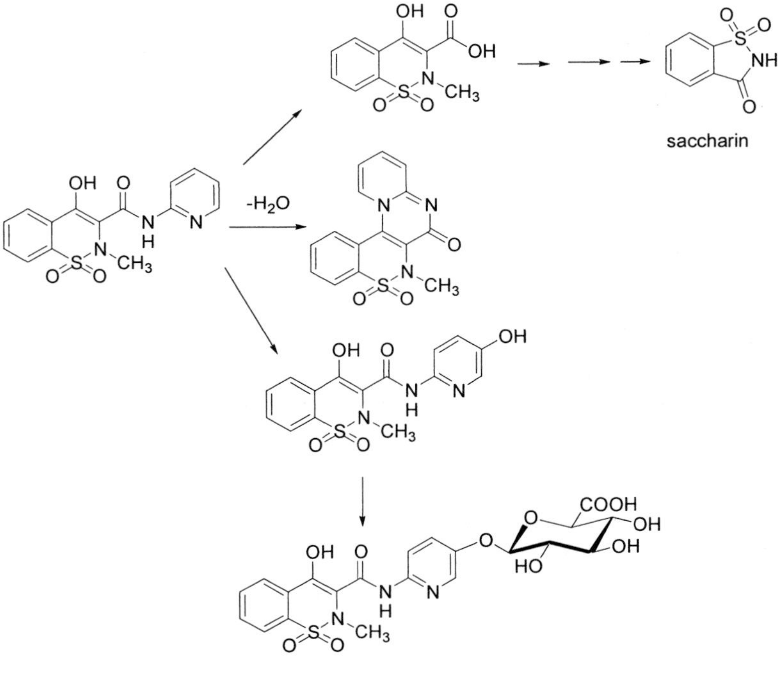

COX selectivity

IC_{50} [μM]	COX-1	COX-2	ratio
purified enzyme (1)	13	>100	<0.1
cell culture (2)	0.45	0.77	0.6
whole blood (3)	2.9	0.93	3
whole blood (4)	0.76	8.9	0.08

(1) Gierse et al. (1995)

(2) Berg et al. (1997)

(3) Patrignani et al. (1997)

(4) Brideau et al. (1996)

Scheme 75: Metabolic pathway of piroxicam.

: Feldéne (F),
(Ger), Feldene (UK,
US)

Beside COX inhibition, piroxicam weakly inhibits the accumulation of nitric oxide generated by inducible nitric oxide synthase (iNOS, IC_{50} 240 μM) and LPS-induced interleukin-6 formation (IC_{50} 470 μM; Berg et al., 1999). These activities were measured not in whole blood, but in LPS-stimulated cell lines and occur only at high concentrations. Another COX-independent activity of piroxicam is a neuroprotective role against hypoxia and reperfusion by modulation of molecules from the intercellular signaling cascade (Vartiainen et al., 2001). Since all these activities are seen in the high concentration range, the anti-inflammatory potential of piroxicam, which is evident at a mean serum concentration (i.e. not the target compartment of local inflammation) of 16.6 μM after a standard dose of 20 mg/day (Cryer and Feldman, 1998), is questionable.

Propacetamol

Propacetamol

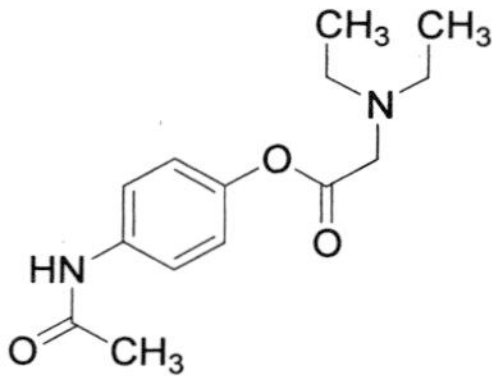

([*66532-85-2*], *N,N*-diethylglycine-4-(acetylamino)phenyl-ester, $C_{14}H_{20}N_2O_3$, M_r 264.33). It is used as hydrochloride ([*66532-86-3*] , $C_{14}H_{20}N_2O_3$ HCl, M_r 300.79)

Synthesis (Dittert et al., 1968; Kleemann et al., 1999): 4-Hydroxyacetaniline is coupled with chloroacetylchloride to yield *p*-acetamidophenyl-chloroacetate, which is finally reacted with diethylamine to produce propacetamol.

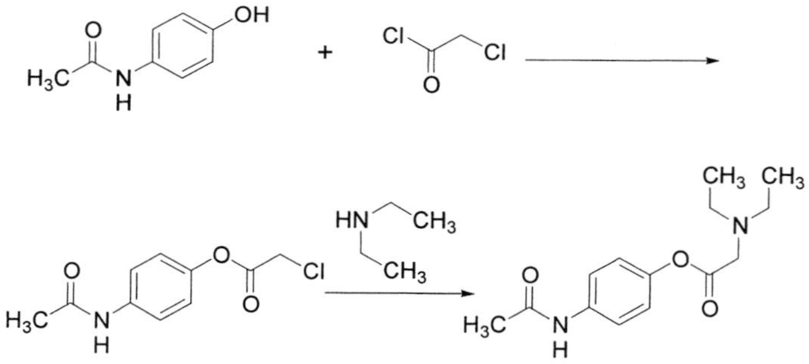

Scheme 76: Synthesis of propacetamol.

Trade name: Pro-Dafalgan (Belg, Fr, Switz), Pro-Efferalgan (Italy)

Propacetamol is a soluble glycine prodrug derivative of paracetamol. It is administered by the intramuscular or intravenous route and is rapidly metabolized to free paracetamol (Depre et al., 1992).

Propacetamol is given in doses of 1 to 2 g per day.

Propyphenazone

Synthesis (Hoffmann-La Roche, 1931; Volk (Riedel-de Haen), 1954; Kleemann et al., 1999):

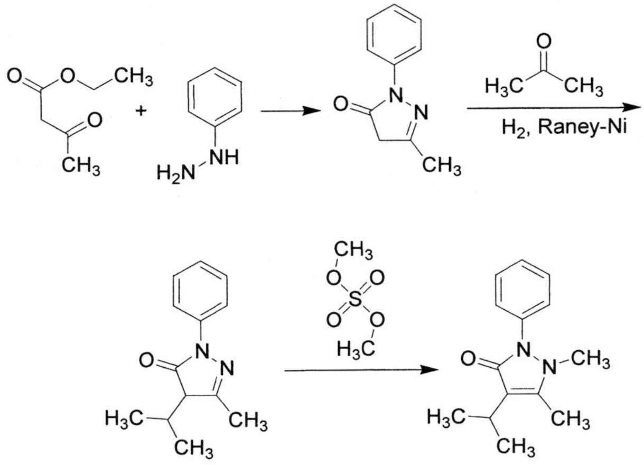

Propyphenazone

Scheme 77: Synthesis of propyphenazone.

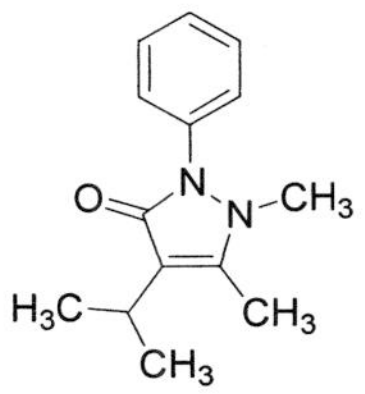

[479-92-5], 1,2-Dihydro-1,5-dimethyl-4-(1-methylethyl)-2-phenyl-3*H*-pyrazol-3-one, $C_{14}H_{18}N_2O_3$, M_r 230.31, *mp* 103 °C

Clinical use: Propyphenazone is a derivative of phenazone and has similar analgesic and antipyretic properties.

Propyphenazone is also used in multi-ingredient preparations.

Trade name: Demex (Ger)

Rofecoxib

Synthesis: The condensation of phenylacetic acid with ethyl bromoacetate by means of triethylamine in THF yields 2-(phenylacetoxy)acetic ethyl ester, which is cyclized to the hydroxyfuranone by means of potassium *tert*-butoxide in *tert*-butanol. The reaction with triflic anhydride and diisopropylethylamine in CH_2Cl_2 affords the corresponding triflate, which by reaction with LiBr in hot acetone yields the bromofuranone. Condensation with 4-(methylsulfanyl)phenylboronic acid by means of Na_2CO_3 and $Pd[(C_6H_5)_3P]_4$ in hot toluene gives 4-[4-(methylsulfanyl)-phenyl]-3-phenylfuran-2(5*H*)-one, which is finally oxidized with $2KHSO_5 \cdot KHSO_4 \cdot K_2SO_4$ (oxone) (Drugs Fut., 1998).

Rofecoxib

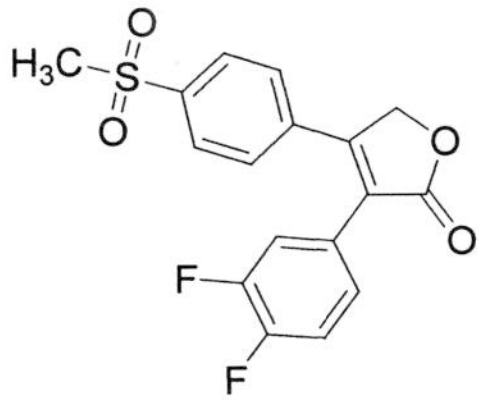

[162011-90-7], 4-[4-(Methylsulfonyl)phenyl]-3-phenylfuran-2(5*H*)-one, $C_{17}H_{14}O_4S$, M_r 314.36

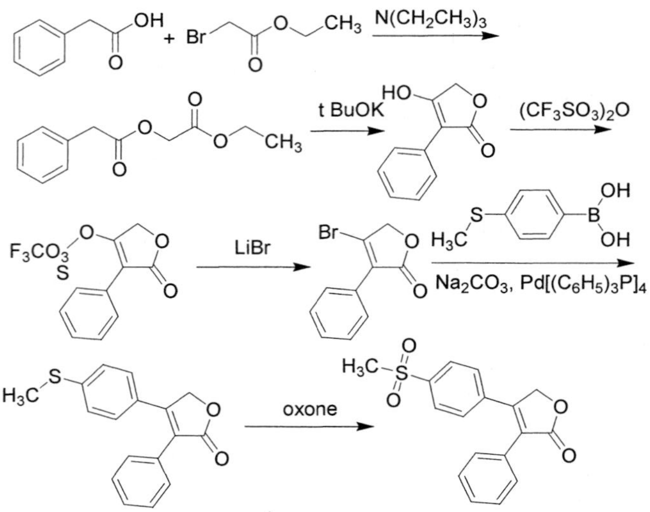

Christoph and Buschmann

Scheme 78: Synthesis of rofecoxib.

The synthesis of rofecoxib can be achieved by several different routes (Drugs Fut., 1998). A highly efficient synthesis for rofecoxib was recently described (Thérien et al., 2001). As illustrated in Scheme 79, acetophenon (**i**) is prepared according to the literature, by Friedel-Crafts acylation with thioanisole. Oxidation with MMPP (magnesium monoperoxyphthalate hexahydrate) affords the sulfone (**ii**), which is reacted with bromine in chloroform in the presence of a trace amount of AlCl₃, to give (**iii**). Bromoketone (**iii**) is than coupled and cyclized in a second step, one-pot procedure with phenylacetic acid. Firstly, the mixture of bromoacetophenone (**iii**) and phenylacetic acid in acetonitrile is treated with triethylamine at room temperature, to provide the ester intermediate, subsequent cooling and addition of DBU effected the cyclization to provide rofecoxib as the final product.

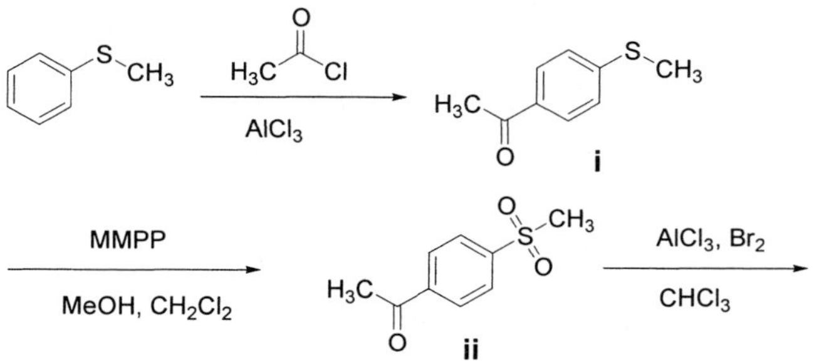

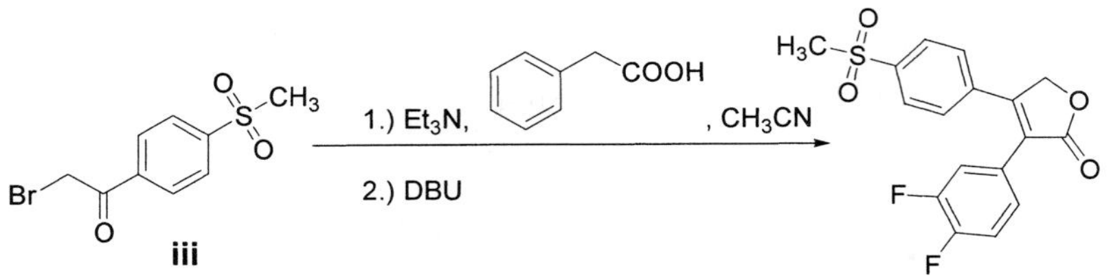

Scheme 79: Alternative synthesis of rofecoxib.

Clinical use: Rofecoxib (Sorbera et al., 1998) is a second generation COX-2 selective inhibitor. It was the second COX-2 selective drug to reach the market in 1999. Rofecoxib is used for the treatment of rheumatoid arthritis, osteoarthritis and pain.

The selectivity for COX-2 compared to COX-1 is more than 800-fold in cellular assays and more than 10-fold in whole blood assays.

Rofecoxib is used for a once-daily treatment of rheumatoid arthritis, osteoarthritis (12.5-25 mg/day) and pain (50 mg/day).

Rofecoxib reaches peak plasma concentrations between 2 to 9 h after oral administration. It is bound ~87% to plasma protein and has an elimination half-life of about 17 h. Its main metabolites in the liver are the *cis*-dihydro and *trans*-dihydro derivatives which are excreted mainly in the urine (72%) with some unchanged drug excreted in the faeces (14%).

Rofecoxib shows significantly less gastrointestinal toxicity compared to ibuprofen in studies with osteoarthritis patients (Laine et al., 1999) and compared to naproxen in patients with rheumatoid arthritis (Bombardier et al., 2000).

COX selectivity

IC50 [µM]	COX-1	COX-2	ratio
recomb. enzyme (1)	26	0.34	76
cell culture (1)	>15	0.018	>833
whole blood (2)	63	0.84	75

(1) Chan et al. (1999)

(2) Warner et al. (1999)

Trade name: Vioxx (EC, US)

Salicylamide

Synthesis (Hoffenberg und Hauser, 1955; Kleemann et al., 1999):

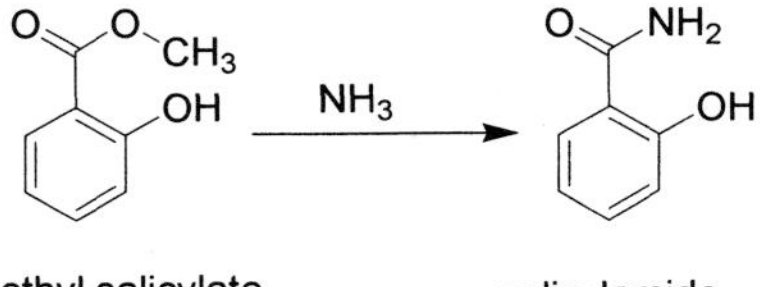

methyl salicylate   salicylamide

Scheme 80: Synthesis of salicylamide.

Salicylamide

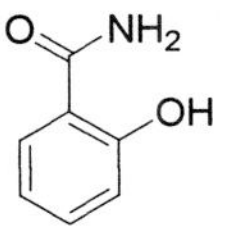

[*65-45-2*], 2-Hydroxy-benzamide, $C_7H_7NO_2$, M_r 137.14, *mp* 140 °C

Clinical use: Salicylamide has analgesic and antipyretic effects and is used in multidrug combinations for the treatment of a variety of mild pain conditions including musculoskeletal, soft tissue and joint disorders.

Trade name: Percutalgine (F), Glutisal (Ger), Intralgin (UK), Anabar (US)

Salicylamide is given orally in daily doses of 1 to 2.5 g or applied topically in concentrations of about 5%. It is metabolized to inactive metabolites during absorption or in the liver.

Sulindac

Sulindac

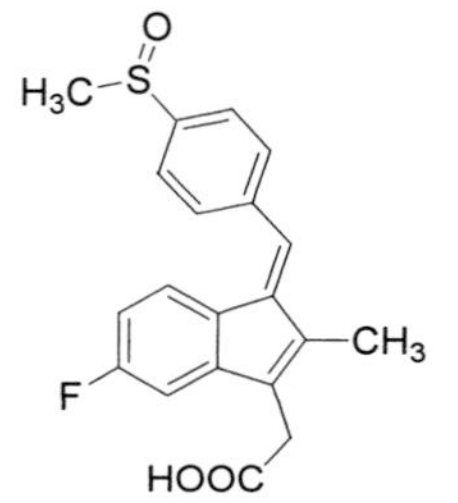

[*38194-50-2*], (*Z*)-[6-Fluoro-3-(4-methanesulfinyl-benzylidene)-2-methyl-3*H*-inden-1-yl]-acetic acid, $C_{20}H_{17}FO_3S$, 356.41, *mp* 182-185 °C (decomp.)

Synthesis (Tull et al. (Merck & Co.), 1975; 1976) Friedel-Crafts reaction of fluorobenzene and α-bromoisobutyryl bromide gives 5-fluoro-2-methylindan-1-one, which is treated with 4-methylthiobenzylmagnesium chloride to yield 5-fluoro-2-methyl-1-(4-methylthiobenzyl)indene. Condensation with glyoxylic acid in the presence of *N*-benzyltrimethyl ammonium hydroxide (Triton B) gives 3-carboxy methylene-5-fluoro-2-methyl-1-(4-methylthio-ben-zyl) indene, which is isomerized in acid to 5-fluoro-2-methyl-1-(4-methylthiobenzylidene)indene-3-acetic acid. Oxidation with hydrogen peroxide affords sulindac.

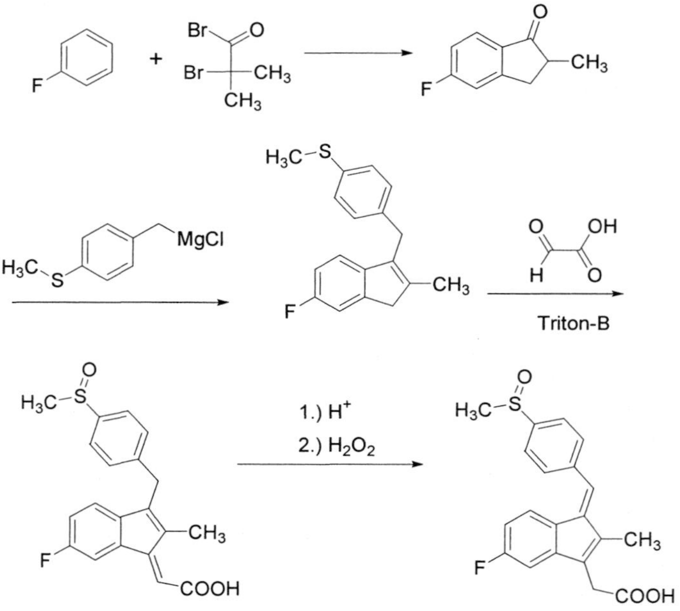

Scheme 81: Synthesis of sulindac.

Another synthesis starting from *p*-fluorobenzaldehyde is shown:

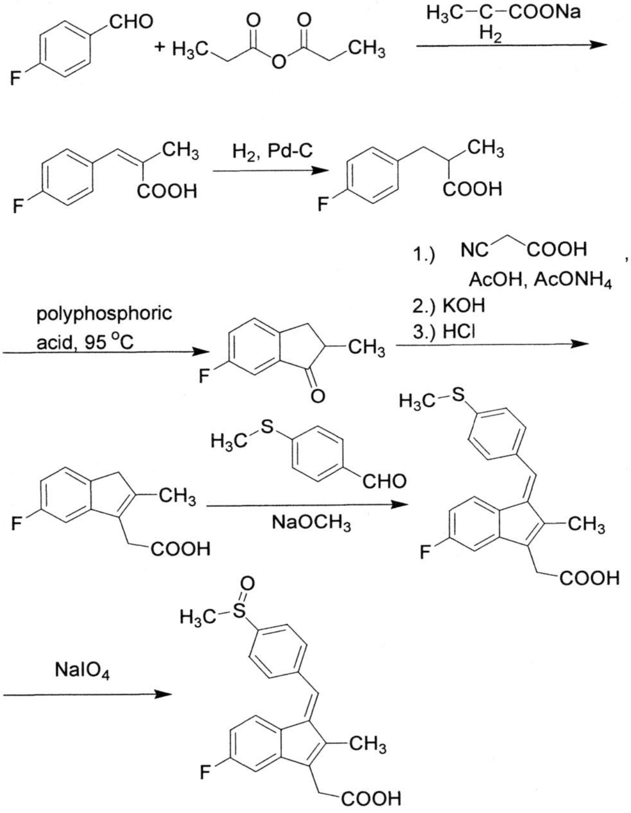

Scheme 82: Synthesis of sulindac.

Clinical use: Sulindac (Brogden, 1978a) is a nonsteroidal anti-inflammatory drug used in the treatment of mild to moderate pain including musculoskeletal and joint disorders such as rheumatoid arthritis, osteoarthritis and gout.

Sulindac shows no relevant inhibition of cyclooxygenase (Warner et al., 1999), whereas the active metabolite sulindac sulfide shows inhibition of both isoenzymes with a preference for COX-1 in a whole blood assay (see also Brideau et al., 1996; ratio COX-1/COX-2 = 0.1). Sulindac is one of the NSAIDs, extensively studied in cancer reseach (Haanen, 2001). The metabolite sulindac sulfone induces apoptosis in tumor cells.

Sulindac is absorbed from the gastrointestinal tract and reversibly metabolised to sulindac sulfide and irreversibly metabolised to sulindac sulfone. Peak plasma

COX selectivity of the active metabolite sulindac sulfide

IC50 [µM]	COX-1	COX-2	ratio
cell culture (1)	0.028	0.004	7
whole blood (2)	1.9	55	0.03

(1) Riendeau et al. (1997)

(2) Warner et al. (1999)

concentrations of sulindac sulfone are reached within 2 h. Sulindac as well as the sulfone and sulfide metabolites show extensive plasma protein binding. The plasma elimination half-life of sulindac and sulindac sulfide is 7 to 8 h and 16 to 18 h, respectively. Sulindac and its sulfone metabolite as well as the respective glucuronates are excreted mainly in the urine, whereas only a small amount of sulindac sulphide is excreted in the urine.

Trade name: Arthrocine (F), Clinoril (UK, US)

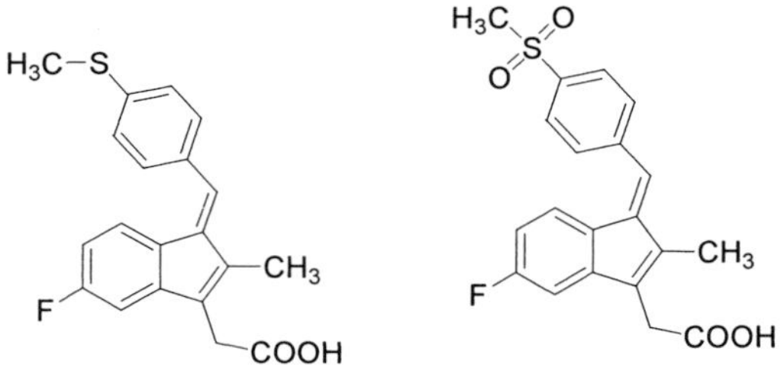

Structures of the metabolites sulindac sulfide and sulindac sulfone

Figure 23: Metabolites of sulindac.

The main side effects are gastro-intestinal disturbances and renal stones (Whelton et al., 1983).

Tenoxicam

Tenoxicam

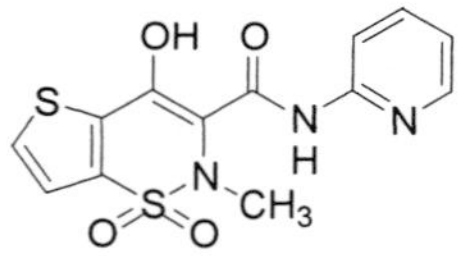

[59804-37-4], 4-Hydroxy-2-methyl-1,1-dioxo-1,2-dihydro-1λ^6thieno[2,3-e][1,2]thiazine-3-carboxylic acid pyridin-2-ylamide, 4-hydroxy-2-methyl-N-2-pyridinyl-2H-thieno[2,3-e]-thiazine-3-carboxamide-1,1-dioxide, $C_{13}H_{11}N_3O_4S_2$, M_r 337.38, mp 209-213 °C (decomp.)

Synthesis: The reaction of methyl 3-hydroxythiophen-2-carboxylate with PCl_5 in refluxing CCl_4 gives 3-chlorothiophene-2-carboxylic acid, which by treatment with $NaHSO_3$ and Cu in basic water at 143 °C in a pressure vessel is converted into 3-sulfothiophene-2-carboxylic acid. The first esterification with refluxing methanol affords methyl-3-sulfothiophene-2-carboxylate, which by reaction with refluxing $SOCl_2$ yields methyl-3-chlorosulfonyl thiophene-2-carboxylate. The following condensation with sarcosine ethyl ester in hot $CHCl_3$ gives 3-(N-ethoxycarbonylmethyl-N-methylsulfamoyl)thiophene-2-carboxylate, which is cylized by treatment with sodium methoxide in refluxing methanol affording 3-ethoxycarbonyl-4-hydroxy-2-methyl-2H-thieno-[2,3-e]-1,2-thiazine 1,1-dioxide. Finally this compound is condensed with 2-aminopyridine in refluxing toluene (Hromatka et al. (Hoffmann-La Roche), 1975; Arrigoni-Martelli, 1982; Kleemann et al., 1999).

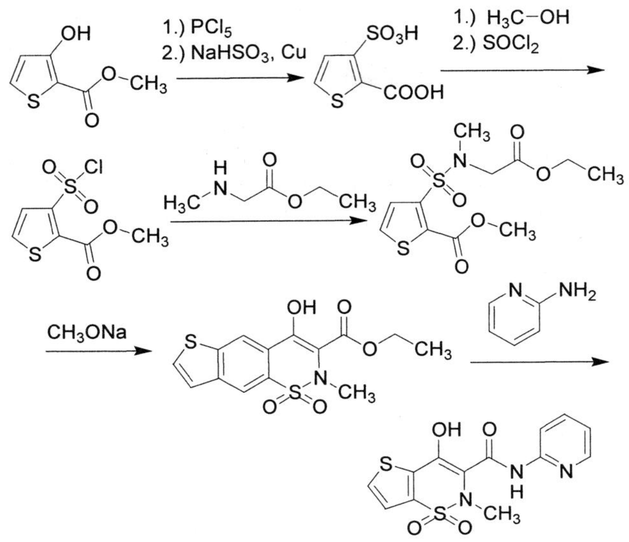

Scheme 83: Synthesis of tenoxicam.

Clinical use: Tenoxicam (Todd and Clissold, 1991) is a nonsteroidal anti-inflammatory drug used for the treatment of mild to moderate pain states in musculoskeletal, soft tissue and joint disorders such as rheumatoid arthritis, osteoarthritis and gout.

Tenoxicam shows a balanced inhibition of both, COX-1 and COX-2.

Tenoxicam is given by oral, rectal or intramuscular routes (20 mg/day, maximal dose 40 mg/day).

Peak plasma concentration appears within 1 to 6 h depending on fasted or fed status. There is 99% binding of tenoxicam to plasma proteins and a long plasma elimination half-life of 49 to 81 h. Tenoxicam is eliminated by liver metabolism. The main metabolites are 5'-hydroxy-tenoxicam and the 6-O-glucuronidate which are excreted in urine and bile, respectively (Nilsen, 1994). The hydroxylated metabolites of tenoxicam are shown in Scheme 84:

COX selectivity

IC50 [µM]	COX-1	COX-2	ratio
cell culture (1)	0.32	0.13	2.5
whole blood (2)	2.3	14.2	0.2

(1) Berg et al. (1999)

(2) Brideau et al. (1996)

Trade name: Tilcotil (Aust, Austral, Belg, F, Ger, Ital, Neth, Spain), Mobiflex (Canad, Irl, UK)

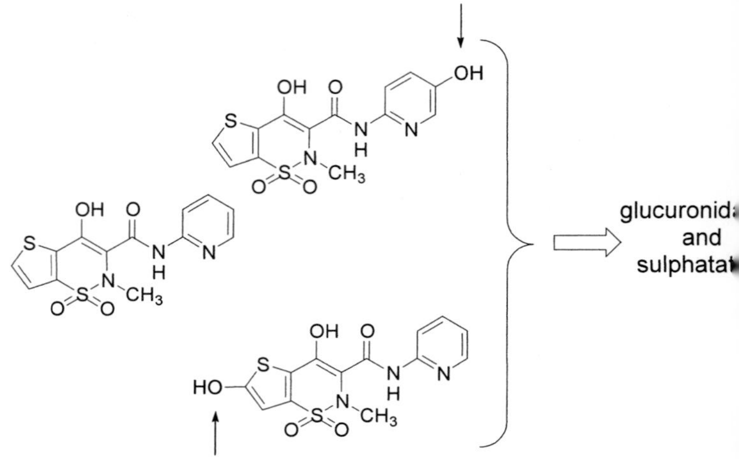

Scheme 84: Hydroxylated metabolites of tenoxicam.

Tiaprofenic Acid

Tiaprofenic Acid

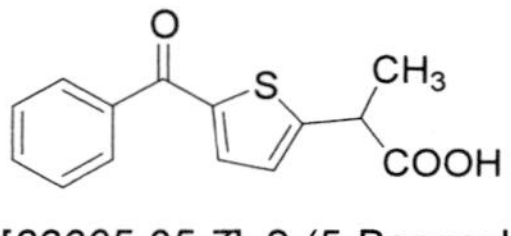

[*33005-95-7*], 2-(5-Benzoyl-
thiophen-2-yl)-propionic
acid, $C_{14}H_{12}O_3S$, M_r 260.31,
mp 96 °C

Synthesis (Clemence (Roussel-Uclaf), 1970; Kleemann et al., 1999):

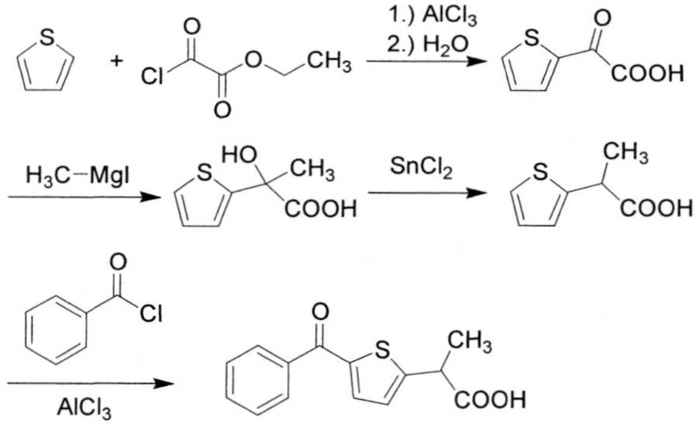

Scheme 85: Synthesis of tiaprofenic acid.

Clinical use: Tiaprofenic acid (Plosker and Wagstaff, 1995) is a nonsteroidal anti-inflammatory drug used for the treatment of mild to moderate pain states in musculoskeletal, soft tissue and joint disorders as well as for postoperative pain.

Tiaprofenic acid is a racemate and given as oral or rectal preparations (600 mg/day) and as an intramuscular injection of the trometamol salt.

After oral administration, tiaprofenic acid reaches peak plasma concentrations after 1.5 h. Tiaprofenic acid binds efficiently to plasma proteins (~98%) and has a short elimination half-life of about 2 h. Tiaprofenic acid and its metabolites are excreted mainly in urine (Davies, 1996).

The main side-effects are urinary tract symptoms such as cystitis and bladder irritation (Mayall et al., 1994).

Trade name: Surgam (Austr, Belg, F, Ger, Irl, Neth, UK, Switz), Suralgan (Ital), Surgamic (Spain)

Tolmetin

Synthesis (Carson et al., 1971; Carson (McNeil), 1973; Kleemann et al., 1999):

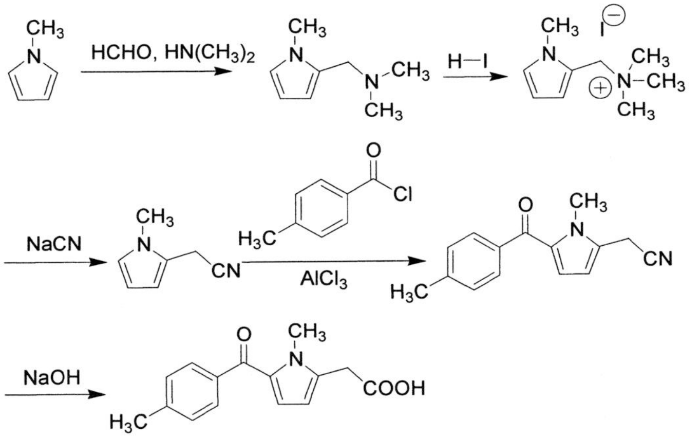

Tolmetin

Scheme 86: Synthesis of tolmetin.

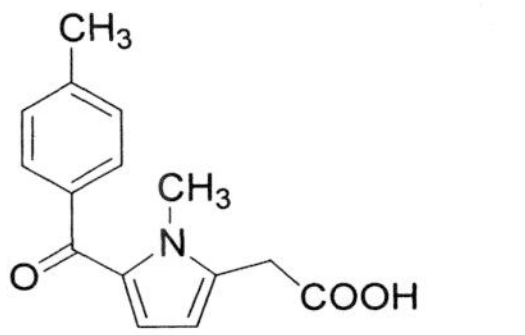

[*26171-23-3*], [1-Methyl-5-(4-methyl-benzoyl)-1*H*-pyrrol-2-yl-acetic acid, $C_{15}H_{15}NO_3$, M_r 257.28, *mp* 155-157 °C; sodium salt [35711-34-3], $C_{15}H_{14}NNaO_3$, M_r 279.27; sodium salt dihydrate [64490-92-2], $C_{15}H_{14}NNaO_3 \cdot 2\ H_2O$, M_r 315.30

Clinical use: Tolmetin (Brogden et al., 1978b) is a nonsteroidal anti-inflammatory drug used for the treatment of mild to moderate pain states in musculoskeletal, soft tissue and joint disorders such as rheumatoid arthritis, osteoarthritis and gout as well as juvenile rheumatoid arthritis.

Tolmetin inhibits both isoforms of cyclooxygenase with a preference for COX-1 in whole blood assays (see also COX-1/COX-2 ratios of 0.2, 0.4 and 0.5 in Brideau et al., 1996; Young et al., 1996 and Cryer and Feldman, 1998, respectively).

COX selectivity

IC_{50} [µM]	COX-1	COX-2	ratio
whole blood	0.35	0.82	0.4

Warner et al. (1999)

Tolmetin is given as oral, rectal (600-1800 mg/day) or topical preparation (5% topical gel).

The peak plasma concentrations are reached within 30 to 60 min after oral administration. Tolmetin shows a high plasma protein binding of 99% and a biphasic plasma half-life of 1 to 2 and 5 h, respectively. Tolmetin and its metabolites and conjugates are excreted in the urine (Grindel, 1981).

Trade name: Tolectin (Austria, Switz., UK, US)

Valdecoxib

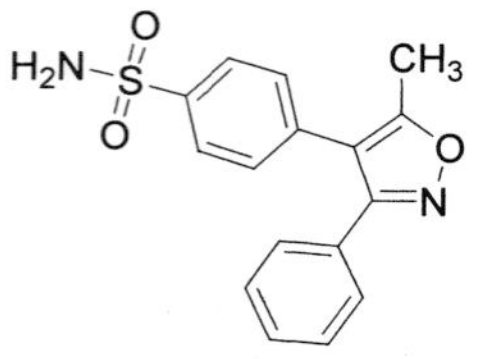

Valdecoxib

[*181695-72-7*], 4-(5-Methyl-
3-phenylisoxazol-4-yl)ben-
zenesulfonamide
$C_{16}H_{14}N_2O_3S$, 314.366; mp
172-173 °C

COX selectivity

IC50 [µM]	COX-1	COX-2	ratio
recomb. enzyme (1)	140	0.005	28000
	1120 (2)	0.18 (2)	6222 (2)
whole blood (1)	25.4	0.89	28.5
	>50 (2)	0.329 (2)	>152 (2)

Talley et al. (2000a)

activity of the active
metabolite of valdecoxib

Synthesis: Deoxybenzoin is converted to the corresponding oxime by treatment with hydroxylamine under basic conditions with sodium acetate in aqueous ethanol or in toluene in the presence of potassium hydroxide in absolute ethanol. Treatment of the oxime under nitrogen with two equivalents of butyllithium in tetrahydrofurane is followed by cyclization in ethyl acetate or acetic anhydride to the isoxazoline derivative. Finally, treatment of the isoxazoline with cold chlorosulfonic acid followed by reaction of the intermediate with aqueous ammonia affords the desired product. (Talley, 2000a; Sorbera, 2001b).

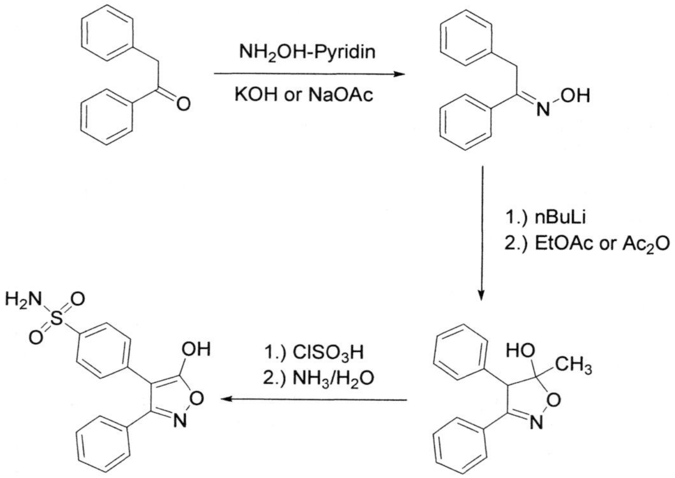

Scheme 87: Synthesis of valdecoxib.

Clinical use: Valdecoxib (Sorbera et al., 2001b) is a third generation COX-2 inhibitor in clinical development. It shows about 30-fold selectivity for COX-2 in a whole blood assay (see also Riendeau et al., 2001; COX-1/COX-2 = 30). Valdecoxib shows efficacy in a variety of animal models of inflammation (Talley et al., 2000a).

Valdecoxib is converted in rodents and dogs, and in a low abundance in humans, by hydroxylation of the methyl group to an active metabolite (4-(5-Hydroxymethyl-3-phenyl-isoxazol-4-yl)-benzenesulfonamide) (Talley et al., 2000a). Pharmacological evaluation of the independently synthesized metabolite showed that it possessed oral activity in the acute anti-inflammatory assay (carrageenan paw edema, ED_{50}=1.06 mg/kg). Chronic inflammatory activity was achieved with the metabolite in the rat adjuvant arthritis model (ED_{50}=1.49 mg/kg/day). *In vitro* the metabolie showed an IC_{50} of 1120 μM against COX-1 and an IC_{50} of 0.18 μM against COX-2.

Structure of the active metabolite of valdecoxib

Trade name: Bextra (US)

Valdecoxib is a substrate for cytochrome P450 3A4 and 2C9 (Cheer and Goa, 2001; Gotta, 2001).

References

Aarbakke, J.: *Clinical pharmacokinetics of phenylbutazone*, Clin. Pharmacokinet. **1978**, *3*, 369-380.

Alvarez, F. (Syntex): *Di-(6-methoxy-2-naphtyl)zinc and 6-methoxy-2-naphtylzinc halide*, US 3 663 584, **1972**.

Ameer, B. and Greenblatt D.J.: *Acetaminophen*, Ann. Intern. Med. **1977**, *87*, 202-209.

Arrigoni-Martelli, E., Drugs of the Future **1978a**, *3*, 28-33.

Arrigoni-Martelli, E., Drugs of the Future **1978b**, *3*, 307-310.

Arrigoni-Martelli, E., Drugs of the Future **1978c**, *3*, 539-542.

Arrigoni-Martelli, E., Drugs of the Future **1982**, *7*, 493-494.

Arrigoni-Martelli, E., Drugs of the Future **1983**, *8*, 871-874.

Auclair, J., Georges, M., Grapton, X., Gryp, L., D'Hooghe, M., Meiser, R. G., Noto, R., Schmidtmayer, B.: *A double-blind controlled multicenter study of percutaneous niflumic acid gel and placebo in the treatment of achilles heel tendinitis*, Curr. Ther. Res. **1989**, *46*, 782-788.

Azab, A., Fraifeld, V., Kaplanski, J.: *Nimesulide prevents lipopolysaccharide-induced elevation in plasma tumor necrosis factor-alpha in rats,* Life Sci. **1998**, *63*, PL 323-327.

Balfour, J. A., and Buckley, M. M.: *Etodolac. A reappraisal of its pharmacology and therapeutic use in rheumatic diseases and pain states*, Drugs **1991**, *42*, 274-299.

Balfour, J. A., Fitton, A., Barradell, L. B.: *Lornoxicam. A review of its pharmacology and therapeutic potential in the management of painful and inflammatory conditions*, Drugs **1996**, *51*, 639-657.

Barnett, J. W., Dunn, D. J., Kertesz, D.J., Morgans, A. B.; Ramesha, C. S.; Sigal, C. E.; Sjogren, E. B., Smith, D. B.; Talamas, D. B.: *Pyrrole derivatives*, EP 714895 (**1996**).

Bayly, C.I., Black, W.C., Léger, S., Ouimet, N., Uuellet, M., Percivall, M.D.: *Structure-based design of COX-2 selectivity into flurbiprofen*, Bioorg. Med. Chem. Lett. **1999**, *9*, 307-312.

Bayly, C. I., Black, W. C., Ouimet, N., Percival, M. D., Léger, S., Ouellet, M.: *Biaryl-acetic acid derivatives and their use as COX-2 inhibitors* (Merck Frosst Canada Inc.), WO 9941224, **1999**.

v. Bebenburg, W., Steinmetz, G., Thiele, K.: *Substituted polyaminopyridines*, Chem.-Ztg. 1979, *103*, 387-399.

v. Bebenburg, W., Thiele, K., Engel, J., Sheldrick, W.S.: *Synthesis and molecular structure of the structurally novel analgesic Flupirtin*, Chem.-Ztg. **1981**, *105*, 217-219.

Bellamy, N.: *Etodolac in the management of pain: a clinical review of a multipurpose analgesic*, Inflammopharmacology **1997**, *5*, 139-152.

Berg, J., Christoph, T., Widerna, M., Bodenteich, A.: *Isoenzyme-specific cyclooxygenase inhibitors: a whole cell assay system using the human erythroleukemic cell line HEL and the human monocytic cell line Mono Mac 6*, J. Pharmacol. Toxicol. Methods **1997**, *37*, 179-186.

Berg, J., Fellier, H., Christoph, T., Grarup, J., Stimmeder, D.: *The analgesic NSAID lornoxicam inhibits cyclooxygenase (COX)-1/-2*, inducible *nitric oxide synthase (iNOS), and the formation of interleukin (IL)-6 in vitro*, Inflamm. Res. **1999**, *48*, 369-79.

Bianchi Porro, G., Caruso, I., Petrillo, M., Montrone, F., Ardizzone. S.: *A double-blind gastroscopic evaluation of the effects of etodolac and naproxen on the gastrointestinal mucosa of rheumatic patients*, J. Intern. Med. **1991**, *229*, 5-8.

Black, W. C., Bayly, C., Belly, M.; Chan, C. C., Charleson, S., Denis, D., Gauthier, J. Y., Gordon, R., Guay, D., Kargman, S., Lan, C.K., Leblanc, Y., Mancini, J., Quellet, M., Percival, D., Roy, P., Skorey, K., Tagari, P., Vickers, P., Wong, E., Xu, L.; Prasit, P., Bioorg. Med. Lett. **1996**, *6*, 725-730.

Boltze, K. H. and Kreisfeld, H.: [On the chemistry of etofenamate, a novel anti-inflammatory agent from the series of N-arylanthranilic acid derivatives (author's transl)], Arzneim.-Forsch./Drug Res. **1977**, *27(I)*, 1300-1312.

Bombardier, C., Laine, L., Reicin, A., Shapiro, D., Burgos-Vargas, R., Davis, B., Day, R., Ferraz, M. B., Hawkey, C. J., Hochberg, M. C., Kvien, T. K., Schnitzer, T. J.: *Comparison of upper gastrointestinal toxicity of rofecoxib and naproxen in patients with rheumatoid arthritis. VIGOR Study Group*, New Engl. J. Med. **2000**, *343*, 1520-1528.

Bonica, J. J.: *Biochemistry and Modulation of Nociception and Pain.* in: The Management of Pain, J.J. Bonica ed., 2nd Edition, **1990**, p.96 Lea & Febiger, USA.

Boskmühl, M. and Schwarz, A. (I.G. Farben): *Verfahren zur Darstellung von N-methylschwefligsauren Salzen sekundärer aromatisch-aliphatischer Amine*, DRP 476 663, **1922**.

Bottiger, L. E. and Westerholm, B.: *Drug-induced blood dyscrasias in Sweden*, Br. Med. J. **1973**, *3*, 339-343.

Brideau, C., Kargman, S., Liu, S., Dallob, A. L., Ehrich, E. W., Rodger, I. W., Chan, C. C.: *A human whole blood assay for clinical evaluation of biochemical efficacy of cyclooxygenase inhibitors*, Inflamm. Res. **1996**, *45*, 68-74.

Brochier, M. L.: *Evaluation of flurbiprofen for prevention of reinfarction and reocclusion after successful thrombolysis or angioplasty in acute myocardial infarction. The Flurbiprofen French Trial*, Eur. Heart J. **1993**, *14*, 951-957.

Brocks, D. R. and Jamali, F.: *Etodolac clinical pharmacokinetics*, Clin. Pharmacokinet. **1994**, *26*, 259-274.

Brogden, R. N., Pinder, R. M., Sawyer, P. R., Speight, T. M., Avery, G. S.: *Bufexamac: a review of its pharmacological properties and therapeutic efficacy in inflammatory dermatoses*, Drugs **1975**, *10*, 351-356.

Brogden, R. N., Pinder, R. M., Speight, T. M., Avery, G. S.: *Fenoprofen: a review of its pharmacological properties and therapeutic efficacy in rheumatic diseases*, Drugs **1977** *13*, 241-265.

Brogden, R. N., Heel, R. C., Speight, T. M., Avery, G. S.: *Sulindac: a review of its pharmacological properties and therapeutic efficacy in rheumatic diseases*, Drugs **1978a**, *16*, 197-114.

Brogden, R. N., Heel, R. C., Speight, T. M., Avery, G. S.: *Tolmetin: a review of its pharmacological properties and therapeutic efficacy in rheumatic diseases*, Drugs **1978b**, *15*, 429-450.

Brogden, R. N., Heel, R. C., Pakes, G. E., Speight, T. M., Avery, G. S.: *Diflunisal: a review of its pharmacological properties and therapeutic use in pain and musculoskeletal strains and sprains and pain in osteoarthritis*, Drugs **1980**, *19*, 84-106.

Brogden, R. N., Heel, R. C., Speight, T.M., Avery, G.S.: *Piroxicam: a review of its pharmacological properties and therapeutic efficacy*, Drugs **1981b**, *22*, 165-187.

Brogden, R. N., Heel, R. C., Speight, T. M., Avery, G. S.: *Fenbufen: a review of its pharmacological properties and therapeutic use* in *rheumatic diseases and acute pain.* Drugs **1981a** *21*, 1-22.

Brogden, R. N., Heel, R. C., Speight, T.M., Avery, G. S.; *Piroxicam. A reappraisal of its pharmacology and therapeutic efficacy*, Drugs **1984**, *28*, 292-323.

Brogden, R. N.: *Pyrazolone Derivatives*, Drugs **1986**, *32*, 60-70.

Brooks, C. D. W., Kolasa, T., Lee, W., Stewart, A. O.: *Oxime derivatives of indoles and indenres as inhibitor compounds of prostaglandin biosynthesis* (Abbott Laboratories), US 5750558, **1998**.

Brooks, C. D. W., Craig, R. A., Kolasa, T., Lee, W., Stewart, A. O.: *Oxime derivatives of fenamates as inhibitors of prostaglandin biosynthesis* (Abbott Laboratories) US 5840758, **1998**.

Brooks, C. D. W., Craig, R. A., Kolasa, T., Stewart, A. O.: *Iminoxy derivatives of fenamates as inhibitors of prostaglandin biosynthesis* (Abbott Laboratories) US 5863946, **1999**.

Brown, K. (John Wyeth and Brothers, ltd): *Oxazoles*, US 3578671 (**1971**).

Büchi, J., Ammann, J., Lieberherr, R., Eichenberger, E.: *New 3,5-dioxopyrazolidines*, Helv. Chim. Acta **1953**, *36*, 75-85.

Buckley, M. M. and Brogden, R. N.: *Ketorolac. A review of its pharmacodynamic and pharmacokinetic properties, and therapeutic potential*, Drugs **1990**, *39*, 186-109.

Busson, M.: *Update on ibuprofen: review article*, J. Int. Med. Res. **1986**, *14*, 53-62.

Buu-Hoi, N. P., Lambelin, G., Lepoivre, C., Gillet, C., Gautier, M., Thiriaux, J.: *[A new anti-inflammatory agent of non-steroid structure: p-butoxyphenylacethydroxamic acid]*, Hebd. Seances Acad. Sci. **1965**, *261*, 2259-2262.

Campos, C., de Gregorio, R., Garcia-Nieto, R., Gago, F., Ortiz, P., Alemany, S.: *Regulation of cyclooxygenase activity by metamizol*, Eur. J. Pharmacol. **1999**, *378*, 339-347.

Carson, J. R., McKinstry, D. N., Wong, S.: 5-Benzoyl-1-methylpyrrole-2-acetic acids as antiinflammatory agents, J. Med. Chem. **1971**, *14*, 646-647.

Carson, J. R. (McNeil): *Aroyl-substituted pyrroles*, US 3 752 826, **1973**; GB 1 428 272, **1973**.

Castaner, L., Arrigoni-Martelli, E., Drugs of the Future **1977a**, *2*, 21-23.

Castaner, L., Arrigoni-Martelli, E., Drugs of the Future **1977b**, *2*, 124-127.

Chan, C. C., Boyce, S., Brideau, C., Charleson, S., Cromlish, W., Ethier, D., Evans, J., Ford-Hutchinson, A. W., Forrest, M. J., Gauthier, J. Y., Gordon, R., Gresser, M., Guay, J., Kargman, S., Kennedy, B., Leblanc, Y., Leger, S., Mancini, J., O'Neill, G.P., Ouellet, M., Patrick, D., Percival, M. D., Perrier, H., Prasit, P., Rodger, I., Tagari, P., Therien, M., Vickers, P., Visco, P., Wang, J., Webb, J., Wong, E., Xu, L.-J., Young, R. N., Zamboni, R., Riendeau, D.: *Rofecoxib [Vioxx, MK-0966; 4-(4'-methylsulfonylphenyl)-3-phenyl-2-(5H)-furanone]: a potent and orally active cyclooxygenase-2 inhibitor. Pharmacological and biochemical profiles*, J. Pharmacol. Exp. Ther. **1999**, *290*, 551-560.

Chauret, N., Yergey, J. A., Brideau, C., Friesen, R. W., Mancini, J., Riendeau, D., Silva, J., Styhler, A., Trimble, L. A., Nicoll-Griffith, D. A.: *In vitro metabolism considerations, including activity testing of metabolites, in the discovery and selection of the COX-2 inhibitor etoricoxib (MK-0663)*, Bioorg. Med. Chem. Lett. **2001**, *11*, 1059-1062.

Cheer, S. M., Goa, K. L.: *Parecoxib (parecoxib sodium)*, Drugs **2001**, *61*, 1133-1141; discussion 1142-1143.

Chin, B., Wallace: *ML-3000*, J., Curr. Opin. CPNS Invest. Drugs **1999**, *1*, 148-152.

Churchill, L., Graham, A. G., Shih, C. K., Pauletti, D., Farina, P. R., Grob, P. M.: *Selective inhibition of human cyclo-oxygenase-2 by meloxicam*. Inflammopharmacol. **1996**, *4*, 125-135.

Civelli, M., Vigano, T., Acerbi, D., Caruso, P., Giossi, M., Bongrani, S., Folco, G. C.: *Modulation of arachidonic acid metabolism by orally administered morniflumate in man*, Agents Actions **1991**, *33*, 233-239.

Cleij, M., Archelas, A., Furstoss, R.: *Microbiological Transformations 43. Epoxide Hydrolases as Tools for the Synthesis of Enantiopure Methylstyrene Oxides: A New and Efficient Synthesis of (S)-Ibuprofen*, J. Org. Chem. **1999**, *64*, 5029-5035.

Clemence, F. (Roussel-Uclaf): *Neue Derivate der Thiophenessigsäure und Verfahren zu deren Herstellung*, DOS 2 055 264, **1970**.

Clissold, S. P.: *Paracetamol and phenacetin*, Drugs **1986**, *32*, Suppl. *4*, 46-59.

Coletta, R., Maggiolo, F., Di Tizio, S.: *Etofenamate and transcutaneous electrical nerve stimulation treatment of painful spinal syndromes*, Int. J. Clin. Pharmacol. Res. **1988**, *8*, 295-298.

Comm. Farmaceutica Milanese: *Preparation of 4-n-butyl-2-phenyl-pyrazolidine-3,5-dione and 1-alkyl substituents thereof*, GB 839 057, **1957**.

Courade, J. P., Chassaing, C., Bardin, L., Alloui, A., Eschalier, A.: *5-HT receptor subtypes involved in the spinal antinociceptive effect of acetaminophen in rats*, Eur. J. Pharmacol. **2001**, *432*, 1-7.

Crofford, L. J., Wilder, R. L., Ristimaki, A. P., Sano, H., Remmers, E. F., Epps, H. R., Hla, T.: *Cyclooxygenase-1 and -2 expression in rheumatoid synovial tissues. Effects of interleukin-1 beta, phorbol ester, and corticosteroids*, J. Clin. Invest. **1994**, *93*, 1095-1101.

Cryer, B., Feldman, M.: *Cyclooxygenase-1 and cyclooxygenase-2 selectivity of widely used nonsteroidal anti-inflammatory drugs*. Am. J. Med. **1998**, *104*, 413-421.

Dannhardt, G.; Laufer, S.: *Structural Approaches to Explain the Selectivity of COX-2 Inhibitors: Is There a Common Pharmacophore?* Curr. Med. Chem. **2000**, *7*, 1101-1112.

Davies, N. M. and Anderson, K. E.: *Clinical pharmacokinetics of naproxen*, Clin. Pharmacokinet. **1997**, *32*, 268-293.

Davies, N. M.: *Clinical pharmacokinetics of ibuprofen. The first 30 years*, Clin. Pharmacokinet. **1998a**, *34*, 101-154.

Davies, N. M.: *Clinical pharmacokinetics of nabumetone. The dawn of selective cyclo-oxygenase-2 inhibition?*, Clin. Pharmacokinet. **1997**, *33*, 404-416.

Davies N. M. *Clinical pharmacokinetics of oxaprozin*, Clin. Pharmacokinet. **1998b**, *35,* 425-436.

Davies, N. M.: *Clinical pharmacokinetics of tiaprofenic acid and its enantiomers*, Clin Pharmacokinet. **1996**, *31*, 331-347.

Davies, I. W., Marcoux, J. F., Corley, E. G., Journet, M., Cai, D.-W., Palucki, M., Wu, J., Larsen, R. D., Rossen, K., Pye, P. J., DiMichele, L., Dormer, P., Reider, P. J.: *A Practical Synthesis of a COX-2-Specific Inhibitor*, J. Org. Chem. **2000**, *65*, 8415-8420.

Davis, R. and Brogden, R. N.: *Nimesulide. An update of its pharmacodynamic and pharmacokinetic properties, and therapeutic efficacy*, Drugs **1994**, *48*, 431-454.

Demerson, C. A., Humber, L. G., Dobson, T. A., Jirkovsky, I. L. (American Home Products): *1-Carboxamido pyrano (thiopyrano) [3,4-6]indole derivatives*, US 3 843 681, **1974**.

Demerson, C. A., Humber, L. G., Dobson, T. A., Martel, R. R.: *Chemistry and antiinflammatory activities of prodolic-acid and related 1,3,4,9-tetrahydropyrano[3,4-b]indole-1-alkanoic acids*, J. Med. Chem. **1975**, *18*, 189-191.

Depre, M., van Hecken, A., Verbesselt, R., Tjandra-Maga, T. B., Gerin, M., de Schepper, P. J.: *Tolerance and pharmacokinetics of propacetamol, a paracetamol formulation for intravenous use*, Fundam. Clin. Pharmacol. **1992**, *6*, 259-262.

Dinchuk, J. E., Car, B. D., Focht, R. J., Johnston, J. J., Jaffee, B. D., Covington, M. B., Contel, N. R., Eng, V. M., Collins, R. J., Czerniak, P. M., Gorry, S. A., Trzaskos, J. M.: *Renal abnormalities and an altered inflammatory response in mice lacking cyclooxygenase II*, Nature **1995**, *378*, 406-409.

Dittert, L. W., et al., J. Pharm. Sci. **1968**, *57*, 774.

Dittrich, P., Radhofer-Welte, S., Magometschnigg, D., Kukovetz, W. R., Mayerhofer, S., Ferber, H. P.: *The effect of concomitantly administered antacids on the bioavailability of lornoxicam, a novel highly potent NSAID*, Drugs Exp. Clin. Res. **1990**, *16*, 57-62.

Dong, X.: *Genetic dissection of systemic acquired resistance*, Curr. Opin. Plant Biol. **2001**, *4*, 309-314.

Dorfman, R. L.: *Chemistry and pharmacology of naproxen*, Arzneim.-Forsch./Drug Res. **1975**, *25*, 278-281.

Downie, W. W., Gluckman, M. I., Ziehmer, B. A., Boyle, J. A.: *Isoxicam*, Clin. Rheum. Dis. **1984**, *10*, 385-399.

Dubach, U. C., Rosner, B., Pfister, E.: *Epidemiologic study of abuse of analgesics containing phenacetin. Renal morbidity and mortality (1968-1979)*, New Engl. J. Med. **1983**, *308*, 357-362.

Dube, D., Fortin, R., Friesen, R., Wang, Z., Gauthier, J. Y.: *Substituted pyridines as selective cyclooxygenase-2 inhibitors* (Merck Frosst Canada Inc.), WO 9803484, (US 5861419, EP 0912518).

Ehrhart, G., Ruschig, H.: *Arzneimittel, Entwicklung, Wirkung, Darstellung*, Verlag Chemie, Weinheim **1972**, Vol. I, 171-172.

Engelhardt, G., Homma, D., Schlegel, K., Utzmann, R., Schnitzler, C.: *Anti-inflammatory, analgesic, antipyretic and related properties of meloxicam, a new non-steroidal anti-inflammatory agent with favourable gastrointestinal tolerance*, Inflamm. Res. **1995**, *44*, 423-433.

Faich, G. A.: *Risks and indications of phenylbutazone: another look*. Pharmacotherapy **1987**, *7*, 25-27.

Failli, A. A., Stefan, R. J., Kreft, A. F., Caggiano, T. J., Caufield, C. E.: *Pyranoiddole and tetrahydrocarbazole inhibitors of COX-2* (American Home Products Corp.), US5830911, **1998**.

Failli, A. A.: *Indene inhibitors of COX-2* (American Home Products Corp.), WO 9821195, **1998**.

Failli, A. A.: *Indene inhibitors of COX-2* (American Home Products Corp.), US 5869524, **1999**.

Farge, D., Messer, M. N., Moutonnier, C. (Rhône-Poulenc): *(3-Benzoylphenyl) alkanoic acids*, US 3 641 127, **1972**.

Faure, A. and Hoffmann, C. (Labs. U.P.S.A.): *Derivatives of 2-anilino-nicotinic acid and process for their preparation,* US 3 415 834, **1968**.

Ferreiro, C., Vivas, S., Jorquera, F., Dominguez, A. B., Espinel, J., Munoz, F., Herrera, A., Fernandez, M. J., Olcoz, J. L., Ortiz de Urbina, J.: *[Toxic hepatitis caused by nimesulide, presentation of a new case and review of the literature]*, Gastroenterol. Hepatol. **2000**, *23*, 428-430.

FitzGerald, G. A., Patrono, C.: The *coxibs, selective inhibitors of cyclooxygenase-2*, New Engl. J. Med. **2001**, *345*, 433-442.

Fletcher, M. R., Loebl, W., Scott, J. T., *Feprazone, a new anti-inflammatory agent. Studies of potency and gastrointestinal tolerance*, Ann. Rheum. Dis. **1975** *34*, 190-194.

Franco, F. F., Greenhouse, R., Muchowski, J. M., *Novel syntheses of 5-aroyl-1,2-dihydro-3H-pyrrolo[1,2-a]pyrrole-1-carboxylic acids,* J. Org. Chem. **1982**, *47*, 1682-1688.

Friedel, H. A., Langtry, H. D., Buckley, M. M.: *Nabumetone. A reappraisal of its pharmacology and therapeutic use in rheumatic diseases*, Drugs **1993**, *45*, 131-156.

Friesen, R. W., Brideau, C., Chan, C. C.: *2-Pyridinyl-3-(4-methylsulfonyl)phenylpyridines: Selective and orally active cyclooxygenase-2 inhibitors*, Bioorg. Med. Chem. Lett. **1998**, *8*, 2777-2780.

Fujimoto, R. A., Mcquire, L. W., Mungrage, B. B., Van Duzer, J. H., Xu, D.: *Certain 5-alkyl-2-arylaminophenylacetic acids derivatives* (Novartis-Erfindungen Verwaltungsgesellschaft mbH), WO 9911605, **1999**.

Fujimoto, R.: *Flobufen*, Current Opinion in CPNS Investigational Drugs **1999**, *1*, 142-147.

Funk, C. D., Funk, L. B., Kennedy, M. E., Pong, A. S., Fitzgerald, G. A.: *Human platelet/erythroleukemia cell prostaglandin G/H synthase: cDNA cloning, expression, and gene chromosomal assignment*, FASEB J. **1991**, *5*, 2304-2312.

Gierse, J. K., Hauser, S. D., Creely, D. P., Koboldt, C., Rangwala, S. H., Isakson, P. C., Seibert, K.: *Expression and selective inhibition of the constitutive and inducible forms of human cyclooxygenase*, Biochem. J. **1995**, *305*, 479-484.

Gillis, J. C. and Brogden, R. N.; *Ketorolac. A reappraisal of its pharmacodynamic and pharmacokinetic properties and therapeutic use in pain management*, Drugs **1997**, *53*, 139-188.

Glaser, K., Sung, M.L., O´Neil, K., Belfat, M., Hartmann, B., Carlson, R., Kreft, A., Kubrak, D., Hgio, C.L., Weichmann, B.: *Etodolac selectively inhibits human prostaglandin G/H synthase-2 (PGHS-2) versus human PGHS-1*, Eur. J. Pharmacol. **1995**, *281*, 107-111.

Gögelein, H., Dahlem, D., Englert, H. C., Lang, H. J.: *Flufenamic acid, mefenamic acid and niflumic acid inhibit single nonselective cation channels in the rat exocrine pancreas*, FEBS Lett. **1990**, 268, 79-82.

Goldstein, J. L., Correa, P., Zhao, W. W., Burr, A. M., Hubbard, R. C., Verburg, K. M., Geis, G. S.: *Reduced incidence of gastroduodenal ulcers with celecoxib, a novel cyclooxygenase-2 inhibitor, compared to naproxen in patients with arthritis*, Am. J. Gastroenterol. **2001**, *96*, 1019-1027.

Gotta, A. W.: *Parecoxib*, IDrugs **2001**, *4*, 939-944.

Goudie, A. C., Gaster, L. M., Lake, A. W., Rose, C. J., Freeman, P. C., Hughes, B. O., Miller, D.: 4-(6-Methoxy-2-naphthyl)butan-2-one and related analogues, a novel structural class of antiinflammatory compounds, J. Med. Chem. **1978**, *12*, 1260-1264.

Graul, A., Martel, A. M., Castaner, J.: *Celecoxib*, Drugs Fut. **1997**, *22*, 711-714.

Grindel, J. M.: *The pharmacokinetic and metabolic profile of the antiinflammatory agent tolmetin in laboratory animals and man*, Drug Metab. Rev. **1981**, *12*, 363-377.

Grover, G. J., D'Alonzo, A. J., Sleph, P. G., Dzwonczyk, S., Hess, T. A., Darbenzio, R. B.: *The cardioprotective and electrophysiological effects of cromakalim are attenuated by meclofenamate through a cyclooxygenase-independent mechanism*, J. Pharmacol. Exp. Ther. **1994**, *269*, 536-540.

Gruber, C. M., *Clinical pharmacology of fenoprofen: a review.* J. Rheumatol. **1976**; 2, 8-17.

Guzman, A., Yuste, F., Toscana, R. A., Young, J. M., Van Horn, A. R., Muchowski, J. M., *Absolute configuration of (-)-5-benzoyl-1,2-dihydro-3H-pyrrolo[1,2-alpha]pyrrole-1-carboxylic acid, the active enantiomer of ketorolac*, J. Med. Chem. **1986**, *29*, 589-591.

Haanen, C.: *Sulindac and its derivatives: a novel class of anticancer agents*, Curr. Opin. Inv. Drugs. **2001**, 2, 677-683.

Häflinger, F. (Geigy): *Substituted 1,2-diphenyl-3,5-dioxopyrazolidines*, US 2 745 783, **1956**.

Hannah, J., Ruyle, W. V., Jones, H., Matzuk, A. R., Kelly, K. W., Witzel, B. E., Holtz, W. J., Houser, R. A., Shen, T. Y., Sarett, L. H.: *Novel analgesic-antiinflammatory salicylates*, J. Med. Chem. **1978**, *21*, 1093-1100.

Harks, E. G., de Roos, A. D., Peters, P. H., de Haan, L. H., Brouwer, A., Ypey, D. L., van Zoelen, E. J., Theuvenet, A. P.: *Fenamates: a novel class of reversible gap junction blockers*, J. Pharmacol. Exp. Ther. **2001**, *298*, 1033-1041.

Hennig, J., Malamy, J., Grynkiewicz, G., Indulski, J., Klessig, D.F.: *Interconversion of the salicylic acid signal and its glucoside in tobacco*, Plant J. **1993**, *4*, 593-600.

Higgs, G. A., Salmon, J. A., Henderson, B., Vane, J. R.: *Pharmacokinetics of aspirin and salicylate in relation to inhibition of arachidonate cyclooxygenase and antiinflammatory activity*, Proc. Natl. Acad. Sci. USA **1987**, *84*, 1417-1420.

Hitzenberger, G., Radhofer-Welte, S., Takacs, F., Rosenow, D.: *Pharmacokinetics of lornoxicam in man*, Postgrad. Med. J. **1990**, *66*, Suppl. 4, S22-27.

Hla, T., Neilson, K.: *Human cyclooxygenase-2, cDNA*, Proc. Natl. Acad. Sci. USA **1992**, *89*, 7384-7388.

Ho, L., Pieroni, C., Winger, D., Purohit, D. P., Aisen, P. S., Pasinetti, G. M.: *Regional distribution of cyclooxygenase-2 in the hippocampal formation in Alzheimer's disease*, J. Neurosci. Res. **1999**, *57*, 295-303.

Hoffenberg, D. S., Hauser, C. R.: *Dehydration or Beckmann rearrangement of aldoximes with boron fluoride. Conversion of aldoximes to corresponding amides*, J. Org. Chem. **1955**, *20*, 1496-1500.

Hoffmann-La Roche: *Verfahren zur Herstellung von 1-Phenyl-3-methyl-4-alkyl- und –4-aralkylpyrazolonen*, DRP 565 799, **1931**.

Hromatka, O., Binder, D., Pfister, R., Zeller, P. (Hoffmann-La Roche): *Thiazinderivate*, DOS 2 537 070, **1975**.

Hommeril, J. L., Bernard, J. M., Gouin, F., Pinaud, M.: *Ketoprofen for pain after hip and knee arthroplasty*, Br. J. Anaesth. **1994**, *72*, 383-387.

Huber, R., Zech, K., Dittmann, E. C., Luhmann, R., Petitet, A.: *[Pharmacokinetics of the antirheumatic lonazolac-Ca in humans]* Arzneimittelforschung **1990**, *40*, 918-925.

in t' Veld, B. A., Ruitenberg, A., Hofman, A., Launer, L. J., van Duijn, C. M., Stijnen, T., Breteler, M. M., Stricker, B. H.: *Nonsteroidal antiinflammatory* drugs *and the risk of Alzheimer's disease*, New Engl. J. Med. **2001**, *345*, 1515-1521.

Inagaki, M.; Tsuri, T.; Joyama, H.; Ono, T.; Yamada, K.; Kobayashi, M.; Hori, Y.; Arimura, A.; Yasui, K.; Ohno, K.; Kakudo, S.; Koizami, K.; Suzuki, R.; Kato, M.; Kawai, S.; Matsumoto, S.: *Novel Antiarthritic Agents with 1,2-Isothiazolidine-1,1-dioxide (Sultam) Skeleton: Cytokine Suppressive Dual Inhibitors of Cyclooxygenase-2 and 5-Lipoxygenase*. J. Med. Chem. **2000**, *43*, 2040-2048.

Jacobi, H. and Dell, H. D.: *[On the pharmacodynamics of acemetacin (author's transl)]* Arzneimittelforschung **1980**, *30*, 1348-1362.

Jamali, F., Brocks, D.R.: *Clinical pharmacokinetics of ketoprofen and its enantiomers*. Clin. Pharmacokinet. **1990**, *19*, 197-217.

Jett, M. F., Ramesha, C. S., Brown, C. D., Chiu, S., Emmett, C., Voronin, T., Sun, T., O'Yang, C., Hunter, J. C., Eglen, R. M., Johnson, R. M.: *Characterization of the analgesic and anti-inflammatory activities of ketorolac and its enantiomers in the rat*, J. Pharmacol. Exp. Ther. **1999**, *288*, 1288-1297.

Jiménez, J.-M., Crespo, M. I., Godessart, N.: *Progress with selective COX-2 inhibitors*. Idrugs **2000**, *3*, 907-919.

Jones, H., Houser, R. (Merck & Co.), US 3 415 834, **1980**, see also US 3 992 495 (Merck & Co.) and US 4 131 618 (Merck & Co.) for alternative synthesis.

Juby, P. F., Hudyma, T. W., Brown, M.: *Preparation and antininflammatory properties of some 5-(2-anilinophenyl)tetrazoles*, J. Med. Chem. **1968**, *11*, 111-117.

Kalgutkar, A. S., Crews, B. C., Rowlinson, S. W., Garner, C., Seibert, K., Marnett, L. J.: *Aspirin-like molecules that covalently inactivate cyclooxygenase-2*, Science **1998a**, *280*, 1268-1270.

Kalgutkar, A. S., Kozak, K. R., Crews, B. C., Hochgesang, G. P., Mamett, L. J., *Covalent modification of cyclooxygenase-2 (COX-2) by 2-acetoxyphenyl alkyl sulfides, a new class of selective COX-2 inactivators.* J. Med. Chem. **1998b**, *41*, 4800-4818.

Kalgutkar, A. S., Crews, B. C., Rowlinson, S. W., Marnett, A. B., Kozak, K. R., Remmel, R. P., Marnett, L. J.: *Biochemically based design of cyclooxygenase-2 (COX-2) inhibitors: facile conversion of nonsteroidal antiinflammatory drugs to potent and highly selective COX-2 inhibitors*, Proc. Natl. Acad. Sci. USA **2000**, *97*, 925-930.

Kalgutkar, A. S.; Marnett, A. B.; Crews, B. C.; Remmel, R. P.; Marnett, L. J.: *Ester and amide derivatives of the nonsteroidal antiinflammatory drug, indomethacin, as selective cyclooxygenase-2 inhibitors*, J. Med. Chem. **2000**, *43*, 2860-2870.

Kassahun, K., McIntosh, I. S., Shou, M., Walsh, D. J., Rodeheffer, C., Slaughter, D. E., Geer, L. A., Halpin, R. A., Agrawal, N., Rodrigues, A. D.: *Role of human liver cytochrome P4503A in the metabolism of etoricoxib, a novel cyclooxygenase-2 selective inhibitor*, Drug Metab. Dispos. **2001**, *29*, 813-820.

Kawai, S., Nishida, S., Kato, M., Furumaya, Y., Okamoto, R., Koshino, T, Mizushima, Y.: *Comparison of cyclooxygenase-1 and -2 inhibitory activities of various nonsteroidal anti-inflammatory drugs using human platelets and synovial cells*, Eur. J. Pharmacol. **1998**, *347*, 87-94.

Kerwar, S. S., *Pharmacologic properties of fenbufen*, Am. J. Med. **1983** 75, 62-69.

Kiefer, J. R., Pawlitz, J. L., Moreland, K. T., Stegeman, R. A., Hood, W. F., Gierse, J. K., Stevens, A. M., Goodwin, D. C., Rowlinson, S. W., Marnett, L. J., Stallings, W. C., Kurumbail, R. G.: *Structural insights into the stereochemistry of the cyclooxygenase reaction*, Nature **2000**, *405*, 97-101.

Kleemann, A., Engel, J. Kutscher, B., Reichert, D.: *Pharmaceutical Substances, Synthesis, Patents, Applications, Thieme*, Stuttgart, New York, 1999 (available in print and CD-ROM).

Komhoff, M., Wang, J. L., Cheng, H. F., Langenbach, R., McKanna, J. A., Harris, R. C., Breyer, M. D.: *Cyclooxygenase-2-selective inhibitors impair* glomerulogenesis *and renal cortical development*, Kidney Int. **2000**, *57*, 414-422.

Koup, J. R., Tucker, E., Thomas, D. J., Kinkel, A. W., Sedman, A. J., Dyer, R., Sharoky, M.: *A single and multiple dose pharmacokinetic and metabolism study of meclofenamate sodium*, Biopharm. Drug Dispos. **1990**, *11*, 1-15.

Kreft, A. F., Caufield, C. E., Failli, A. A., Caggiano, T. J., Greenfield, A. A., Kubrak, D. M.: *Pyranoindole inhibitors of COX-2* (American Home Products Corp.), US 5776967, **1998**.

Kreft, A. F., Caufield, C. E., Failli, A. A., Caggiano, T. J., Greenfield, A. A., Kubrak, D. M.: *Pyranoindole and carbazole inhibitors of COX-2* (American Home Products Corp.), WO 9804527, **1998**.

Kujubu, D. A., Fletcher, B. S., Varnum, B. C., Lim, R. W., Herschman, H. R.: *TIS10, a phorbol ester tumor promoter-inducible mRNA from Swiss 3T3 cells, encodes a novel prostaglandin synthase/cyclooxygenase homologu*, J. Biol. Chem. **1991**, *266*, 12866-12872.

Kuhnert, N., *Hundredth anniversary of Aspirin*, Chem. i. u. Zeit **1999**, *33*, 213-220.

Kurumbail, R. G., Stevens, A. M., Gierse, J. K., McDonald, J. J., Stegeman, R. A., Pak, J. Y., Gildehaus, D., Miyashiro, J. M., Penning, T. D., Seibert, K., Isakson, P. C., Stallings, W. C.: *Structural basis for selective inhibition of cyclooxygenase-2 by anti-inflammatory agents*, Nature **1996**, *384*, 644-648.

Laine, L., Harper, S., Simon, T., Bath, R., Johanson, J., Schwartz, H., Stern, S., Quan, H., Bolognese, J.: *A randomized trial comparing the effect of rofecoxib, a cyclooxygenase 2-specific inhibitor, with that of ibuprofen on the gastroduodenal mucosa of patients with osteoarthritis.Rofecoxib Osteoarthritis Endoscopy Study Group*, Gastroenterology **1999**, *117*, 776-783.

Lake, A. W. and Rose, C. J. (Beecham*): Naphthalene derivatives*, US 1474377, **1974** US 4 420 639, **1983**.

Langenbach, R., Loftin, C. D., Lee, C., Tiano, H.: *Cyclooxygenase-deficient mice. A summary of their characteristics and susceptibilities to inflammation and carcinogenesis*, Ann. NY Acad. Sci. **1999**, *889*, 52-61.

Laufer, S. A., Augustin, J., Dannhardt, G., Kiefer, W.: *(6,7-diaryldihydropyrrolizin-5-yl)acetic acids, a novel class of potent dual inhibitors of both cyclooxygenase and 5-lipoxygenase*, J. Med. Chem. **1994**, *37*, 1894-1897.

Lazer, E. S., Cywin, C. L., Sorcek, R.: *2-Benzyl-4-sulfonyl-4H-isoquinolin-1,3-diones and their use as anti-inflammatory agents* (Boehringer Ingelheim Pharmaceuticals Inc.), WO 9746532, **1997**; US-05741798, **1998**.

Leblanc, Y., Black, W. C., Chan, C. C., Charleson, S., Delorme, D., Denis, D., Gauthier, J. Y., Grimm, E. L., Gordon, R., Guay, D., Hamel, P., Kargman, S., Lan, C. K., Mancini, J., Quellet, M., Percival, D., Roy, P., Skorey, K., Tagari, P., Vickers, P., Wang, E., Xu, L., Prasit, P., Bioorg. Med. Lett. **1996**, *6*, 731-736.

Lee, Y. T. and Wang, Q.: *Inhibition of hKv2.1, a major human neuronal voltage-gated K+ channel, by meclofenamic acid*, Eur. J. Pharmacol. **1999**, *378*, 349-356.

Levy, M., Zylber-Katz, E., Rosenkranz, B.: *Clinical pharmacokinetics of dipyrone and its metabolites*, Clin. Pharmacokinet. **1995**, *28*, 216-234.

Lewis, R. K. and Paloucek, F. P.: *Assessment and treatment of acetaminophen overdose*, Clin. Pharm. **1991**, *10*, 765-774.

Lombardino, J. G. (Pfizer): *Benzothiazine dioxides*, US 3 591 584, **1971**; US 4 469 866, **1984**.

Lombardino, J. G., Wisemann, E. H., Chiaini, J.: *Potent anti-inflammatory N-heterocyclic 3-carboxamides of 4-hydroxy-2-methyl-2H-1,2-benzothiazine 1,1-dioxide*, J. Med. Chem. **1973**, *5*, 493-496.

Loew, D., Schuster, O., Knoell, H. E., Graul, E. H..: *[Pharmacology, toxicology and pharmacokinetics of mofebutazone]*, Z. Rheumatol. **1985**, *44*, 186-192.

Lombardino, J. G., Wisemann, E. H., *Antiinflammatory 3,4-dihydro-2-alkyl-3-oxo-2H-1,2-benzothiazine-4-carboxamide 1,1-dioxides*, J. Med. Chem. **1971**, *14*, 973.

Lopez-Garcia, J. A. and Laird, J. M.: *Central antinociceptive effects of meloxicam on rat spinal cord in vitro*, Neuroreport **1998**, *9*, 647-651.

Lora, M., Denault, J. B., Leduc, R., de Brum-Fernandes, A. J.: *Systematic pharmacological approach to the characterization of NSAIDs*, Prostaglandins Leukot. Essent. Fatty Acids **1998**, *59*, 55-62.

Lundbeck, *Improvements in and relating to the manufacture of 2-ethoxy benzamide*, GB 656 746, **1948**.

Marks, J. S. and Gleeson, M. H.: *Steatorrhoea complicating therapy with mefenamic acid*, Br. Med. J. **1975**, *4*, 442.

Marshall, W. S. (Eli Lilly & Co.): *Substituted phenylalkanoic acids and derivatives thereof*, US 3600437, **1971**.

Martel, R. R., Demerson, C.A., Humber, L.G., Philipp, A.H., Etodolic acid and related compounds. Chemistry and antiinflammatory actions of some potent di- and trisubstituted 1, 3, 4, 9-tetrahydropyrano[3, 4-b]indole-1-acetic acids, J. Med. Chem. **1976**, *19*, 391-395.

Masferrer, J. L., Koki, A., Seibert, K.: *COX-2 inhibitors. A new class of antiangiogenic agents*, Ann. NY Acad. Sci. **1999**, *889*, 84-86.

Matsuoka, H., Maruyama, N., Kashiwagi, H.: *Indole derivatives and mono and diazaindole derivatives* (Chugai Seiyku Kabushiki Kaisha), WO 9851667, **1998**.

Matsuoka, H., Kato, N., Takahashi, T., Maruyama, N., Ishizawa, T., Suzuki, Y.: *Heterocyclic Indole derivatives and mono or diazaindole derivatives* (Chugai Seiyku Kabushiki Kaisha), WO 9961436, **1999**.

Mayall, F. G., Blewitt, R. W., Staff, W. G.: *Cystitis and ureteric obstruction in patients taking tiaprofenic acid*, Br. Med. J. **1994**, *309*, 599-600.

Mayer, J. M., Testa, B., Drugs Fut. **1997**, *22*, 1347-1366.

McCarthy, C. J., Crofford, L. J., Greenson, J., Scheiman, J. M.: *Cyclooxygenase-2 expression in gastric antral mucosa before and after eradication of Helicobacter pylori infection*, Am. J. Gastroenterol. **1999**, *94*, 1218-1223.

McCormick, P. A., Kennedy, F., Curry, M., Traynor, O.: *COX 2 inhibitor and fulminant hepatic failure*, Lancet **1999**, *353*, 40-41.

McLean, J. R. and Gluckman, M. I.: *On the mechanism of the pharmacologic activity of meclofenamate sodium*, Arzneimittelforschung **1983**, *33*, 627-631.

Miller, L. G.: *Oxaprozin: a once-daily nonsteroidal anti-inflammatory drug*, Clin. Pharm. **1992**, *11*, 591-603.

Mitchell, J. A., Akarasereenont, P., Thiemermann, C., Flower, R. J., Vane, J. R.: *Selectivity of nonsteroidal antiinflammatory drugs as inhibitors of constitutive and inducible cyclooxygenase*, Proc. Natl. Acad. Sci. USA **1993**, *90*, 11693-11697.

Moffett, R. B., Aspergren, B. D.: *Aminoalkylphenothiazines*, J. Am. Chem. Soc. **1960**, *82*, 1605.

Morham, S. G., Langenbach, R., Loftin, C. D., Tiano, H. F., Vouloumanos, N., Jennette, J. C., Mahler, J. F., Kluckman, K. D., Ledford, A., Lee, C. A., Smithies, O.: *Prostaglandin synthase 2 gene disruption causes severe renal pathology in the mouse*, Cell **1995**, *83*, 473-482.

Moser, P., Sallmann, A., Wiesenberg, I.: *Synthesis and quantitative structure-activity relationships of diclofenac analogues,* J. Med. Chem. **1990**, *33*, 2358-2368.

Muchowski, J. M. and Greenhouse, R. (Syntex): *Process for preparing 5-aroyl 1,2-dihydro-3-H pyrrolo[1,2-A]pyrrole-1-carboxylic acids and novel intermediates therein*, US 4 347 186, **1982**; US 4 458 081, **1984**; US 4 873 340, **1989**.

Muchowski, J. M., Unger, S. H., Ackrell, J., Cheung, P., Cooper, G. F., Cook, J., Gallegra, P., Halpern, O., Koehler, R., Kluge, A. F., et al.: *Synthesis and antiinflammatory and analgesic activity of 5-aroyl-1,2-dihydro-3H-pyrrolo[1,2-a]pyrrole-1-carboxylic acids and related compounds*, J. Med. Chem. **1985**, *28*, 1037-1049.

Mukherjee, D., Nissen, S. E., Topol, E. J.: *Risk of cardiovascular events associated with selective COX-2 inhibitors*: J. Am. Med. Assoc. **2001**, *286*, 954-959.

Nakao, K., Stevens, R. W., Kawamura, K., Uchida, C., Koike, H., Caron, S.: *2,3-Substituted Indole compounds as COX-2 inhibitors* (Pfizer Inc.), WO-09935130, **1999**.

Needs, C. J. and Brooks, P. M.: *Clinical pharmacokinetics of the salicylates*, Clin. Pharmacokinet. **1985**, *10*, 164-177.

Neuman, M., Drugs Fut. **1981**, *6*, 35-36.

Nilsen, O. G.: *Clinical pharmacokinetics of tenoxicam*, Clin. Pharmacokinet. **1994**, *26*, 16-43.

Ogino, K., Hatanaka, K., Kawamura, M., Katori, M., Harada, Y.: *Evaluation of the pharmacological profile of meloxicam as an anti-inflammatory agent, with particular reference to ist relative selectivity for cyclooxygenase-2 over cyclooxygenase-1*, Pharmacology **1997**, *55*, 44-53.

O'Banion, M. K., Winn, V. D., Young, D. A.: *cDNA cloning and functional activity of a glucocorticoid-regulated inflammatory cyclooxygenase*, Proc. Natl. Acad. Sci. USA **1992**, *89*, 4888-4892.

Okumura, Y., Murata, Y., Mano, T.: *Benzimidazole derivatives as cyclooxygenase-2 inhibitors* (Pfizer Inc.), EP-0937722, **1999**.

Olkkola, K. T., Brunetto, A. V., Mattila, M. J.: *Pharmacokinetics of oxicam nonsteroidal anti-inflammatory agents*, Clin. Pharmacokinet. **1994**, *26*, 107-120.

Patrignani, P., Panara, M. R., Sciulli, M. G., Santini, G., Renda, G., Patrono, C.: *Differential inhibition of human prostaglandin endoperoxide synthase-1 and -2 by nonsteroidal anti-inflammatory drugs*, J. Physiol. Pharmacol. **1997**, *48*, 623-631.

Patrignani, P., Santini, G., Panara, M. R., Sciulli, M. G., Greco, A., Rotondo, M. T., di Giamberardino, M., Maclouf, J., Ciabattoni, G., Patrono, C.: *Induction of prostaglandin endoperoxide synthase-2 in human monocytes associated with cyclo-oxygenase-dependent F2-isoprostane formation*, Br. J. Pharmacol. **1996**, *118*, 1285-1293.

Patrono, C.: *Aspirin as an antiplatelet drug*, New Engl. J. Med. **1994**, *330*, 1287-1294.

Parke Davis: *Un medicament nouveau, l'acide N-(3-trifluoromethylphenyl)-anthranilique*, FR 1 341 M, **1961**.

Paulson, S. K., Engel, L., Reitz, B.Y., Bolten, S., Burton, G., Maziasz, T. J., Yan, B., Schoenhard, G.: *Evidence for Polymorphism in the Canine Metabolism of the Cyclooxygenase 2 Inhibitor*, Celecoxib, Drug Metabolism and Distribution **1999**, *27*, 1133-1142.

Paulson, S. K., Hribar, J. D., Liu, N. W. K., Hajdu, E., Bible Jr., R. H., Piergies, A., Karim, A.: *Metabolism and Excretion of (^{14}C)-Celecoxib in Healthy Male Volunteers*, Drug Metabolism and Distribution **2000**, *28*, 308-314.

Penning, T. D., Talley, J. J., Bertenshaw, S. R., Carter, J. S., Collins, P. W., Docter, S., Graneto, M. J., Lee, L. F., Malecha, J. W., Miyashiro, J. M., Rogers, R. S., Rogier, D. J., Yu, S. S., Anderson, G. D., Burton, E. G., Cogburn, J. N., Gregory, S. A., Koboldt, C. M., Perkins, W. E., Seibert, K., Veenhuizen, A. W., Zhang, Y. Y., Isakson, P. C.: *Synthesis and biological evaluation of the 1,5-diarylpyrazole class of cyclooxygenase-2 inhibitors: identification of 4-[5-(4-methylphenyl)-3-(trifluoromethyl)-1H-pyrazol-1-yl]benze nesulfonamide (SC-58635, celecoxib)*, J. Med. Chem. **1997**, *40*, 1347-1365.

Picot, D., Loll, P.J., Garavito, R.M.: *The X-ray crystal structure of the membrane protein prostaglandin H2 synthase-1*, Nature **1994**, *367*, 243-249.

Pierce, K. L., Gil, D. W., Woodward, D. F., Regan, J. W.: *Cloning of human prostanoid receptors*, Trends Pharmacol. Sci. **1995**, *16*, 253-256.

Plosker, G. L. and Wagstaff, A. J.: *Tiaprofenic acid. A reappraisal of its pharmacological properties and use in the management of rheumatic diseases*, Drugs **1995**, *50*, 1050-1075.

Prabhakar, C., Reddy, G. B., Reddy, C. M., Nageshwar, D., Devi, A. S., Babu, J. M., Vyas, K., Sarma, M. R., Reddy, G.O., Organic Process Res. & Dev. **1999**, *3*, 121-125.

Pruss, T.P., Stroissnig, H., Radhofer-Welte, S., Wendtlandt, W., Mehdi, N., Takacs, F., Fellier, H.: *Overview of the pharmacological properties, pharmacokinetics and animal safety assessment of lornoxicam*, Postgrad. Med. J. **1990**, *66*, S18-21.

Rainer, G., Riedel, R., Klemm, K. (Byk Gulden): *Pyrazolderivate und Verfahren zu deren Herstellung*, DE 1 946 370, **1969** US 4 4 325 962, **1982**.

Rainer, G., Krüger, U., Klemm, K.: [Synthesis and physico-chemical properties of lonazolac-Ca, a new antiphlogistic/antirheumatic agent], *Arzneim.-Forsch./Drug Res.* **1981**, *31*, 649-655.

Rautio, J., Nevalainen, T., Taipale, H., Vepsäläinen, J., Gynther, J., Laine, K., Järvinen, T.: *The synthesis and in vitro evaluation of novel morpholinyl- and methylpiperazinylacyloxyalkyl prodrugs af 2-(6-*

methoxy-2-naphthyl)propionic acid (naproxen) for topical drug delivery, J. Med. Chem. **2000**, *43*, 1489-1494.

Ravi, S., Keat, A.C., Keat, E.C.: *Colitis caused by non-steroidal anti-inflammatory drugs*, Postgrad. Med. J. **1986**, *62*, 773-776.

Rejholec, V.: *Flobufen (general review of flobufen, summarizing ist synthesis, antiinflammatory and immunomodulatory effects, pharmacokinetics, and toxicological studies)*, Drugs Fut. **1989**, *14*, 24-25.

Riedel, R.: *[Lonazolac-Ca = Calcium [3-(p-chlorophenyl)-1-phenylpyrazole-4[-acetate 1 Pharmacological properties of a new antiinflammatory/antirheumatic drug (author's transl)]*, Arzneimittelforschung **1981**, *31*, 655-665.

Riendeau, D., Percival, M. D., Boyce, S., Brideau, C., Charleson, S., Cromlish, W., Ethier, D., Evans, J., Falgueyret, J.P., Ford-Hutchinson, A.W., Gordon, R., Greig, G., Gresser, M. , Guay, J., Kargman, S., Leger, S., Mancini, J.A., O'Neill, G., Ouellet, M., Rodger, I.W., Therien, M., Wang, Z., Webb, J.K., Wong, E., Xu, L., Young, R.N., Zamboni, R., Prasit, P., Chan, C.C.: *Biochemical and pharmacological profile of a tetrasubstituted furanone as a highly selective COX-2 inhibitor*, Br. J. Pharmacol. **1997**, *121*, 105-117.

Riendeau, D., Percival, M. D., Brideau, C., Charleson, S., Dube, D., Ethier, D., Falgueyret, J.P., Friesen, R.W., Gordon, R., Greig, G., Guay, J., Mancini, J., Ouellet, M., Wong, E., Xu, L., Boyce, S., Visco, D., Girard, Y., Prasit, P., Zamboni, R., Rodger, I.W., Gresser, M., Ford-Hutchinson, A.W., Young, R.N., Chan, C.C.: *Etoricoxib (MK-0663): preclinical profile and comparison with other agents that selectively inhibit cyclooxygenase-2*, J. Pharmacol. Exp. Ther. **2001**, *296*, 558-566.

Riker: *Substituierte Sulfonamidodiphenyläther*, DOS 2 333 643, **1973**; US 3 840 597, **1974**.

Rotstein, D.M., Sjorgen, E.B.: *5-Aroylnaphthalene derivatives* (Hoffmann-La Roche AG), WO-09832732, **1998**.

Sawaoka, H., Kawano, S., Tsuji, S., Tsuji, M., Sun, W., Gunawan, E. S., Hori, M.: *Helicobacter pylori infection induces cyclooxygenase-2 expression in human gastric mucosa*, Prostaglandins Leukot. Essent. Fatty Acids **1998**, *59*, 313-316.

Scherrer, R. A., Short, F. W. (Parke Davis): *Anthranilic acids and derivatives,* US 3 313 848, **1967**; DE 1 149 015, **1961**.

Scherrer, R. A. (Parke Davis): *Verfahren zur Herstullung von neuen Anthranilsäurederivaten*, DE 1 163 846, **1961**, US 3 138 636, **1964**;.

Schloemer, G. C. (Syntex): *Preparation of α-arylalkanoic acids*, US 4 605 758, **1986**.

Shen, T.-Y. (Merck & Co.): *Verfahren zur Herstullung von Indolyl-(3)-alkancarbonsäuren und ihren Salzen*, DE 1 232 150, **1962**, US 3 161 654, **1964**.

Shen, T. Y., Windholz, T. B., Rosegay, A., Witzel, B. E., Wilson, A. N., Willett, J. D., Holtz, W. J., Ellis, R. L., Matzuk, A. R. et al.: *Nonsteroid antiinflammatory agents*, J. Am. Chem. Soc. **1963**, *85*, 488-489.

Shen, T.Y., Perspectives in nonsteroidal anti-inflammatory agents, Angew. Chem. Int. Ed. Engl. **1972**, *11*, 460-472.

Sherlock, M. H. and Sperber, N. (Schering Corp.): *Substituted nicotinic acids and method for the manufacture thereof*, US 3 337 570, **1967**.

Silverstein, F. E., Faich, G., Goldstein, J. L., Simon, L. S., Pincus, T., Whelton, A., Makuch, R., Eisen, G., Agrawal, N. M., Stenson, W.F., Burr, A. M., Zhao, W. W., Kent, J. D., Lefkowith, J. B., Verburg, K. M., Geis, G. S.: *Gastrointestinal toxicity with celecoxib vs nonsteroidal anti-inflammatory drugs for osteoarthritis and rheumatoid arthritis: the CLASS study: A randomized controlled trial. Celecoxib Long-term Arthritis Safety Study*, J. Am. Med. Assoc. **2000**, *284*, 1247-1255.

Singla, A. K., Chawla, M., Singh, A.: *Review - Nimesulide: Some Pharmaceutical and Pharmacological Aspects - An Update*, J. Pharm. Pharmacol. **2000**, *52*, 467-486.

Sonawane, H. R., Bellur, N. S., Ahuja, J. R., Kulkarni, D. G.: *Recent developments in the synthesis of optically active arylpropanoic acids: an important class of non-steroidal anti-inflammatory agents*, Tetrahedron: Asymmetry **1992**, *3*, 163-192.

Sonawane, H. R., Nanjundiah, B. S.: *Nazerruddin, G.M., An efficient synthesis of fenoprofen, an important antiinflammatory agent,* Ind. J. Chem. **1994**, *33B*, 705-706.

Song, Y.; Connor, D. T.; Doubleday, R.; Sorenson, R. J.; Sercel, A. D.; Unangst, P. C.; Roth, B. D.; Gilbertsen, R. B.; Chan, R. D.; J. Med. Chem. **1999**, *42*, 1151-1160.

Sorbera, L. A., Castaner, R. M., Silvestre, J., Castaner, J.: *Etoricoxib.* Drugs Fut. **2001a**, *26*, 346-353.

Sorbera, L. A., Leeson, P. A., Castaner, J., Castaner, R. M.: *Valdecoxib and Parecoxib Sodium,* Drugs Fut. **2001b**, *26*, 133-140.

Sorbera, L. A., Leeson, P. A., Castaner, J.: *Rofecoxib.* Drugs Fut. **1998**, *23*, 1287-1296.

Steinbach, G., Lynch, P. M., Phillips, R. K., Wallace, M. H., Hawk, E., Gordon, G. B., Wakabayashi, N., Saunders, B., Shen, Y., Fujimura, T., Su, L. K., Levin, B.: *The effect of celecoxib, a cyclooxygenase-2 inhibitor, in familial adenomatous polyposis,* New Engl. J. Med. **2000**, *342*, 1946-1952.

Stenzl, H. (Geigy): *Derivatives of 3,5-dioxo-pyrazolidine and process for their manufacture,* US 2 562 830, **1951**.

Stevens, R. W., Nakao, K., Kawamura, K., Uchida, C., Fujiwara, S.: *Indole compounds as COX-2 inhibitors* (Pfizer Inc.), WO9905104.

Stock, J. L., Shinjo, K., Burkhardt, J., Roach, M., Taniguchi, K., Ishikawa, T., Kim, H. S., Flannery, P. J., Coffman, T. M., McNeish, J. D., Audoly, L. P.: *The prostaglandin E2 EP1 receptor mediates pain perception and regulates blood pressure,* J. Clin. Invest. **2001**, *107*, 325-331.

Symposium on new perspectives on aspirin therapy (various authors), Am. J. Med. **1983**, *74* no. 6A, 1-109.

Taha, A. S., McLaughlin, S., Holland, P. J., Kelly, R. W., Sturrock, R. D., Russel, R. I.: *Effect of repeated therapeutic doses of naproxen and etodolac on gastric and duodenal mucosal prostaglandins (PGs) in rheumathoid arthritis (RA):* Gut **1989**, *30*, A751.

Talley, J. J., Penning, T. D., Collins, P. W., Rogier, D. J., Malecha, J. W., Miyashiro, J. M., Bertenshaw, S. R., Khanna, I. K., Granets, M. J., Carter, J. S., Docter, S. H. (Searle & Co.): Substituted pyrazolyl benzenesulfonamides for the treatmennt of inflammation, WO 9515316 (US 5 521 207, EP 731 795).

Talley, J. J., Brown, D. L., Nagarajan, S., Carter, J.S., Weier, R. M., Stealey, M. A., Collins, P. W., Seibert, K., Graneto, M. J., Xu, X., Partis, R. (Pharmacia Corp.): *Substituted isoxazoles for the treatment of inflammation,* WO 9625405

Talley, J. J.: *Selective Inhibitors of Cyclooxygenase-2 (COX-2).* Progress in Medicinal Chemistry - Vol. 36, King, F.D., Oxford, A.W. (Ed.), Elsevier, **1999**.

Talley, J. J., Bertenshaw, S. R., Brown, D. L., Carter, J. S., Graneto, M. J., Kellogg, M. S., Koboldt, C. M., Yuan. J., Zhang, Y. Y., Seibert, K.: *N-[[(5-methyl-3-phenylisoxazol-4-yl)-phenyl]sulfonyl]propanamide, sodium salt, parecoxib sodium: A* potent *and selective inhibitor of COX-2 for parenteral administration,* J. Med. Chem. **2000b**, *43*, 1661-1663.

Talley, J. J., Brown, D. L., Carter, J. S., Graneto, M. J., Koboldt, C. M., Masferrer, J. L., Perkins, W. E., Rogers, R. S., Shaffer, A. F., Zhang, Y. Y., Zweifel, B. S., Seibert, K.: *4-[5-Methyl-3-phenylisoxazol-4-yl]- benzenesulfonamide, valdecoxib: a potent and selective inhibitor of COX-2,* J. Med. Chem. **2000a**, *43*, 775-777.

Tegeder, I., Pfeilschifter, J., Geisslinger, G.: *Cyclooxygenase-independent actions of cyclooxygenase inhibitors,* FASEB J. **2001**, *15*, 2057-2072.

Thérien, M., Gauthier, J.Y., Leblanc, Y., Léger, S., Pertrier, H., Prasit, P., Wang, Z.: *Synthesis of Rofecoxib, (MK 0966, Vioxx 4-(4-Methylsulfonylphenyl)-3-Phenyl-2(5H)-Furanone), a Selective and Orally Active Inhibitor of Cycooxygenase-2,* Synthesis **2001**, 1778-1779.

Thiele, K. and v. Bebenburg, W. (Degussa): *Verfahren zur Herstellung neuer substituierter Aminopyridine,* DE 1 670 522, **1966**; US 3 513 171, **1970**.

Trummlitz, G., Engel, W., Seeger, E., Engelhardt, G. (Thomae GmbH): *Neue 4-Hydroxy-2H-1,2-benzothiazin-3-carboxamid-1,1-dioxide, Verfahren zu ihrer Herstellung und diese enthaltende Arzneimittel,* DE 2 756 113, **1979**.

Todd, P. A. and Clissold, S. P.: *Naproxen. A reappraisal of its pharmacology, and therapeutic use in rheumatic diseases and pain states*, Drugs **1990**, *40*, 91-137.

Todd, P. A. and Clissold, S. P.: *Tenoxicam. An update of its pharmacology and therapeutic efficacy in rheumatic diseases*, Drugs **1991**, *41*, 625-646.

Todd, P. A. and Sorkin, E. M.: *Diclofenac sodium. A reappraisal of its pharmacodynamic and pharmacokinetic properties, and therapeutic efficacy*, Drugs **1988**, *35*, 244-285.

Tomiyama, T., Tomiyama, A., Yokota, M., Uchibori, S.: *Derivatives of carboxalkyl azulenes and azulene-1-carboxylic acid* (Kotobuki Seiaku Co. LTD), GB-02320715, **1998**.

Tomcufcik, R .A., Child, S.G., Sloboda, A. E. (American Cyanamid Co.): *Substituierte Benzoylpropionsäuren enthaltende Mittel und ihre Verwendung*, DE 2147111, **1972**.

Trummlitz, G., Engelhardt, G., Busch, U. Drugs Fut. **1989**, *14*, 1047-1048.

Tull, R. J.,Czaja, R. F.,Shuman, R. F.,Pines,S. H. (Merck & Co.): *Process for preparing indenyl acetic acids,* US 3870753, **1975**.

Tull, R. J.,Czaja, R. F.,Shuman, R. F.,Pines, S. H., Merck & Co., US 3994600, **1976**.

Unterhalt, B., Drugs Fut. **1982**, *7*, 110-111.

Vane, J. R., Bakhle Y. S., Botting, R. M.: *Cyclooxygenases 1 and 2*, Ann. Rev. Pharmacol. Toxicol. **1998**, *38*, 97-120.

Vane, J.R.: *Inhibition of prostaglandin synthesis as a mechanism of action for aspirin-like drugs*, Nat. New Biol. **1971**, *231*, 232-235.

Vartiainen, N., Huang, C. Y., Salminen, A., Goldsteins, G., Chan, P. H., Koistinaho, J.: *Piroxicam and NS-398 rescue neurones from hypoxia/reoxygenation damage by a mechanism independent of cyclooxygenase inhibition*, J. Neurochem. **2001**, *76*, 480-489.

von Mering, J.: *Beiträge zur Kenntniss der Antipyretica*, Ther. Monatsh. **1893**, *7*, 577-587.

Volk, H. (Riedel-de Haen): *Verfahren zur Herstellung von in 4-Stellung durch einen Kohlenwasserstoffrest substituierten 1-Phenyl-2-alkyl-3-methyl-pyrazolonen-(5)*, DE 962 254, **1954**.

Waldman, R. J., Hall, W. N., McGee, H., Van Amburg, G.: *Aspirin as a risk factor in Reye's syndrome*, J. Am. Med. Assoc. **1982**, *247*, 3089-3094.

Wallace, J. and Chin, B.: *Celecoxib*, Cur. Op. CNPS Inv. Drugs **1999**, *1*, 132-141.

Warner, T. D., Giuliano, F., Vojnovic, I., Bukasa, A., Mitchell, J. A., Vane, J. R.: *Nonsteroid drug selectivities for cyclo-oxygenase-1 rather than cyclo-oxygenase-2 are associated with human gastrointestinal toxicity: a full in vitro analysis*, Proc. Natl. Acad. Sci. USA **1999**, *96*, 7563-7568.

Wasfi, I. A., Abdel Hadi, A. H., Zorob, O., Osman, M.al-G., Boni, N. S.: *Pharmacokinetics of phenylbutazone in camels*, Am. J. Vet. Res. **1997**, *58*, 636-640.

Wechter, W. J., Leipold, D. D., Murray, E. D. Jr., Quiggle, D., McCracken, J. D., Barrios, R. S., Greenberg, N. M.: *E-7869 (R-flurbiprofen) inhibits progression of prostate cancer in the TRAMP mouse*, Cancer Res. **2000**, *60*, 2203-2208.

Weithmann, K. U., Alpermann, H.-G.: *Biochemical and Pharmacological effect of Dipyrone and ist Metabolites in Model Systems Related to Arachidonic Acid Cascade*, Arzneim.-Forsch./Drug Res. **1983**, *35*, 947-952.

Whelton, A., Bender, W., Vaghaiwalla, F., Hall-Craggs, M,. Solez, K.: *Sulindac and renal impairment*, J. Am. Med. Assoc. **1983**, *249*, 2892-2893.

White, M. M. and Aylwin, M.: *Niflumic and flufenamic acids are potent reversible blockers of Ca2(+)-activated Cl- channels in Xenopus oocytes*, Mol. Pharmacol. **1990**, *37*, 720-724.

Wiseman, E. H., Chang, Y. H., Lombardino, J. G.: *Piroxicam, a novel anti-inflammatory agent*, Arzneim.-Forsch./Drug Res. **1976**, *26*, 1300-1303.

Wilbert, G., De Angelis, J., .Warner-Lambert US 2 998 450, **1961**.

Willoughby, D. A., Moore, A. R., Colville-Nash, P. R.: *COX-1, COX-2, and COX-3 and the future treatment of chronic inflammatory disease*, Lancet **2000**, *355*, 646-648.

Woods, K. M., McCroskey, R. W., Michaelides, M. R. (Abbott Laboratories): *Heterocyclic compounds as COX-2 inhibitors,* WO 9839330.

Yamamoto, H.: 1-Acyl-indoles. II. A new syntheses of 1-(p-chlorobenzoyl)-5-methyoxy-3-indolyacetic acid and its polymorphism, Chem. Pharm Bull. **1968**, *16*, 17; *ibid* **1968**, *16*, 647.

Yasojima, K., Schwab, C., McGeer, E. G., McGeer, P. L.: *Distribution of cyclooxygenase-1 and cyclooxygenase-2 mRNAs and proteins in human brain and peripheral organs,* Brain Res. **1999**, *830*, 226-236.

Young, J. M., Panah, S., Satchawatcharaphong, C., Cheung, P. S.: *Human whole blood assays for inhibition of prostaglandin G/H synthases-1 and -2 using A23187 and lipopolysaccharide stimulation of thromboxane B2 production,* Inflamm. Res. **1996**, *45*, 246-253.

Zinnes, H., Sircar, J. C., Lindo, N., Schwartz, M. L., Fabian, A. C., Shavel, J. Jr, Kasulanis, C. F., Genzer, J. D., Lutomski, C., DiPasquale, G.: *Isoxicam and related 4-hydroxy-N-isoxazolyl-2H-1,2-benzothiazine-3-carboxamide 1,1-dioxides. Potent nonsteroidal antiinflammatory agents,* J. Med. Chem. **1982**, *25*, 12-18.

Zinnes, H., Schwartz, M., Shavel, J. (Warner-Lambert): *4-Hydroxy-3-(3-isoxazolocarbamyl-2H-1,2-benzothiazin-1,1-dioxyde und Verfahren zu ihrer Herstellung,* DOS 2 208 351, **1972**.

3 Opioids

3.1 Introduction

Elmar Friderichs

Opioids is the common name for all compounds which have the same mode of action as the constituents of opium, the dried milky liquid of the poppy seed, *Papaver somniferum* (Brownstein, 1993). All opioids interact in biological systems with the same type of receptor, the so-called opioid receptor.

Definition

With respect to structural features (Casy and Parfitt, 1986) opioids can be divided into three groups:

Natural and synthetic opioids, opioid peptides

- The first group contains the natural products morphine, codeine and thebaine, which have been isolated from the natural product opium. In addition, the group contains various semi-synthetic derivatives of morphine, codeine and thebaine, which are prepared by chemical modifications of these natural products

- The second group comprises fully synthetic compounds which often have a totally different chemical structure as compared to the semi-synthetic analogs, but interact with the same opioid receptors and show the same spectrum of analgesia and side-effects as the natural compounds. The older name 'opiates' is still in use to describe both groups

Opiates is the older name for non-peptidic opioids

- The third group consists of naturally occurring and synthetic peptides with opioid-like properties. The opioid peptides were discovered during the search for endogenous ligands of the opioid receptors and share the same action and side-effect profile as the non-peptidic compounds

The endogenous opioid system (Akil et al., 1984) is widely distributed within the body, it is phylogenetically very old and is expressed in all vertebrates. A high density of opioid receptors is found in the brain (Mansour et al., 1995) and spinal cord, where these receptors are involved in pain inhibition and additionally in many other central regulatory processes. In addition to localisation in the CNS, opioid receptors are expressed in many peripheral organs (Herz, 1983). Of great importance are the opioid receptors of the gastrointestinal system, which regulate stomach emptying, gut motility and intestinal fluid secretion. Opioid receptors are found in cells of the immune system and peripheral opioids seem to be involved in the regulation of inflammatory and immunological processes (Stefano et al., 1996). In addition to the outstanding role in central pain inhibition,

Functions of the endogenous opioid system:

1. Central and (peripheral) pain processing

2. Regulation of autonomous functions

3. Regulation of immune and inflammatory processes

action at peripheral opioid receptors, which are expressed in high density during inflammation and immune stimulation, may add to central pain inhibition (Stein et al., 1999).

Opioid Receptor Types

The action profile of synthetic opioids reinforced speculation, that more than one type of opioid receptor exists and is involved in the analgesic activity of these compounds. Martin and co-workers in 1960 investigated these differences in a specially developed test model, the chronic spinal dog (Martin et al., 1976). According to the analgesia and side-effect profile they postulated three types of opioid receptors, the μ-receptor (ligand = morphine), the κ-receptor (ligand = ketazocine) and the σ-receptor (ligand = SKF 10081).

Table 1:   Differentiation of opioid receptors in the chronic spinal dog by Martin et al. (1984).

Prototypic compound	Action profile	Receptor type
Morphine	Analgesia, miosis, respiratory depression, bradycardia, hypothermia, inattention to external stimuli	μ-receptor
Ketazocine	Miosis, strong sedation, inhibition of flexor reflex	κ-receptor
N-Allylnormetazocine (SKF-10047)	Mydriasis, respiratory stimulation, tachycardia, delirium	σ-receptor

Opioid receptor subtypes:
μ, κ, and δ

This was later confirmed by binding experiments with radioactively labeled ligands and by the different binding and action profiles of the endogenous opioid peptides, the enkephalins and endorphines (Fowler and Fraser, 1994), which led to the identification of the δ-opioid receptor. Since the σ-receptor today is no longer considered to be an opioid receptor, three opioid receptor subtypes, the μ-, κ-, and δ-opioid receptor, had been confirmed (Martin, 1983; Dhavan et al., 1996).

ORL1- receptor

More recently, a fourth opioid receptor type, named ORL1-receptor has been added (Meunier et al., 1995). It was detected as an cDNA, which coded for a protein with opioid receptor-like properties. Within a short time, the endogenous ligand, a peptide named nociceptin, was isolated, which depending on the place and route of administration, induced pro-nociceptive or anti-nociceptive actions. The full spectrum of biological activity of nociceptin and the physiological role of the ORL-1 opioid receptor in pain processing is still under evaluation.

Subtypes of the Different Opioid Receptors

Corresponding to other receptor systems, binding studies as well as functional investigations indicate that subtypes of opioid receptors exist (Wood, 1982; Pasternak and Wood, 1986). Within the μ- and δ-receptor type 2 subtypes, the μ-1 and μ-2 and δ-1 and δ-2 have been described. The κ-receptor contains an additional κ-3 subtype. It was postulated by some investigators, that analgesia and opioid-side effects occur at different receptor subtypes, this would therefore make it possible to separate analgesia from the unwanted opioid side effects. According to Pasternak and Wood (1986) analgesia should be mediated by the μ-1 receptor site, whereas respiratory depression and addiction is mediated via the μ-2 receptor subtype. But in contrast to binding experiments, the functional separation of the μ-1 and μ-2 and other subtypes is more equivocal and a clear separation of analgesia from respiratory depression and addiction potential has never been found among the μ-opioids. Therefore, an attempt to differentiate μ-opioid analgesics according to subtype specificity is no longer maintained.

Functional significance of subtypes of opioid receptors still contoversial

It is interesting, that the subtypes of opioid receptors could not be confirmed in cloning experiments (Gaveriaux-Ruff and Kieffer, 1999), since for each receptor only one individual gene with an homogenous transcript was detected. Therefore, possible heterogeneity of opioid receptor subtypes must result from a later modification which is independent from the gene level. Possible variations could include splice variants, receptor association, posttranslational modifications (e.g. glycosidation) or coupling with different transduction mechanisms.

Molecular Pharmacology of Opioid Receptors

The development of the polymerase chain reaction (PCR) technique made it possible to amplify isolated opioid receptor cDNA and to synthesize small amounts of the receptor protein necessary to identify their amino acid

sequence. The first successfully cloned opioid receptor
was the δ-opioid receptor of the mouse, which was
described in parallel by Kieffer et al. (1992) and Evans et
al. (1992). Both used neuroblastoma-glioma hybridoma
cells which express a high density of δ-receptors in their
membranes. The isolated receptor protein consisted of
372 amino acids and had a molecular mass of 40.644.
The amino acid sequence showed a partial overlap with
the receptors of somatostatin (37%), angiotensin (31%)
and interleukin-8 (22%). Similar to the somatostatin
receptor, seven hydrophobic domains were identified by
which the receptor is inserted into the lipid bilayer of the
cell membrane. Shortly thereafter the rat and human δ-
receptors were cloned and they showed nearly total
homology with the rat receptor (mouse - rat homology:
97%; rat - human homology: 99%).

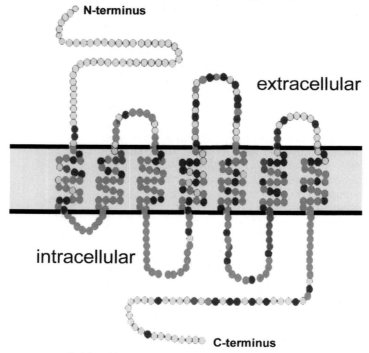

Figure 1: Common model for the μ-, κ- and δ-opioid receptor (modified from
Gaveriaux-Ruff and Kieffer, 1999).

Using the same technique a novel opioid-like cDNA was
isolated (Reinscheid et al., 1995), which coded for an
unknown opioid receptor. The new receptor had many
similarities with the classical opioid receptors (Calo et al.,
2000) and was added as the fourth member to the opioid

receptor family under the name ORL-1 ('opioid receptor–like' protein). In addition to rat and mouse receptors, the human types of all four opioid receptors have now been identified. They show a high degree of structural identity, which corresponds to their widely overlapping biological functions (Knapp et al., 1995; Gaveriaux-Ruff and Kieffer, 1999).

All opioid receptors belong to the group of pertussis toxin-sensitive G protein coupled receptors of the rhodopsine family with seven transmembrane spanning hydrophobic domains. The N-terminal is oriented to the outer side of the cell membrane and is involved in the selection and binding of the receptor-specific ligands. Studies with chimeric or point-mutated receptors indicate that predominantly the second and third extracellular loop determine receptor selectivity. The N-terminal sequence contains several free amino groups which can be conjugated with sugar residues. The carboxy terminal is directed towards the interior of the cell and is involved in the signal transduction cascade. The carboxy terminal contains groups which can be phosphorylated and which are involved in receptor internalization and inactivation. The seven transmembrane regions are connected by extracellular and intracellular loop regions of different length. Comparing the sequences of the μ-, δ- and κ-receptor reveals that the highest degree of similarity is located in the transmembrane regions and in the intracellular loop, whereas the external loops and both terminal regions are more heterogeneous. The external loops and the terminal moiety are involved in the selection and binding of ligands and contain the structural elements which determine the receptor selectivity.

Molecular structure of opioid receptors and receptor homology

Structure-Activity Relationship of Opioid Receptor Interaction

The structural and conformational prerequisites for opioid receptor binding have been most extensively studied for the μ-opioid receptor. These investigations, which were aimed at finding clinically improved opioid analgesics were initiated long before the receptor binding technique was elaborated. The basic concept dates back to the middle of the last century when Beckett and Casy (1954) developed a receptor model with three binding sites. This model was refined by Janssen and Jageneau (1957) to include the binding characteristic of the phenylpiperidine opioids. As essential elements the receptor ligand must contain an aromatic ring system, a central quarternary carbon atom and a side chain of two carbon atoms with a terminal basic

Structural elements for opioid receptor binding

nitrogen group which should be substituted with at least one methyl group (Janssen and van der Eycken, 1968). An hydroxyl group in the meta-position of the aromatic ring increases receptor binding and analgesic potency. In the morphine molecule, the side chain is incorporated into ring D and corresponds to atoms C15 - C16. Synthetic opioids of the fentanyl and oripavine type indicate, that a second aromatic ring system is advantageous, provided that both rings are at an optimal distance to each other and to the basic nitrogen group.

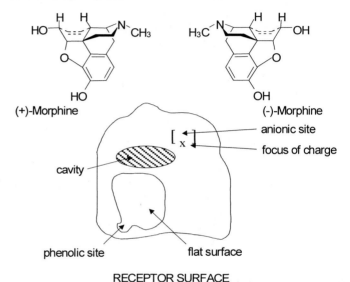

(+)-Morphine   (-)-Morphine

RECEPTOR SURFACE

Figure 2: The classical opioid receptor model developed by Casy (modified from Casy and Parfitt, 1986).

A more recent modeling (Brandt et al., 1993) of the three-dimensional structure of the µ-opioid ligands resulted in a binding model with seven essential binding areas. This model fits peptidic and non-peptidic µ-opioid structures. Area A represents the anionic center of the binding pocket which interacts with the protonated nitrogen of the opioid ligand. Area B contains a hydrophilic binding area which interacts with the phenolic hydroxyl or analogous groups via hydrogen bridges. Binding area C is a lipophilic site which interacts with the aromatic ring system. Area D is a further lipophilic site, where the second aromatic ring of molecules with more than one aromatic group is bound. Areas E, F and G are hydrophilic regions of possible interactions with corresponding polar groups of the ligand. Essential for a high receptor binding affinity is the appropriate distance between the aromatic rings and the basic nitrogen. It was shown in modeling experiments, that the optimal distance between the two aromatic rings is in the range of 10 Å. An optimal receptor interaction results when all seven areas are occupied by corresponding structural or electrically charged counterparts.

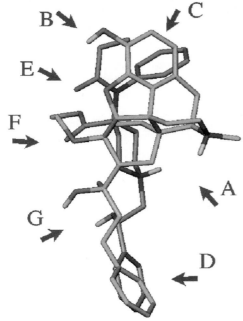

Figure 3: The refined model according to Portoghese et al. (1981) and Brandt et al. (1993, 2002).

Transduction Mechanisms of Opioid Receptor Interaction

Functional studies of the opioid receptors (Childers, 1991) revealed that all four receptor types belong to the group of G protein coupled receptors (GPCRs). Agonistic binding at the receptor induces association of the α-, β- and γ-subunit of the G protein which triggers several biochemical reactions within the cell (McFadzean, 1988; Simonds, 1988; Blake et al., 1997; Law and Loh, 1999). The pharmacological properties of the opioids depend mostly on the following three mechanisms:

Cellular effects of opioid receptor activation (see Fig. 4)

- Activation of a hyperpolarizing K^+ channel (inward rectifying K^+ channel)

- Inactivation of voltage dependent Ca^{++} channels (N-, P- and R-type)

- Inhibition of adenylate cyclase

A further relevant mechanism involved in the inhibition of synaptic transmission by opioids is a direct impairment of the exocytotic release of neurotransmitters, induced by stabilization of the presynaptic membrane.

Additional actions, with only partially understood relevance, are activation of phospholipases (PLH2, PLC7), activation of MAP-kinases and activation of some voltage dependent Ca^{2+} channels (L-type and T-type).

As a result of these actions opioids inhibit neurotransmission at the presynaptic and postsynaptic sites. Presynaptic inhibition depends mostly on the direct inhibitory effect on transmitter exocytosis from membrane-associated storage vessels. This direct effect is increased by the inhibition of Ca^{2+} channels, since Ca^{2+} ions trigger the transmitter release. Activation of K^+ ions induces membrane hyperpolarization which is the most important action component of postsynaptic inhibition.

Activation of K^+ channels, inactivation of Ca^{2+} channels and direct inhibition of neurotransmitter release are powerful mechanisms by which opioids inhibit the neuronal transmission of the pain signal.

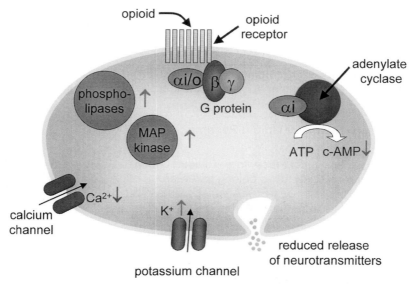

Figure 4: Cellular effector system, activated by opioid receptor binding.

Inhibitory and excitatory mechanisms of opioids

Opioid receptors are not only located at excitatory synapses, but are also expressed at inhibitory neurons. At these synapses, opioids inhibit the transmission of the inhibitory signal, which as result, induces excitation and an increased release of neurotransmitters in the innervated neuron.This explains why opioids, in addition to their prominent inhibitory actions, also have some stimulant effects.

Relationship of the Biological Effect to the Opioid Receptor Type

The peptide structure of the four different opioid receptors is very similar (Gaveriaux-Ruff and Kieffer, 1999) and this is the reason why most of the opioid receptor ligands show affinity for more than one type of receptor. In most cases, one type is preferred and the action and side-effect profile is dominated by the properties of this receptor. Intensive research was necessary to find out receptor-specific 'selective' ligands, but several selective agonists and antagonists for each type of opioid receptor have now been developed. With the aid of these selective compounds it was possible to differentiate receptors via binding properties, to dissect their physiological functions and to allocate analgesic properties and side-effects to the individual type of receptor.

Table 2:   Receptor-selective opioid agonists and antagonists.

Receptor type	Agonist	Antagonist
μ-receptor	Sufentanil *Endomorphine 1;2* *DAMGO*	CTAP
δ-receptor	SNC-80 *DPDPE*	Naltrindole ICI-174 864
κ-receptor	Enadoline U-50488 U-62593	Norbinaltorphimine
ORL1-receptor	*Nociceptin* Ro 64-6198	J-113397
	Peptides are in italics.	

Table 3: Pharmacological actions of opioids at different receptors.

μ-receptor	κ-receptor	δ-receptor	ORL1-receptor
Analgesia	Analgesia	Analgesia?	Analgesia?
Respiratory depression	Diuresis	Anxiolysis?	Pro-nociception
Constipation	Dysphoria		Anxiolysis?
Euphoria	Hallucinations		

μ-Opioid Receptors

Morphine-like analgesics are
μ-selective

Binding experiments and investigations in pain models have shown that the μ-receptor and to a lesser degree the κ-and δ-receptors predominates in the mediation of pain inhibition.

Table 4: Binding affinities of μ-selective opioid analgesics at recombinant human opioid receptor membranes expressed in CHO-K1 or HEK293 cells (Grünenthal, Dep. of Molecular Pharmacology).

Compound	Opioid Receptor Affinity (Ki / nM)			
	μ-OR (^{3}H-Naloxone)	κ-OR (^{3}H-Cl-977)	δ-OR (^{3}H-Deltorphin II)	ORL1 (^{3}H-Nociceptin)
Sufentanil	0.00085	0.34	0.047	0.12
Fentanyl	0.0079	3.71	1.1	2.45
Buprenorphine	0.00032	0.0004	0.0017	0.034
Hydromorphine	0.004	0.35	0.13	>10
Morphine	0.025	1.7	0.95	>> 10
Levomethadone	0.0070	12.9	0.83	>> 10
Ketobemidone	0.023	1.15	0.27	>> 10
Pethidine	2.0	>> 10	27	>> 10
Meptazinol	0.23	~10	~3	24.7
Detropropoxyphene	0.34	19.7	2.4	>> 10
Codeine*	1.78	1.0	3.2	>> 10
Tilidine*	2.42	> 10	>> 10	>> 10
Tramadol*	32.6	>> 10	>> 10	>> 10

Most of the opioid analgesics in clinical use (Cherny, 1996) have a prevalence for the μ-opioid receptor and this confirms that μ-receptor activation is the common mechanism of these compounds. Since morphine is the prototype, they are called 'morphine-like' analgesics.

Their common side-effect profile includes respiratory depression, constipation and addiction and dependence. All these side-effects, corresponding to analgesia, are mediated via μ-opioid receptor activation. This is the reason why the primary goal of the development of synthetic opioids, i.e. the separation of analgesia from the addiction and dependence potential, has never been achieved. The involvement of the same receptor population in the analgesia and side-effect profile of morphine and morphine-like opioids was impressively confirmed in μ-knock-out mice (Matthes et al., 1996; Kieffer, 1999). In these animals, morphine had no analgesic effect and no side effects. There was no respiratory depression and no inhibition of gastrointestinal motility and secretion. In behavioral models in μ-knock-outs, morphine did not induce liking or any other signs of addiction and repeated treatment with morphine did not produce signs of tolerance or physical dependence.

κ-Opioid Receptors

Activation of κ-receptors induces clinically-relevant pain inhibition (Scopes, 1993; Barber and Gottschlich, 1997), which seem to be less efficacious than μ-receptor-mediated analgesia. The most prominent side-effects of κ-activation are sedation and diuresis. In contrast to μ-agonists, which induce well-being and euphoria, activation of κ-receptors in the limbic system induces dysphoria and other unpleasant psychic effects such as e.g. hallucinations and spatial disorientation. The dose range of analgesia and psychic side-effects partly overlap and this causes problems in the potential medical use of κ-receptor agonists. This may explain why despite an intensive search for κ-selective analgesics, no selective κ-agonist has been successfully developed up to clinical use.

Clinical failure of κ-agonists because of psychotomimetic side-effects

κ-Receptor interaction is a common action component of the so called partial opioid agonists or agonists-antagonists like e.g. pentazocine, nalbuphine, butorphanol and buprenorphine (Hoskin and Hanks, 1991; Jacobs and Youngblood, 1992; Archer, 1992). In contrast to buprenorphine, which has κ-antagonistic activity, the other compounds have an agonistic or partial agonistic κ-action, which is responsible for analgesia and the often unpleasant side-effects of these compounds. Most of them

κ-component induces analgesia in mixed agonists-antagonists

have an additional µ-partial agonistic or µ-antagonistic action. The combination of both components results in a moderate to marked analgesia, weak respiratory depression, and a weak abuse and dependence potential.

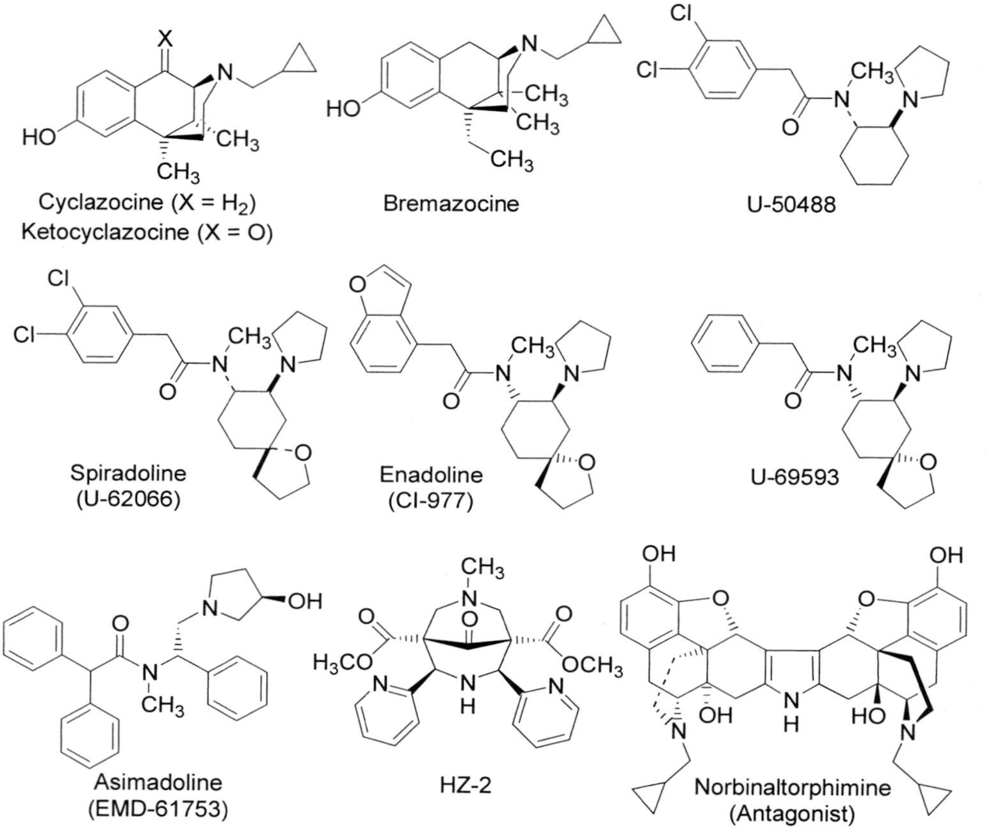

Cyclazocine (X = H$_2$)
Ketocyclazocine (X = O)

Bremazocine

U-50488

Spiradoline
(U-62066)

Enadoline
(CI-977)

U-69593

Asimadoline
(EMD-61753)

HZ-2

Norbinaltorphimine
(Antagonist)

Scheme 1: Selective κ-opioid agonists and norbinaltorphimine (antagonist).

In compounds with stronger µ-agonistic activity (buprenorphine and pentazocine), the abuse potential is marked and in contrast to earlier estimations, both compounds had to be subjected to narcotic control. In compounds with a marked κ-agonistic component (cyclazocine, nalorphine) the dysphoric side effects are so prominent that the compounds could not be used for therapeutic purposes.

Pain-relevant peripheral opioid receptors – even now an unverified therapeutic option

The investigations of Stein (1991) and Stein et al. (1999) have shown that pain-relevant opioid receptors are not only situated in the central nervous system but also in peripheral organs and tissues. Investigations in pain models with peripherally-acting opioids indicate that κ-receptors may predominantly mediate peripheral pain inhibition.

Table 5:   Receptor binding profile of mixed agonists-antagonists.

Compounds	κ-receptor	μ-receptor
Cyclazocine, Nalorphine, Nalbuphine	+	-
Butorphanole, Pentazocine, Dezocine	+	(+)
Buprenorphine	-	(+)
Meptazinole, Propiram		(+)
+ = Agonist; (+) = partial Agonist; - = Antagonist		

Expression of peripheral opioid receptors and peptides seems to be triggered by immunological and inflammatory processes, and it is speculated that these opioid receptors represent a second peripheral pain inhibitory system. This has triggered an intensive search for peripherally-acting κ-agonists, which are devoid of the centrally-mediated psychogenic side-effects and which are believed to be attractive new compounds for the treatment of traumatic, inflammatory and burn-induced pain.

δ-Opioid Receptors

In contrast to μ-, and κ-receptors, indications for a prominent role of δ-receptors in the pain process are less obvious (Dondio et al., 1997; Scheideler, 2000).There is an on-going broad but still controversial discussion concerning a genuine analgesic effect mediated by δ-1 or δ-2 receptors, since analgesia is scarcely observed in compounds having purely δ-agonistic activity. Many δ-agonists have an additional μ-action component or they are metabolized to a μ-agonistic metabolite (SNC-80), which is responsible or at least involved in the analgesic effect (Thomas et al., 2001)

Other investigations show that δ-active compounds increase the analgesic effect of μ-opioids, which is explained by 'cross-talk' between μ- and δ-receptors (Vaught et al., 1982). By this cross-talk δ-agonists inhibit the spinal release of pronociceptive cholecystokinin (CCK-

Cross-talk of μ- and δ-receptors may increase analgesic effect

8), which is induced by µ-receptor activation (Noble et al., 1994). The µ-, δ-receptor interaction was confirmed in δ-knock-out mice (Gomes et al., 2000) and although no δ-selective analgesic has been developed so far, mixed µ-, δ-agonists may become clinically-relevant pain inhibitors.

ORL-1 Receptors

Pain relevance of ORL1-receptors

The ORL-1 receptor (Calo et al., 2000; Mollereau and Mouledous, 2000) is more diverse in its peptide sequence compared to the classical opioid receptors. In contrast to these, ORL-1 receptor activation by the endogenous ligand nociceptin, at least at the supraspinal level, has a pro-nociceptive effect and induces pain. Release of CCK-8, NMDA or PGE-2 is discussed as the mechanism of pronociceptive activity. Spinal administration, in contrast, induces antinociception. With the systemically not bioavailable peptidic ligand nociceptin the question whether peripheral administration of an ORL-1 agonist would induce analgesia or a pain reaction can not be answered. To circumvent the restrictions of peptidic compounds, non-peptidic ORL-1 agonists and antagonists are in development which will elucidate whether ORL-1 agonists or antagonists are the better compound for pain inhibition. In addition to interaction with pain processing, ORL-1 agonists have a broad spectrum of somatic and vegetative effects, e.g. sedation, anxiolysis, anticonvulsant activity, memory impairment, inhibition of food consumption and cardiovascular stimulation. With the aid of the non-peptidic agonists and antagonists, which are currently under development, it will be possible to elucidate the contribution of the ORL-1 opioid system to pain processing and to other physiological processes (Bertorelli et al., 2000).

Location of Opioid Receptors in the Pain Pathway

The endogenous opioid system (Mansour et al., 1995) is the most important component of the pain inhibitory system of the body. Opioids act at different levels in the pain pathway and their action effects different aspects of pain processing (Lipp, 1991; Yaksh, 1997). This results in:

• Inhibition of the transmission of the pain signal

• Inhibition of the emotional aspect of pain

• Inhibition of pain realization

Pain pathway

Pain processing is inhibited at the spinal and supraspinal level. Spinal opioid receptors are located pre- and post synyptically at interneurons of the substantia gelatinosa of the dorsal horn. The opioid interneurons inhibit the release of excitatory transmitters and reduce the transmission of the pain signal from the primary afferents to the secondary neurons of the ascending spinal pain pathway. Supraspinally, opioids are located in different regions of the brainstem, in the periaquaeductal gray matter, in the limbic system, in the thalamic nuclei, in the basal ganglia and in the cortex. Cortical and thalamic localization is involved in the perception of the pain stimulus; the cortical regions are also involved in identifying the source of the pain.

Opioids in the different parts of the limbic system suppress the emotional component of pain and the pain suffering. Opioids in the formatio reticularis inhibit the pain-induced activation of autonomous functions, e.g. increase in respiration, increase in blood pressure and sweating. The inhibitory actions at the formatio reticularis are responsible for the major side-effects of the opioids such as respiratory depression, bradycardia and the central component of gastrointestinal inhibition.

In addition to the inhibitory effect at the ascending pain transmission, opioids activate a descending pain inhibitory system, which originates from different centers of the pons and medulla, e.g. nucleus coeruleus, areas of the periaquaeductal gray matter and areas of the raphe nuclei. The descending nerve fibers terminate at the spinal interneurones in noradrenergic and serotoninergic inhibitory synapses, which suppress the ascending pain signal. Thus, opioids inhibit the spinal pain processing by two mechanisms, one is a direct pre- and postsynaptic inhhibition of the ascending pain pathway and the other is a centrally-mediated activation of the descending pain inhibitory system.

Use of Opioids in Pain Treatment

Opioids are used for the treatment of moderate to severe or very severe pain of acute or chronic type (Stein, 1999). Nearly all forms of pain are sensitive to opioid treatment and in contrast to traditional opinions even neuropathic pain is reasonably sensitive to higher doses of opioids. This was clearly shown in well-controlled clinical studies (Watson, 2000). The most important use of opioids in acute pain treatment is postoperative pain, whereas treatment of cancer pain, often accompanied by a neuropathic pain component, is the classical domain of chronic opioid treatment.

Opioids are potent therapeutic options for almost all acute and chronic pain states

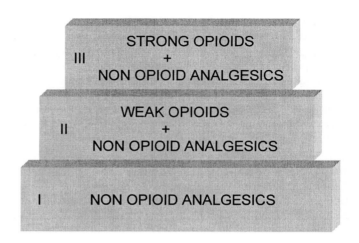

Figure 5: The WHO analgesic ladder.

WHO Guidelines for cancer pain treatment

(WHO, 1986)

To improve the world-wide under-treatment of chronic cancer pain, especially in underdeveloped countries, a guideline for chronic cancer pain treatment was published by the WHO in 1986. Meanwhile these guidelines have become the standard not only for malignant pain but also for benign chronic and acute pain states. The WHO proposal is often described as treatment 'by mouth, by the clock and by the ladder' (Jadad and Browman, 1995). This means that for repeated administration of the analgesic, the oral route should be used. The dosing interval should be regular and selection of the compounds should follow an increase in potency and efficacy as indicated in the three-step analgesic ladder. The first step starts with the single use of a non-opioid analgesic. If pain control is not sufficient, a weak opioid may be added. If a further increase in analgesic efficacy is needed, the weak opioid should be replaced by a strong opioid and the non-opioid may be omitted. Each stage of the treatment may be supplemented by the use of co-analgesics and other pharmacological and non-pharmacological interventions to improve pain control and to reduce side-effects.

Opioid Side-effects

Table 6:   Side-effect profile of μ-opioids (Martin, 1983).

1. Respiratory system • respiratory depression • chest wall rigidity	**3. Cardiovascular system** • bradycardia • impairment of cardiac conduction
2. Gastrointestinal system • inhibition of gastric emptying • inhibition of gut motility • inhibition of intestinal fluid secretion • constipation • nausea and emesis	**4. CNS effects** • sedation and tranquilization • deepening of anesthesia • euphoria • addiction **5. Systemic adaption** • induction of tolerance and physical dependence

Respiratory Depression

Opioids induce respiratory depression via inhibition of the respiratory center of the medulla oblongata, which respond to the pCO_2 content of the blood (Etches et al., 1989; Shook et al., 1990). The inhibitory effect is more prominent with respect to the respiratory frequency than to the volume of respiration. At higher opioid dosages, respiration becomes irregular and gasping occurs. Opioid-induced respiratory depression is augmented by other CNS-depressant compounds, like e.g. sedatives and hypnotics. In patients who are awake, respiratory depression by opioids can be voluntarily compensated over a broad dose range. Respiratory impairment is not a prominent feature in pain patients who are awake, since pain itself is a strong stimulus for respiration.

Respiratory depression - the most dangerous side effect of postoperative opioid use

Respiratory depression becomes an important side-effect when opioids are used for postoperative pain treatment, since the anesthetic agent and most adjuncts of anesthesia induce a long-lasting depressant effect on respiration, which can increase the opioid effects up to respiratory arrest. Therefore careful supervision of respiration during the postoperative period is mandatory (Mulroy, 1996). Opioid-induced respiratory depression can be interrupted by the opioid antagonist naloxone. Naloxone has a short duration of action and repeated administration may be necessary to successfully counteract the effect of longer-acting opioids. The degree of respiratory depression corresponds to opioid receptor affinity and highly potent opioids induce severe respiratory depression in the higher dose range. In addition, they induce a stiffness of the chest musculature (Jackson, 1994), called chest rigidity or 'wooden chest', which is mediated via stimulation of dopamine release in the nucleus caudatus. Chest rigidity further increases the respiration impairment caused by these compounds. Therefore use of higher doses of potent opioids such as fentanyl and analogs, as used for anesthesia, must be accompanied by artificial or at least assisted ventilation.

Respiratory depression is most prominent with μ-type opioid compounds and less so with κ-agonists and δ-agonists. δ-Agonists seem to have a compensatory stimulant action component, which counteracts respiratory depression.

Cardiovascular Effects

Nearly all opioids induce bradycardia (Bowdle, 1998), most likely mediated via central stimulation of the vagus nerve. Cardiovascular depression associated with most opioids is moderate and only the stronger opioids of the fentanyl group induce a more severe effect. Morphine and some of its analogs induce a non-opioid receptor-mediated release of histamine, which can result in a decrease in blood pressure and compensatory tachycardia.

Gastrointestinal Effects

Gastrointestinal side-effects of opioids are used for treatment of diarrhea

Opioids induce an inhibitory effect on gastrointestinal motility and fluid secretion (Kromer, 1990). The effect is peripherally and centrally mediated. The peripheral component is related to μ- and κ-receptors in intestinal organs, which are densely equipped with opioid receptors. They are located at parasympathic ganglia and inhibit the release of acetylcholine, which stimulates the contraction of smooth muscles. Inhibition of the intestinal fluid secretion is mediated via inhibition of adenylate cyclase. The intestinal effects of opioids extend to all parts of the gut and results in inhibition of stomach emptying and inhibition of secretion and motility of duodenum, jejunum, colon and rectum.

Reduced motility and secretion can lead to constipation, which is the most common side-effect of chronic opioid treatment (Mancini and Bruera, 1998). Opioid-induced constipation can increase to the stage of megacolon or paralytic ileus. Therefore chronic opioid treatment should be accompanied by concomitant use of laxatives. Besides their peripheral actions, opioids are involved in the central regulation of intestinal functions which are located in the formatio reticularis. This explains why the intestinal side-effects of opioids are not restricted to the more hydrophilic compounds like morphine, but are also seen with the use of more centrally active lipophilic analogs. During chronic opioid treatment a varying degree of tolerance towards the intestinal side-effects may occur.

The intestinal inhibitory action of opioids can be used for treatment of diarrhea (De Luca and Coupar, 1996). The clinically most important anti-diarrheal opioid is loperamide (Heel et al., 1978). After oral administration, loperamide acts locally within the gastro-intestinal tract. After parenteral administration, the compound is rapidly inactivated and does not reach the CNS. Therefore loperamide does not show the typical central opioid side-effects, has no analgesic action and has no abuse potential.

Emetic Activity

Nausea and emesis are common unpleasant side-effects of opioids (Campora et al., 1991; Aparasu et al., 1999). They are most intensively experienced at the beginning of the treatment. During chronic administration, tolerance may occur, which reduces the emetic sequelae. Nausea and emesis are induced via activation of chemoreceptors which are located in the trigger zone of the area postema of the formatio reticularis. The receptors are at the tissue surface and in contact with the circulating blood. Thus the emetic effect of opioids is not mediated centrally, i.e. after penetration of the blood-brain barrier, but rather peripherally via the amount of the compound, which is distributed in the circulating blood.

Opioids in the circulating blood induce nausea and emesis and an anti-emetic effects after penetration of the blood brain barrier

After passage through the blood brain barrier, opioids have an anti-emetic effect (Blancquaert et al., 1986). Emesis inhibition is induced via blockade of an emesis centre located in a more central area of the formatio reticularis. This explains why the emetic effect of opioids is most apparent immediately after anministration, especially after rapid intravenous administration and is reduced or terminated when the compound has reached the CNS. The more hydrophilic opioids like morphine have stronger emetic side-effects than lipophilic compounds like methadone or fentanyl (Barnes et al., 1991), which are rapidly transported into the CNS.

Tolerance and Dependence

μ-Opioid compounds induce a feeling of well-being and euphoria, which is mediated by the release of dopamine within the limbic system. κ-Opioids induce an opposite effect with dysphoria, disorientation and hallucinations (Pfeifer et al., 1986). Repeated activation of the μ-opioid rewarding system may induce a psychological dependence, which leads to addiction and compulsive drug seeking behavior (Brown and Lo, 2000). In addition, higher opioid dosages, as used for non-medicinal purposes, induce tolerance and as a consequence a further increase of the dose is needed to achieve the intended effect. In the course of tolerance development opioid users becomes physically dependent on a supply of the compound (Taylor and Fleming, 2001) and suspension of the treatment or blocking of the opioid receptors with an antagonist induces withdrawal reactions, characterized by strong dysphoria, restlessness, pain and various symptoms of autonomic dysregulation such as diarrhea, shivering, chills and cardiovascular collapse.

Opioid kick

The euphorigenic effect of opioids, the 'opioid kick', is more intensely induced by lipophilic compounds such as diacetylmorphine (heroine), which rapidly penetrates the CNS. The feeling of euphoria at one site and the absence of well-being at another site is increased by rapidly changing brain concentrations of the opioid and this intensifies drug seeking behavior and psychological as well as physical dependence.

Regular use and adequate dosing of opioids minimizes tolerance and dependence development in the treatment of chronic pain

In contrast to recreational use, the treatment of chronic pain with opioids has only a limited risk of inducing psychological dependence and drug addiction (Heit, 2001). Regular dosing can often postpone tolerance development for longer time periods. The most important precaution for avoiding tolerance and dependence development is to ensure constant plasma levels of the opioid, which should be high enough to give complete pain relief. This can be reasonably achieved by oral administration of retarded formulations or by using a patch (Reder, 2001). Breakthrough pain, which is often induced by a fluctuation in pain intensity, should be rapidly addressed by the administration of additional treatment with an immediate-release formulation of the same or a similar opioid.

References

Akil, H., Watson, S.J., Young, E., Lewis, M.E., Khachaturian, H., Walker, J.M.: *Endogenous opioids: biology and function*, Ann. Rev. Neurosci. **1984**, 7, 223-255.

Aparasu, R., McCoy, R.A., Weber, C., Mair, D., Parasuraman, T.V.: *Opioid-induced emesis among hospitalized nonsurgical patients: effect on pain and quality of life,* J. Pain Symptom Manage. **1999**, *18*, 280-188.

Archer, S.: *State-of-the-art analgesics from the agonist-antagonist concept.* NIDA Res. Monogr. **1992**, *119*, 71-75.

Barber, A.,Gottschlich, R.: *Novel developments with selective, non-peptidic kappa-opioid receptor agonists,* Exp. Opin. Invest. Drugs **1997**, *6*, 1354-1368.

Barnes, N.M., Bunce, K.T., Naylor, R.J., Rudd, J.A.: *The actions of fentanyl to inhibit drug-induced emesis,* Neuropharmacology **1991**, *30*, 1073-1083.

Beckett, A.H. and Casy, A.F.: *Synthetic analgesics: Stereochemical considerations,* J. Pharm. Pharmacol. **1954**, *6*, 986-1000.

Bertorelli, R., Calo, G., Ongini, E., Regoli, D.: *Nociceptin/orpanin FQ and its receptor: a potential target for drug discovery;* Trends Pharmacol. Sci. **2000**, *21*, 233-234.

Blake, A.D., Bot, G., Tallent, M., Law, S.F., Li, S., Freeman, J.C., Reisine, T.: *Molecular regulation of opioid receptors,* Receptors Channels **1997**, *5*, 231-235.

Blancquaert, J.P., Lefebvre, R.A., Willems, J.L.: *Emetic and antiemetic effects of opioids in the dog,* Eur. J. Pharmacol. **1986**, *128*, 143-150.

Bowdle, T.A.: *Adverse effects of opioid agonists and agonist-antagonists in anaesthesia.* Drug Saf. **1998**, *19*, 173-189.

Brandt, W.: *Struktur-Wirkungs-Beziehungen von Opioiden (Structure-activity relationships of opioids),* Pharm. i. u. Zeit **2002**, *31*, 60-68.

Brandt, W., Barth, A., Höltje, H.D.: *A new consistent model explaining structure (conformation)-activity relationships of opiates with mu-selectivity,* Drug Des. Discov. **1993**, *10*, 257-283.

Brown, R. and Lo, R.: *The physical and psychosocial consequences of opioid addiction: an overview of changes in opioid treatment,* Aust. NZ J. Ment. Health Nurs. **2000**, *9*, 65-74.

Brownstein, M.J.: *A brief history of opiates, opioid peptides, and opioid receptors,* Proc. Natl. Acad. Sci. USA. **1993**, *15*, 5391-5393.

Calo, G., Bigoni, R., Rizzi, A., Guerrini, R., Salvadori, S., Regoli, D.: *Nociceptin/orphanin FQ receptor ligand*s, Peptides **2000**, *21*, 935-947.

Campora, E., Merlini, L., Pace, M., Bruzzone, M., Luzzani, M., Gottlieb, A., Rosso, R.: *The incidence of narcotic-induced emesis,* J. Pain Symptom. Manage. **1991**, *6*, 428-430.

Casy, A.F. and Parfitt, R.T.: *Opioid analgesics. Chemistry and receptors,* Plenum Press, New York and London; **1986**.

Cherny, N.I.: *Opioid analgesics: comparative features and prescribing guidelines,* Drugs **1996**, *51*, 713-737.

Childers, S.R., Creese, I., Snowman, A.M., Synder, S.H.: *Opiate receptor binding affected differentially by opiates and opioid peptides,* Eur. J. Pharmacol. **1979**, *55*, 11-18.

Childers, S.R.: *Opioid receptor-coupled second messenger systems,* Life Sci. **1991**, *48*, 1991-2003.

De Luca, A. and Coupar, I.M.: *Insights into opioid action in the intestinal tract,* Pharmacol. Ther. **1996**, *69*, 103-115.

Dhawan, B.N., Cesselin, F., Raghubir, R., Reisine, T., Bradley, P.B., Portoghese, P.S., Hamon, M.: *International Union of Pharmacology. XII. Classification of opioid receptors,* Pharmacol. Rev. **1996**, *48*, 567-592.

Dondio, G., Ronzoni, S., Petrillo, P.: *Non-peptide δ opioid agonists and antagonists*, Exp. Opin. Ther. Patents **1997**, *7*, 1075-1098.

Evans, C.J., Keith, D.E., Jr., Morrison, H., Magendzo, K., Edwards, R.H.: *Cloning of a delta opioid receptor by functional expression*, Science **1992**, *258*, 1952-1955.

Etches, R.C., Sandler, A.N., Daley, M.D.: *Respiratory depression and spinal opioids*, Can. J. Anaesth. **1989**, *36*, 165-185.

Fowler, C.J. and Fraser, G.L.: *Mu-, delta-, kappa-opioid receptors and their subtypes. A critical review with emphasis on radioligand binding experiments*, Neurochem. Int. **1994**, *24*, 401-426.

Gaveriaux-Ruff, G. and Kieffer, B.: *Opioid receptors: Gene structure and function*, in: Opioids in pain control. Basic and clinical aspects, edited by C. Stein, **1999**, Cambridge University Press, Cambridge.

Gomes, I., Jordan, B.A., Gupta, A., Trapaidze, N., Nagy, V., Devi, L.A.: *Heterodimerization of mu and delta opioid receptors: A role in opiate synergy*, J. Neurosci. **2000**, *20*, RC110.

Heel, R.C., Brogden, R.N., Speight, T.M., Avery, G.S.: *Loperamide: a review of its pharmacological properties and therapeutic efficacy in diarrhoea*, Drugs **1978**, *15*, 33-52.

Heit, HA.: *The truth about pain management: the difference between a pain patient and an addicted patient*, Eur. J. Pain. **2001**, *5*, Suppl. A, 27-29.

Herz, A.: *Multiple opiate receptors and their functional significance*, J. Neural. Transm. Suppl. **1983**, *18*, 227-233.

Hoskin, P.J., Hanks, G.W.: *Opioid agonist-antagonist drugs in acute and chronic pain states*, Drugs **1991**, *41*, 326-344.

Jackson, F.W.: *Fentanyl and the wooden chest*, Gastroenterology **1994**, *106*, 820-821.

Jacobs, A.M. and Youngblood, F.: *Opioid receptor affinity for agonist-antagonist analgesics*, J. Am. Paediatr. Med. Assoc. **1992**, *82*, 520-524.

Jadad, A.R. and Browman, G.P.: *The WHO analgesic ladder for cancer pain management. Stepping up the quality of its evaluation*, JAMA **1995**, *274*, 1870-1873.

Janssen, P.A. and Jageneau, A.H.: *A new series of potent analgesics: Dextro 2:2 diphenyl-3-methyl-4-morpholino-butyrylpyrrolidine and related amides*, J. Pharm. Pharmacol. **1957**, *9*, 381-400.

Janssen, P.A. and Van der Eycken, C.A.: *The chemical anatomy of potent morphine-like analgesics*, in: Drugs affecting the central nervous system, edited by A. Burger, **1968**, 25-60, Marcel Decker, New York.

Kieffer, B.L., Befort, K., Gaveriaux-Ruff, C., Hirth, C.G.: *The delta-opioid receptor: isolation of a cDNA by expression cloning and pharmacological characterization*, Proc. Natl. Acad. Sci. USA **1992**, *89*, 12048-12052.

Kieffer, B.L.: *Opioids: first lessons from knockout mice*, Trends Pharmacol. Sci. **1999**, *20*, 19-26.

Knapp, R.J., Malatynska, E., Collins, N., Fang, L., Wang, J.Y., Hruby, V.J., Roeske, W.R., Yamamura, H.I.: *Molecular biology and pharmacology of cloned opioid receptors*, FASEB J. **1995**, *9*, 516-525.

Kromer, W.: *Endogenous opioids, the enteric nervous system and gut motility*, Dig. Dis. **1990**, *8*, 361-373.

Law, P.Y. and Loh, H.H.: *Regulation of opioid receptor activities*, J. Pharmacol. Exp. Ther. **1999**, *289*, 607-624.

Lipp, J.: *Possible mechanisms of morphine analgesia*, Clin. Neuropharmacol. **1991**, *14*, 131-147.

Mancini, I. and Bruera, E.: *Constipation in advanced cancer patients*, Support. Care Cancer **1998**, *6*, 356-364.

Mansour, A., Fox, C.A., Akil, H., Watson, S.J.: *Opioid-receptor mRNA expression in the rat CNS: anatomical and functional implications*, Trends Neurosci. **1995**, *18*, 22-29.

Mansour, A., Watson, S.J., Akil, H.: *Opioid receptors: past, present and future*, Trends Neurosci. **1995**, *18*, 69-70.

Martin, W.R., Eades, C.G., Thompson, J.A., Huppler, R.E., Gilbert, P.E.: *The effects of morphine- and nalorphine- like drugs in the nondependent and morphine-dependent chronic spinal dog*, J. Pharmacol. Exp. Ther. **1976**, *197*, 517-532.

Martin, W.R.: *Pharmacology of opioids*, Pharmacol. Rev. **1983**, *35*, 283-323.

Matthes, H.W., Maldonado, R., Simonin, F., Valverde, O., Slowe, S., Kitchen, I., Befort, K., Dierich, A., Le Meur, M., Dolle, P., Tzavara, E., Hanoune, J., Roques, B.P., Kieffer, B.L.: *Loss of morphine-induced analgesia, reward effect and withdrawal symptoms in mice lacking the mu-opioid-receptor gene*, Nature **1996**, *383*, 819-823.

McFadzean, I.: *The ionic mechanisms underlying opioid actions*, Neuropeptides **1988**, *11*, 173-180.

Meunier, J.C., Mollereau, C., Toll, L., Suaudeau, C., Moisand, C., Alvinerie, P., Butour, J.L., Guillemot, J.C., Ferrara, P., Monsarrat, B.: *Isolation and structure of the endogenous agonist of opioid receptor-like ORL1 receptor*, Nature **1995**, *377*, 532-535.

Mollereau, C. and Mouledous, L.: *Tissue distribution of the opioid receptor-like (ORL1) receptor*, Peptides **2000**, *21*, 907-917.

Mulroy, M.F.: *Monitoring opioids*, Reg. Anesth. **1996**, *21*, Suppl, 89-93.

Noble, F., Smadja, C., Roques, B.P: *Role of endogenous cholecystokinin in the facilitation of mu-mediated antinociception by delta-opioid agonists*, J. Pharmacol. Exp. Ther. **1994**, *271*, 1127-1134.

Pasternak, G.W. and Wood, P.J.: *Multiple mu opiate receptors*, Life Sci. **1986**, *38*, 1889-1898.

Pfeiffer, A., Brantl, V., Herz, A., Emrich, H.M.: *Psychotomimesis mediated by kappa opiate receptors*, Science **1986**, *233*, 774-776.

Portoghese, P.S., Alreja, B.D., Larson, D.L.: *Allylprodine analogues as receptor probes. Evidence that phenolic and nonphenolic ligands interact with different subsites on identical opioid receptors*, J. Med. Chem. **1981**, *24*, 782-787.

Reder, R.F.: *Opioid formulations: tailoring to the needs in chronic pain*, Eur. J. Pain. **2001**, *5*, Suppl A, 109-111.

Reinscheid, R.K., Nothacker, H.P., Bourson, A., Ardati, A., Henningsen, R.A., Bunzow, J.R., Grandy, D.K., Langen, H., Monsma, F.J. Jr., Civelli, O.: *Orphanin FQ: a neuropeptide that activates an opioidlike G protein-coupled receptor*, Science **1995**, *270*, 792-794.

Scheideler, M.A.: *Evidence for the role of δ opioid agonists in pain signaling*, Curr. Opin. CPNS Invest. Drugs **2000**, *2*, 171-177.

Scopes, D.I.: *Recent developments in non-peptide kappa receptor agonists*, Drug Fut. **1993**, *18*, 933-947.

Shook, J.E., Watkins, W.D., Camporesi, E.M.: *Differential roles of opioid receptors in respiration, respiratory disease, and opiate-induced respiratory depression*, Am. Rev. Respir. Dis. **1990**, *142*, 895-909.

Simonds, W.F.: *The molecular basis of opioid receptor function*, Endocr. Rev. **1988**, *9*, 200-212.

Stefano, G.B., Scharrer, B., Smith, E.M., Hughes, T.K. Jr., Magazine, H.I., Bilfinger, T.V., Hartman, A.R., Fricchione, G.L., Liu, Y., Makman, M.H.: *Opioid and opiate immunoregulatory processes*, Crit. Rev. Immunol. **1996**, *16*, 109-144.

Stein, C., Cabot, P.J., Schafer, M.: *Peripheral opioid analgesia: Mechanisms and clinical implications,* in: Opioids in pain control. Basic and clinical aspects, edited by C. Stein, **1999**, Cambridge University Press, Cambridge.

Stein, C.: *Opioids in pain control. Basic and clinical aspects,* **1999**, Cambridge University Press, Cambridge.

Stein, C.: *Peripheral analgesic actions of opioids,* J. Pain Symptom. Manage. **1991**, *6*, 119-124.

Taylor, D.A. and Fleming, W.W.: *Unifying perspectives of the mechanisms underlying the development of tolerance and physical dependence to opioids,* J. Pharmacol. Exp. Ther. **2001**, *297*, 11-18.

Thomas, J.B., Herault, X.M., Rothman, R.B., Atkinson, R.N., Burgess, J.P., Mascarella, S.W., Dersch, C.M., Xu, H., Flippen-Anderson, J.L., George, C.F., Carroll, F.I.: *Factors influencing agonist potency and selectivity for the opioid delta receptor are revealed in structure-activity relationship studies of the 4-[(N-substituted-4-piperidinyl)arylamino]-N,N-diethylbenzamides,* J. Med. Chem. **2001**, *44*, 972-987.

Vaught, J.L., Rothman, R.B., Westfall, T.C.: *Mu and delta receptors: their role in analgesia in the differential effects of opioid peptides on analgesia,* Life Sci. **1982**, *30*, 1443-1455.

Watson, C.P.: *The treatment of neuropathic pain: antidepressants and opioids,* Clin. J. Pain **2000**, *16*, S49-55.

WHO. *Cancer pain relief,* **1986**, World Health Organisation, Geneva.

Wood, P.L.: *Multiple opiate receptors: support for unique mu, delta and kappa sites,* Neuropharmacology **1982**, *21*, 487-497.

Yaksh, T.L.: *Pharmacology and mechanisms of opioid analgesic activity,* Acta Anaesthesiol. Scand. **1997**, *41*, 94-111.

3.2 Opioid Peptides

Bernd Sundermann and Corinna Maul

Introduction

Opioids, the most important analgesics for the treatment of moderate to severe pain, can be divided into three groups (Buschmann et al., 2002):

- Morphine and codeine as well as their natural and synthetic derivatives ultimately derived from opium ('opiates')

- Purely synthetic non-peptidic compounds with opioid properties but non-morphinan structure

- Naturally-occurring and synthetic opioid peptides

Classification of µ-opioids

Discovery of Endogenous Opioids

While morphine as a component of opium has been in use for centuries and the first synthetic opioid, pethidin, was prepared as early as 1939, opioid peptides, the endogenous pentapeptides Met- and Leu-enkephalin (YGGFM and YGGFL), were identified in brain extracts only in 1975 by Kosterlitz and Waterfield (Hughes et al., 1975; also see: Cox et al., 1975; Hughes, 1975; Lord et al., 1977).

Discovery of Met- and Leu-enkephalin

Met- (X = Met) & Leu-enkephalin (X = Leu)
(YGGFX = H-Tyr-Gly-Gly-Phe-X-OH)

These peptides were characterized *in vitro* and found to be powerful opioid agonists in the mouse vas deferens (MVD) and guinea pig ileum (GPI) assay. In vivo (rat tail-flick) they are only active when administered directly to the brain – a general limitation of simple linear peptides consisting of natural L-amino acids – but with less potency and shorter duration of action than morphine (Casy and Parfitt, 1986).

Simple linear peptides consisting of natural L-amino acids are rapidly broken down *in vivo* (and in many *in vitro* systems) by ubiquitously occurring aminopeptidases

This discovery was the starting point for further investigations that led to the identification of more endogenous opioids. Remarkably, not all endogenous opioids have been isolated from animal brains: the

Discovery of further endogenous opioid peptides

Amino acid sequences of prominent endogenous opioid peptides are given in Table 1

dermorphins and deltorphins (see below) have been identified in skin extracts of the South African frogs *Phyllomedusa sauvagei* and *Phyllomedusa bicolor*, respectively (Montecucchi et al., 1981; Erspamer et al., 1989). The opioid peptides β-casomorphine-5 (YPFPG) and morphiceptin (YPFP-amid) are fragments of bovine β-casein (Brandt et al., 1979; Holzgrabe et al., 1997).

Table 1: Selected human opioid peptide sequences.
(with modifications from Straßburger and Friderichs, 2002)

Peptide	Amino acid sequence	Selectivity
Endomorphin-1[1]	**Y** *P* W **F**-amid	μ
Endomorphin-2[1]	**Y** *P* F **F**-amid	μ
β-Endorphin[2]	**YGGF** *M* T S E **K** S Q T P L V T L F K N A I I K N A Y K K G E	μ = δ
Met-Enkephalin[3]	**YGGF** *M*	δ > μ
Leu-Enkephalin[3]	**YGGFL**	δ > μ
Methorphamid[3]	**YGGF** *M* **R R** V-amid	μ >> δ > κ
Dynorphin A[4]	**YGGFLRR** I **R** P **K** L **K** W **D N Q**	κ >> μ, δ
Dynorphin B[4]	**YGGFLRR** Q F **K** V V T	κ >> μ, δ
α-Neoendorphin[4]	**YGGFLR** K Y P *K*	κ >> μ, δ
Nociceptin[5]	F **GGF** T G A R **K** S A R **K** L A N **Q**	ORL1

Corresponding amino acids are shown in bold or italic.
Precursor peptides: [1]pro-endomorphin*, [2]pro-opiomelanocortin, [3]pro-enkephalin, [4]pro-dynorphin, [5]pro-nociceptin (* presumed to exist).

Amino acid one letter code:

A: alanine	F: phenylalanine	K: lysine	P: proline	T: threonine
C: cysteine	G: glycine	L: leucine	Q: glutamine	V: valine
D: asparagic acid	H: histidine	M: methionine	R: arginine	W: tryptophane
E: glutamic acid	I: isoleucine	N: asparagine	S: serine	Y: tyrosine

Biological role of endogenous opioids

Endogenous opioids influence a variety of biological functions (reviewed yearly, see Vaccarino and Kastin, 2001), but particularly pain perception: while acute pain in itself has a protective function for the organism, in a 'fight or flight' situation - as an extreme example - endogenous opioids may render even excruciating pain tolerable and thus assure survival. Furthermore, endogenous opioids are released in stressful situations and are assumed to be at least partly responsible for the euphoria sometimes experienced by athletes. The biological functions of the heptadecapeptide nociceptin (Meunier et al., 1995; Reinscheid et al., 1995), the endogenous agonist of ORL1, the latest member of the opioid receptor family to be identified, are still a topic of intensive investigation.

Opioid peptides with the common N-terminal sequence YGGF, the so-called 'opioid message area', do not show a very pronounced selectivity for μ, δ or κ receptors. β-Endorphin for example is non-selective with respect to μ and δ receptors while the enkephalins bind an order of magnitude more potently to δ receptors. The highly selective endomorphins and nociceptin on the other hand differ specifically in the classical 'message area'. In this respect today the N-terminal tetrapeptide sequence YGGF is considered to be necessary and sufficient for μ and δ receptor affinity, Y (Tyr^1) and F (Phe^4) being essential, while additional C-terminal amino acids are necessary for κ receptor affinity.

Subtype selectivity of endogenous opioids

The μ selectivity of the endomorphins (and morphiceptin) is thought to arise from the substitution of Gly^2 by the cyclic amino acid proline which significantly increases rigidity of the peptide backbone. With an N-terminal F instead of Y, nociceptin (NC) lacks the aromatic hydroxy function common among natural as well as many synthetic opioids. Although NC has some structural similarity to dynorphin A and β-endorphin, this major difference sets NC apart from all other known endogenous opioids and thus is believed to give rise to its selectivity.

Endomorphins and nociceptin – subtype selective endogenous opioids

Synthetic Peptidic Tool Compounds

Endogenous opioid peptides and structurally related tool compounds have played an important role in the differentiation and characterization of opioid receptor subtypes as well as in the elucidation of opioid receptor function. A selection of prominent opioid peptides is given below (review: Hruby and Gehrig, 1989):

...derived from enkephalin; deltorphins and dermorphin

- **DALAMID**: [D-Ala^2]Leu-enkephalin   H-Tyr-D-Ala-Gly-Phe-Leu-OH
- **DADL(E)**: [D-Ala^2,D-Leu^5]enkephalin   H-Tyr-D-Ala-Gly-Phe-D-Leu-OH
- **DSL(E)T**: [D-Ser^2,Thr^6]enkephalin   H-Tyr-D-Ser-Gly-Phe-Leu-Thr-OH
- **DTLET**: [D-Thr^2,Leu^5,Thr^6]enkephalin   H-Tyr-D-Thr-Gly-Phe-Leu-Thr-OH
- **DA(M)GO**: [D-Ala^2,MePhe^4,Gly-ol^5]enkephalin   H-Tyr-D-Ala-Gly-N(CH$_3$)Phe-Gly-ol
- **DALCE**: [D-Ala^2,D-Leu^5,Cys^6]enkephalin   H-Tyr-D-Ala-Gly-Phe-D-Leu-Cys-OH
- **DAMME**: [D-Ala^2,MePhe^4,Met(O)-ol^5]enkephalin H-Tyr-D-Ala-Gly-N(CH$_3$)Phe-Met(O)-ol
- **[D-Met^2,Pro^5]enkephalinamide**   H-Tyr-D-Met-Gly-Phe-Pro-NH$_2$
- **[D-Ala^2]deltorphin I**   H-Tyr-D-Ala-Phe-Asp-Val-Val-Gly-NH$_2$
- **[D-Ala^2]deltorphin II**   H-Tyr-D-Ala-Phe-Glu-Val-Val-Gly-NH$_2$
- **[D-Ala^2]dermorphin**   H-Tyr-D-Ala-Phe-Gly-Tyr-Pro-Ser-NH$_2$
- **DALDA**:   H-Tyr-D-Arg-Phe-Lys-NH$_2$

Unfavorable pharmacokinetic properties of opioid peptides (very short half-life; inability to cross the blood-brain barrier) prohibit their therapeutic use as analgesics.

While opioid peptides have been very useful for investigating the pharmacology of different opioid receptor subtypes, pharmacological investigations have established that no pharmacodynamic advantage is to be expected from opioid peptides with respect to analgesic activity or side-effects. Furthermore, they have their own shortcomings with respect to potential clinical applications. Most importantly their peptidic structure usually prohibits administration by the oral or transdermal route, which are the routes of choice for pain treatment.

Strategies for the design and synthesis of more stable opioid peptides

Therefore, until the present time not a single opioid peptide has become a marketed drug, although many attempts have been made to overcome their serious disadvantages in comparison to non-peptidic opioids. Among others, the following strategies have been followed:

- Incorporation of 'unnatural' D-amino acids (e.g. D-Ala instead of Gly^2)
- Incorporation of derivatized L-amino acids (e.g. N-methylated Phe^4 or Met^5 with an oxidized sulfide side chain)
- Conversion of the terminal COOH to an amide (e.g. $CONH_2$) or reduction to CH_2OH
- Formation of cyclic peptides (e.g. DPDPE) less prone to enzymatic degradation by aminopeptidases
- Formation of peptide dimers or oligomers (e.g. biphalin)
- Incorporation of β-amino acids

Parenterally-active Opioid Peptides

FK 33-824 (DAMME)

The first significant advances towards parenterally-active opioid peptides were made by a Sandoz group (Roemer et al., 1977; Pless et al., 1979). Within the pentapeptide [D-Ala^2,$MePhe^4$,$Met(O)$-ol^5]enkephalin (FK 33-824, DAMME) several approaches towards a stable enkephalin analog have been combined. FK 33-824 has been reported to be several orders of magnitude more potent than morphine when applied i.c.v. and to be orally active.

[D-Met^2,Pro^5]enkephalin-amide

[D-Met^2,Pro^5]enkephalinamide has been shown to be nearly equipotent to FK 33-824 when administered i.v. (Casy and Parfitt, 1986, p. 352).

Biphalin
(H-Tyr-D-Ala-Gly-Phe-NH_2)$_2$

The dimeric tetrapeptide hydrazide biphalin, essentially an abbreviated enkephalin dimer, is a potent μ and δ receptor agonist preclinically evaluated as a potential analgesic (Horan et al., 1993). When administered via the i.c.v. route in mice it was found to be two orders of magnitude more potent than morphine. Although biphalin crosses the blood-brain barrier, its clinical development was halted due to low plasma stability.

The agonistic δ_1 selective enkephaline analog DPDPE is conformationally constrained through the formation of a disulfide bond between Pen^2 and Pen^5 (Mosberg et al., 1983) and is reported to have an enhanced stability in blood ($t_{1/2}$ > 500 min; Weber et al., 1991). While DPDPE - as well as its even more potent [p-Cl-Phe^4] derivative - crosses the blood-brain barrier in mice after systemic and oral administration, DPDPE is also a substrate for the P-glycoprotein efflux mechanism (Witt et al., 2000) and is rapidly excreted biliarily (Weber et al., 1992; Chen and Pollack, 1997).

DPDPE

[D-Pen^2,D-Pen^5]enkephalin

(H-Tyr-D-Pen-Gly-Phe-D-Pen-OH)

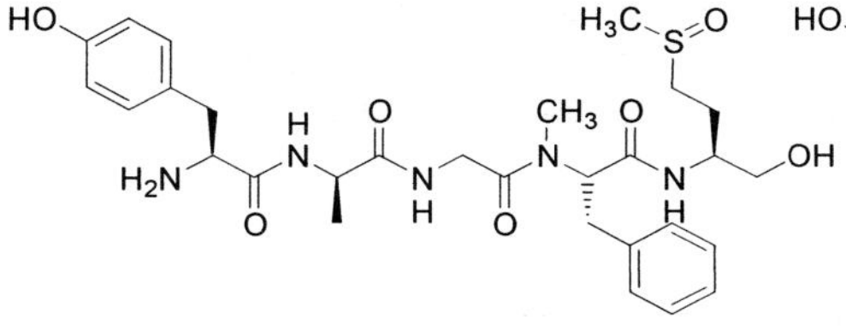

FK 33-824 (DAMME)

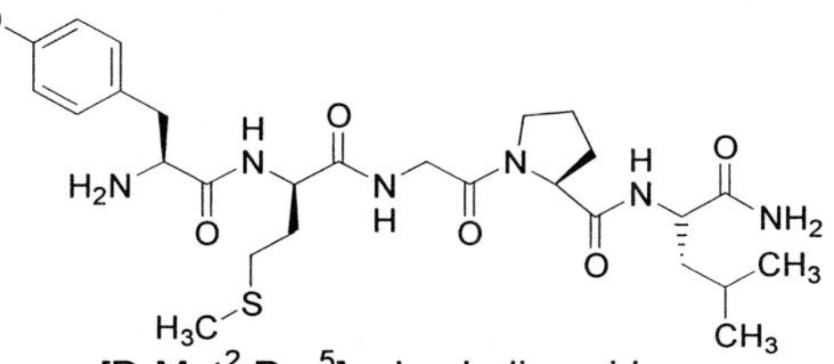

[D-Met^2,Pro^5]enkephalinamide

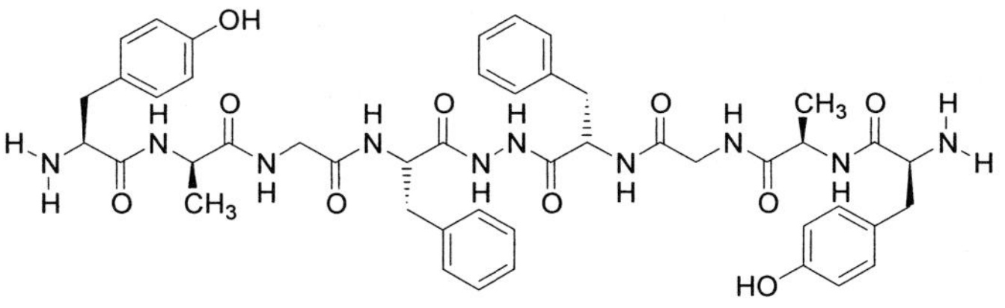

Biphalin

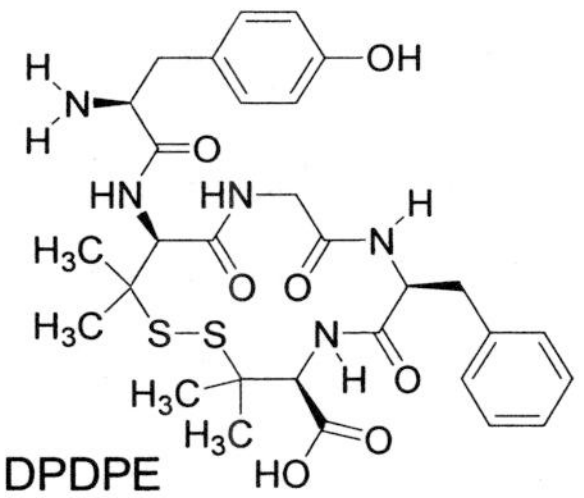

DPDPE

While no further development of FK 33-824, Biphalin, DPDPE or other prominent opioid peptides has been reported, opioid peptides are still among the most important tool compounds in opioid receptor pharmacology. An overview is given in Table 2 (Corbett et al., 2002):

Important peptidic tool compounds for opioid receptors

Table 2: Peptidic opioid receptor tool compounds.

	μ	δ		κ	ORL1
agonists	DA(M)GO Endomorphin I Endomorphin II	δ_1:	DPDPE (DADL(E))	-	nociceptin
		δ_2:	[D-Ala2]deltorphin I [D-Ala2]deltorphin II (DSLET)		
antagonists	-	δ_1:	(DALCE)	-	-

Patent applications disclosed in the last several years reveal further activities directed towards the discovery and potential development of opioid peptides as analgesics (e.g. Kim et al. (Biomeasure Inc.), 1994; Dooley and Houghten (Torrey Pines Institute for Molecular Studies), 1996-1999; Grandy et al. (Oregon Health Sciences University), 1998; Kahn et al. (Molecumetics Ltd.), 1998; Moreau et al. (Biomeasure Inc.), 1997; Wang (Astra Aktiebolag), 1997); Junien et al. (Ferring B.V.), 1999; Persons et al. (Sepracor Inc.), 1999; Sakurada et al. (Daiichi Pharmaceutical Co.), 1999; Szeto (Cornell Research Foundation), 2002). Selected examples include:

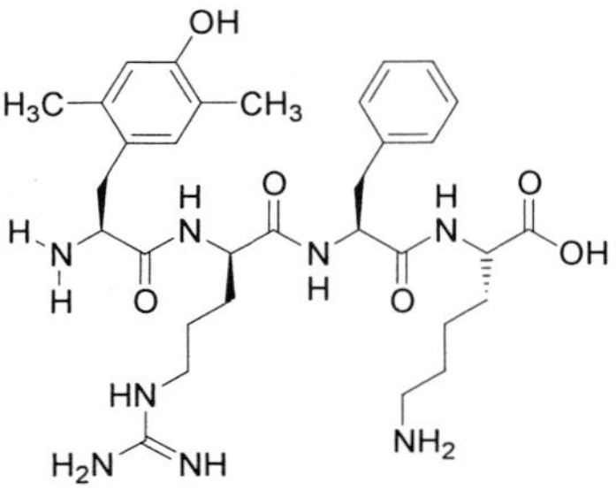

cpd. 1 - [Dmt[1]]DALDA (Szeto, 2002)

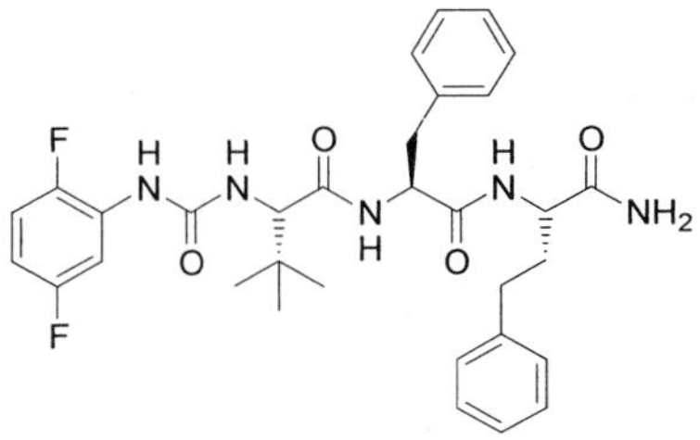

cpd. 2 (Persons et al., 1999)

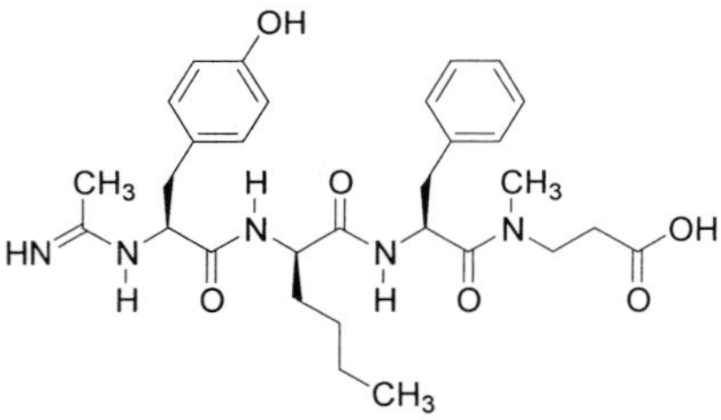

cpd. 3 (Sakurada et al., 1999)

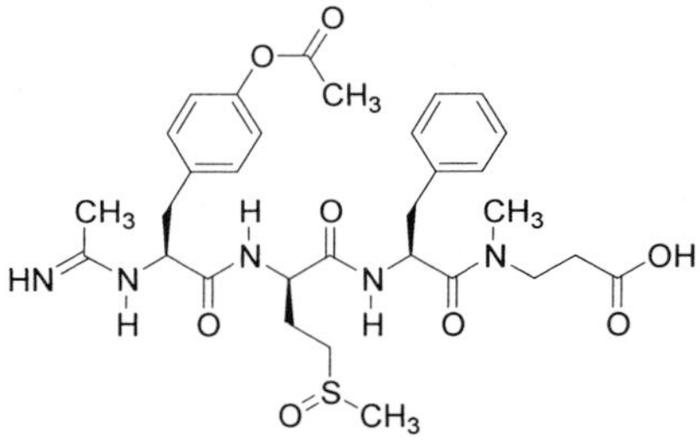

cpd. 4 (Sakurada et al., 1999)

Cpds. 3 and 4 have been described to be orally active in a tail pressure-stress assay in mice with ED_{50} values of 7.9 and 1.2 mg/kg, respectively, compared to 22 mg/kg for morphine.

Summary

Opioid peptides have an action and side-effect profile identical to non-peptidic opioids, but in general have significantly less favorable physicochemical and pharmacokinetic properties. Considering the numerous attempts to overcome these drawbacks undertaken since the mid-1970s that have not resulted in a single opioid peptide being successfully developed for clinical use, it seems unlikely to expect opioid peptides to ever reach the market. Nevertheless, recent patent activity discloses opioid peptides still to be considered as potential analgesics (see above).

References

Brandt, V. and Teschemacher, H.: *A material with opioid activity in bovine milk and milk products*, Naunyn-Schmiedeberg's Arch. Pharmacol. **1979**, *306*, 301-304.

Brandt, V., Teschemacher, H., Henschen, A., Lottspeich, F.: *Novel opioid peptides derived from casein (beta-casomorphins). I. Isolation from bovine casein peptone*, Hoppe-Seyler's Z. Physiol. Chem. **1979**, *360*, 1211-1216.

Buschmann, H., Sundermann, B., Maul, C.: *μ-Selektive Opioide ohne Morphinanstruktur (μ-selective opioids without morphinan structures)*, Pharmazie i. u. Zeit **2002**, *31*, 44-50.

Casy, A.F. and Parfitt, R.T.: *Enkephalins, endorphins, and other opioid peptides*, in *Opioid analgesics – chemistry and receptors*, **1986**, 333-384, Plenum Press, New York.

Chen, C. and Pollack, G.M.: *Extensive biliary excretion of the model opioid peptide [D-Pen^{2,5}] enkephalin in rats*, Pharm. Res. (NY) **1997**, *14*, 345-350.

Corbett, A., McKnight, S., Henderson, G.: *Opioid receptors*, http://opioids.com/receptors, **2002**.

Cox, B.M., Opheim, K.E., Teschemacher, H., Goldstein, A.: *A peptide-like substance from pituitary that acts like morphine*, Life Sci. **1975**, *16*, 1777-1782.

Dooley, C. and Houghten, R. (Torrey Pines Institute for Molecular Studies): *Novel mu opioid receptor ligands: agonists and antagonists*, WO9640208 (**1996**); US5641861 (**1997**); US5919897 (**1999**).

Dooley, C. and Houghten, R. (Torrey Pines Institute for Molecular Studies): *Novel kappa receptor selective opioid peptides*, WO9640206 (**1996**), US5610271 (**1997**).

Erspamer, V., Melchiorri, P., Falconieri-Erspamer, G., Negri, L., Corsi, R., Severini, C., Barra, D., Simmaco, M., Kreil, G.: *Deltorphins: a family of naturally occurring peptides with high affinity and selectivity for δ opioid binding sites*, Proc. Natl. Acad. Sci. USA **1989**, *86*, 5188-5192.

Grandy, D.K., Bunzow, J.R., Civelli, O., Reinscheid, R.K., Nothacker, H.-P., Monsma, F.J. (Oregon Health Sciences University): *Mammalian opioid receptor ligand and uses*, US5837809 (**1975**).

Horan, P.J., Mattia, A., Bilsky, E.J., Weber, S., Davis, T.P., Yamamura, H.I., Malatynska, E., Appleyard, S.M., Slaninova, J., Misicka, A.: *Antinociceptive profile of biphalin, a dimeric enkephalin analog*, J. Pharmacol. Exp. Ther. **1993**, *265*, 1446-1454.

Holzgrabe, U., Nachtsheim, C., Siener, T., Drosihn, S., Brandt, W.: *Opioid-Agonisten und -Antagonisten, Opioid-Rezeptoren (Opioid-agonists and -antagonists, opioid-receptors)*, Pharmazie **1997**, *52*, 4-22.

Hughes, J.: *Isolation of an endogenous compound from the brain with pharmacological properties similar to morphine*, Brain Res. **1975**, *88*, 205-308.

Hughes, J., Smith, T.W., Kosterlitz, H.W., Fothergill, L.A., Morgan, B.A., Morris, H.R.: *Identification of two related pentapeptides from the brain with potent opiate agonist activity*, Nature **1975**, *258*, 577-580.

Hruby, V. and Gehrig, C.A.: *Recent developments in the design of receptor specific opioid peptides*, Med. Chem. Res. **1989**, *9*, 343-401.

Junien, J.L., Riviere, P.J.M., Schteingart, C., Diaz, J.S., Trojnar, J.A., Vanderah, T.W. (Ferring B.V.): *Kappa receptor opioid peptides*, WO9932510 (**1999**).

Kahn, M.S., Eguchi, M., Kim, H.-O. (Molecumetics Ltd.): *Reverse-turn mimetics and methods relating thereto*, WO9849168 (**1998**).

Kim, S.H., Moreau, J.-P., Taylor, J.E. (Biomeasure Inc.): *Opioid peptides*, WO9411018 (**1994**).

Lord, J.A.H., Waterfield, A.A., Hughes, J., Kosterlitz, H.W.: *Endogenous opioid peptides: multiple agonists and receptors*, Nature **1977**, *267*, 495-499.

Meunier, J.-C., Mollereau, C., Toll, L., Suaudeau, C., Moisand, C., Alvinerie, P., Butour, J.-L., Guillemot, J.-C., Ferrara, P., Monsarrat, B., Mazargil, H., Vassart, G., Parmentier, M., Costentin, J.: *Isolation and structure of the endogenous agonist of the opioid receptor-like ORL1 receptor*, Nature **1995**, *377*, 532-535.

Montecucchi, P.C., de Castiglione, R., Piani, S., Gozzini, L., Erspamer, V.: *Amino acid composition and sequence of dermorphin, a novel opiate-like peptide from the skin of Phyllomedusa sauvagei*, Int. J. Peptide Protein Res. **1981**, *17*, 275-283.

Moreau, J.-P., Kim, S.H., Taylor, J.E. (Biomeasure Inc.): *Opioid peptides*, US5663295 (**1997**).

Mosberg, H.I., Hurst, R., Hruby, V.J., Gee, K., Akiyama. K., Yamamura, H.I., Galligan, J.J., Burks, T.F.: *Cyclic penicillamine containing enkephalin analogs display profound delta receptor selectivities*, Life Sci **1983**, *33 Suppl. 1*, 447-50.

Persons, P.E., Hauske, J., Hussoin, R.A. (Sepracor Inc.): *Tetrapeptides, analogs and peptidomimetics which bind selectively mammalian opioid receptors*, WO9965932 (**1999**).

Pless, J., Bauer, W., Cardinaux, F., Closse, A., Hauser, D., Hugenin, R., Roemer, D., Buescher, H.-H., Hill, R.C.: *Synthesis, opiate receptor binding and analgesic activity of enkephalin analogues*, Helv. Chim. Acta **1979**, *62*, 398-411.

Reinscheid, R.K., Nothacker, H.-P., Bourson, A., Ardati, A., Hennigsen, R.A., Bunzow, J.R., Grandy, D.K., Langen, H., Monsma, F.J. Jr., Civelli, O.: *Orphanin FQ: A neuropeptide that activates an opioid like G protein-coupled receptor*, Science **1995**, *270*, 792-794.

Roemer D., Buescher H. H., Hill R. C., Pless J., Bauer W., Cardinaux F., Closse A., Hauser D., Huguenin R., *A synthetic enkephalin analogue with prolonged parenteral and oral analgesic activity*, Nature **1977**, *268*, 547-549

Sakurada, S., Hagiwara, M., Miyamae, T., Okayama, T., Ogawa, T., Oya, T., Nukui, E., Yagisawa, M., (Daiichi Pharmaceutical Co.): *Preparation of peptide derivatives as opioid peptides for prevention and treatment of pains*, WO9933864 (**1999**).

Straßburger, W. and Friderichs, E.: *Ironman, Muttermilch und Krötenhaut (Ironman, mother's milk and frog skin)*, Pharmazie i.u. Zeit. **2002**, *31*, 52-58.

Szeto, H. (Cornell Research Foundation): *Mu-opioid receptor agonist peptide*, WO0205748 (**2002**).

Vaccarino, A.L. and Kastin, A.J.: *Endogenous opiates: 2000*, Peptides **2001**, *22*, 2257-2328.

Wang, W. (Astra Aktiebolag): *Novel opioid peptides*, WO9707130 (**1997**).

Weber, S.J., Greene, D.L., Sharma, S.D., Yamamura, H.I., Kramer, T.H., Burks, T.F., Hruby, V.J., Hersh, L.B., Davis, T.P.: *Distribution and analgesia of [³H] [D-Pen², D-Pen⁵]enkephalin and two halogenated analogs after intravenous administration*, J. Pharmacol. Exp. Ther. **1991**, *259*, 1109-1117.

Weber, S.J., Greene, D.L., Hruby, V.J., Yamamura, H.I., Porreca, F., Davis, T.P.: *Whole body and brain distribution of [³H]cyclic [D-Pen², D-Pen⁵]enkephalin after intraperitoneal, intravenous, oral and subcutaneous administration*, J. Pharmacol. Exp. Ther. **1992**, *263*, 1308-1316.

Witt, K.A., Slate, C.A., Egleton, R.D., Huber, J.D., Yamamura, H.I., Hruby, V.J., Davis, T.P.: *Assessment of stereoselectivity of trimethylphenylalanine analogues of δ-opioid [D-Pen², Pen⁵]-enkephalin*, J. Neurochem., **2000**, *75*, 424-435.

3.3   Synthetic Opioids

Corinna Maul, Helmut Buschmann, and Bernd Sundermann

Introduction

Morphine has always been an accepted standard analgesic, the medicament without which, until recently, no one could practice medicine effectively. Its use, however, bears some risks of side-effects. If the dose is only a little too high, breathing may be depressed to a life-threatening degree. Nausea, vomiting, sweating, dizziness, and sluggishness occur frequently. The heart rate is slowed and the blood pressure may fall. With repeated use of morphine, the analgesic effects wane and the dose has to be increased. Furthermore, morphine can cause addiction, an accommodation of the cells of the body to its presence so that its use must be continued or a withdrawal syndrome appears. Thus the search for a better analgesic is a search for a better morphine, a substance with morphine's beneficial properties and with attenuated or no harmful side-effects including tolerance and dependence (Eddy and May, 1973).

Following the isolation of morphine by Sertürner in 1805 further alkaloids were isolated from opium, for example narcotine in 1817, codeine in 1832, thebaine in 1835 and papaverine in 1848.

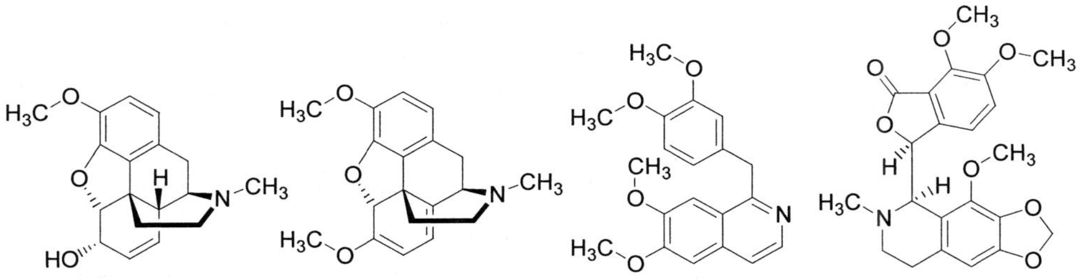

1805	Morphine
1874	Heroin
1925	Oxycodone
1939	**Pethidine**
1946	**Methadone**
1961	**Fentanyl**
1962	**Tramadol**
1965	**Tilidine**

Scheme 1: Opium alkaloids isolated in the 19th century.

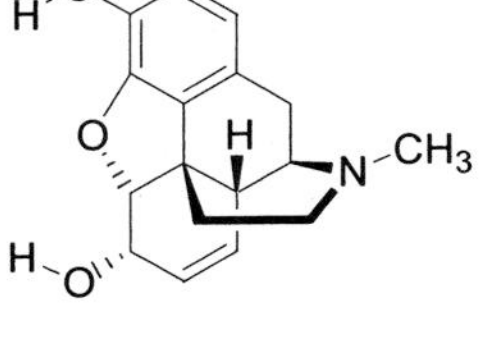

The earliest attempts to develop a non-dependence-inducing morphine derivative resulted in the preparation of heroin (3,6-diacetylmorphine) by acetylation of morphine (Wright, 1874, Dreser, 1898). The potency of heroin was soon recognized. It underwent more investigation than any other product of the time, and was introduced into clinical medicine in 1898. Reports of its reduced respiratory depression and dependence liability were soon shown to be unfounded, but its analgesic effects in animals and man (twice morphine) were confirmed. Pharmacological examination of acyl derivatives of morphine showed that

Morphine

heroin and its higher and lower acyl homologs have similar analgesic potencies in rodents and have high physical dependence liability (May and Jacobson, 1977).

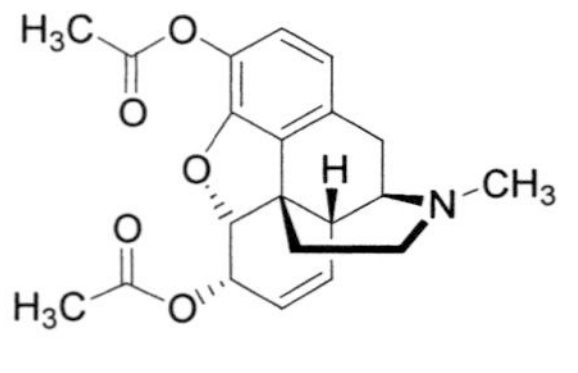

The introduction of heroin, although based on inaccurate observations and interpretation, undoubtedly influenced the trend and objectives of morphine research and marked the beginning of the search for an improved analgesic. During the 25 years after the introduction of heroin, other morphine derivatives were incorporated into medical practice some of which are still being used today. These include dihydrocodeine, differing from codeine only in the saturation of one double bond, hydrocodone (dihydrocodeinone) which is very similar in activity, having in addition one hydroxyl replaced by a keto group and an effective dose one-sixth that of codeine, and thebacon (acetyldihydrocodeinone) an acetylation product of hydrocodone and similar to it in activity. All of these are analgesics, but mainly used as antitussives. Also introduced in that period was hydromorphone (dihydromorphinone) which is very similar to heroin in its action.

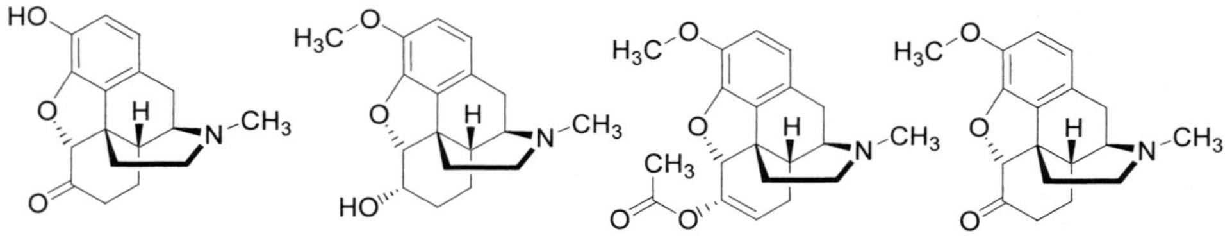

Heroin

Hydromorphone   Dihydrocodeine   Thebacon   Hydrocodone

Scheme 2: Opioids introduced into clinical practice at the beginning of the 20th century.

The Search for Opioids with Reduced Side-Effects

In the 1920s a most significant change in analgesic research came about: the beginning of the first systematic study of structure-action relationships which endeavored to separate analgesic effectiveness from side-effects and addiction liability.

In the USA, this plan was directed from 1929-1939 by the Committee on Drug Addiction of the National Research Council (NRC) with financial support from the Rockefeller Foundation. The program consisted of modification of the morphine molecule at all accessible points and also targeted (modified) partial structures of the morphine molecule, such as phenanthrene, hydrogenated phenanthrene, isoquinoline, dibenzofuran, and carbazole. More than 150 derivatives of morphine and more than 300 synthetic products were tested for analgesic, respiratory, gastrointestinal, sedative, and other central nervous system effects. The significance of the phenolic and alcoholic hydroxyls for intensity of analgesic action was established. Removal of the latter, as in desomorphine, resulted in the most rapidly acting and potent analgesic known at that time (Eddy and May, 1973).

After 10 years of intensive research, no significant dissociation of potent analgesia and dependence liability was accomplished. As an indirect result of the systematic program the identification of the 17-hydroxy-7,8-dihydro compounds oxycodone (patented in 1925 by E. Merck AG, Germany) and oxymorphone, derived from thebaine, are of particular note.

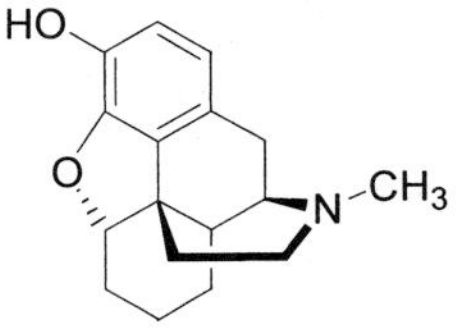

Desomorphine

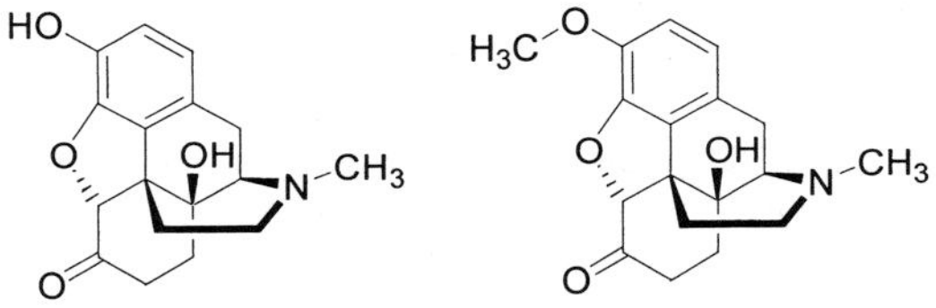

Oxymorphone   Oxycodone

Scheme 3: Structures of oxymorphone and oxycodone.

During the late 1930s some 4-phenylpiperidine derivatives were examined as potential spasmolytics on the basis of their chemical relationship to atropine. The antinociceptive properties of one member, ethyl 1-methyl-4-phenyl-piperidine-4-carboxylate, was detected in screening tests and the compound was subsequently introduced into clinical use by Eisleb and Schaumann in 1939. The compound, well known as pethidine in Europe and meperidine in North America (proprietary names include Demerol, Dolantin, and Dolosal), was soon in widespread use for the relief of pain, and it is remarkable how pethidine, the original non-opioid-derived opioid analgesic, has retained its popularity for many years in the face of competition from other synthetic analgesics introduced since 1939.

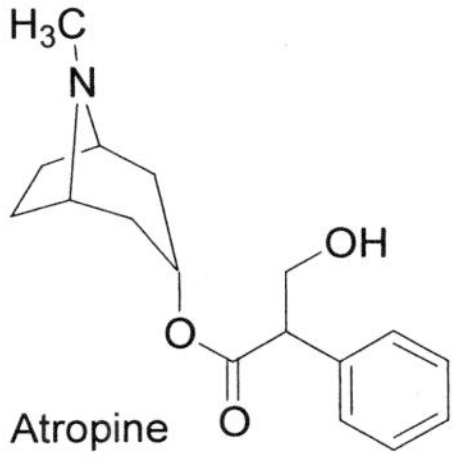

Atropine

Thousands of phenylpiperidines, related to pethidine, were synthesized during the following years. Some of these variations and other drugs which were developed are shown in scheme 4. But again there has been no significant progress in relating specific structural features with analgesia or side-effects and dependence.

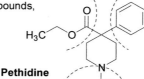

Ketobemidone

structural variation:
- other esters (bulky esters usually reduce activity, except adamantyl
- inversed esters (usually leads to an increase in potency)
- ether or keto oxygen functions (leads to analgesic compounds, e.g. ketobemidone)

replacement by other aromatic groups:
- gross increase in size leads to inactive compounds
- replacement of phenyl by heteroaromatic groups is usually disadvantageous in analgesics (*exception: 2-furyl, 2-thienyl*)
- substitution generally leads to fall in activity (*exception: the presence of a meta phenolic hydroxyl in ketobemidone elevates activity 13-14 times*)

Pethidine

structural variation:
alkyl, phenalkyl, N- or O-containing alkyl substituents lead to various new analgesics; some of them have been used clinically but have only a historical role
examples: anileridine, piminodine, phenoperidine, furethidine

Anileridine   Piminodine   Phenoperidine   Furethidine

further variations:
- alkyl substitution in the piperidine ring (examples: α-prodin (nisentil), trimeperidine (γ-promedol))
- ring size (examples: profadol, meptazinol)

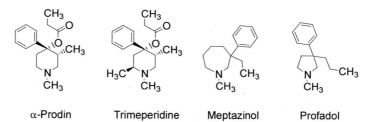

α-Prodin   Trimeperidine   Meptazinol   Profadol

Scheme 4: Variations of the pethidine structure. Ketobemidone and pethidine itself are the only compounds which are still in frequent clinical use.

During World War II, chemists working in the Hoechst Laboratories of I.G. Farbenindustrie discovered that certain derivatives of 3,3-diphenyl-N,N-dimethylpropyl-amine have analgesic properties. The best known member of this group, 6-dimethylamino-4,4-diphenylheptan-3-one (methadone), was introduced into clinical practice in 1946. The path from pethidine to the methadone structure was never clearly revealed, but both contain several features in common with morphine and with each other. Methadone matched the pharmacological profile of morphine qualitatively, but there are significant differences in the time-courses of action. It is as effective as morphine as an analgesic but longer acting when administered orally. Compared with morphine and heroin, the methadone abstinence syndrome is slower in onset, longer in duration, and much less intense.

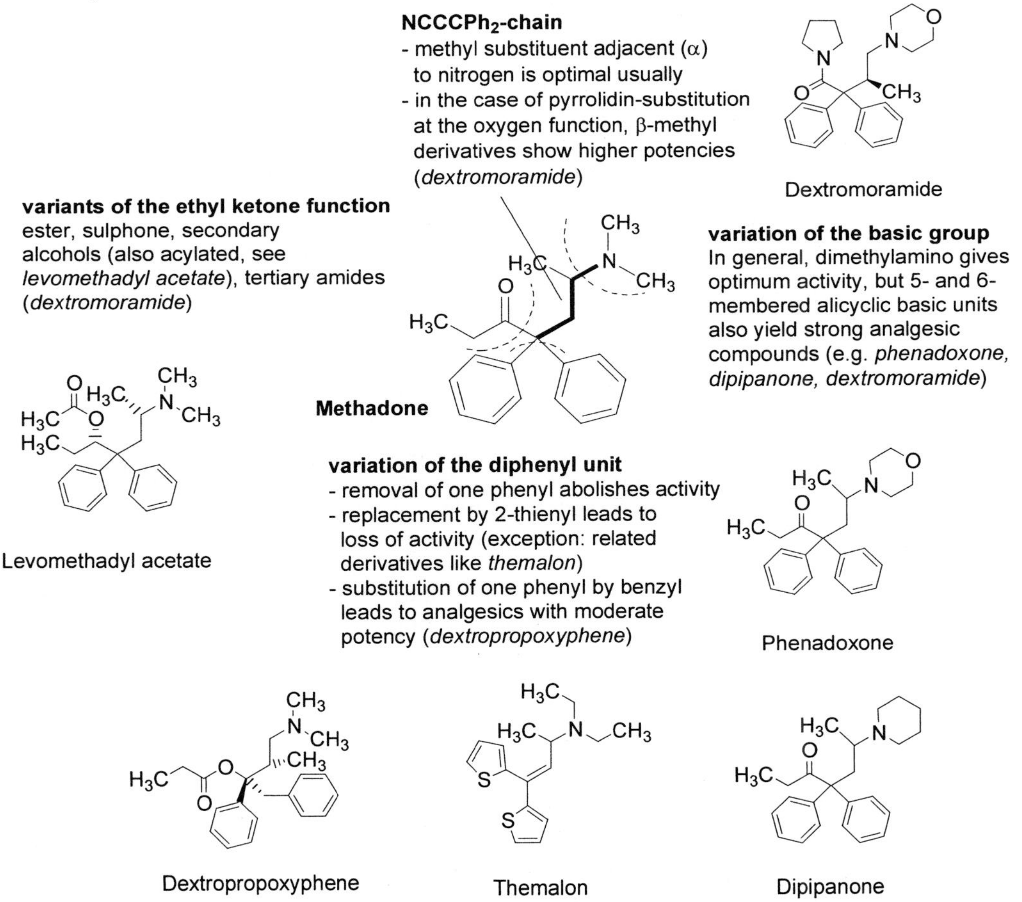

NCCCPh₂-chain
- methyl substituent adjacent (α) to nitrogen is optimal usually
- in the case of pyrrolidin-substitution at the oxygen function, β-methyl derivatives show higher potencies (*dextromoramide*)

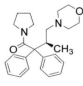

Dextromoramide

variants of the ethyl ketone function
ester, sulphone, secondary alcohols (also acylated, see *levomethadyl acetate*), tertiary amides (*dextromoramide*)

variation of the basic group
In general, dimethylamino gives optimum activity, but 5- and 6-membered alicyclic basic units also yield strong analgesic compounds (e.g. *phenadoxone, dipipanone, dextromoramide*)

Methadone

Levomethadyl acetate

variation of the diphenyl unit
- removal of one phenyl abolishes activity
- replacement by 2-thienyl leads to loss of activity (exception: related derivatives like *themalon*)
- substitution of one phenyl by benzyl leads to analgesics with moderate potency (*dextropropoxyphene*)

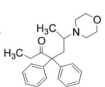

Phenadoxone

Dextropropoxyphene

Themalon

Dipipanone

Scheme 5: Variations of methadone. Levomethadyl acetate, levomethadone, dextropropoxyphene and dextromoramide are still in clinical use

Many methadone derivatives have been prepared with varying degrees of analgesic potency and duration of action. Variations of the methadone structure and some derivatives are shown in scheme 5.

The attempts to synthesize morphine led to the synthesis of its basic skeleton by Grewe, published in 1946. This work, continued by Schnider et al. (1950; 1951), yielded the significant discovery that the complete morphine structure is not essential for potent analgesic activity. N-Methylmorphinan is analgesic, and (-)-3-hydroxy-N-methylmorphinan (levorphanol) is an effective therapeutic agent, more potent than morphine.

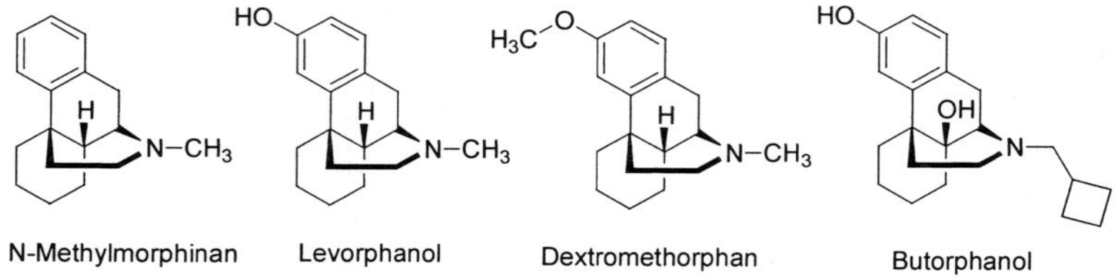

| N-Methylmorphinan | Levorphanol | Dextromethorphan | Butorphanol |

Scheme 6: Selected morphinanes

The activity of levorphanol prompted the synthesis of two even simpler modifications, phenylmorphans and 6,7-benzomorphans starting in 1953. Levorphanol, a morphinan, has one ring less than morphine, and benzomorphan has one ring less than levorphanol. The first of the benzomorphans to be brought to general attention was phenazocine. When administered orally, it is an effective analgesic with a significantly lower dependence capacity in monkeys and a somewhat lower dependence liability in man. The attachment of a phenethyl group to the nitrogen atom led to a systematic study of the role of the tertiary amine in opioid action, which showed that although activity was reduced by N-ethyl substitution, it began to be restored and increased with increasing size of the N-alkyl group (from propyl up to phenacyl).

Ketocyclazocine, an analog with an oxidized C-1 methylene, although active in antinociceptive tests, differs from most other opioids in failing to elicit a 'Straub tail' reaction and mydriasis in mice. It was found that the main activity of the compound is κ-agonism (Casy and Parfitt, 1986). Another derivative, bremazocine, carrying an hydroxy substituent in its alkyl side chain, is a potent, long-acting κ-agonist with activity at μ-sites as well. However, it was found to possess strong psychomimetic side effects, a problem which frequently occurs with κ-agonists.

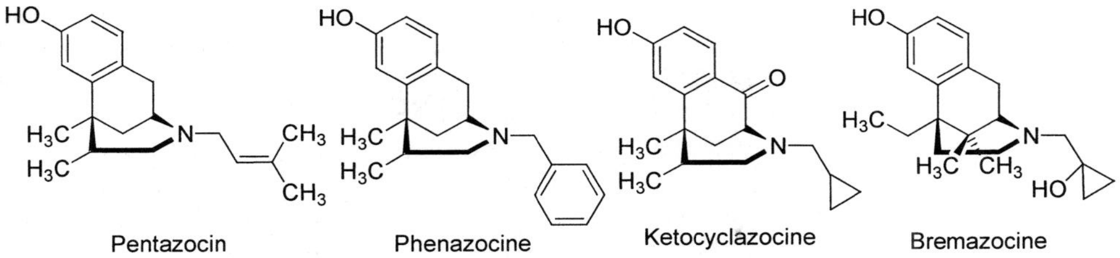

Scheme 7: Selected benzomorphanes

The morphinanes and benzomorphanes are structurally derived from morphine as it is shown in figure 8. Furthermore, the opioids known by the end of the 1950s from the pethidine group and the methadone group retrospectively incorporate substructures of the morphine skeleton. All active compounds possess at least one aromatic ring. The most common aromatic entity is the phenyl ring, where substituents are generally disadvantageous with the exception of a correctly placed hydroxy group. The other important substructure is the basic nitrogen atom, where a methyl substituent is most commonly associated with agonism.

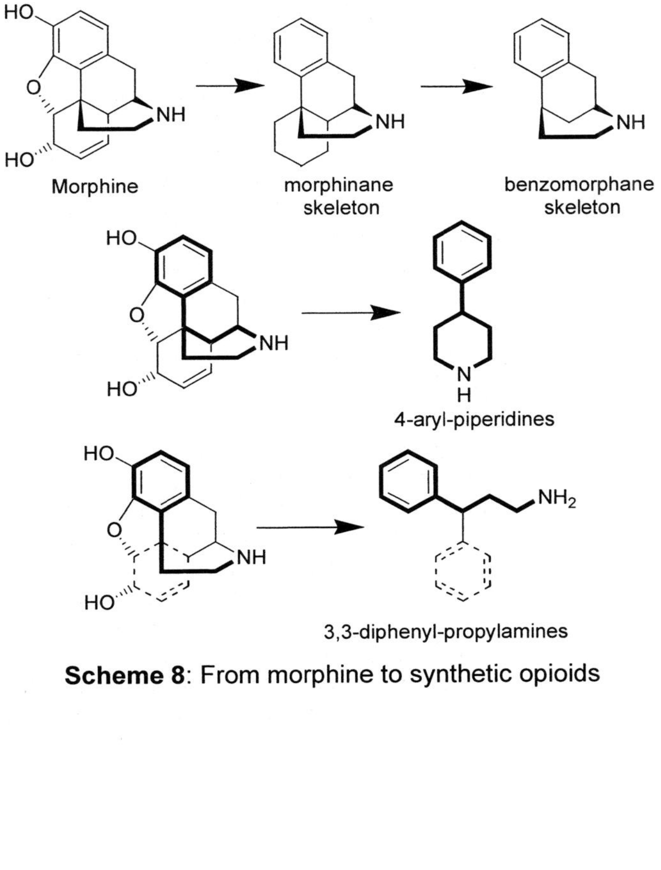

Scheme 8: From morphine to synthetic opioids

An important step for the treatment of severe pain was made in the early 1960s: Paul Janssen's exploitation of 4-piperidone chemistry proved remarkably successful in that it led to the clinical use of both a major tranquilizer (haloperidol) and a potent narcotic analgesic, fentanyl. Fentanyl is related to pethidine and also to basic anilides with analgesic properties and is characterized by high potency and short duration of action. Again, a series of derivatives was synthesized over the following decades which led to several products for clinical use, however fentanyl is still very important for the treatment of severe pain.

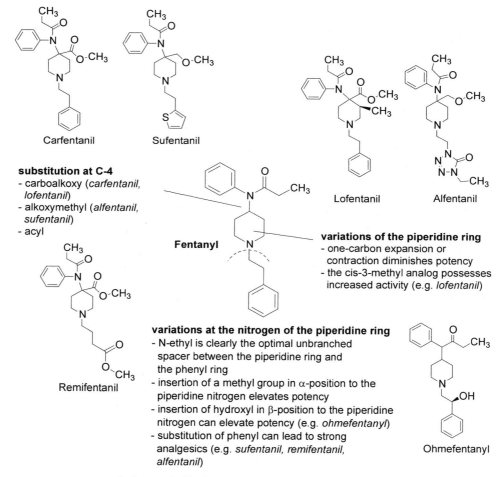

Carfentanil   Sufentanil   Lofentanil   Alfentanil

substitution at C-4
- carboalkoxy (*carfentanil, lofentanil*)
- alkoxymethyl (*alfentanil, sufentanil*)
- acyl

Fentanyl

variations of the piperidine ring
- one-carbon expansion or contraction diminishes potency
- the cis-3-methyl analog possesses increased activity (e.g. *lofentanil*)

Remifentanil

variations at the nitrogen of the piperidine ring
- N-ethyl is clearly the optimal unbranched spacer between the piperidine ring and the phenyl ring
- insertion of a methyl group in α-position to the piperidine nitrogen elevates potency
- insertion of hydroxyl in β-position to the piperidine nitrogen can elevate potency (e.g. *ohmefentanyl*)
- substitution of phenyl can lead to strong analgesics (e.g. *sufentanil, remifentanil, alfentanil*)

Ohmefentanyl

Scheme 9: Variations of the fentanyl structure.

Several compounds have been prepared with the probable aim of combining the most attractive features of both diphenylpropylamine and 4-phenylpiperidine analgesics. The derivatives diphenoxylate and loperamide have limited access to the brain and are used for the prevention of diarrhea, whereas benzitramide and piritramide represent potent analgesics.

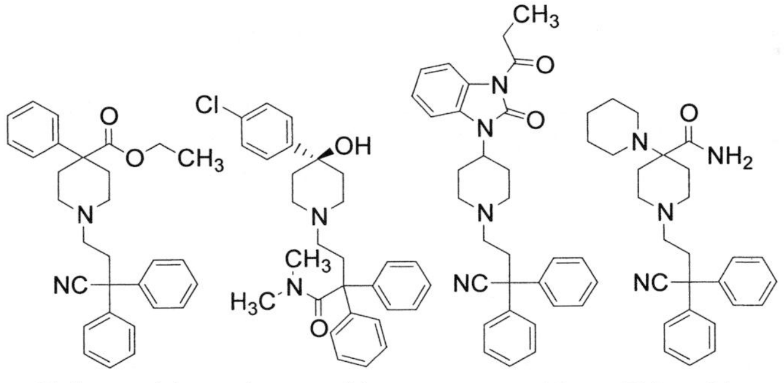

| Diphenoxylate | Loperamide | Benzitramide | Piritramide |

Scheme 10: Combined diphenylpropylamine/4-phenyl-piperidine opioids.

From a structural point of view, cyclohexane forms the common element of a variety of opioid analgesics that are otherwise difficult to classify.

In 1962, Flick (Grünenthal, Germany) aimed to synthesize a new antitussive compound. He took codeine as a model and simplified the complex structure as shown in figure 11, which can be regarded as an early rational design (Flick et al., 1978). The resulting compound, tramadol, did have antitussive properties, but due to its outstanding combination of analgesic properties and low potential for abuse or dependence (Scott and Perry, 2000) became one of the most important drugs for moderate to severe pain by the late 1990s.

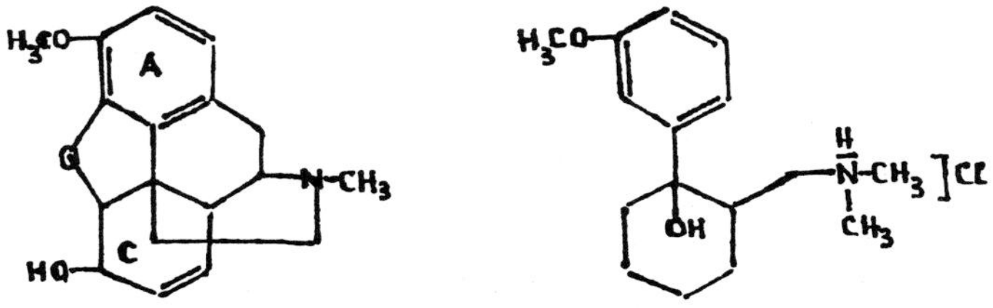

Scheme 11: Reaction scheme taken from the original notes of Kurt Flick (1962): early rational design of a new opioid (left: codeine; right: tramadol).

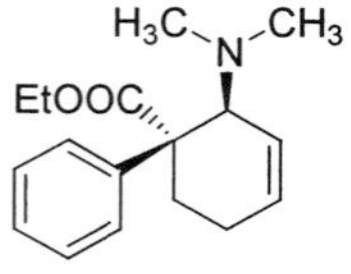

Tilidine

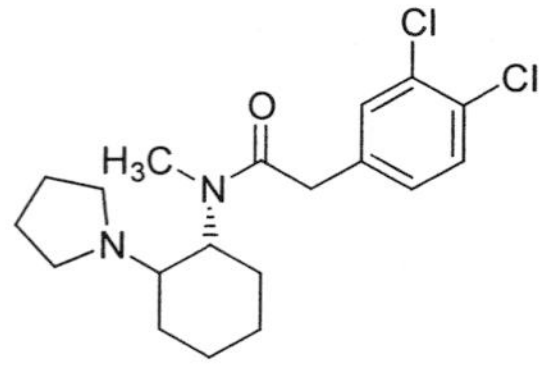

U-50488

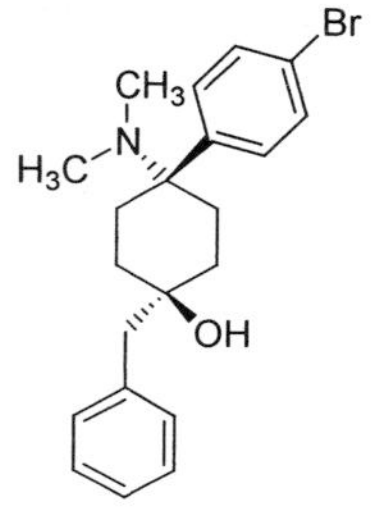

1-Benzyl-4-(4-bromo-phenyl)-
4-dimethylamino-cyclohexanol

A number of cyclohexane derivatives with tertiary amino substituents, especially dimethylamine, have proven to be opioid analgesics. Tilidine, which was synthesized at the beginning of the 1960s, is one of these compounds. Its trans NMe$_2$/CO$_2$Et configuration is important for activity since the corresponding cis-isomer is less potent.

Another aminocyclohexane with relevant analgesic properties is the 1,2-diaminocyclohexane derivative U-50488 and its analogs. Biological evaluation suggests that they are κ- rather than μ-agonists. The 3,4-dichlorophenyl unit is also present in other cyclohexane derivatives showing κ-agonistic activity (Holzgrabe et al., 1997)

The discovery of 1-aryl-1-dimethylamino-cyclohexanes resulted from a surrey of compounds in which aromatic and basic features, both critical structural requirements of opioid analgesics, but usually separated by two or three carbon atoms, are linked to the same quaternary carbon. The synthesis of these compounds yielded a series of highly potent opioids (e.g. 1-Benzyl-4-(4-bromo-phenyl)-4-dimethylamino-cyclohexanol), however none of them are in clinical use (Lednicer et al., 1981).

Reduction of the morphine structure (via tramadol) to the known essential substructures of efficient opioids (basic nitrogen atom plus a m-phenol) led to the synthesis of a series of open-chained potent analgesics. Moreover, the removal of the tertiary hydroxy group further increased analgesic potency. The (+)-enantiomer of the resulting derivative is, to the best of our knowledge, the smallest μ-opioid agonist at least equipotent to morphine ever described. The (-)-enantiomer, having a dual mechanism of action like tramadol, is being investigated in clinical trials (Buschmann et al., 2002).

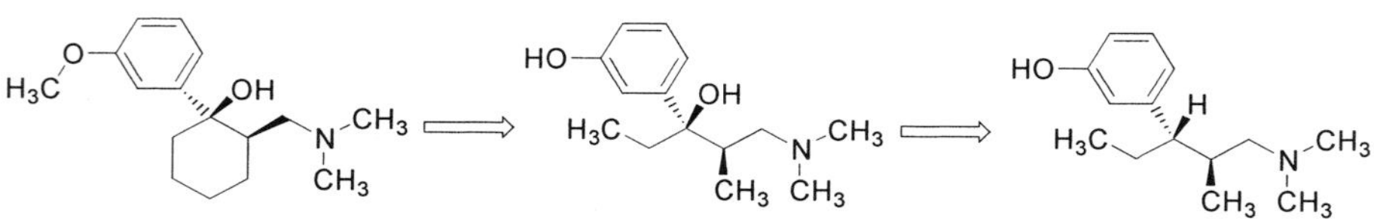

Scheme 12: Small but potent new μ-opioid agonists.

Starting from morphine, the search for an ideal opioid analgesic has resulted in a huge number of μ-opioids - many of them are in clinical use today. Over recent decades, efforts to find further μ-opioids with attenuated side-effects were clearly reduced, but with respect to the fact that μ-opioids are still the only drugs for the treatment of severe pain there may be a renewed interest in novel μ-opioids in the near future.

References

For compound-specific and mechanism-directed literature see corresponding chapters.

Buschmann, H., Sundermann, B., Maul, C.: *μ-Selektive Opioide ohne Morphinanstruktur*, Pharmazie in unserer Zeit **2002**, *31*, 44-50.

Casy, A.F. and Parfitt, R.T.: *Opioid analgesics*, Plenum Press, New York, **1986**, 333-384.

Dreser, H.: *Pharmacologisches über einige Morphinderivate*, Deut. Med. Wochenschr. **1898**, *24*, 185.

Eddy, N. B. and May, E. L., *The search for a better analgesic*, Science **1973**, *181*, 407-414.

Eisleb, O. and Schaumann, O.: *Dolantin, ein neuartiges Spasmolytikum und Analgetikum*, Dtsch. Med. Wschr. **1939**, *65*, 967-968.

Flick, K., Frankus, E., Friderichs, E.: *Studies on chemical structure and analgetic activity of phenyl substituted aminomethylcyclohexanoles*, Arzneim.-Forsch./Drug Res. **1978**, *28 (I)*, 107-113.

Grewe, R.: *Das Problem der Morphin-Synthese*, Naturwissenschaften **1946**, *33*, 333-337.

Holzgrabe, U., Nachtsheim, C., Siener, T., Drosihn, S., Brandt, W.: *Opioid-Agonisten und -Antagonisten, Opioid-Rezeptoren,* Pharmazie **1997**, *52*, 4-22.

Krauß, W. (E. Merck AG): *Verfahren zur Herstellung von Oxykodeinon*, DRP 411 530, **1925**.

Lednicer, D., von Voigtlander, P.F., Emmert, D.E.: *4-Aryl-4-aminocyclohexanones and their derivatives, a novel class of analgesics. 3. m-Hydroxyphenyl derivatives*, J. Med. Chem. **1981**, *24*, 341-346.

May, E. L., and Jacobson, A. E.: *Chemistry and pharmacology of homologs of 6-acetyl-and 3,6-diacetylmorphine*, J. Pharm. Sci. **1977**, *66*, 285-286.

Schnider, O. and Hellerbach, J.: *Optisch aktive 3-Oxymorphinane*, Helv. Chim. Acta **1950**, *33*, 1437-1448.

Schnider, O. and Grüssner, A.: *Oxy-morphinane - Optisch aktive 3-Oxymorphinane*, Helv. Chim. Acta **1951**, *34*, 2211-2217.

Scott, L. J. and Perry, C. M.: *Tramadol*, Drugs **2000**, *60*, 139-176.

Wright, C. R. A.: *On the action of organic acids and their anhydrides on the natural alkaloids*, J. Chem. Soc. **1874**, *27*, 1031.

3.4 Opioids with Clinical Relevance

Elmar Friderichs and Helmut Buschmann

Alfentanil

Synthesis: The cyclization of ethyl isocyanate with sodium azide by means of AlCl$_3$ in refluxing THF gives 1-ethyl-1,4-dihydro-5*H*-tetrazol-5-one, which is alkylated with 1-chloro-2-bromo-ethane in the presence of Na$_2$CO$_3$ and KI in refluxing 4-methyl-2-pentanone to afford 1-ethyl-4-(2-chloroethyl)1,4-dihydro-5*H*-tetrazol-5-one **i** (Janssen (Janssen), 1978; Janssens et al., 1986; Hopkins, 1981; Kleemann et al., 1999).

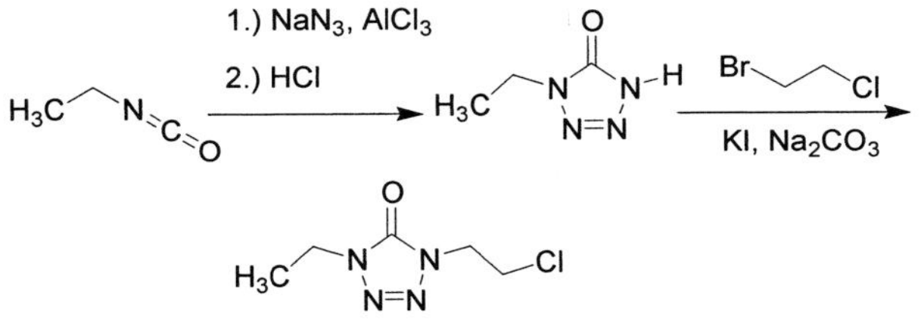

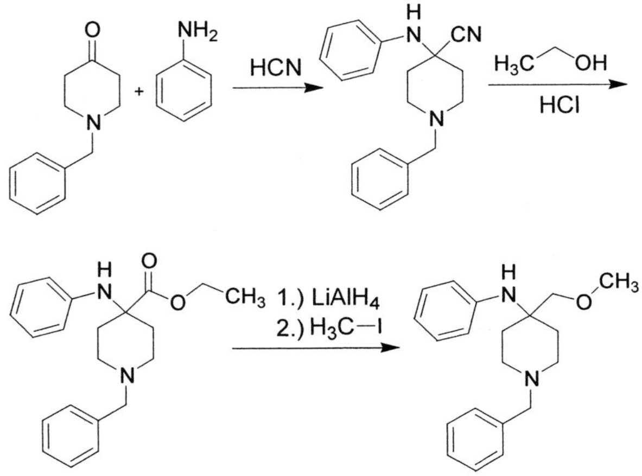

Alfentanil

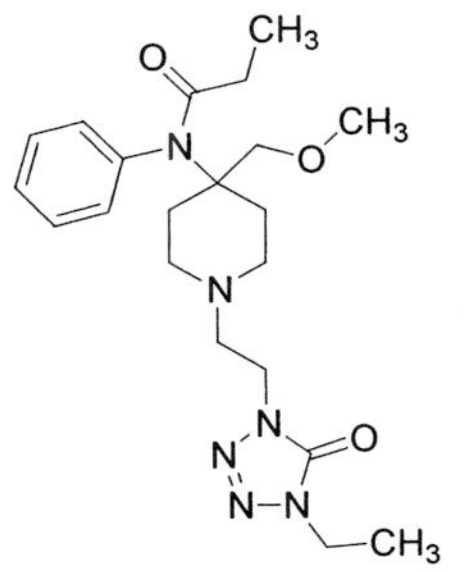

[71195-58-9], N-{1-[2-(4-Ethyl-5-oxo-4,5-dihydro-tetrazol-1-yl)-ethyl]-4-methoxymethyl-piperidin-4-yl}-N-phenyl-propion-amide, C$_{21}$H$_{32}$N$_6$O$_3$, M$_r$ 416,25; hydrochloride monohydrate [70879-28-6], C$_{21}$H$_{32}$N$_6$O$_3$ · HCl · H$_2$O, M$_r$ 470.99, mp 138.4-140.8 °C

Scheme 1: Synthesis of 1-ethyl-4-(2-chloroethyl)-1,4-dihydro-5*H*-tetrazol-5-one.

N-(4-methoxymethyl-4-piperidinyl)-N-phenyl-propionamide **ii** is synthesized according the following scheme starting from 1-benzyl-4-piperidone:

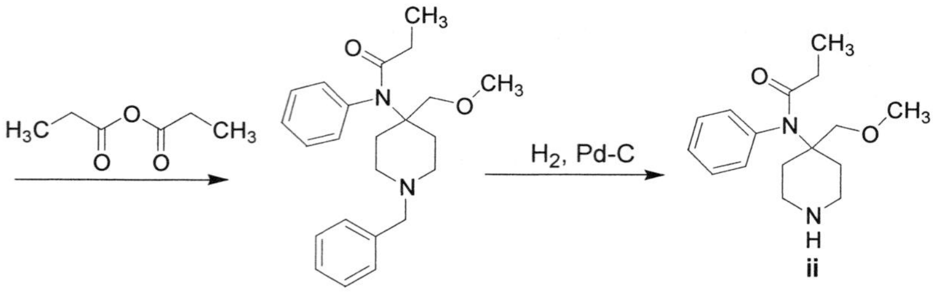

Scheme 2: Synthesis of *N*-(4-methoxymethyl-4-piperidinyl)-*N*-phenyl-propionamide

Finally the tetrazole derivative **i** is condensed with the propionamide **ii** by means of Na_2CO_3 and KI in refluxing 4-methyl-2-pentanon.

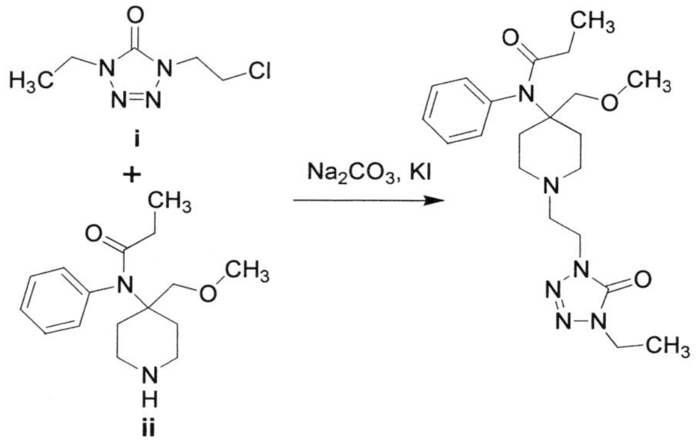

Scheme 3: Synthesis of alfentanil.

An alternative synthetic route is described in the literature (Kleemann et al., 1999): the reaction of 4-oxopiperidine 1-carboxylic acid ethyl ether with chloroform, benzyltriethylammonium chloride and NaOH in THF/water gives the corresponding spirooxetane, which is treated with aniline and NaOH to yield the anilide. The methylation of the amide nitrogene by means of sodium hydide and methyliodide in THF affords the methylated anilide. The following reaction with KOH in refluxing isopropanol causes elimination of its ethoxycarbonyl group, providing compound **i**, which is reduced with lithium triethyl-borohydride in THF to yield 4-(hydroxymethyl)-4-(phenyl-amino)piperidine. Condensation with the tetrazolone derivative **ii** by means of KI in refluxing acetonitrile yields the adduct **iii**, which is methylated with NaH and methyliodide in THF to afford the methoxy derivative. Finally, this compound is acylated with propionyl chloride in chloroform to provide the target compound. The intermediate tetrazolone derivative **ii** has been obtained by reaction of 1-ethyl-4,5-dihydro-1H-tetrazol-5-one with 1,2-dibromoethane by means of TEA in acetonitrile.

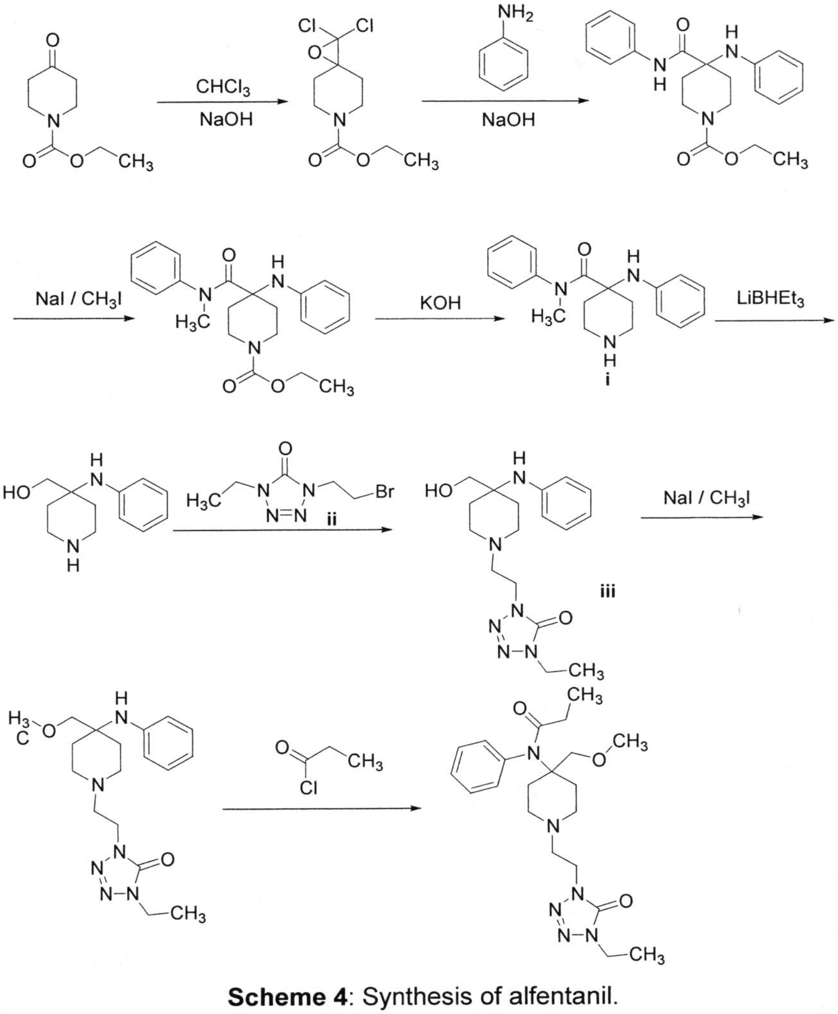

Scheme 4: Synthesis of alfentanil.

Opioid receptor binding: Alfentanil is a μ-selective opioid (Cookson et al., 1983) with a receptor affinity in the range of morphine and fentanyl.

Analgesic efficacy and clinical use: Alfentanil is a short-acting potent opioid with analgesic and anesthetic properties (Larijani and Goldberg, 1987). It is less potent than fentanyl but administration can be better controlled. It is mostly used as a supplement to general anesthesia or as a primary anesthetic e.g. in cardiac surgery. Intravenous or epidural bolus or on-demand administration can be used for postoperative pain treatment.

Dosages and routes of administration: Alfentanil is only used parenterally. Because of strong respiratory depression administration under spontaneous respiration has to be confined to a dose range up to 200 µg/h. Higher doses as used in anesthesia need assisted ventilation.

Pharmacokinetic properties: Intravenous alfentanil (Hull, 1983) has a rapid onset and a short duration of action. It has a shorter elimination time (terminal half-life 1-2 h) than fentanyl. It is less lipid-soluble and the short duration of action is more dependent on metabolic inactivation than on redistribution. Alfentanil has a high (90%) plasma protein binding. Metabolic inactivation is effected by oxidative N- and O-demethylation.

Trade name: Rapifen (Ger, Fr, UK); Alfenta (USA)

Side-effects: Alfentanil has a strong respiratory depressant action and high doses induce chest wall rigidity. The compound has a µ-type addiction and dependence potential.

Buprenorphine

Buprenorphine

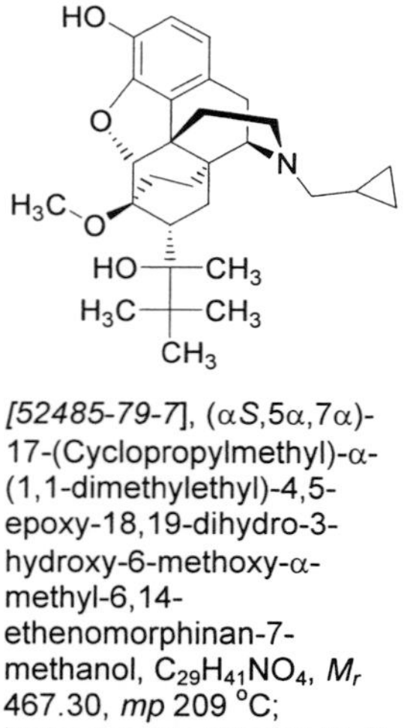

[52485-79-7], (αS,5α,7α)-17-(Cyclopropylmethyl)-α-(1,1-dimethylethyl)-4,5-epoxy-18,19-dihydro-3-hydroxy-6-methoxy-α-methyl-6,14-ethenomorphinan-7-methanol, $C_{29}H_{41}NO_4$, M_r 467.30, *mp* 209 °C; hydrochloride [53152-21-9], $C_{29}H_{41}NO_4 \cdot HCl$, M_r 504.10

Synthesis (Bentley (Reckitt & Sons), 1963; 1966; 1969; Dorner, 1986, Kleemann et al., 1999; Husbands and Lewis, 2000; Christoph, 2002): condensation of thebaine and but-3-en-2-one yields 7-acetyl-6,14-endoetheno-6,7,8,14-tetrahydrothebaine, which is hydrogenated to the corresponding *endo*-ethano derivative. The reaction of the *endo*-ethano-derivative with tertbutyl-magnesium chloride in ether-benzene yields 7-α-(2-hydroxy-3,3-dimethyl-2-butyl)-6,14-*endo*-ethano-6,7,8,14-tetrahydrothebaine. The following reaction with BrCN in methylene chloride affords 7-α-(2-hydroxy-3,3-dimethyl-2-butyl)-6,14-*endo*-ethano-N-cyano-6,7,8,14-tetrahydrothebaine, which is treated with potassium hydroxide in ethylene glycol to give 7-α-(2-hydroxy-3,3-dimethyl-2-butyl)-6,14-*endo*-ethano-N-cyano-6,7,8,14-tetrahydronorthebaine. This compound is treated with cyclopropylcarbonyl chloride in methylene chloride containing triethylamine, followed by reduction with $LiAlH_4$ in refluxing THF yielding 7-α-(2-hydroxy-3,3-dimethyl-2-butyl)-6,14-*endo*-ethano-6,7,8,14-tetrahydronorthebaine. In the final step this compound is demethylated with KOH in diethylene glycol at 210-220°C.

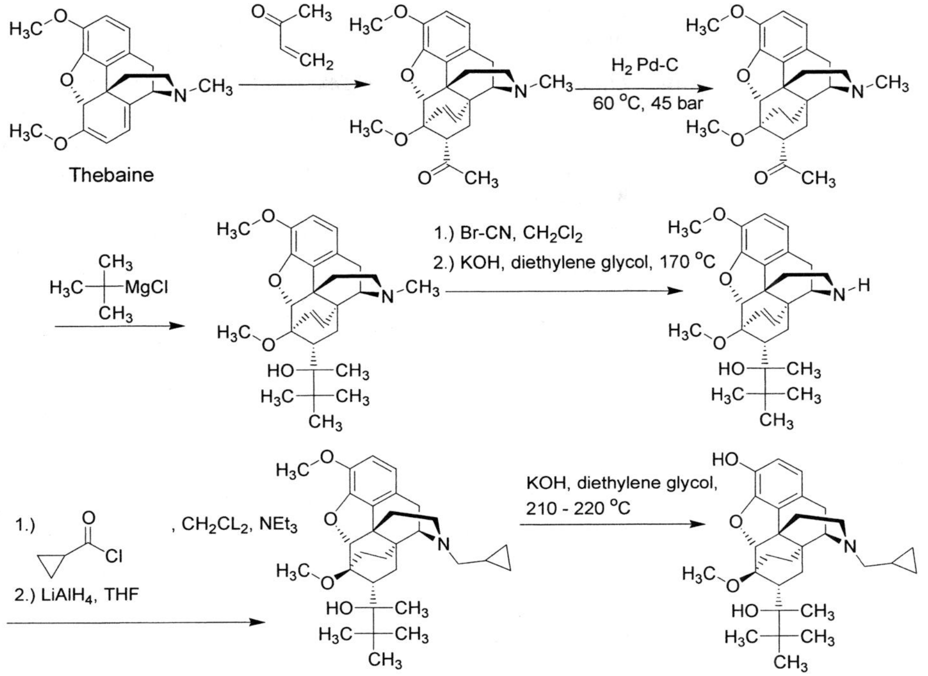

Scheme 5: Synthesis of buprenorphine.

Opioid receptor binding: Buprenorphine has a mixed agonistic-antagonistic action profile with a high affinity for the μ-, κ-, and δ-opioid receptors (Huang et al., 2001). An approximately 100-fold lower affinity was observed for the ORL1-receptor. The compound dissociates slowly from the receptor which may explain some peculiarities in its pharmacological actions.

Analgesic efficacy and clinical use: Buprenorphine (Heel et al.,1979) is a potent mixed agonistic-antagonistic opioid analgesic, which is used for the treatment of moderate to severe pain. The potency is about 20-30 times higher than that of morphine. No ceiling of analgesia is observed in clinical dosages (Zenz et al.,1985). Buprenorphine may be used for premedication or as adjunct to anesthesia. The compound has a long duration and a slow offset of action and is used in the treatment of opioid addiction as well. Due to its partial agonistic properties it can act in combination with full agonists as an antagonist, reducing their effect and precipitating a withdrawal reaction in opioid agonist-dependent persons. Antagonistic properties are seen in doses much higher than the analgesic dose range.Therefore no precautions are necessary when

Friderichs and Buschmann

changing the treatment from a standard opioid agonist to buprenorphine or vice-versa (Atkinson et al.1990).

Dosages and routes of administration: Buprenorphine is given parenterally, orally (sublingual) or by the trans-cutanous route as a patch. The doses for slow intravenous or intramuscular administration are 300-600 µg, the sublingual doses 200-400 µg, both given every 6-8 h. A transdermal formulation of buprenorphine is available as an advanced matrix patch with release rates of 35; 52.5 and 70 µg/h, corresponding to daily dosages of about 0.8, 1.2 and 1.6 mg, respectively and providing 3 days pain control.

Pharmacokinetic properties: Buprenorphine (Kuhlman et al., 1996) is subject to considerable first-pass metabolism after oral application, but sublingual administration results in a high rate of transmucosal absorption and good bioavailabilty. Buprenorphine is highly lipophilic and about 96% is bound to plasma proteins. Plasma elimination half-lives are between 1 and 7 h. There is only a weak correlation between plasma levels and analgesic effect. The compound is metabolized by N-dealkylation to norbuprenorphine, which has a reasonable µ-opioid receptor affinity and may be involved in the analgesic action (Huang et al., 2001). An essential part of the drug is excreted unchanged in the faeces.

Side-effects: Buprenorphine induces µ-opioid-type side effects including respiratory depression, drowsiness, nausea and vomiting. In the clinical literature, however, there are only few cases of significant respiratory depression. Reversal of respiratory depression may need higher doses of naloxone (Gal, 1989). Buprenorphine has a limited abuse potential and withdrawal reactions, due to slow receptor dissociation, are mild and delayed.

Trade name: Temgesic (Ger, Fr, UK); Bupenex (USA); Transtec

Butorphanol

Synthesis (Monkovic and Conway (Bristol-Myers), 1973; Monkovic, 1973; 1987; Kleemann et al., 1999): Condensation of 7-methoxy-3,4-dihydro-1(2H)-naphthalenone with tetramethylene dibromide by means of NaH in benzene or *tert* amyl alcohol gives 3,4-dihydro-7-methoxy-2,2-tetramethylene-1(2H)-naphthalene (bp (0,05 mbar) 120-123 °C), which is treated with acetonitrile and butyllithium in THF yielding 1-hydroxy-7-methoxy-1,2,3,4-tetrahydro-2,2-tetramethylene-1-naphthalene-acetonitrile (mp 140-142 °C). This compound is reduced with LiAlH$_4$ in THF to afford hydro-2,2-tetramethylene-1-naphthol (mp 178-180 °C), and isomerized to 4a-(2-aminoethyl)-1,2,3,4,4a,9-hexahydro-6-methoxy-phenantrene **i** (mp 187 °C).

This amine **i** is cyclized by reaction with bromine in CHCl₃ giving 3-methoxy-9a-bromonorhasybanan hydrobromide (mp 207.0-208.5 °C (decomp.)), and isomerized with dehydrobromination by treatment with NaHCO₃ in DMF affording 3-methoxy-δ(8,14)-morphinan (mp 180-184 °C). The acetylation of this compound with trifluoroacetic anhydride yields 3-methoxy-N-trifluoroacetyl-δ(8,14)-morphinan (mp 94-96 °C) which is epoxidized with m-chloroperbenzoic acid in methylene chloride giving 8,14-epoxy-3-methoxy-N-trifluoroacetylmorphinan (mp 102-105 °C). The deacetylation of this intermediate with NaSH₄ in ethanol gives 8,14-epoxy-3-methoxymorphinan, an oily product that is treated with LiAlH₄ in THF to open the epoxide ring and yield 14-hydroxy-3-methoxymorphinan (HCl salt, mp 243-244 °C (decomp.)). The condensation of this derivative with cyclobutylcarbonyl chloride by means of pyridine in CH₂Cl₂ affords N-cyclobutylcarbonyl-14-hydroxy-3-methoxymorphinan (mp 183-185 °C), which is reduced with LiAlH₄ in refluxing THF giving N-cyclobutylmethyl-14-hydroxy-3-methoxymorphinan (HCl salt, mp 248- 250 °C (decomp.)). Finally the methoxy ether is demethylated by treatment with refluxing 48% HBr. Resolution of the racemic mixture is achieved by crystallization of the diastereomeric tartaric acid salt.

[42408-82-2], 11-Cyclobutyl-methyl-1,2,3,4,9,10-hexa-hydro-4a,10-propano-phenanthrene-6,10a-diol, C₂₁H₂₉NO₂, M_r 327.22, mp 215-217 °C, [α]_D -70° (c = 0.1, CH₃OH); tartrate[58786-99-5], C₂₁H₂₉NO₂·C₄H₆O₆, M_r 477.55, mp 217-219 °C, [α]_D -64.0° (c = 0.4, CH₃OH)

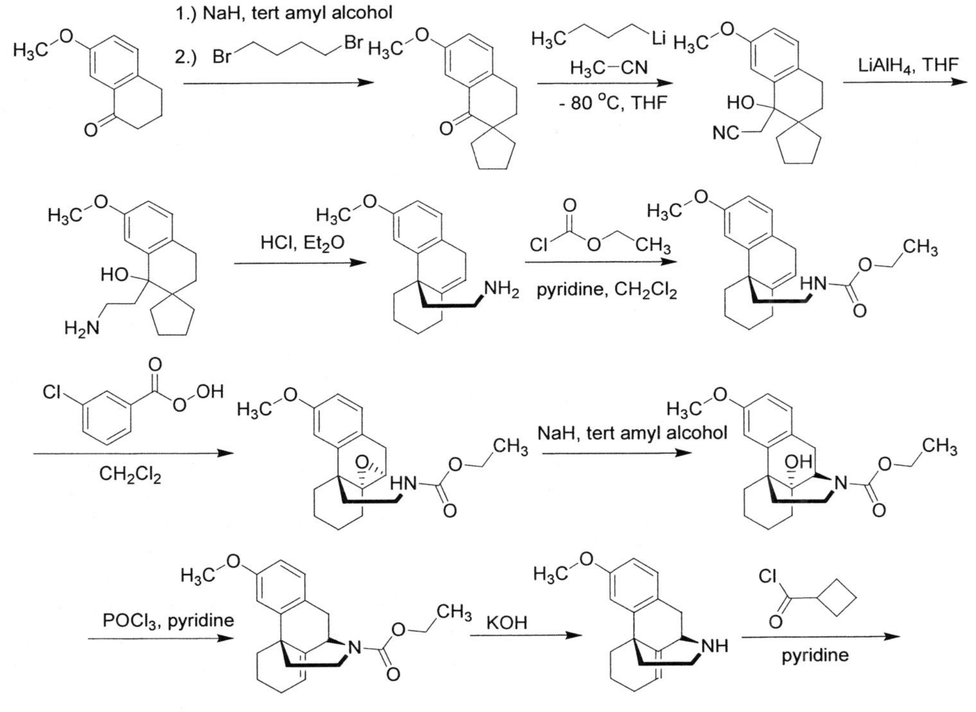

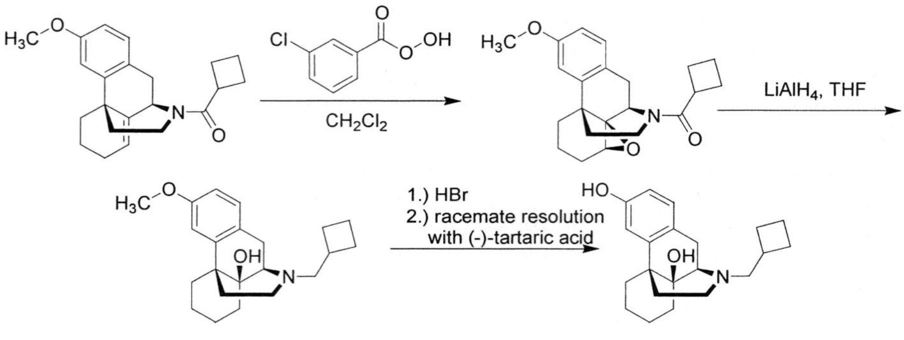

Scheme 6: Synthesis of butorphanol.

Alternatively the cyclization of the amine **i** to the methoxy ether derivative **ii** can be performed by the following reaction sequence.

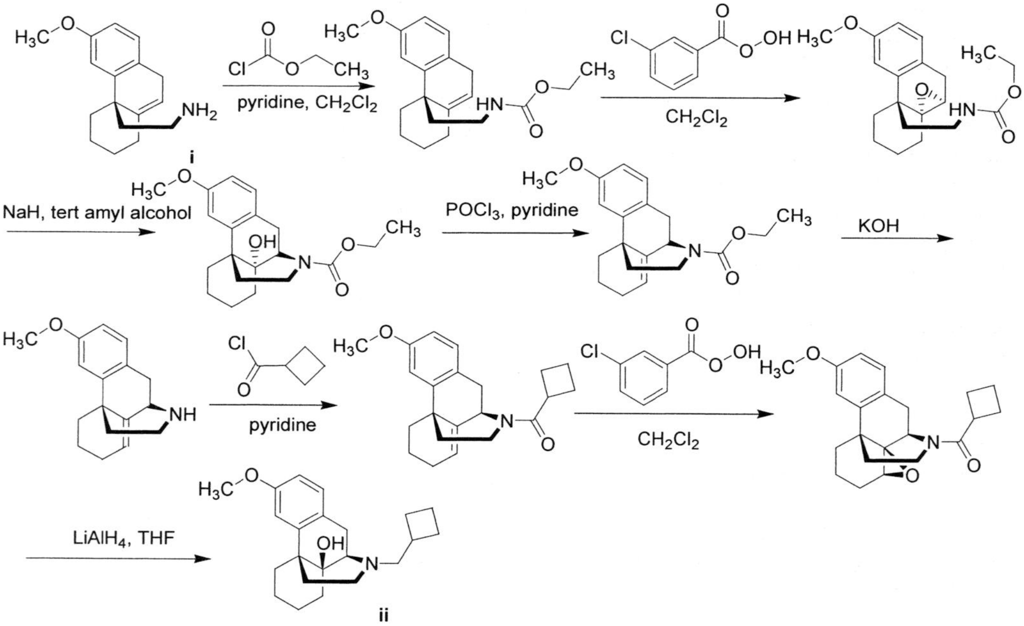

Scheme 7: Synthesis of butorphanol.

Opioid receptor binding: Butorphanol (Rosow, 1988) is a mixed agonist-antagonist opioid with full agonistic activity at the κ-receptor and partial agonistic-antagonistic effect at the μ-receptor. The compound has a high μ- and κ-receptor affinity.

Analgesic efficacy and clinical use: Butorphanol (Heel et al., 1978; Ameer and Salter, 1979) is a fairly potent opioid analgesic, the analgesic properties are effected by activation of μ- and κ-opioid receptors. It is used for the treatment of moderate to severe pain, for migraine and headache (Homan, 1994) and as an adjunct to anesthesia.

Dosages and routes of administration: Butorphanol is orally inactive but can be given by the nasal route (Homan 1994). The usual administration is via the intramuscular or intravenous route. The intramuscular doses are 1-4 mg every 3-4 h, the intravenous doses are 0.5-2 mg. Nasal doses are ~ 1mg/spray in each nostril.

Pharmacokinetic properties: Butorphanol (Vachharajani et al., 1997) is rapidly inactivated by first pass metabolism in the gut. Intramuscular and nasal administration induces a peak effect between 0.5–1hr and a duration of action of about 3 h, corresponding to the plasma half-life time of the compound. Butorphanol has a plasma protein binding of about 80%, metabolic inactivation includes hydroxylation, N-dealkylation and glucuronidation and only about 5% remain unchanged.

Side-effects: Butorphanol (Rosow, 1988) has a side-effect profile combining morphine- and pentazocine-like symptoms. They include drowsiness, weakness, sweating, feelings of floating, and nausea. It has respiratory depressant properties similar to morphine but with a ceiling effect. Naloxone can be used as an antidote. Overt hallucinations or other psychotic effects are rare and less often reported than with pentazocine. The compound has a very low abuse potential and has not been submitted to narcotic control.

Trade name: Stadol (USA)

Codeine

Preparation: Codeine is extracted from opium (present in opium from 0.7 to 2.5 % depending on the source), but mostly prepared by methylation of morphine in a phase transfer reaction (Boehringer, 1912; Ehrhart and Ruschig, 1972; Casy and Parfitt, 1986).

Codeine

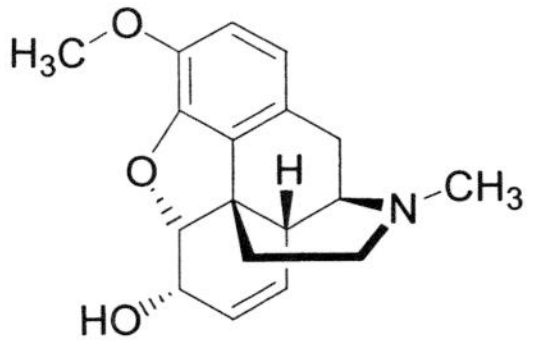

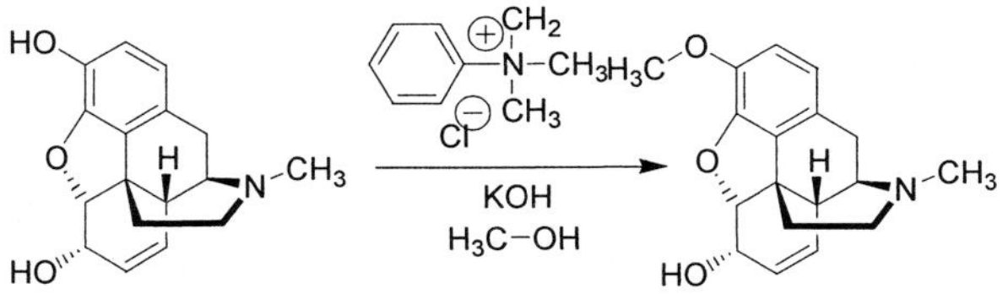

Scheme 8: Synthesis of codeine.

[76-57-3], $C_{18}H_{21}NO_3$, M_r
299.36, *mp* 154-156 °C
(monohydrate from water or
diluted alcohol), sublimes
when anhydrated at 140-
145 °C under 1.5 mm
pressure, $[\alpha]_D^{25}$ -136° (*c* = 2,
CH_3CH_2OH); monohydrate
[6059-47-8], $C_{18}H_{21}NO_3$
H_2O, M_r 317.38, *mp* 154-156
°C; hydrochloride dihydrate
$C_{18}H_{21}NO_3 \cdot HCl \cdot 2H_2O$, M_r
371.86, *mp* 280 °C
(decomp.), $[\alpha]_D$ -108° ;
hydrobromide dihydrate
[125-25-7], $C_{18}H_{21}NO_3 \cdot HBr \cdot$
$2H_2O$, M_r 416.31, *mp* 190-
192 °C (anhydrous), $[\alpha]_D$ -
96.6°; phosphate *[52-28-8]*

Opioid receptor binding : Codeine has a low affinity at μ-,
δ-, and κ-opioid receptors and the *in vivo* effects are
predominantly induced by morphine, formed by metabolic
O-demethylation.

Analgesic efficacy and clinical use: Codeine (Honig and
Murray, 1984) has a morphine-like action profile with
analgesic and antitussive properties. As compared to
morphine the analgesic potency is 5–10fold lower. The
compound is used for the treatment of mild to moderate
pain and for cough inhibition (Eccles,1996).

Dosages and routes of administration: Codeine is used
orally in single doses of 30 to 60 mg up to a total dose of
240 mg per day for pain relief. Codeine is used in the form
of different salts such as hydrochloride, phosphate and
sulfate. To increase the duration of action, slow-release
preparations have been developed. Codeine is often
combined with other analgesics e.g. acetyl salicylic acid or
paracetamol. For cough inhibition lower doses are
sufficient.

The following scheme shows the codeine consumption in
different European countries and the United States.

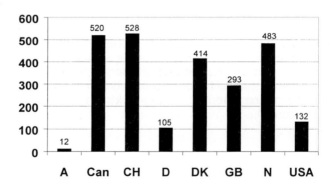

Figure 1: Codeine consumption (1995) in different
countries in kg compound /Mio inhabitants (Sohn and
Zenz, 1998).

Pharmacokinetic properties: Codeine (Sindrup and
Brosen, 1995) has a good oral bioavailability. The
compound is extensively metabolized by O- and N-
demethylation followed by glucuronidation. The main
metabolites are norcodeine, morphine and hydrocodeine
and their glucuronides. There are indications (Yue et al.,
1997), that the analgesic effect is reduced in persons with
low CYP2D6 activity (poor metabolizers).

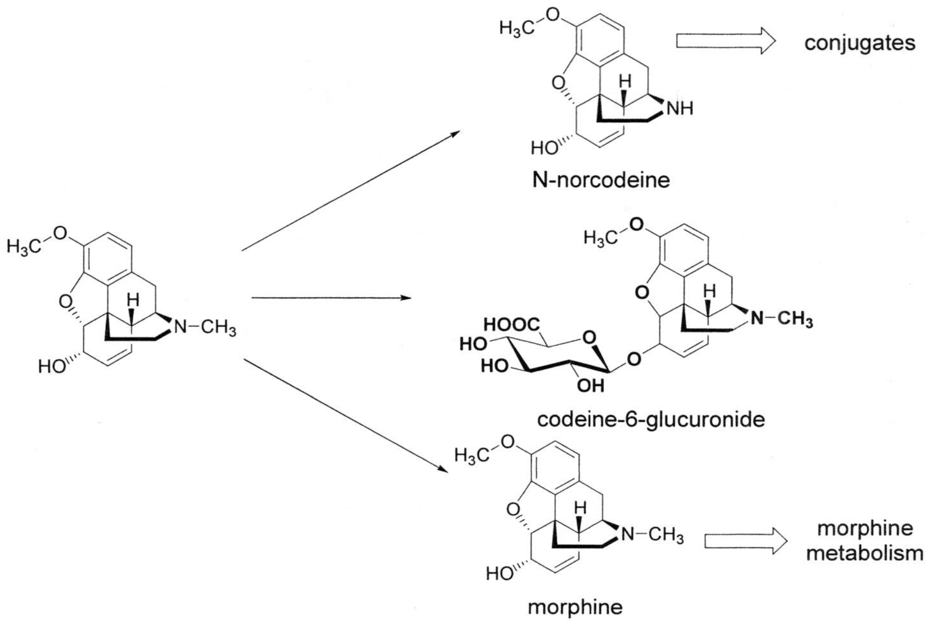

Scheme 9: Metabolic pathway of codeine.

Side-effects: Codeine has a similar spectrum of side-effects as morphine including nausea, vertigo and somnolence, but with a lower intensity. Most prominent are constipation, excitement and convulsions in the higher dose range. Abuse and dependence are less prevalent as compared to morphine, which can be explained by the fact that the opioid principle is only available after metabolic activation.

Trade name:
Codipront (Gerri);
Codicaps (Ger), Codimal (USA)

Dextromoramide

Synthesis (Janssen and Karel (Janssen), 1956; Kleemann et al., 1999).

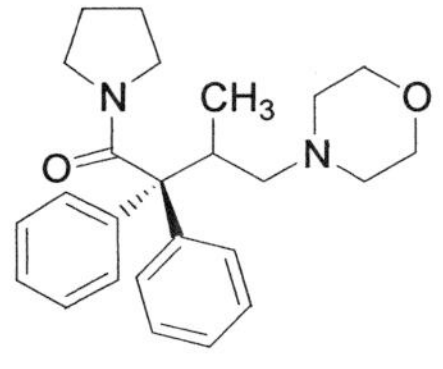

Opioid receptor binding: Dextromoramide is a μ-selective opioid with a higher receptor affinity than morphine.

Analgesic efficacy and clinical use: Dextromoramide tartrate (Kay, 1973) is a strong opioid related to methadone and is used in the treatment of severe pain (Judd et al., 1981).

Dosages and routes of administration: Dextromoramide is administered orally and rectally. The parenteral potency is in the range of morphine, but the duration of action is shorter.

Dextromoramide

[*357-56-2*], (+)-(*S*)-3-Methyl-4-morpholin-4-yl-2,2-diphenyl-1-pyrrolidin-1-yl-butan-1-one, $C_{25}H_{32}N_2O_2$, M_r 392.55, *mp* 183-184 °C, $[\alpha]_D^{25}$ +25.5° (*c* = 5, benzene), $[\alpha]_D^{25}$ +16° (*c* = 5, ethanol), D-tartrate [*2922-44-3*], $C_{25}H_{32}N_2O_2 \cdot C_4H_6O_6$ M_r 542.64, *mp* 189-192 °C, $[\alpha]_D^{25}$ +25.5° (*c* = 5, water), $[\alpha]_D^{25}$ +30.5° (*c* = 5, CH_3OH)

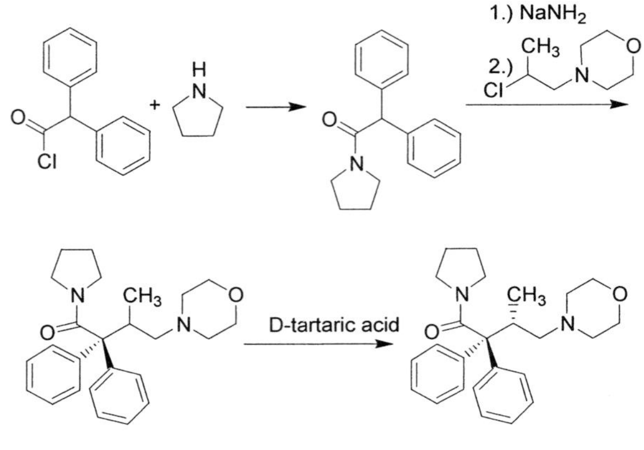

Scheme 10: Synthesis of dextromoramide

Side-effect profile: The compound has a morphine-type abuse and dependence potential.

Trade name: Palfium (Fr, UK, NL)

Dextropropoxyphene

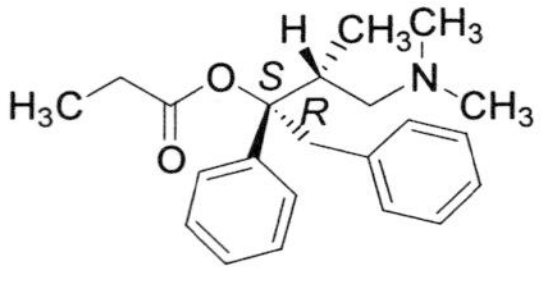

[*469-62-5*], Propionic acid 1-benzyl-3-dimethylamino-2-methyl-1-phenyl-propyl ester, [*S*-(*R**,*S**)]-α-[2-(di-methylamino)-1-methyl-ethyl]-α-phenylbenzene-ethanol propanoate (ester), $C_{22}H_{29}NO_2$, M_r 339.47, *mp* 75-76 °C, $[\alpha]_D^{25}$ +67.3° (*c* = 0.6, $CHCl_3$); hydrochloride [1639-60-7], $C_{22}H_{29}NO_2 \cdot$ HCl, M_r 375.93, *mp* 163-168.5 °C, $[\alpha]_D^{25}$ +59.8° (*c* = 0.6, water)

Synthesis (Pohland, 1953; 1955; 1963; janssen and Karel (Janssen)1956; Sullivan et al., 1963): In the Grignard reaction of 3-dimethylamino-2-methyl-1-phenyl-propan-1-one with benzylmagnesium chloride 4-dimethylamino-3-methyl-1,2-diphenyl-butan-2-ol is formed. The preferred product is the a-diastereomer(75 % α-form, 15 % β-form). The α-form crystallizes and the diastereomeric β-form remains in solution, because of its better solubility. Racemic resolution to obtain the analgetically (+) enantiomer can be achieved on the pure α-Grignard product via fractional crystallization of the salts with *D*-camphorsulfonic acid. Alternatively the resolution can be achieved by treating the racemic mannich product 3-dimethylamino-2-methyl-1-phenyl-propan-1-one with (-)-dibenzoyltartaric acid in acetone as solvent.

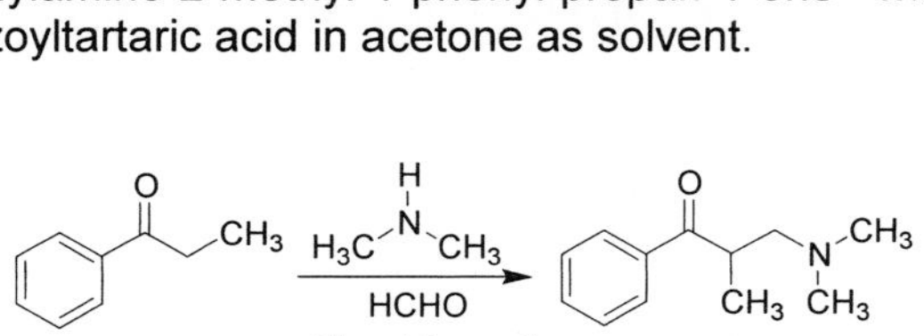

Mannich reaction

Opioid receptor binding: Dextropropoxyphene has a lower µ-opioid receptor binding capacity than morphine. Binding at other opioid receptors is even weaker.

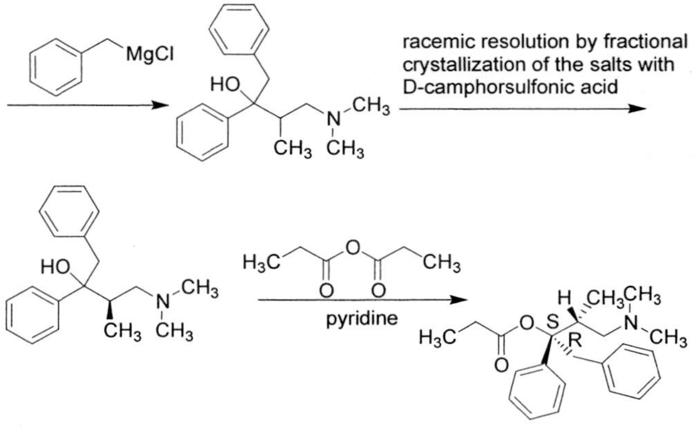

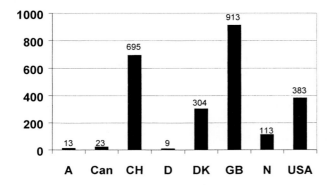

Scheme 11: Synthesis of dextropropoxyphene.

Analgesic efficacy and clinical use: Dextropropoxyphene (Grover,1988) is a moderately potent opioid analgesic often combined with paracetamol or acetylsalicylic acid or other NSAIDs (Collins et al., 2000). As the hydrochloride or napsylate it is used orally for the treatment of mild, moderate, or severe pain (Beaver, 1984).

Dosages and routes of administration: Dextropropoxyphene is mostly administered by the oral route. Parenteral injection and rectal administration is painful and induces tissue damage. The ordinary oral doses are 65 mg of the hydrochloride and 100 mg of the napsylate.

The following scheme shows the dextropropoxyphene consumption in different European countries and the United States.

Figure 2: Dextropropoxyphene consumption (1995) in different countries in kg compound /Mio inhabitants (Sohn and Zenz, 1998).

Pharmacokinetic properties: Dextropropoxyphene (Pearson, 1984) has a reasonable oral bioavailability and is readily absorbed from the gastrointestinal tract. Peak plasma concentrations are reached within 1–2 hrs. It is rapidly distributed and about 80% are bound by plasma proteins. The compound is metabolized by N-demethylation to the active metabolite nordextropropoxyphene and other inactive metabolites which are excreted in the urine. Accumulation of the compound and the metabolites may occur with chronic use and the nor-metabolite may contribute to toxicity (Inturrisi et al., 1982).

Trade name: Develin (Ger), Darvon (USA), Doloxene (UK), Antalvic (Fr)

Side-effects: Adverse reactions in the therapeutic range are mild and include drowsiness, dizziness, sedation and nausea. Overdosage can induce serious adverse reactions including profound sedation, respiratory depression, cardiovascular disturbances, convulsions and psychotic reactions, often with fatal outcome (Lawson and Northridge, 1987). Oral dextropropoxyphene has a relatively low abuse liability. Abuse by injection is impeded by severe irritation at the injection side.

Dezocine

Dezocine

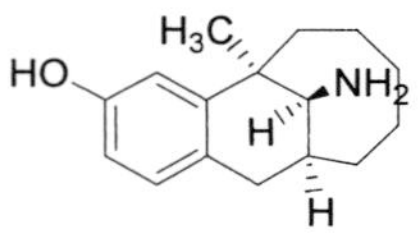

[53648-55-8], 15-Amino-1-methyl-tricyclo[7.5.1.0^{127,255}] pentadeca-2-4-6-trien-4-ol, [5R-(5α,11α,13S*)]-13-amino-5,6,8,9,10,11,12-octahydro-5-methyl-5,11-methanobenzocyclodecen-3-ol, $C_{16}H_{23}NO$, M_r 245.36; hydrobromide [57236-36-9], $C_{16}H_{23}NO \cdot HBr$, M_r 326.27, mp 269-270 °C

Synthesis (Freed and Potoski (American Home), 1971; Freed, 1973; Kleemann et al., 1999,): Dezocine is prepared through the following sequence: The condensation of 1-methyl-7-methoxy-2-tetralone with 1,5-dibromopentane by means of NaH or potassium tertbutylate affords 1-(5-bromopentyl)-1-methyl-7-methoxy-2-tetralone; this product is cyclized with NaH to give 5-methyl-3-methoxy-5,6,7,8,9,10,11,12-octahydro-5,11-methano-benzocyclodecen-13-one **i**. The ketone **i**, by reaction with hydroxylamine hydrochloride in pyridine, is converted into its oxime **ii**, which is reduced with H_2 over Raney Ni to a mixture of isomeric amines which were separated by crystallization of the HCl salts giving 5-α-methyl-3-methoxy-5,6,7,8,9,11α,12-octahydro-5,11-methanobenzo-cyclodecen-13β-amine, which is finally cleaved with concentrated HBr.

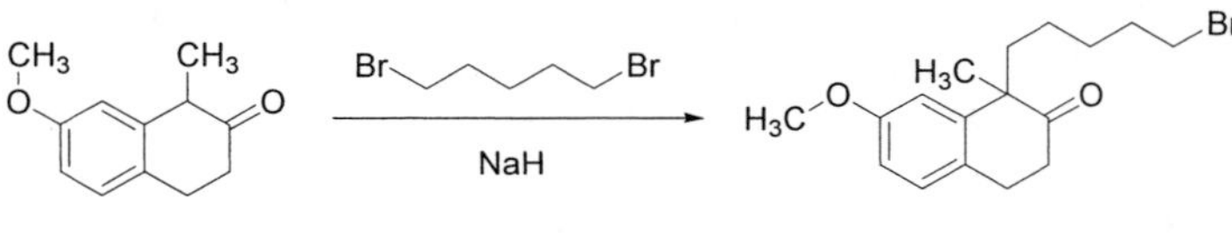

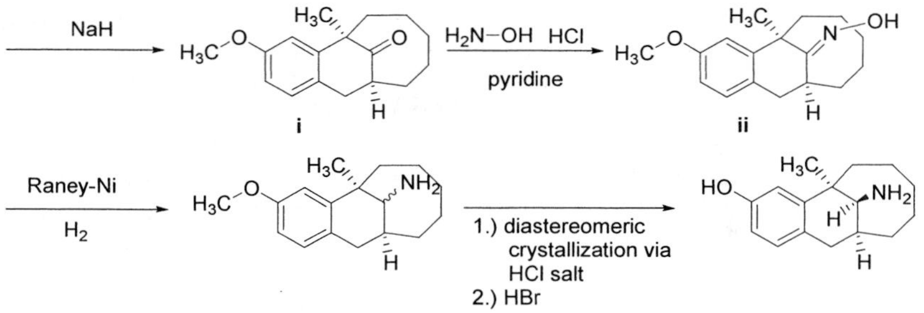

Scheme 12: Synthesis of dezocine.

Another synthetic pathway to dezocine is shown in the following scheme:

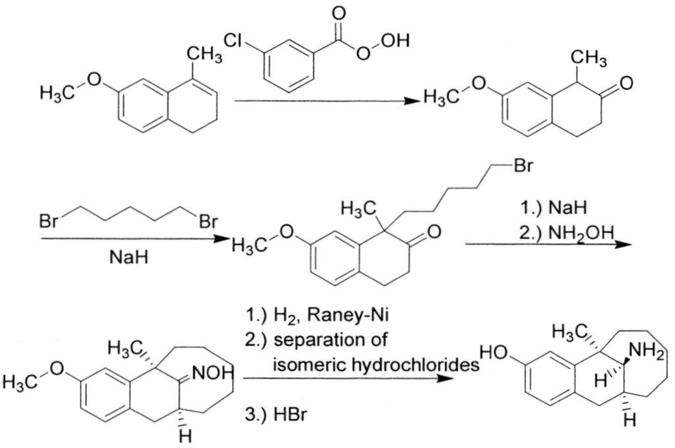

Scheme 13: Synthesis of dezocine.

Opioid receptor binding: Dezocine (Chen et al., 1993) is a mixed agonist-antagonist with binding affinity to the μ-receptor in the range of morphine. The δ- and κ-affinity is 10-100-fold lower (O'Brien and Benfield, 1989).

Analgesic efficacy and clinical use: Dezozine has medium opioid analgesic potency and is used for treatment of moderate to moderately severe pain.

Dosages and routes of administration : The compound is only used parenterally in single dosed of 5-20 mg.

Pharmacokinetic properties: The compound is subject to an intensive first-pass metabolism via glucuronidation of the free phenolic hydroxyl group (Wilson et al.,1995; Strain et al.,1996). This strongly reduces oral bioavailability and induces a short duration of action.

Trade name: Dalgan (USA)

Side-effects: Dezocin induces μ-opioid-type side-effects with nausea, vomiting and drowsiness. Overdoses may be treated with naloxone. The compound has a low abuse potential and is not under narcotic control. Because of its partial antagonistic properties dezocine can precipitate withdrawal in opioid-dependent subjects (Strain et al., 1996).

Diamorphine (Heroin)

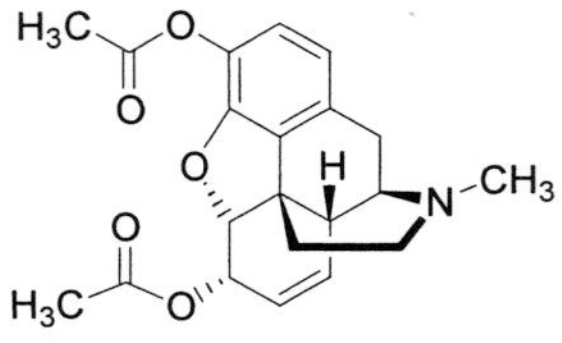

[561-27-2], $C_{21}H_{23}NO_5$, M_r 369.41, *mp* 173 °C, $[\alpha]_D^{25}$ -166° (*c* = 1.49, CH_3OH); hydrochloride monohydrate [561-27-2], $C_{21}H_{23}NO_5 \cdot HCl$ H_2O, M_r 423.89, *mp* 243-244 °C, $[\alpha]_D^{25}$ -156° (*c* = 1.044)

Diamorphine (Diacetylmorphine, Heroin)

Synthesis: morphine is acetylated with acetic anhydride (Ehrhart and Ruschig, 1972).

Opioid receptor binding: Diamorphine (Inturrisi et al.,1983) has a 10-100fold lower μ-opioid receptor binding affinity than morphine. The relevant opioid properties originate from the high μ-receptor affinity of the metabolites 6-acetylmorphine and morphine (Umans and Inturrisi, 1981).

Analgesic efficacy and clinical use: Diamorphine is a strong opioid analgesic used for the treatment of severe pain, especially in terminally ill cancer patients (Sawynok, 1986). In addition it can be used for the treatment of cough associated with terminal lung cancer.

Dosages and routes of administration: Diamorphine is given by the oral as well as by parenteral (i.m., s.c) or intrathecal routes. Diamorphine is about twice as potent as morphine. The parenteral doses are 5-10 mg every 4 h, oral doses are up to two-fold higher.

Pharmacokinetic properties: Diamorphine is a lipophilic morphine derivative, which is well absorbed from the intestinal tract and rapidly penetrates into the CNS. It is already metabolized during the transport to the CNS yielding the active metabolites 6-acetylmorphine and morphine. The rapid brain access induces a quick onset of action and seems to be the reason for its high abuse potential (Inturrisi et al., 1984).

Trade name: Diagesil (UK)

Side-effects: Diamorphine has in principle the same side-effect profile as morphine. High doses as used by addicts may cause fatal pulmonary edema (Darke and Zadol, 1996). Because of its high abuse potential therapeutic administration is prohibited in many countries including Germany and the USA, in other countries like the UK it is used for severe pain mostly among terminally ill patients.

Dihydrocodeine

Synthesis (Stein, 1955, Ehrhart and Ruschig, 1972; Kleemann et al., 1999): Hydrogenation of codeine yields Dihydrocodeine (Kleemann et al., 1999).

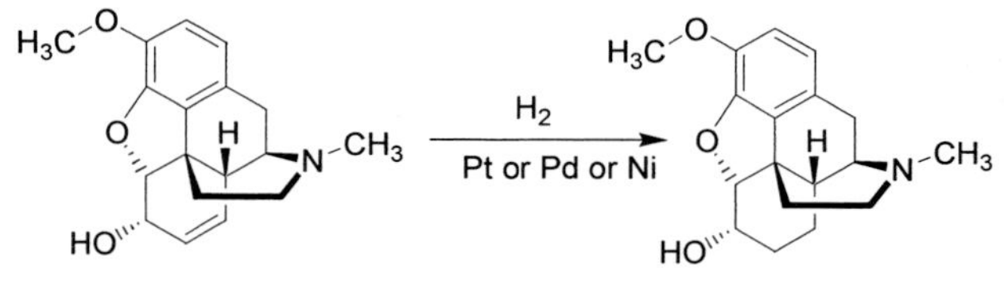

Scheme 14: Synthesis of dihydrocodeine.

Dihydrocodeine

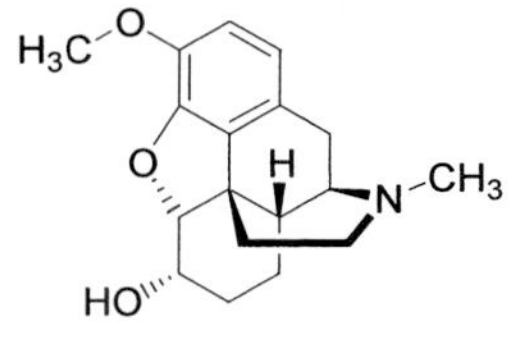

[*125-28-0*], (5α,6α)-4,5-epoxy-3-methoxy-17-methylmorphinan-6-ol, $C_{18}H_{23}NO_3$, M_r 301.38, *mp* 112-113 °C; tartrate (1 : 1) [*5965-13-9*], $C_{18}H_{23}NO_3$ $C_4H_6O_6$, M_r 451.47, *mp* 192-193 °C (commercial medicinal grade usually melts at 186-190 °C), $[\alpha]_D^{25}$ -72° to -75° (*c* = 1.0, water)

Opioid receptor binding: Dihydrocodeine has a low μ-opioid receptor binding and its opioid properties are mostly due to metabolic activation to dihydromorphine.

Analgesic efficacy: Dihydrocodeine has codeine-like analgesic and antitussive properties and is used for the treatment of moderate to severe pain (Edwards et al., 2000) and as antitussive (Matthys et al., 1985).

Dosages and routes of administration: Dihydrocodeine is mostly used in the form of immediate or sustained release oral formulations (Lloyd et al., 1992). For pain treatment the dose range is 30-80 mg, for cough inhibition doses are in the range of 10 mg.

The following scheme shows the dihydrocodeine consumption in different European countries and the United States.

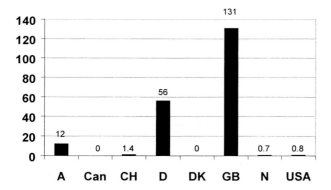

Figure 3: Dihydrocodeine consumption (1995) in different countries in kg compound /Mio inhabitants (Sohn and Zenz, 1998)

Pharmacokinetic properties: Like codeine, dihydrocodeine is metabolized by CYP2D6 yielding the active metabolite dihydromorphine (Ammon et al., 1999). N-Demethylation to nordihydrocodeine and nordihydromorphine takes place to a lesser extent.

Trade name: Paracodin (Ger), Dicodin (Fr), DHC Continus (UK), Synalgos (USA)

Side-effects: Dihydrocodeine induces morphine-type side-effects with a lower intensity than morphine. Chronic treatment may produce dependence and abuse has been reported. On the other hand, the compound has been used as substitution therapy for morphine dependence (Banbery et al., 2000)

Diphenoxylate

Diphenoxylate

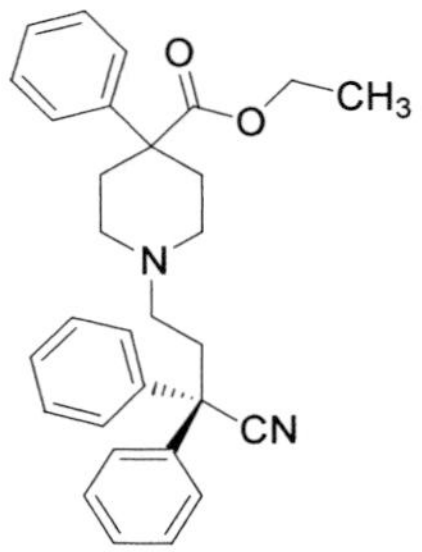

[*915-30-0*], 1-(3-Cyano-3,3-diphenyl-propyl)-4-phenyl-piperidine-4-carboxylic acid ethyl ester, $C_{30}H_{32}N_2O_2$, M_r 452.59; hydrochloride [*3810-80-8*], $C_{30}H_{32}N_2O_2 \cdot HCl$, M_r 489.06, *mp* 220.5-222.0 °C

Synthesis (Janssen, 1959; Dryden and Erickson (Searle), 1978, Kleemann et al., 1999): The reaction of 4-phenyl-piperidine-4-carboxylic acid ethyl ester with 4-bromo-2,2-diphenyl-butyronitrile yields diphenoxylate (Kleemann et al., 1999, p. 250).

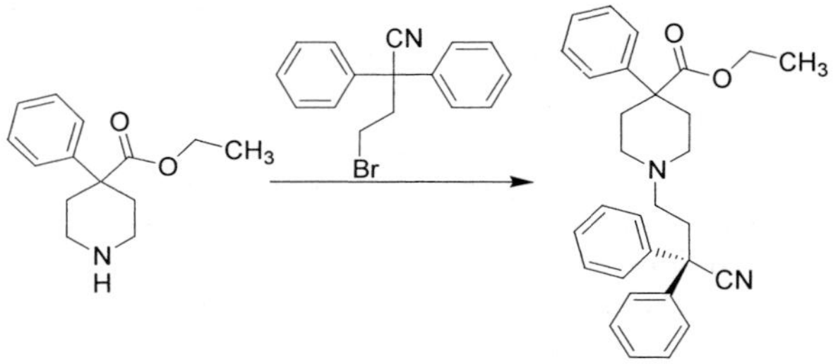

Scheme 15: Synthesis of diphenoxylate.

Alternatively the condensation of diphenylacetonitrile with 1-(2-chloro-ethyl)-4-phenyl-piperidine-4-carboxylic acid ethyl ester by means of sodium amide can be carried out.

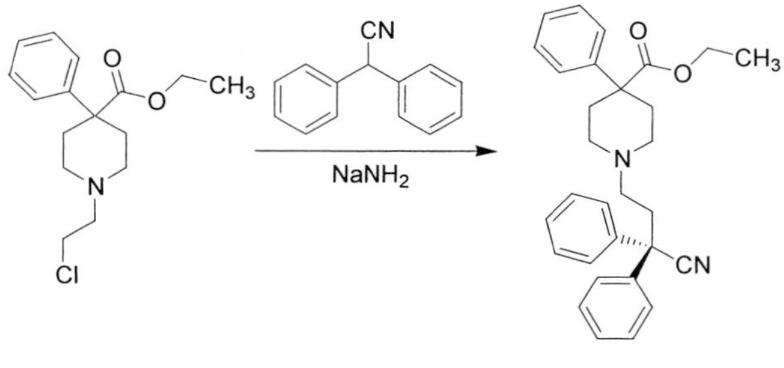

Scheme 16: Synthesis of diphenoxylate.

Opioid receptor binding: Diphenoxylate and its active metabolite difenoxine (Niemegeers et al., 1972) has a high affinity and selectivity for the μ-type of opioid receptor.

Analgesic efficacy and clinical use: Diphenoyxlate is a synthetic pethidine analog with a limited access to the brain and minimal analgesic activity. It has mainly peripheral opioid activity and oral administration induces inhibition of gastrointestinal motility and secretion. The compound is used for the treatment of acute and chronic diarrhea (Shee and Pounder, 1980; Lustman et al., 1987).

Dosages and routes of administration: Diphenoxylate is used orally at initial doses of 10 mg, followed by 5 mg every 5 h. The standard formulation contains 1% atropine to inhibit parenteral misuse.

Pharmacokinetic properties: The compound is readily absorbed from the gastrointestinal tract, but rapidly and extensively metabolized in the liver (Karim et al.,1972), which strongly reduces systemic and CNS availability. The main metabolite is the free diphenoxylic acid, which still has anti-diarrheal properties. Other inactive metabolites and their glucuronides are excreted in faeces.

Side-effects: The compound induces mainly peripheral side-effects (Ginsburg, 1973) such as anorexia, nausea and vomiting, and abdominal distension. After higher doses and chronic treatment paralytic ileus and toxic megacolon can occur. Despite restricted access to the CNS, centrally mediated symptoms such as headache, drowsiness, dizziness, euphoria or depression can occur. Diphenoxylate potentiates the effect of CNS depressants and may provoke toxic interactions with MAO inhibitors. Prolonged use of high dosages may induce morphine like addiction and dependence. Illicit use is discouraged by addition of atropine.

Trade name: Reasec (Ger, Ital), Diaserd (Fr), Tropergen (UK), Lomotil (USA)

Ethylmorphine

Synthesis: Ethylation of morphine with ethyl benzenesulfonate (E. Merck, 1902; Ehrhart and Ruschig, 1972; Kleemann et al., 1999).

Ethylmorphine

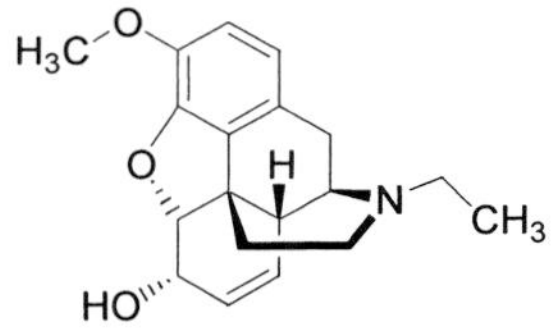

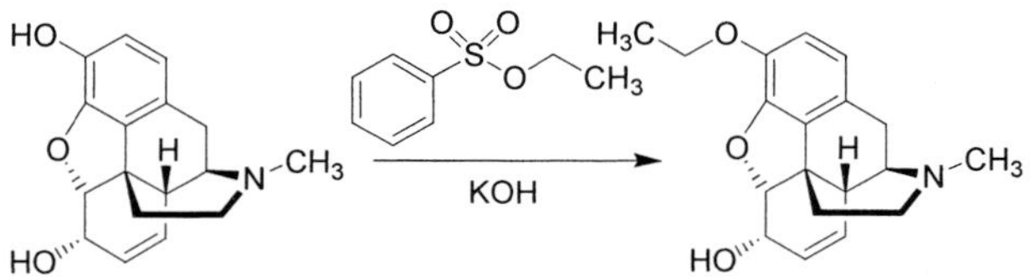

Scheme 17: Synthesis of ethylmorphine

[*76-58-4*], (5α,6α)-7,8-
Didehydro-4,5-epoxy-3-
ethoxy-17-methylmorphinan-
6-ol, $C_{19}H_{23}NO_3$, M_r 313.40,
mp 199-201 °C;
hydrochloride dihydrate
[6746-59-4], $C_{19}H_{23}NO_3$ · HCl
· H_2O, M_r 385.89, *mp* 123 °C
(decomp.), anhydrous form
melts at 170 °C (decomp.)

Opioid receptor binding: Ethylmorphine is an ethyl congener of codeine and has a low opioid receptor affinity (Chen et al., 1991). Like codeine, it is metabolized to the active principle morphine.

Analgesic efficacy and medical use: Ethylmorphine has an action profile similar to codeine with analgesic, antitussive and antidiarrheal properties. It has been used in similar circumstances to codeine as a cough suppressant and analgesic, but today it is mostly out of use.

Pharmacokinetic properties: Ethylmorphine (Aasmundstad et al., 1995) has a reasonable oral bioavailability. Like codeine, it is metabolized by O- and N-desalkylation, leading to nor-ethylmorphine, morphine, nor-morphine, and the respective glucuronides.

Trade name: Codethyline
(B), Trachyl (Fr), Collins
Elixir (UK)

Side-effects: Ethylmorphine has a side-effect profile comparable to codeine (Klinger, 1976) and a low to limited abuse and dependence potential (Jonasson et al., 1999).

Etorphine

[*14521-96-1*], [5α,7α(*R*)]-
4,5-Epoxy-3-hydroxy-6-
methoxy-α,17-dimethyl-α-
propyl-6,14-
ethenomorphinan-7-
methanol, $C_{25}H_{33}NO_4$, M_r
411.53, *mp* 214-217 °C;
hydrochloride [*13764-49-3*],
$C_{25}H_{33}NO_4$ · HCl, M_r 447.99,
mp 266-267 °C

Etorphine

Synthesis (Bentley (Reckitt & Colman), 1963; 1966, Bentley (Reckitt & Sons) 1969, Dorner, 1986; Kleemann et al., 1999): Starting from thebaine etorphine can be synthesized in a similiar way to buprenorphine (see buprenorphine) (Boehringer, 1912; Ehrhart and Ruschig, 1972; Trauner et al., 1983; Mulzer and Trauner, 1999).

Opioid receptor binding: Etorphine (Lee et al., 1999) has a high affinity and selectivity for the μ-opioid receptor.

Analgesic efficacy and medical use: Etorphine (Wallach, 1969) is one of the most potent synthetic opioids with a potency 400-1000-fold higher than morphine. In addition to ist analgesic properties etorphine induces potent CNS depression and is mostly used in veterinary practice for anesthesia, immobilization and pain treatment of large animals (Alford et al.,1974).

Routes of administration: Etorphine is only used parenterally.

Pharmacokinetic properties: Etorphine has an immediate onset of action and an intermediate duration of action (1-1.5 h), indicating rapid absorption and metabolization (Friedrich et al., 1991).

Trade name: Immobilon
(UK)

Side-effects: Etorphine induces potent CNS depression with impairment of respiration leading to coma and death in higher doses. Because of its rapid penetration through skin and mucosa and its outstanding potency, special precautions are necessary to avoid contamination during medical use. As antidote or to terminate anesthesia or immobilization, naloxone or the mixed κ-agonist/μ-antagonist diprenorphine (Alford et al., 1974) can be used. Etorphine has a morphine-type abuse and dependence potential.

Fentanyl

Synthesis (Janssen, P. (Janssen), 1964; 1965; Kleemann et al., 1999):

Fentanyl

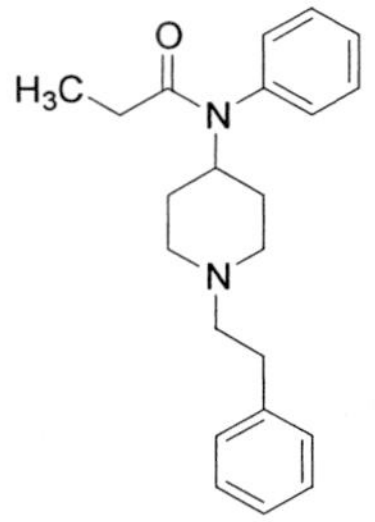

[*437-38-7*], *N*-(1-Phenethyl-piperidin-4-yl)-*N*-phenyl-propionamide, $C_{22}H_{28}N_2O$, M_r 336.47, *mp* 83-85 °C; citrate (1 : 1) [*990-73-8*], $C_{22}H_{28}N_2O \cdot C_6H_8O_7$, M_r 528.60, *mp* 149-151 °C

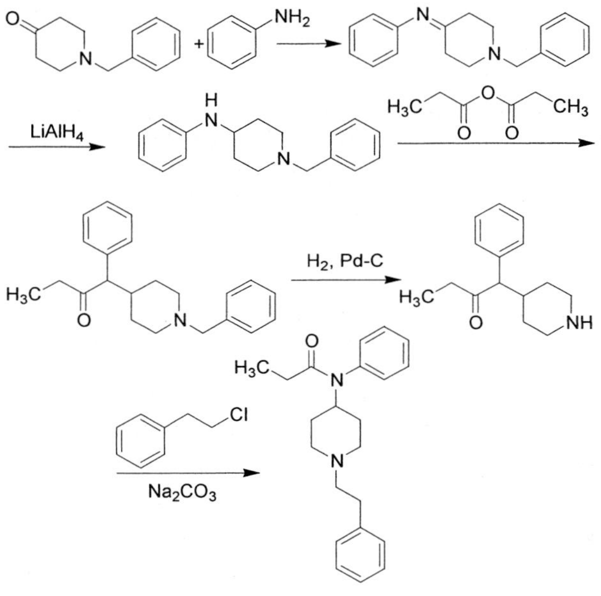

Scheme 18: Synthesis of fentanyl.

Opioid receptor binding: Fentanyl is a μ-selective potent opioid with a similar receptor binding affinity to morphine. The higher *in vivo* potency results from its greater lipophilicity (Subramanian, 2000).

Analgesic efficacy and clinical use: Fentanyl (Clotz and Nahata, 1991) is a potent analgesic and anesthetic compound. It is used for the treatment of severe acute and chronic pain, as a pre-medication or adjunct to anesthesia and as a primary anesthetic for the induction or maintenance of anesthesia. In combinations with neuroleptics e.g. droperidole, it induces a pain free and calm state known as neuroleptanalgesia (Foldes, 1973). In this condition, surgery can be performed in an awake patient, who is able to cooperate with the surgeon.

Dosages and routes of administration: For acute (postoperative) pain and for anesthesia, fentanyl is given by the intravenous route. For pre-medication in anesthesia and for break-through pain the compound can also been given as an oral-transmucosal formulation (Ashburn and Streisand, 1994). A transdermal patch has been developed for chronic pain treatment (Jeal and Benfield, 1997; O'Siordin, 1998). The intravenous doses for premedication are 50-100 μg, oral-transmucosal systems contain 200-400 μg and patch formulations have a delivery rate of 25-100 μg/h.

Pharmacokinetic properties: Fentanyl (Scholz et al., 1996) is a highly lipophilic compound and about 80% binds to plasma proteins. After parenteral administration it has a rapid onset and a short duration of action. The compound is rapidly transported into the CNS and lipid tissues. The short duration of action is due to redistribution rather than metabolic inactivation or excretion. It is released from tissue depots with a half-life of about 4 h and the terminal half-life is up to 7 h. The main metabolites, excreted in urine are 4-N-(N-propionylanilino)-piperidine and the N-hydroxypropionyl derivative.

Trade name: Durogensic (Ger, UK), Fentanyl Janssen (Ger), Sublimase (UK; USA), Duragesic (USA), Thalamonal (combination with Droperidol)

Side-effects: The side-effect profile (Poklis, 1995) is typical of potent μ-opioids with respiratory depression, increased muscle tone (chest wall rigidity during fentanyl anesthesia), strong sedation and emesis being most prominent. Adverse reactions can be antagonized with naloxone.

Fentanyl and fentanyl derivatives (so-called designer drugs) have a fundamental abuse potential (Buchanan and Brown, 1988)) and induce morphine-type physical dependence.

Hydrocodone

Hydrocodone

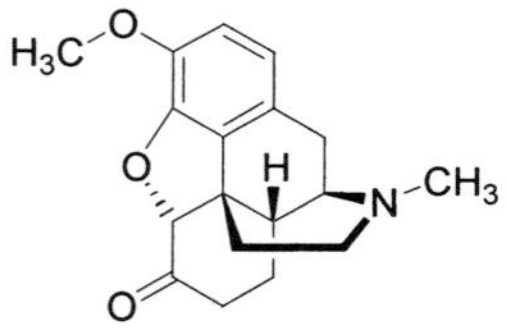

Synthesis (Knoll AG, 1935; Erhart, 1972, Kleemann et al., 1999): Palladium or platin catalyzed isomerization of codeine yields hydrocodone (Kleemann et al., 1999).

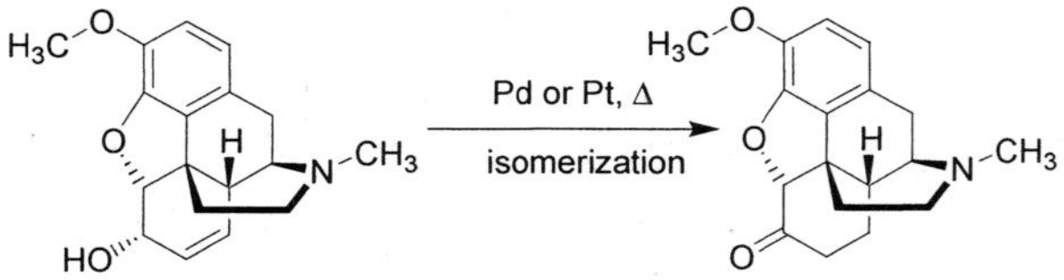

Scheme 19: Synthesis of hydrocodone.

Opioid receptor binding: Hydrocodone has a μ-opioid receptor binding that is 10-100 fold higher than codeine. In contrast to codeine, the compound itself in addition to the active metabolite hydromorphone is responsible for the opioid properties.

Analgesic efficacy and clinical use: Hydrocodone has an action profile similar to codeine, but with higher analgesic and antitussive potency. It is used for the treatment of moderate to moderately severe pain (Palangio et al., 2002) and for cough inhibition (Homsi et al., 2000). Combinations with paracetamol, acetylsalicylic acid or other weak analgesics are common for pain treatment and hydrocodone is added to multi-ingredient cough preparations.

Dosages and routes of administration: Hydrocodone is used orally in doses of 5-10 mg.

Pharmacokinetic properties: Hydrocodone is metabolized by CYP2D6 to the O-desmethyl derivative hydromorphone (Otton et al., 1993). Further steps of metabolization include N-demethylation and glucuronidation.

Side-effects: Hydrocodone induces side-effects similar to codeine and morphine and has an appreciable abuse and dependence potential (Morrison, 1979).

[76-42-6], (5α)-4,5-Epoxy-3-methoxy-17-methylmorphinan-6-one, $C_{18}H_{21}NO_3$, M_r 299.36, mp 198 °C; hydrochloride [25968-91-6], $C_{18}H_{21}NO_3$ · HCl, M_r 335.83; hydrochloride monohydrate [124-90-3], $C_{18}H_{21}NO_3$ · HCl · H_2O, M_r 353.85, mp 185-186 °C (decomp.), $[\alpha]_D^{27}$ -130° (c = 2.877); bitartrate hemipentahydrate [34195-34-1], $C_{18}H_{21}NO_3$ · $C_4H_6O_6$ 5/2 H_2O, M_r 988.99, mp 118-128 °C

Trade name: Dicodid (Ger, UK), Vicodin (USA)

Hydromorphone

Synthesis: Morphine is hydrogenated over a palladium catalyst, and the resulting dihydromorphine is oxidized with benzophenone and potassium *tert*-butoxide. Alternative oxidants are cyclohexanone with aluminium tri(*tert*-butoxide) or aluminium triphenoxide (Rapoport, 1950; Pfister and Tishler (Merck & Co), 1955; Kleemann et al., 1999).

Opioid receptor binding: Hydromorphone has a high affinity and selectivity for the µ-opioid receptor, the µ-affinity is about 10-fold higher than that of morphine.

Analgesic efficacy and clinical use: Hydromorphone is a strong morphine-type analgesic and is used for the treatment of moderate to severe pain and for cough inhibition (Sarhill et al., 2001; Quigley, 2002).

Dosages and routes of administration: Hydromorphone is used in doses of 1-2 mg by subcutaneous, intramuscular, slow intravenous or rectal administration, and in oral doses between 2-4 mg. The doses for cough inhibition are 1 mg, given as a syrup.

Pharmacokinetic properties: Hydromorphone (Hagen et al.,1995) is rapidly but incompletely absorbed from the gastrointestinal tract. It is metabolized in the gut and liver

Hydromorphone

[466-99-9], (5α)-4,5-Epoxy-3-hydroxy-17-methylmorphinan-6-one, $C_{17}H_{19}NO_3$, M_r 285.34, mp 266-267 °C; monohydrochloride [71-68-1], $C_{17}H_{19}NO_3$ · HCl, M_r 321.80

by glucuronidation and N-demethylation, and the conjugates are excreted in urine.

Trade name: Dilaudid (Ger, UK, USA)

Side-effects: Hydromorphone shows the typical morphine-like side-effects, and has a relatively high potential for addiction and dependence (Hill and Zacny, 2000).

Ketobemidone

Ketobemidone

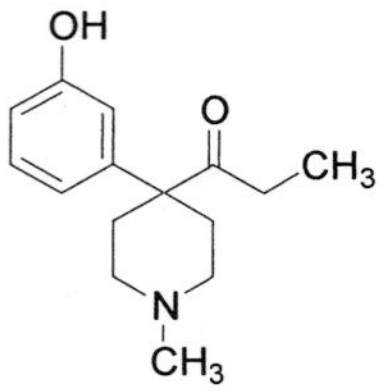

[*469-79-4*], *N*-(3-Hydroxy-phenyl)-*N*-(1-methyl-piperidin-4-yl)-propionamide, $C_{15}H_{21}NO_2$, M_r 247.34, *mp* 150-151 °C; hydrochloride [*5965-49-1*], $C_{15}H_{21}NO_2$. HCl, M_r 283.80, *mp* 201-202 °C

Synthesis: 4-Cyano-4-(3-methoxyphenyl)-1-methyl-piperidine is converted into a ketoethyl group by reaction with ethylmagnesium bromide. Subsequent ether cleavage by means of HBr yields ketobemidone (Eisleb (I. G. Farben, 1941; 1942; Kägi, 1949, Kleemann et al.,1999):

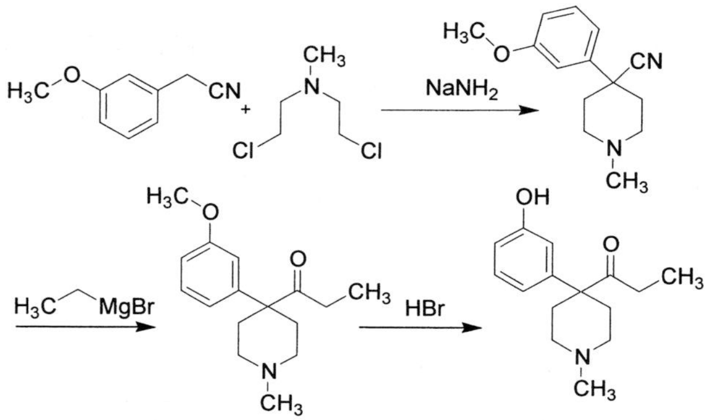

Scheme 20: Synthesis of ketobemidone.

Opioid receptor affinity: Ketobemidone is a μ-selective synthetic opioid with a receptor affinity similar to morphine (Christensen, 1993).

Analgesic efficacy and medical use: Ketobemidone is a potent analgesic and is used for the treatment of moderate to severe pain (Ohqvist et al., 1991).

Dosages and routes of administration: Doses of 5-10 mg are given by mouth, intravenous injection or rectally.

Pharmacokinetic properties: The compound has an acceptable oral bioavailability (Bondesson, 1980). Metabolic inactivation occurs via N-demethylation and glucuronidation at the phenolic hydroxyl.

Trade name: Cliradon (Ger, out of use), Ketogan (Sweden, Norway)

Side-effects: Ketobemidone has morphine-like side-effect and a similar abuse and dependence potential.

Levallorphan

Synthesis: The starting material for the synthesis of levallorphan is 1-(4-Methoxy-benzyl)-1,2,3,4,5,6,7,8-octa-hydro-isoquinoline **6** (*preparation see levorphanol*) (Schnider and Grüssner, 1951; Hellerbach, 1956; Ehrhart and Ruschig, 1972; Patron, 1979; Kleemann et al., 1999):

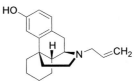

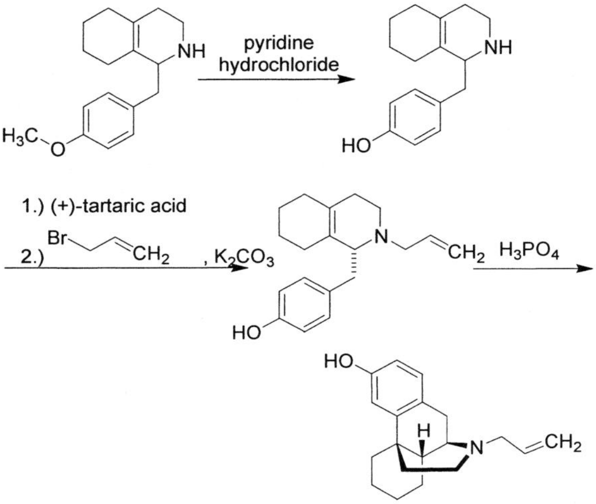

Levallorphan

[*152-02-3*], 17-(2-Propenyl)morphinan-3-ol, 1,*N*-allyl-3-hydroxy-morphinan, $C_{19}H_{25}NO$, M_r 283.42, *mp* 180-182 °C, $[\alpha]_D^{25}$ -88.9° (CH_3OH); hydrogen tartrate (1 : 1) [71-82-9], $C_{19}H_{25}NO \cdot C_4H_6O_6$, M_r 433.50, *mp* 176-177 °C, $[\alpha]_D^{25}$ -39° (water)

Scheme 21: Synthesis of levallorphan.

Opioid receptor binding: Levallorphan has a high binding affinity for the μ-opioid receptor.

Analgesic efficacy and clinical use: Levallorphan (Leimgruber et al., 1973) is an opioid antagonist with a minor agonistic component and practically no analgesic action. It has been used as one of the first relative pure antagonists for the treatment of opioid overdose, to reverse opioid central depression and to antagonize opioid-induced respiratory impairment (Foldes et al.,1969). The compound has now been widely replaced by naloxone (Evans et al., 1974).

Pharmacokinetic properties: The compound has low oral bioavailability because of strong first-pass glucuronidation in the gut and liver.

Side-effects: Levallorphan has virtually no opioid agonistic actions and does not induce analgesia (Blane and Boura, 1968).

Trade name: Lorfan

Levomethadone

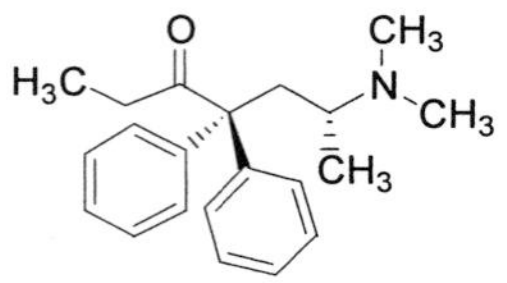

[125-58-6], (R)-6-Dimethylamino-4,4-diphenyl-heptan-3-one, $C_{21}H_{27}NO$, M_r 309.45, mp 98-100 °C (mp racemic form [57-42-1] 78-79 °C), $[\alpha]_D^{20}$ -32° (c = 1.8, CH_3CH_2OH), hydrochloride [5967-73-7], $C_{21}H_{27}NO \cdot HCl$, M_r 345.91, mp 240-241 °C (mp racemic form [1095-90-5] 231 °C), $[\alpha]_D^{20}$ -169° (c = 2.0, water)

Levomethadone

Synthesis (Bockmühl and Ehrhart (Farbw. Hoechst), 1941; 1948; Schultz et al.,1947; Howe and Sletzinger, 1949; Solmssen and Wenis,1948; Larsen et al.,1948, Howe et al. (Merck & Co), 1953; Zaugg (Abott), 1961):

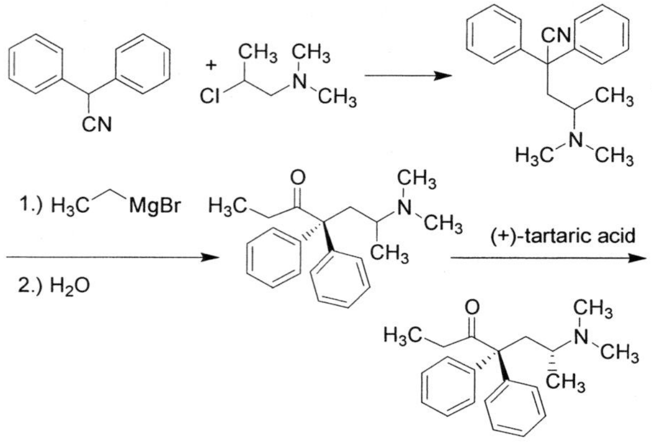

Scheme 22: Synthesis of levomethadone.

Opioid receptor binding: Levomethadone is the more potent and µ-selective levo-enantiomer of racemic methadone (Sim, 1973). It has an opioid receptor affinity in the range of morphine.

Analgesic efficacy and clinical use: Levomethadone like racemic methadone is a potent and long-acting opioid analgesic and can be used for the treatment of moderate to severe pain (Jamison, 2000; Davis and Walsh, 2001). It has an action profile similar to morphine and has significant antitussive properties, for which it is used in terminal lung cancer. The long duration of action makes the compound suitable for substitution treatment of opioid addiction (Joseph et al., 2000; Pallenbach, 2002). For practical and economic reasons the racemate instead of the levo-enantiomer is used in addicts.

Dosages and routes of administration: Levomethadone can be given by mouth or by intravenous, intramuscular, subcutaneous or intraspinal injection. For pain treatment, intravenous doses are between 2.5 and 5 mg and oral doses between 5 and 10 mg. For maintenance treatment in addicts, much higher oral doses up to more than 100 mg are used.

Pharmacokinetic properties: Levomethadone (Olsen et al., 1977) is readily absorbed from the intestinal tract and has high oral bioavailability. The compound is much more lipophilic than morphine and binds to plasma protein in the range of 60-90 %. It undergoes considerable tissue distribution and has a long elimination half-life of around 18 h. Accumulation can occur after repeated administration. Levomethadone is metabolized by N-demethylation to the cyclic derivatives 2-ethylidene-1,5-dimethyl-3,3-diphenyl-pyrrolidine and 2-ethyl-3,3-diphenyl-5-methyl-pyrrolidine, which are both inactive as analgesics (Moody et al., 1997). Together with unmetabolized levomethadone they are excreted in faeces and urine. The metabolic pathway of methadone is shown in the following scheme:

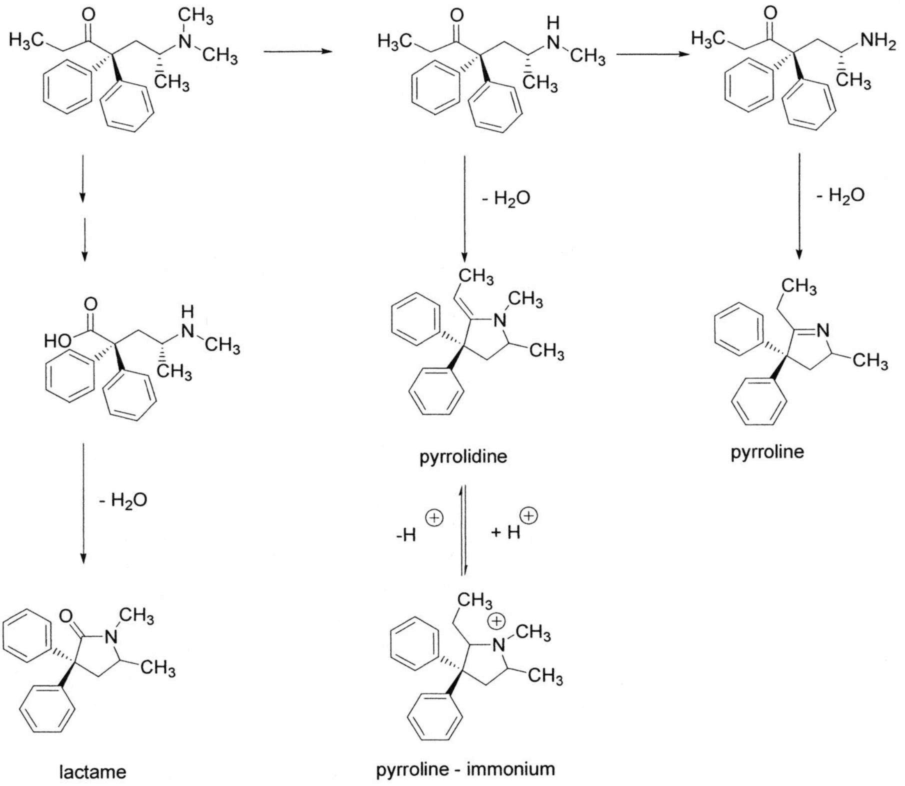

Scheme 23: Metabolic pathway of methadone.

Side-effects: Levomethadone has a morphine-like side-effect profile with stronger respiratory depression and less sedation than morphine (Kreek, 1973). The compound has a morphine-type abuse and dependence potential. Because of its slow elimination withdrawal reactions are more protracted and less severe than with morphine (Lowinson et al., 1978).

Trade name: l-Polamidon (Ger), Dolophine (USA), Physeptone (UK)

Levomethadyl-Acetate

[*34433-66-4*], Acetic acid 4-dimethylamino-1-ethyl-2,2-diphenyl-pentyl ester, [*S*-(*R*,R**)]-β-[2-(Dimethyl-amino)propyl]-α-ethyl-β-phenylbenzeneethanol acetate, $C_{23}H_{31}NO_2$, M_r 353.50; hydrochloride $C_{23}H_{31}NO_2 \cdot HCl$, M_r 389.96, *mp* 215 °C, $[\alpha]_D^{25}$ -60° (*c* = 0.2, water)

Trade name: Orlaam (USA)

Levomethadyl-Acetate (l-α-Acetylmethadol (LAAM))

Synthesis: By reduction of dextromethadon and subsequent acylation (Pallenbach 2002, Carroll et al., 1976, Drugs Fut. 1979).

Opioid receptor binding: Levomethadyl acetate has a moderate affinity for opioid receptors with selectivity for the μ-type. Higher binding affinity is induced by the active metabolites *l*-alpha-nor-acetylmethadol, nor-methadol and methadol (Walczak et al., 1981; Carroll, 1976).

Analgesic efficacy and clinical use: Levomethadyl acetate, a methadone derivative, is a long-acting opioid analgesic, which is mostly used for the treatment of opioid dependence (Blaine et al., 1978; Ling, 1978)

Dosages and routes of administration: The compound is used orally. The initial doses range from 20 to 40 mg every 2-3 days and can be increased up to 140 mg. Due to the slow onset of action, supplementation with other shorter acting opioids is necessary during the first 3 days.

Pharmacokinetic properties: Levomethadyl acetate is well absorbed from the intestinal tract and is extensively metabolized to various active metabolites, which contribute to the long duration of action. The metabolites nor-acytylmethadol, di-nor-acetylmethadol, nor-methadol, and methadol are formed by N-demethylation and hydrolytic cleavage of the ester bond (Moody et al., 1997)

Side-effects: Levomethadyl acetate induces opioid-type side-effects with respiratory depression, bradycardia and impairment of cardiac contractility (Wolven and Archer, 1976). The compound increases the QT-interval and may induce Torsade de pointes (Deamer et al., 2001). Because of the cardiovascular side effects (Q/T interval prolongation) Levomethadyl acetate was recently withdrawn from the market in most of the european countries.

Levorphanol

Levorphanol

Synthesis: The analgesic activity of racemorphan is due to the (-) isomer, levorphanol, which is obtained by resolving the racemate with (+)-*D*-tartaric acid. Resolution can also be carried out on the intermediate 1-(4-Methoxy-benzyl)-1,2,3,4,5,6,7,8-octahydro-isoquinoline **6** prior to *N*-methylation (Grewe 1946, Schnider and Hellerbach, 1950, Schnider and Grüssner, 1951, Ehrhart and Ruschig 1972, Kleemann et al. 1999).

[*77-07-6*], 17-Methylmorphinan-3-ol, (-)-3-hydroxy-*N*-methyl-morphinan, $C_{17}H_{23}NO$, M_r 257.37, *mp* 198-199 °C, $[\alpha]_D^{20}$ -56° (c = 3, CH_3CH_2OH); tartrate dihydrate [*5985-38-6*], $C_{17}H_{23}NO$. $C_4H_6O_6$. 2 H_2O, M_r 257.37, *mp* 113-115 °C (anhydrous *mp* 206-208 °C), $[\alpha]_D^{20}$ -14° (c = 3, water)

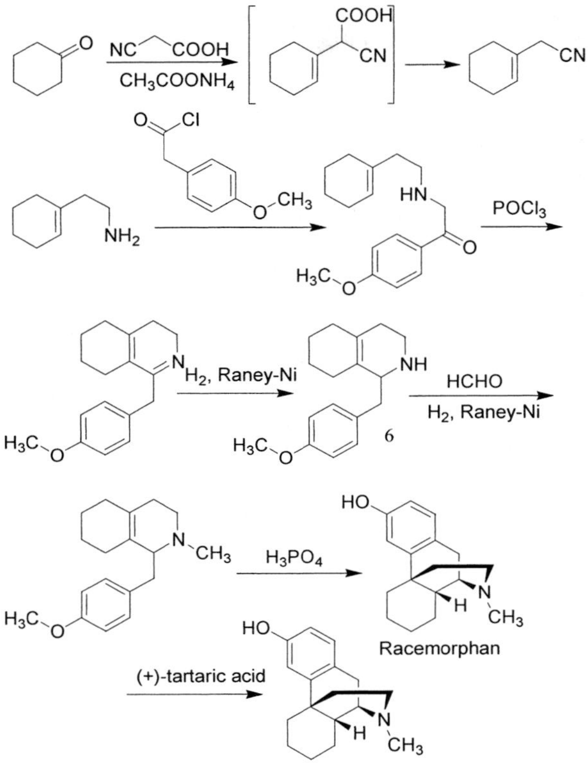

Scheme 24: Synthesis of levorphanol.

Opioid receptor binding: Levorphanol is a µ-selective synthetic opioid with a higher receptor affinity than morphine (Childers et al., 1979).

Analgesic efficacy and clinical use: Levorphanol is a potent and long-acting analgesic used for the treatment of moderate to severe pain (Dixon et al., 1983).

Dosages and routes of administration: The compound is used as the tartrate in doses of 2-4 mg by mouth or 2-3 mg by subcutaneous or slow intravenous injection. In addition, levorphanol can be used as ananesthetic supplement.

Pharmacokinetic properties: After oral administration levorphanol has a relatively slow onset, but a long (up to 8 h) duration of action. Metabolic inactivation occurs via glucuronidation of the phenolic hydroxyl and via N-demethylation (Dixon et al., 1983).

Trade name: Levo-
Dromoran (USA)

Side-effects: Levorphanol has morphine-type side-effects with significant respiratory depression in the high dose range. It induces morphine type addiction and dependence (Coniam, 1991).

Loperamide

Loperamide

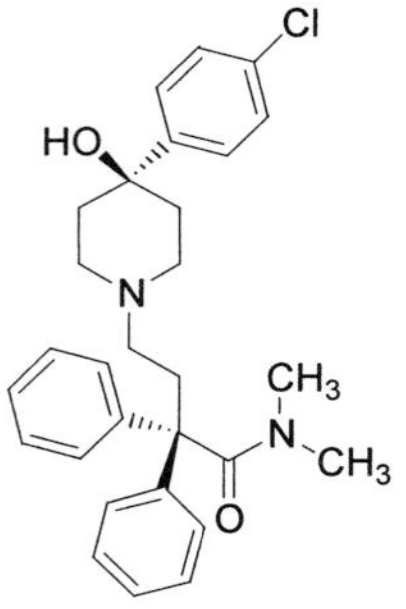

[*53179-11-6*], 4-[4-(4-Chloro-phenyl)-4-hydroxy-piperidin-1-yl]-*N,N*-dimethyl-2,2-diphenyl-butyramide, 4-(4-chlorophenyl)-4-hydroxy-*N,N*-diemethyl-α,α-diphenyl-1-piperidinebutanamide, $C_{29}H_{33}CIN_2O_2$, M_r 477.04; monohydrochloride [*34552-83-5*], $C_{29}H_{33}CIN_2O_2 \cdot HCl$, M_r 513.51, *mp* 222-223 °C (decomp.)

Synthesis (Kleemann et al. 1999, Janssen (Janssen), 1973; Janssen et al. (Janssen), 1973, Stokbroekx et al., 1973, Niemegeers et al., 1974):): Treatment of 2-oxo-3,3-diphenyl-tetrahydrofuran, synthesized by treatment of diphenyl-acetic acid ethyl ester with ethylene oxide, with HBr(gas) yields bromo derivative **i**, which is then converted into butyryl chloride derivative **ii** by means of thionyl chloride in refluxing chloroform. Reaction of derivative **ii** with dimethylamine in toluene affords dimethyl (tetrahydro-3,3-diphenyl-2-furylidene)ammonium bromide, which is then condensed with 4-(4-chlorophenyl)-4-piperidinol by means of Na_2CO_3 and KI in refluxing 4-methyl-2-pentanone to provide loperamide.

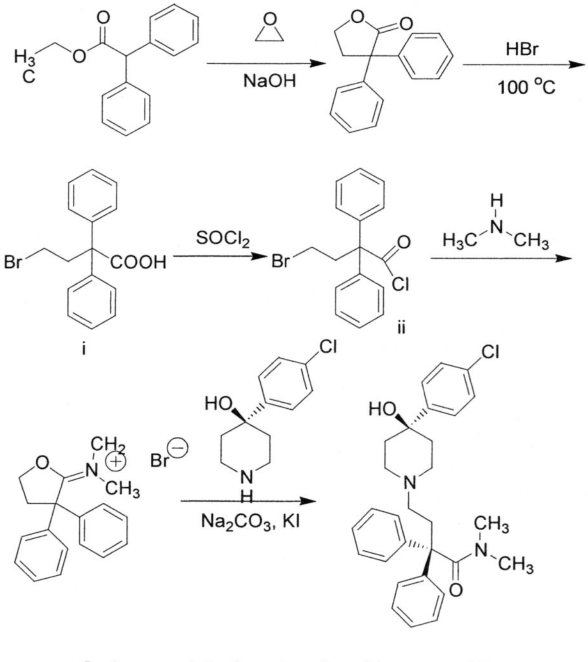

Scheme 25: Synthesis of loperamide.

Opioid receptor binding: Loperamide has a morphine-like affinity and selectivity for the μ-opioid receptor (Dashwood et al., 1990).

Analgesic efficacy and clinical use: Systemic loperamide does not reach the CNS and the compound has no analgesic action. Oral loperamide acts locally in the gut to inhibit intestinal motility and secretion (Awouters et al., 1993). In addition to the strong μ-opioid action, calcium and calmodulin antagonism are involved in the anti-diarrheal activity. The compound is used for the treatment of acute and chronic diarrhea and for the management of colostomies and ileostomies (Heel et al., 1978b, Wheeler 2000).

Dosages and routes of administration: Loperamide is used in various oral formulations with single doses of 4-8 mg and daily doses up to 16 mg.

Pharmacokinetic properties: About 40% of the drug is absorbed from the intestinal tract but nearly completely inactivated by first pass metabolism in the liver (Killinger et al., 1979). The main metabolites are N-desmethyl-loperamide and the di-desmethyl derivative (Yoshida et al., 1979). The elimination half life is about 10 h.

Side-effects: Adverse effects include nausea, dry mouth and dizziness. High doses can induce toxic megacolon and paralytic ileus. The compound has no abuse or dependence potential (Ericsson and Johnson, 1990).

Trade name: Imodium (Ger, Belg., USA, F), Arret (UK)

Meptazinol

Synthesis (Cavalla and White (Wyeth), 1969; 1969; Bradley 1980; Kleemann et al. 1999): By condensation of 2-(m-methoxyphenyl)butyronitrile with ethyl 4-iodobutyrate by means of $NaNH_2$ in liquid NH_3 to give ethyl 5-cyano-5-(m-methoxyphenyl)heptanoate, which is cyclized by hydrogenation with H_2 over Raney Ni in cyclohexane to yield 6-ethyl-6-(m-methoxyphenyl)hexahydro-2H-azepin-2-one; this ketone is reduced with $LiAlH_4$ in THF to 3-ethyl-3-(m-methoxyphenyl)hexahydro-1H-azepine, which in turn, is reductively methylated with HCHO, H_2 and Pd/C in ethanol to give 1-methyl-3-ethyl-3-(m-methoxyphenyl)-hexahydro-1H-azepine, and finally demethylated by reflux-ing with 80% HBr to yield a racemic mixture of the final product.

Meptazinol

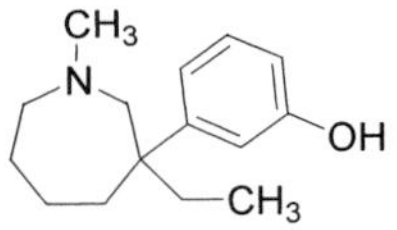

[54340-58-8], 3-(3-Ethyl-1-methyl-azepan-3-yl)-phenol, 3-(3-Ethylhexahydro-1-methyl-1H-azepin-3-yl-phenol, $C_{15}H_{23}NO$, M_r 233.35, *mp* 127.5-133 °C; hydrochloride [59263-76-2], $C_{15}H_{23}NO \cdot HCl$, M_r 269.81

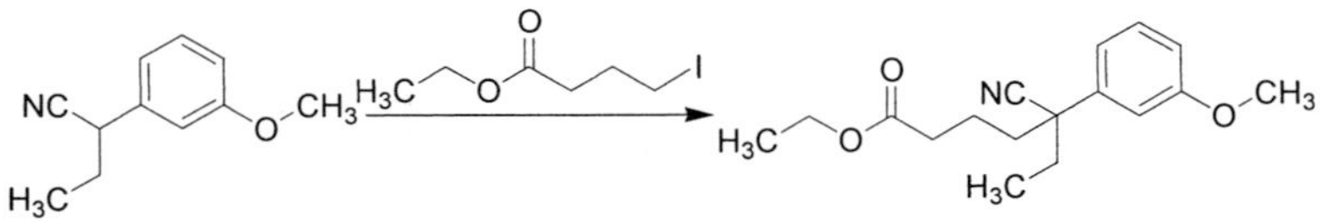

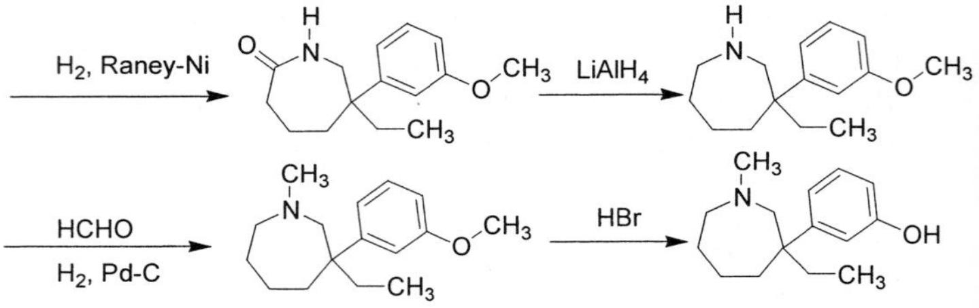

Friderichs and Buschmann

Scheme 26: Synthesis of meptazinol.

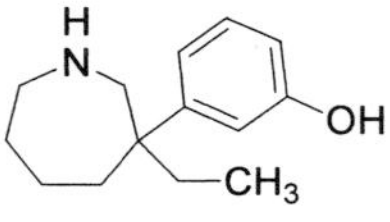

i

The enantiomers are obtained by diastereomeric crystallization of the demethylated methoxyazepine derivative **i** with (D)-(+)-tartaric acid followed by methylation with HCHO, H_2 and Pd/C in ethanol.

Opioid receptor binding: Meptazinol (Holmes and Ward, 1985) is a partial μ-agonist with a high μ-receptor affinity; the selective action at a special μ1-subtype is controversial (Pasternak et al., 1985).

Analgesic efficacy and clinical use: Meptazinol is a medium potent opioid analgesic with an additional cholinergic component. It is used for the treatment of moderate to moderately severe pain. The compound has a shorter duration of action than morphine (Holmes and Ward, 1985; Kay, 1985).

Dosages and routes of administration: Meptazinol is used in parenteral doses of 50-100 mg, given every 2-4 hrs by intramuscular or slow intravenous injection. For short-term treatment of moderate pain, the compound can be given by oral administration in doses of 200 mg every 3-6 h.

Pharmacokinetic properties: Meptazinol has poor oral bio-availability due to extensive first-pass metabolism. Systemic availability is improved after rectal administration. Peak plasma concentrations are reached 30 min after rectal or intramuscular administration and plasma half-life is about 2 h. Plasma protein binding is low (~ 30%). Meptazinole is extensively metabolized in the gut and liver mainly to the glucuronide derivative. Only about 10% is excreted unmetabolised in the faeces (Franklin, 1988).

Side-Effects: The most common side-effects are nausea, vomiting and dizziness. Other vegetative side-effects include sweating, hypotension and drowsiness. The compound is reported to be relatively free of respiratory depressant activity, which was attributed to selective binding to a subtype (μ-1) of the opioid receptor

(Pasternak et al., 1985) , an alternative explanation may be the cholinergic action component (Holmes and Ward, 1985) In accordance with a low κ-receptor affinity, the incidence of psychotomimetic actions and hallucinations is low.

Meptazinole may precipitate withdrawal in persons under long-term opioid treatment. The compound has a low abuse potential (Johnson and Jasinski, 1987) and is not under narcotic control.

Trade name: Meptid (Ger, UK)

Morphine

Preparation: By extraction of poppy capsules or opium (opium contains 9-14 % morphine depending on the source) with water, precipitation with aqueous Na_2CO_3 solution, washing of the precipitate with ethanol and dissolution in dilute acetic acid (Hörner et al. (Knoll), 1977, Trauner et al.,1983, Hudlicky et al.,1996).

The total synthesis of (-)-morphine has been a challenging target for organic chemists for many decades (Casy and Parfitt, 1986; Frackenpohl, 2000). Although a number of successful synthesis have been developed to date (Hudlicky et al., 1996, Casy and Parfitt, 1986, Novak et al., 2000, Bentley 2000) since the first accomplishment by Gates in 1952 (Gates 1952), only a few could produce the alkaloid in an enantio- and diastereocontrolled manner (e.g.: Meuzelaar et al.,1999; Mulzer and Trauner,1999, Davies et al., 2001; Nagata et al., 2001)

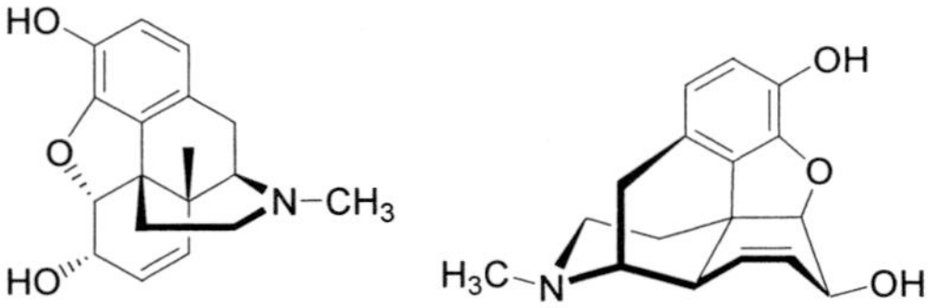

Morphine

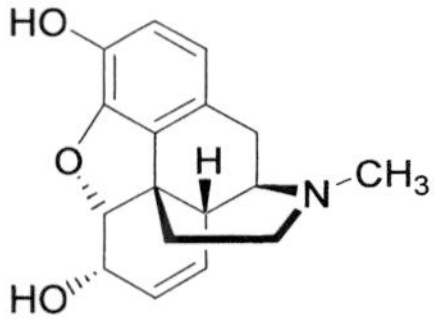

[57-27-2], (5α,6α)-7,8-Didehydro-4,5-epoxy-17-methylmorphinan-3,6-diol, $C_{17}H_{19}NO_3$, M_r 285.34, *mp* 254 °C (decomp., 197 °C is reported for a metastable phase), $[\alpha]_D^{25}$ -132° (c = 1, CH_3OH); hydrochloride [52-26-6], $C_{17}H_{19}NO_3 \cdot HCl$, M_r 321.80, *mp* 200°C (trihydrate), $[\alpha]_D^{25}$ -113.5° (c = 2.2, water); sulfate (2 : 1) [64-31-3], $C_{17}H_{19}NO_3 \cdot 1/2$ H_2SO_4, M_r 668.76; sulfate pentahydrate [6211-15-0], $C_{17}H_{19}NO_3 \cdot 1/2 H_2SO_4 \cdot$ $5H_2O$, M_r 758.85, *mp* 250 °C (decomp.), $[\alpha]_D^{25}$ -108.7° (c = 4, water)

Figure 4: Morphine in the conventional presentation (left) and in a stereoformula according to IUPAC rules (right).

Morphine and codeine biosynthesis (Samuelsson, 1999; Herbert et al., 2000; Novak et al., 2000): Studies on the biosynthesis of morphine have been carried out mainly on cell cultures mainly of *Coptis japonica* and species of *Thalictrum*. Two enzymes (*tyrosine decarboxylase* and *phenolase*) catalyze the formation of dopamine from one molecule tyrosine. Dopamine is also the key intermediate in the biosynthesis of mescaline.

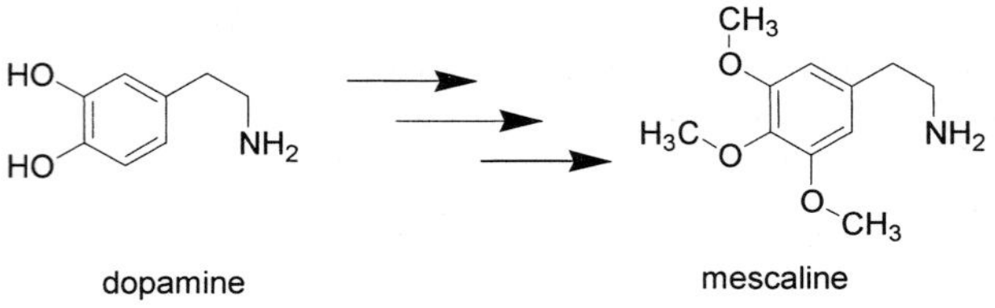

dopamine

mescaline

Scheme 27: Biosynthesis of morphine: conversion of dopamine to mescaline.

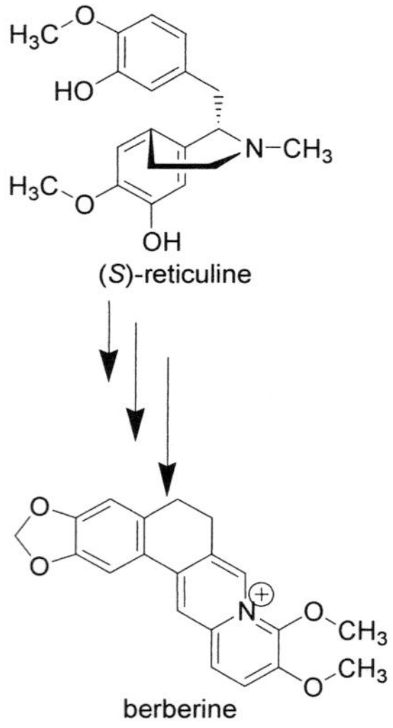

(S)-reticuline

berberine

Scheme 28: Conversion of (S)-reticuline to berberine.

(L)-tyrosine transaminase catalyses the reaction between a second molecule of tyrosine and α-ketoglutaric acid yielding 4-hydroxyphenylpyruvic acid which is decarboxylated by *4-hydroxyphenylpyruvate carboxylase* resulting in the formation of 4-hydroxyphenylacetaldehyde. *(S)-narcoclaurine synthase* catalyzes a stereoselective condensation of dopamine and 4-hydroxy-phenyllacetaldehyde to (S)-norcolaurine. The enzyme has an apparent molecular weight of around 15,000. Methylation of the 6-OH of norcolaurine is catalyzed by *(R,S)-norcolaurine-6-O-methyl-transferase* (6-OMT) yielding (S)-coclaurine. N-methylation of coclaurine is mediated by *(S)-coclaurine-N-methyltransferase* resulting in the formation of (S)-N-methylcoclaurine which is oxidized by a phenolase to yield (S)-3´-hydroxy-N-methylcoclaurine. Methylation of the 4´-OH in this compound, catalyzed by *(S)-3´-hydroxy-N-methyl-(S)-coclaurine-4´-O-methyltransferase* (4-OMT) yields (S)-reticuline. This alkaloid is a key compound in the biosynthesis of other benzylisoquinoline alkaloids such as berberine.

In order to understand the continuation of the biosynthesis of codeine and morphine from reticuline, the structure for (S)-reticuline can be written as follows:

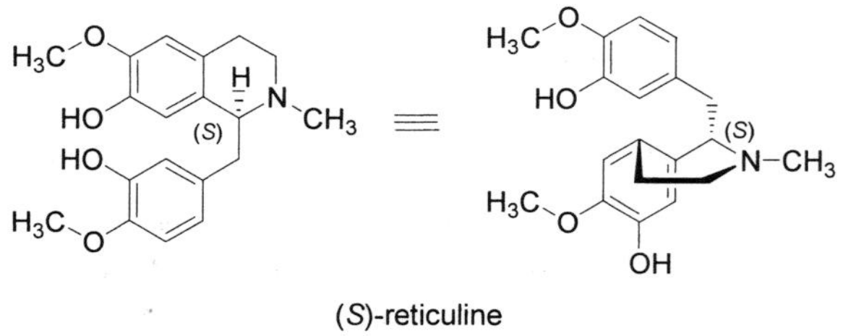

(S)-reticuline

Figure 5: Two different formulas showing the stereochemistry of (S)-reticuline

Reticuline occurs in the two enantiomeric forms: (S)-(+)- and (R)-(-)reticuline. Curiously this compound has the opposite configuration to that found in the morphine family of alkaloids. The two isomers are interconvertable via the 1,2-dehydroreticulinium ion, an intermediate which has been shown to be naturally occuring in *Papaver somniferum*. An enzyme, *1,2-dehydroreticline reductase* (EC 1.5.1.27) has been isolated from seedlings of *Papaver somniferum*. This enzyme stereospecifically reduces 1,2-dehydroreticuline to (*R*)-reticuline. The isolated enzyme is cytosolic, NADPH dependent and constitutes a single polypeptide with a molecular weight of 30,000. It is highly substrate-specific and has been found only in morphinan alkaloid-containing plants. Unlike many other oxireductases, the NADPH-dependent enzyme does not catalyze the physiologically reverse reaction *in vitro*. The 1,2-dihydroreticulinium ion is produced by oxidation of the (*S*)-enantiomer catalyzed by (S)-reticuline-oxidase.

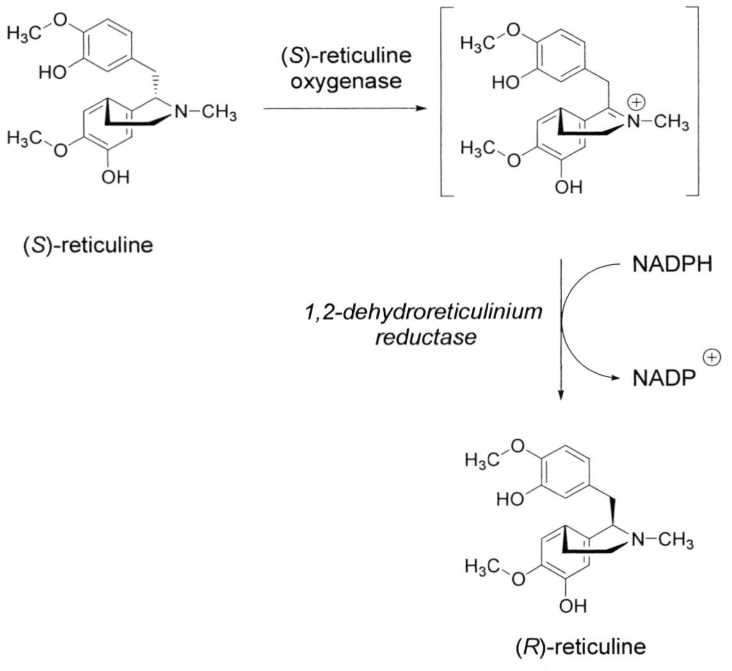

Scheme 29: The stereochemical inversion of (*S*)-(+)- to (*R*)-(-) reticuline via the enzymes *(S)-reticulinium oxygenase* and *1,2-dehydroreticuline reductase*. The 1,2-dehydro-reticulinium ion is proposed as an intermediate.

In the next step (*R*)-reticuline is first transformed to the dienone salutaridine by regioselective *para-ortho* oxidative coupling, catalyzed by a stereo- and regioselective cytochrome P-450-linked microsomal enzyme, which has not yet been isolated. Salutaridine is reduced to salutaridinol by *salutaridine-NADPH 7-oxireductase*. This reaction proceeds at pH 6.0-6.5. The enzyme can also catalyze the reverse reaction - salutaridinol to salutaridine - but the pH optimum for that reaction is much higher, 9.0-9.5. The enzyme is a single polypeptide of molecular mass 52 kDa which is absolutely dependent on NADPH/NADP as pyridine nucleotide cofactors. It was originally isolated from cell cultures of *Papaverum somniferum* but has also been shown to be present in capsules and seedlings of the plant. This enzyme has not been found in any other Papaver species except the thebaine-producing *P. bracteatum.* It is thus highly specific for plants producing the morphinandione skeleton.

The oxide bridge in codeine and morphine is closed in a reaction catalyzed by the enzyme *acetyl-coenzyme A salutaridinol-7O-acetyltransferase* which transfers an acetyl group from acetyl-CoA to the hydroxy group at C-7 of salutaridinol. The product taridinol-7-(O)-acetate under-goes a spontanenous allylic elimination yielding the alkaloid thebaine. The spontaneous elimination reaction has been demonstrated to occur in vitro at pH 8-9 and no enzyme catalyzing this reaction has been found. It is therefore assumed that the elimination reaction also occurs spontaneously *in vivo. Acetyl-coenzyme A salutaridinol-7O-acetyltransferase* was isolated from a cell culture of *Papaver somniferum* and has a molecular mass of 50 kDa. The enzyme is highly substrate specific. The epimer of salutaridinol 7-epi-salutaridinol is not acetylated by this enzyme, thus confirming the previous finding that this compound is not a precursor for thebaine. Thebaine is demethylated to yield neopinone which spontaneously rearranges to codeinone. Codeinone is reduced to codeine by a highly substrate specific and stereoselective enzyme known as *codeine/NADP oxireductase*. Finally, demethylation of codeine yields morphine. The two demethylation reactions are unusual in a biosynthetic pathway. It has been suggested that the methyl groups serve as protecting groups during the biosynthesis, thereby avoiding other possible reactions in which the hydroxy groups in question could participate.

The overall pathway from tyrosine to morphine is illustrated in the following scheme.

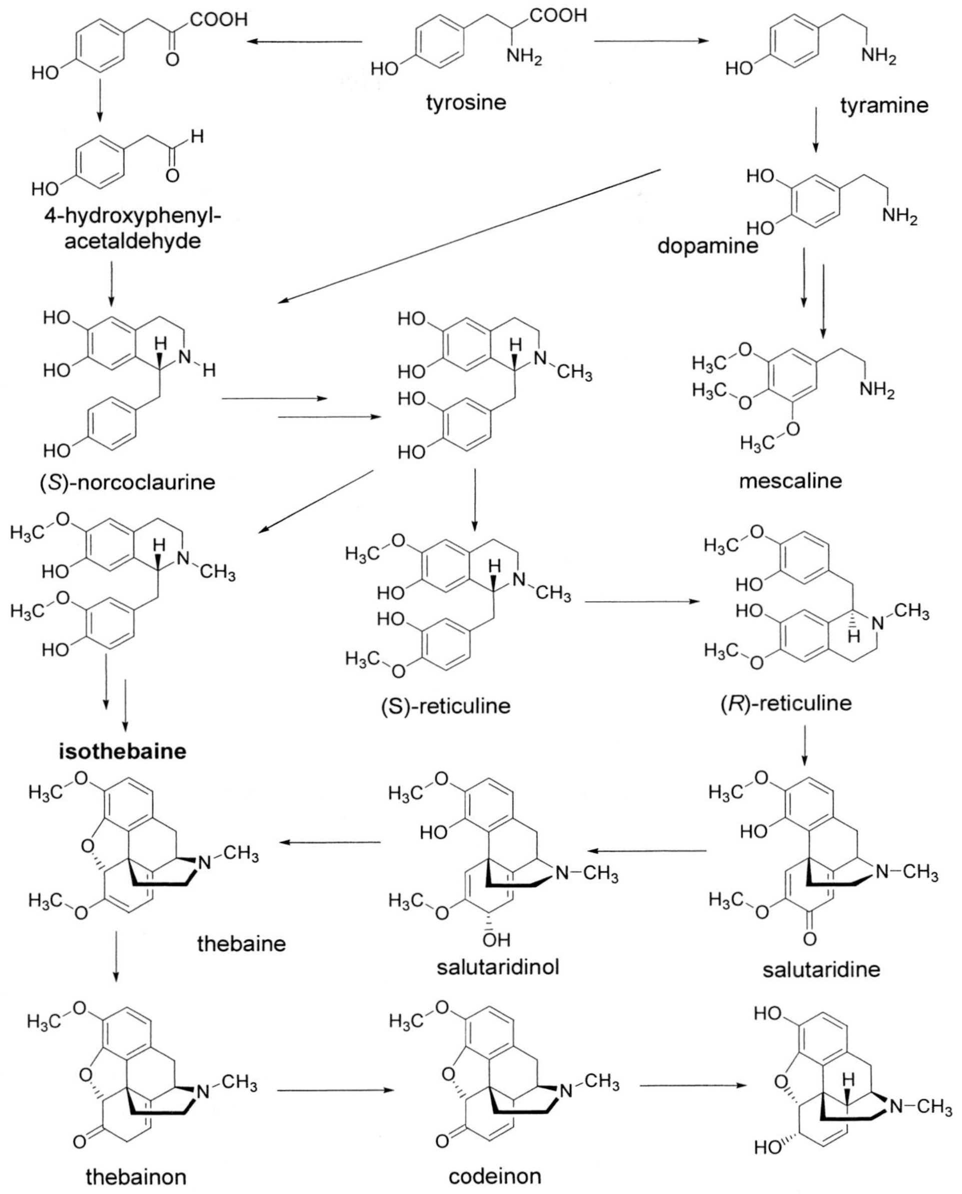

Scheme 30: The overall biosynthetic pathway from tyrosine to morphine

Opioid receptor binding: Morphine has a high (nanomolar) binding affinity for the opioid receptor. The affinity for the δ- and κ- receptor is at least 10-fold lower.

Analgesic efficacy and clinical use: Morphine (Benyhe, 1994) is a very potent analgesic and is used for the treatment of moderate to severe acute and chronic pain of various origins. It is more active in nociceptive and in inflammatory as compared to neuropathic pain and is regarded as the gold standard for pain treatment (Coluzzi,1998).

Dosages and routes of administration: Morphine is available in different salt forms but the hydrochloride and sulfate (Vermeire and Remon, 1999) are used preferentially. The compound can be administered by the oral, parenteral or intraspinal route. Oral application is preferred for chronic pain treatment and various slow release forms have been developed to reduce the administration frequency to 2-3 times per day (Bourke et al., 2000). Parenteral morphine is used in intravenous or intramuscular doses of 10 mg, mostly for postoperative pain and self-administration devices are available for patient-controlled analgesia (PCA). Morphine is additionally used for intraspinal (epidural or intrathecal) administration. Morphine is absorbed reasonably well in the lower gastrointestinal tract and can be given as suppositories.

Pharmacokinetic properties: Morphine is extensively metabolized by glucuronidation at both hydroxyl groups at position 3 and 6 and by N-demethylation (Osborne et al.,1990; Christrup, 1997). The 3-glucuronide has minimal opioid receptor binding affinity and is devoid of analgesic action, whereas the morphine-6-glucuronide (Schwarzinger et al., 2001) has a binding affinity similar to morphine, is analgesically active and seems to be involved in pain inhibition during chronic oral treatment (Lotsch and Geisslinger, 2001). Despite the polar sugar residue the glucuronide can cross the blood-brain barrier. The N-demethyl derivative normorphine is analgesically active, but has a lower μ-receptor affinity than morphine. The main metabolites of morphine are shown in Scheme 31.

Side-effects: Morphine induces a variety of centrally- and peripherally-mediated side-effects. The most important of which is respiratory depression following parenteral administration, especially in the postoperative situation. Chronic oral application induces constipation and chronic treatment with oral morphine must be supplemented with laxatives. Other frequent side-effects are nausea, vomiting, dizziness and sedation.

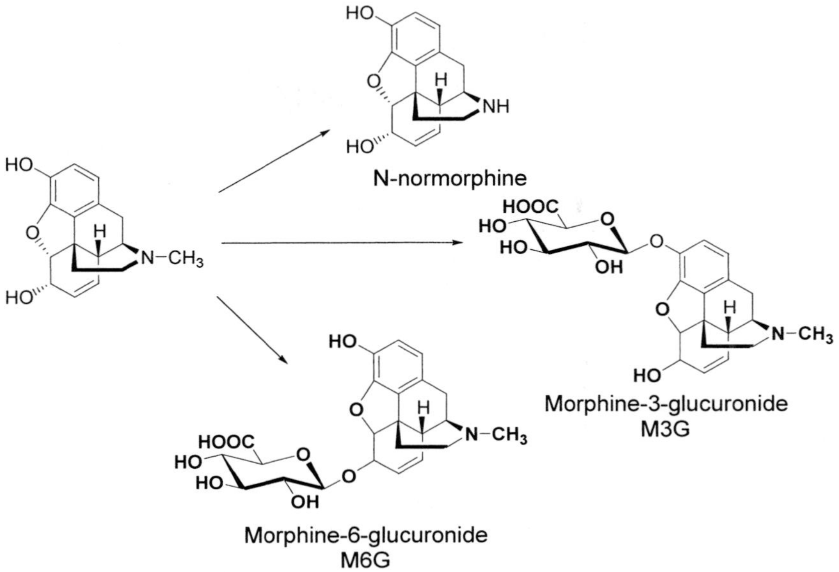

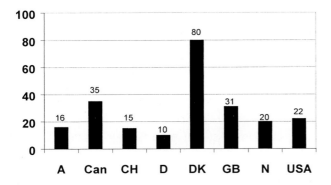

Scheme 31: Metabolic pathway of morphine.

Morphine is a controlled substance since it has a high euphorigenic potential and is liable to abuse and dependence. The euphorigenic effect is less expressed in the context of pain treatment and tolerance and dependence can largely be avoided by appropriate dosing and administration intervals, ensuring constant and pain appropriate plasma levels of the compound.

The following scheme shows the morphine consumption in different European countries and the United States.

Figure 6: Morphine consumption (1995) in different countries in kg compound /Mio inhabitants (Sohn and Zenz, 1998)

Nalbuphine

Nalbuphine

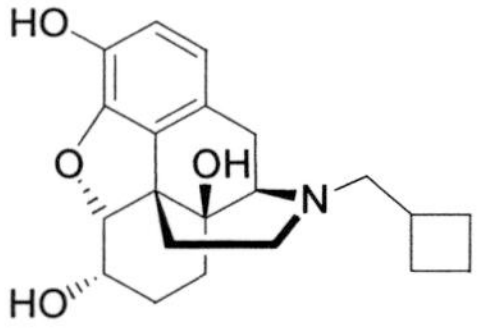

[*20594-83-6*], (5a,6a)-17-
(Cyclobutylmethyl)-4,5-
epoxymorphinan-3,6,14-triol,
$C_{21}H_{27}NO_4$, M_r 357.44, *mp*
230.5 °C; hydrochloride
[*23277-43-2*], $C_{21}H_{27}NO_4$ ·
HCl, M_r 393.91, *mp* 291-292
°C (decomp.)

Synthesis: The starting material for the nalbuphine synthesis is oxycodone (*see oxycodone*). After ether cleavage to oxymorphone the product is acylated and the N-methyl group is removed by treatment with cyanogen bromide. The acetyl groups are hydrolyzed with dilute hydrochloric acid. The resulting 14-hydroxydihydro-normorphinon **i** can be N-alkylated with cyclobutylmethyl bromide, and the carbonyl group at C-6 is reduced (Blumberg et al. (Endo Laboratories), 1967; 1970; Castaner and Roberts, 1977, Kleemann et al. 1999).

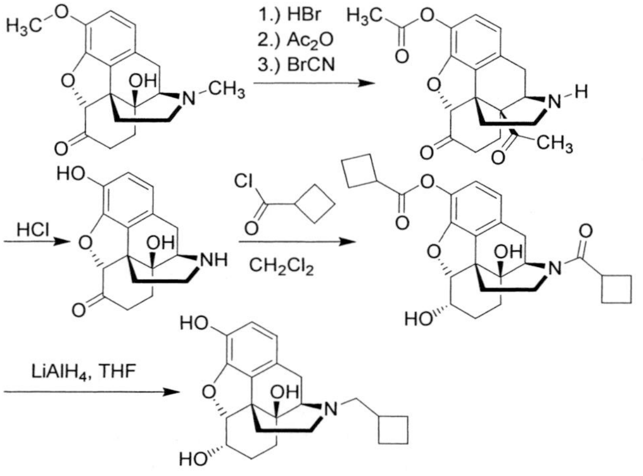

Scheme 32: Synthesis of nalbuphine.

Alternatively the condensation of **i** with cyclobutylmethyl bromide in DMF gives the N-cyclobutylmethyl derivative, which is then reduced with NaBH₄ in ethanol.

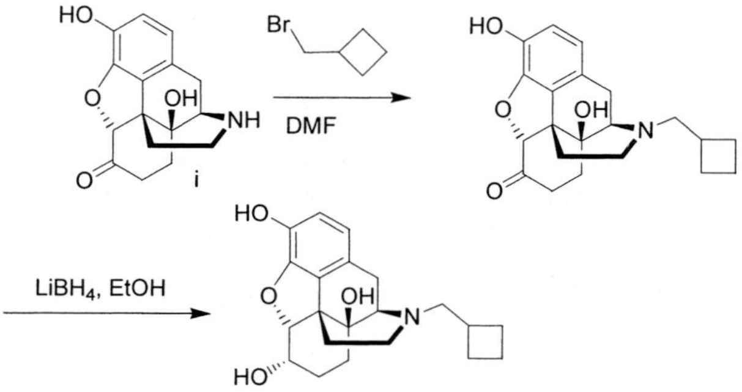

Scheme 33: Synthesis of nalbuphine.

The reduction of **i** with $NaBH_4$ also gives 14-hydroxy-dihydronormophine, which is then alkylated with cyclobutylmethyl bromide in DMF.

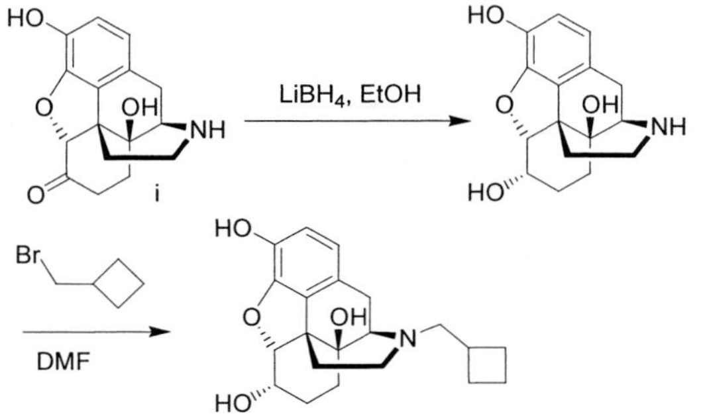

Scheme 34: Synthesis of nalbuphine.

Opioid receptor binding: Nalbuphine is a mixed agonist-antagonist opioid with a high affinity for the μ- and κ-opioid receptor. At the κ-receptor the compound is an agonist, at the μ-receptor a partial agonist with a very low intrisic activity, thus acting more as a μ-antagonist (De Souza et al., 1988).

Analgesic efficacy and clinical use: Nalbuphine (Errick and Heel, 1983; Schmidt et al., 1985) is a medium potent opioid analgesic used for the treatment of moderate to severe pain and inter-operatively as adjunct to anesthesia. Because of its antagonistic action component, analgesia may be subject to a ceiling level.

Dosages and routes of administration: Nalbuphine is used only parenterally by the subcutaneous, intramuscular or intravenous route. Single doses are 10-20 mg and for the treatment of myocardial infarction 30 mg.

Pharmacokinetic properties: Due to intensive first-pass metabolism, nalbuphine has a low oral bioavailability of less than 10%. After intramuscular administration peak plasma concentrations are reached after 30 min, half-life time is about 5 h. The compound is metabolized by glucuronidation and to a minor extent by N-dealkylation, and less than 10% is excreted unmetabolized (Lo et al., 1987).

Side-effects: The most frequent side-effect is drowsiness, others are nausea, vomiting, sweating, dizziness, vertigo, dry mouth and headache. Hallucinations and psychotomimetic reactions are less frequent than with pentazocine, reflecting a relative weak kappa component of the compound. Nalbuphine-induced respiratory depression is less severe than with morphine and is limited by a ceiling level (Pugh et al., 1989).

Trade name: Nubain (Ger, F, UK, USA)

Nalbuphine has a low abuse potential and is not subject to narcotic control.

Nalorphine

Nalorphine

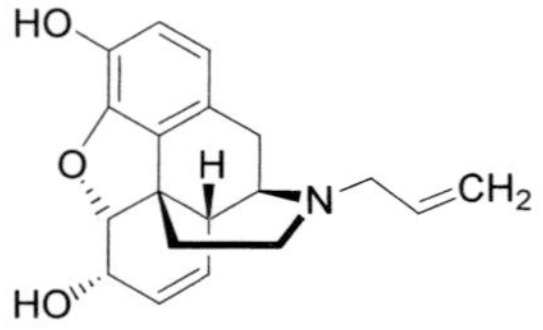

[62-67-9], (5a,6a)-7,8-Didehydro-4,5-epoxy-17-(2-propenyl)morphinan-3,6-diol, $C_{19}H_{21}NO_3$, *M_r* 311.38, *mp* 208-209 °C, $[\alpha]_D^{25}$ -155.3° (*c* = 3, CH_3OH); hydrochloride [*57-29-4*], $C_{19}H_{21}NO_3 \cdot HCl$, *$M_r$* 347.84, *mp* 260-263 °C; hydrobromide [*1041-90-3*], $C_{19}H_{21}NO_3 \cdot HBr$, *$M_r$* 392.29, *mp* 258-259 °C (decomp.)

Synthesis: Diacetylmorphine (Heroin) is demethylated with cyanogene bromide and hydrolyzed to normorphine, which is alkylated to allyl bromide (, Weijlard and Erickson (Merck & Co.), 1944; Weijlard (Merck & Co), 1959; Kleemann et al. 1999).

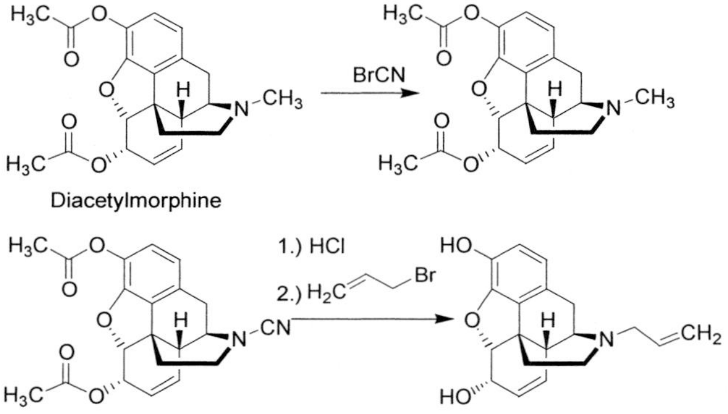

Scheme 35: Synthesis of nalorphine.

Opioid receptor binding: Nalorphine is a mixed agonist-antagonist with high affinity and low intrinsic action at the μ- and κ-opioid receptors.

Analgesic efficacy and clinical use: Nalorphine has substantial analgesic activity and was the first opioid in which a combination of analgesia with antagonistic properties was detected (Eckenhoff et al., 1951; Takemori et al., 1969).

Trade name: Lethidrone (Ger, UK), Nalline (USA), Nalorphine Serb (F)

Side-effects: The compound has prominent κ-type adverse reactions like anxiety, hallucinations and dysphoric mood alterations and is no longer used clinically (Lattin, 1976).

Naloxone

Synthesis: 14-Hydroxydihydronormorphinon (*see nalbuphine*) is *N*-alkylated with allyl bromide (Lewenstein and Fishman, 1962, Olofson et al., 1977, Kleemann et al. 1999, Moser et al., 1990):

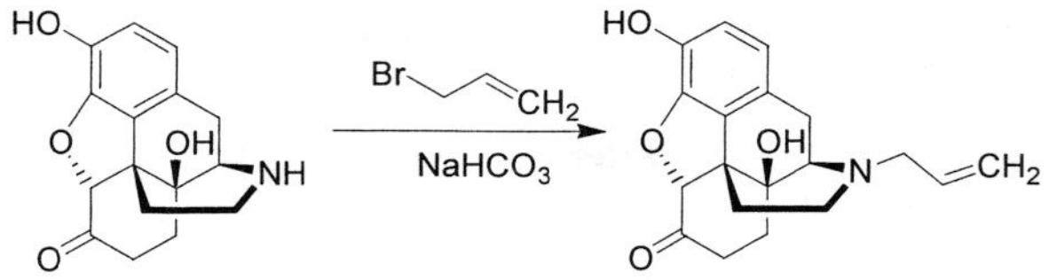

Scheme 36: Synthesis of naloxone.

Naloxone

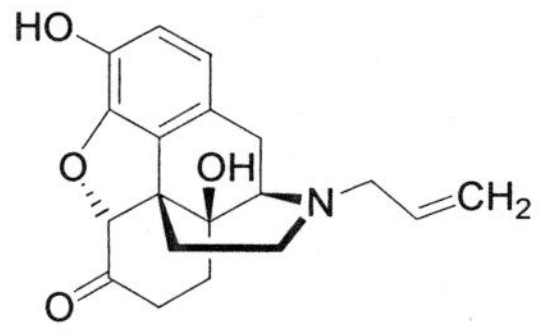

Opioid receptor binding: Naloxone (Simantow and Snyder, 1977) is a pure opioid antagonist with a high affinity and a limited selectivity for the μ-receptor.

Efficacy and clinical use: Naloxone (Handal et al., 1983; Goodrich, 1990) has no analgesic activity. This compound is the standard antidote for treating opioid adverse reactions, opioid overdoses or to terminate a therapeutic use of an opioid compound. Typical indications are inhibition of opioid-induced respiratory depression, termination of opioid anesthesia or protection of neonates following opioid treatment during labor. Naloxone has a short duration of action and repeated administration may be necessary to antagonize longer-acting compounds. To avoid parenteral misuse of non-scheduled oral opioid formulations (tilidine, pentazocine) a small amount of naloxone is added which is inactivated by the oral route, but is fully active after parenteral administration.

Dosages and routes of administration: Naloxone is only used parenterally, mostly as an intravenous bolus or by infusion. The compound is used in single or repetitive doses of 0.4-2 mg up to a total dose of 10 mg.

Pharmacokinetic properties: Oral naloxone is extensively metabolized in the gut and liver, predominantly by glucuronidation of the phenol function (Berkowitz, 1976). The parenteral half-life is about 1 h.

Side-effects: Naloxone induces mainly mild and non-specific side-effects. Higher doses may induce nausea and vomiting and in rare cases a reduction of the seizure threshold.

Trade name: Narcanti (Ger, Austral.), Narcan (F, UK, USA)

Naltrexone

Synthesis: (a) Its preparation is the same as that for naloxone starting from oxycodone via the intermediate **i** except that the nitrogen atom is alkylated with cyclopropyl bromide (Blumberg et al. (Endo Laboratories), 1967; 1973; Drugs Fut. 1977; 2000; Kleemann et al. 1999):

Naltrexone

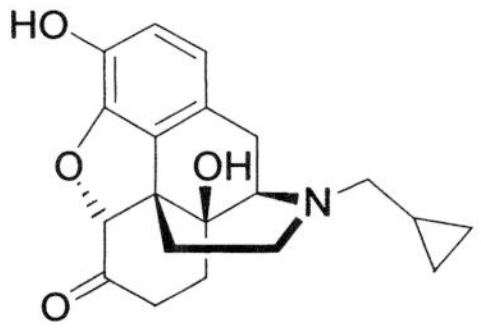

[*16590-41-3*], (5α)-17-(cyclopropylmethyl)-4,5-epoxy-3,14-dihydroxy-morphinan-6-one, $C_{20}H_{23}NO_4$, M_r 341.40, *mp* 168-170 °C; hydrochloride [*16676-29-2*], $C_{20}H_{23}NO_4$ · HCl, M_r 377.87, *mp* 274-276 °C

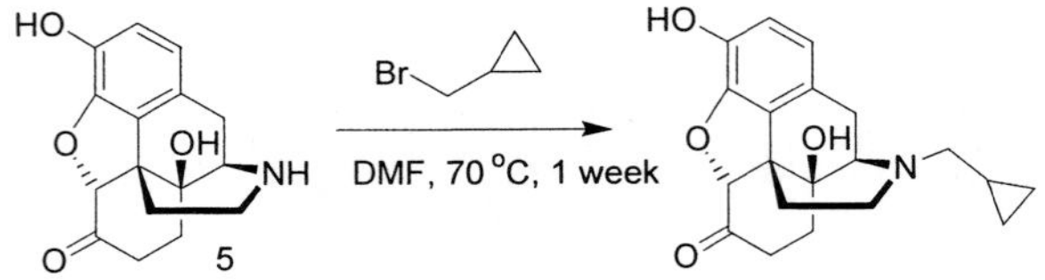

Scheme 37: Synthesis of naltrexone

(b) *Alternative route*: Product **i** is ketalized with ethylene glycol by means of p-toluenesulfonic acid giving the cyclic ketal (mp 311-313 °C); this in turn, is treated with cyclopropyl carbonyl chloride in a mixture of methylene chloride and triethylamine yielding the N,O-dicyclopropyl-carbonyl derivative (mp 219-220 °C). The N,O-dicyclopropylcarbonyl derivative is reduced with $LiAlH_4$, in refluxing THF yielding the ethylene ketal of naltrexone (mp 221-222 °C) which is finally hydrolyzed with aqueous HCl at 100 °C.

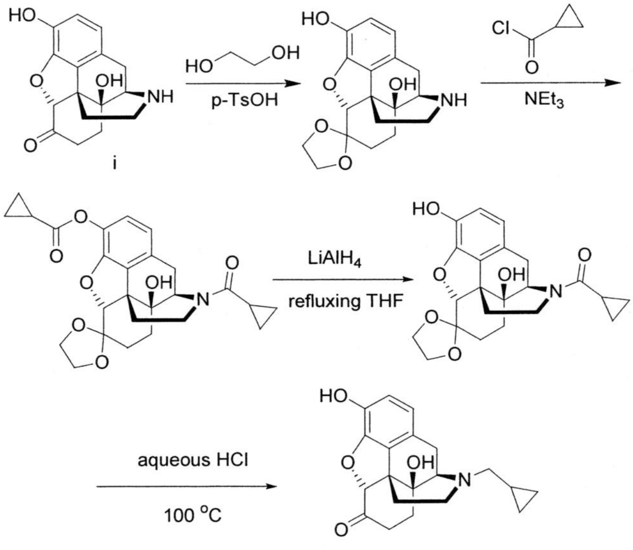

Scheme 38: Synthesis of naltrexone.

Opioid receptor binding: Naltrexone has a high affinity and selectivity for the μ-opioid receptor (Höllt and Herz, 1978).

Efficacy and clinical use: Naltrexone (Crabtree, 1984; Gonzalez and Brogden, 1988) is a pure opioid antagonist and has no analgesic activity. It is used for the treatment of opioid adverse effects, for opioid detoxification and as maintenance treatment for former addicts to avoid a relapse. In chronic opioid users, naltrexone may precipitate an acute withdrawal reaction.

Dosages and routes of administration: Naltrexone (O'Brien et al., 1978) is given orally and parenterally. It is given intravenously as an acute opioid antidote and as a challenge when dependency is suspected. Oral application us used for long-term treatment of former addicts. Naltrexone challenge is started with 200 µg and gradually increased to 1.6 mg, which is repeated until acute abstinence symptoms are no longer seen. Long-term treatment starts with 25 mg and is increased to 50 mg daily. The weekly doses of 350 mg can be given as 100 mg every second day or 150 mg given every third day.

Pharmacokinetic properties: Naltrexone (Misra, 1981) is absorbed from the gastrointestinal tract, but is subject to considerable first-pass metabolism in the liver, yielding the active metabolite 6-beta-naltrexole. Naltrexone has low plasma binding of about 20%. The half-life of naltrexone is ~3 h and of 6-beta-naltrexole is ~13 h.

Side-effects: Naltrexone itself has only weak and uncharacteristic side-effects, stronger effects, as seen in opioid users, are mostly the result of an acute withdrawal reaction.

Trade name: Nemexin (Ger), Nalorex (F, UK), Revia (USA)

Oxycodone

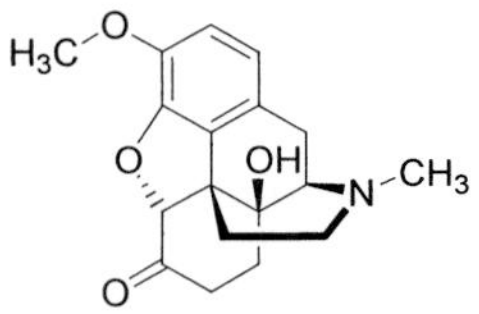

Synthesis (Krauß (E. Merck), 1925, Juby et al., 1968, Ehrhart and Ruschig 1972): Thebaine is oxidized with hydrogene peroxide to 14-hydroxycodeinone (Bentley 1954, Hauser 1974), which is hydrogenated directly or via its oxime, or its bromination products to oxycodone. The reduction of 14-hydroxycodeinone can also be carried out with sodium hydrosulfite. Alternatively 14-hydroxy-codeinone is prepared by oxidation of codeine.

Opioid receptor binding: Oxycodone (Chen et al., 1991) is a µ-selective opioid with a 10-fold higher receptor affinity than codeine. Both the parent compound and the high affinity metabolite oxymorphone mediate the opioid effects of the compound (Cleary et al., 1994).

Analgesic efficacy and clinical use: Oxycodone is a potent opioid and is used for the treatment of moderate to severe pain (Poyhia et al,. 1993).

Dosages and routes of administration: Oxycodone is given by mouth in single doses of 5-10 mg or as controlled release preparations with doses of 40 mg (Cairns, 2001). Rectal administration is also possible. Oral formulations often contain combinations with paracetamol or acetylsalicylic acid.

[*76-42-6*], (5α)-4,5-epoxy-
14-hydroxy-3-methoxy-17-
methylmorphinan-6-one, 14-
hydroxydihydrocodeinone,
dihydrone, dihydrohydroxy-
codeinone, $C_{18}H_{21}NO_4$, M_r
315.36, *mp* 218-220 °C;
hydrochloride [*124-90-3*],
$C_{18}H_{21}NO_4 \cdot HCl$, M_r 351.81,
mp 270-272 °C (decomp.),
$[\alpha]_D^{20}$ -125° (*c* = 2.5, water)

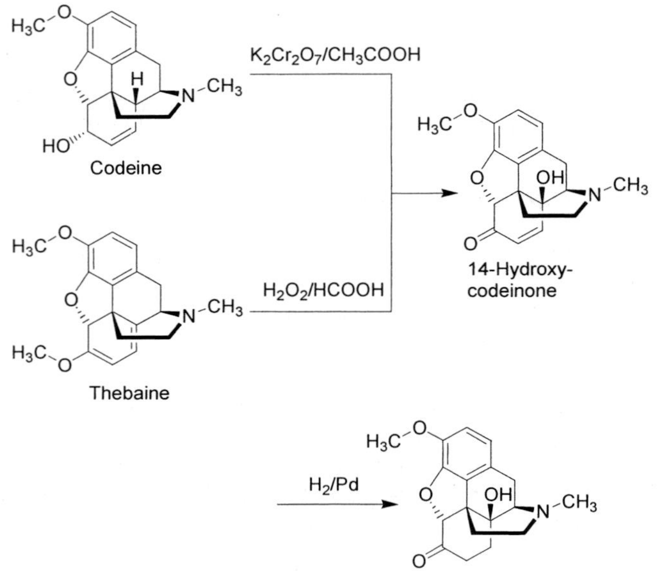

Scheme 39: Synthesis of oxycodon.

Pharmacokinetic properties: Oxycodone (Kaiko et al., 1996) is well absorbed from the gastrointestinal tract. It is metabolized to nor-oxycodone and to a lesser extent to the active metabolite oxymorphone (Poyhia et al., 1993). Metabolites and unchanged parent drug are excreted in the urine.

Trade name: Roxicodone,
OxyContine (USA),
Oxygesic, Eukodal (Ger),
Eubine (F), Proladone (UK)

Side-effects: Oxycodone has a morphine-like side-effect profile. Respiratory depression has been found in children. The compound has a relevant abuse and dependence potential and illicit use of the retarded preparations has been reported.

Oxymorphone

Synthesis (Lewenstein and Weiss, 1955; Weiss 1955): oxycodone is hydrolyzed with boiling concentrated hydrobromic acid.

Opioid receptor binding: Oxymorphone is a μ-selective opioid with a binding affinity in the range of morphine.

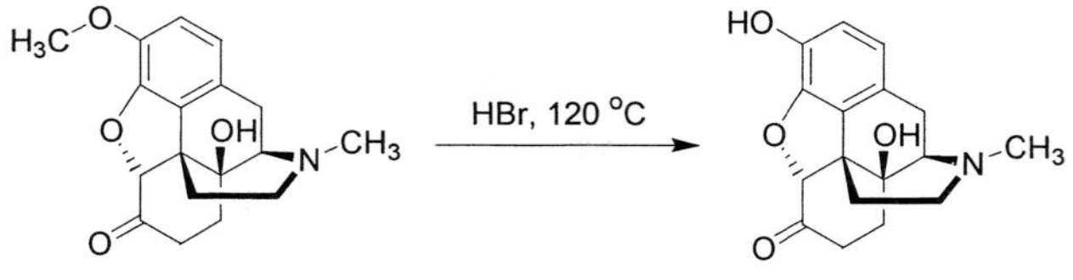

Scheme 40: Synthesis of oxymorphone

Analgesic efficacy and medical use: Oxymorphone is a potent analgesic. It is used for the treatment of moderate to severe pain, including labor pain, and as an adjunct to anesthesia. Oxymorphone has no cough suppressant activity.

Dosages and routes of administration: Oxymorphone is used parenterally by intramuscular or subcutaneous doses of 1-1.5 mg and as suppositories with a content of 5 mg. For patient controlled analgesia (PCA) i.v. bolus doses up to 300 µg are used (Sinatra and Harrison, 1989).

Pharmacokinetic properties: Oxymorphone is excreted into the urine as the unmetabolized drug and to a greater extent as the O-glucuronide (Cone et al., 1983).

Side-effects: Oxymorphone has a morphine-type side-effect profile and can induce addiction and dependence (Copland et al., 1987).

Oxymorphone

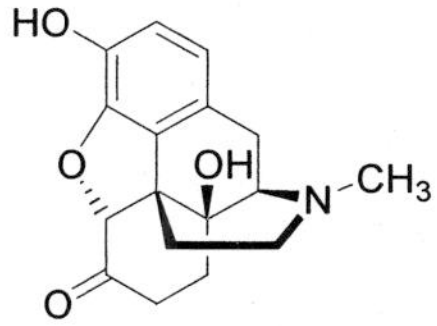

[76-41-5], (5α)-4,5-epoxy-3,14-dihydroxy-17-methylmorphinan-6-one, dihydrohydroxymorphinone, dihydro-14-hydroxymorphinone, 14-hydroxydihydromorphinone, $C_{17}H_{19}NO_4$, M_r 301.34, *mp* 248-249 °C (decomp.); hydrochloride [357-07-3], $C_{17}H_{19}NO_4 \cdot HCl$, M_r 337.80

Trade name: Numorphan (USA, Canad.)

Pentazocine

Synthesis (Archer et al., 1964; Kleemann et al. 1999):

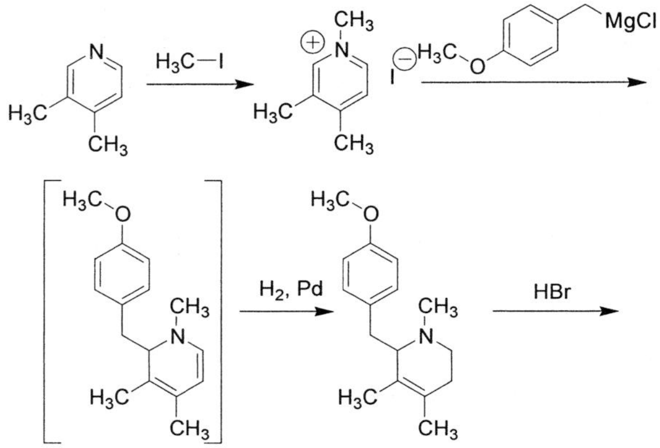

Pentazocine

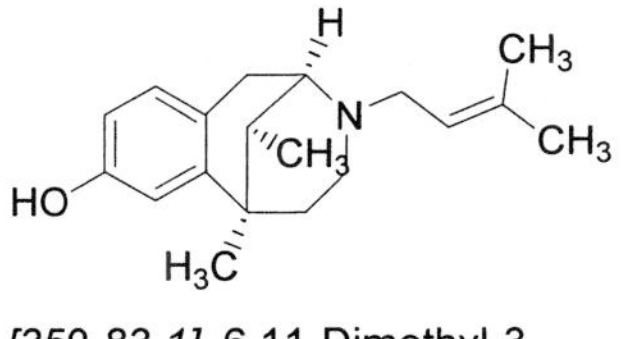

[359-83-1], 6,11-Dimethyl-3-(3-methyl-2-enyl)-1,2,3,4,5,6-hexahydro-2,6-methano-benzo[d]azocin-8-ol, (2α,6α,11R*)-1,2,3,4,5,6-hexahydro-6,11-dimethyl-3-(3-mmethyl-2-butenyl)-2,6-methano-3-benzazocin-8-ol, $C_{19}H_{27}NO$, M_r 285.42, *mp* 145-148 °C; hydrochloride [2276-52-0], $C_{19}H_{27}NO \cdot HCl$, M_r 321.89; lactate (1 : 1) [17146-95-1], $C_{19}H_{27}NO \cdot C_3H_6O_3$, M_r 375.51

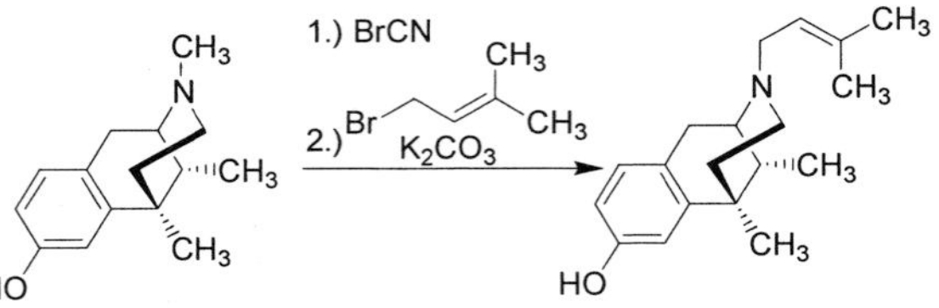

Scheme 41: Synthesis of pentazocine.

Opioid receptor binding: Pentazocine (Brogden et al., 1973) is a mixed opioid agonist-antagonist with agonistic effects at the kappa and partial antagonistic effects at the µ-type of opioid receptor.

Analgesic efficacy and clinical application: Pentazocine is a fairly potent analgesic and is used for the treatment of moderate to severe pain (Goldstein, 1985).

Dosages and routes of administration: Pentazocine is used as the hydrochloride or lactate in oral, parenteral and rectal formulations. Doses for the treatment of moderate to severe pain are in the range of 25-100 mg.

Pharmacokinetic properties: Pentazocine is orally bioavailable but there is a high degree of fluctuation in resorption. The compound is rapidly and extensively metabolized. Metabolites are formed by oxidative demethylation of the methyl residues of the dimethylallyl group and by glucuronidation (Berkowitz, 1973). The metabolic pathway of pentazocine is shown in scheme 42.

Side-effects: Pentazocine induces morphine-type side-effects such as dizziness, nausea, vomiting, sedation and sweating. In high doses seizures may occur (Challoner et al., 1990). In addition, it can cause kappa-agonist type psychotomimetic effects including hallucinations, nightmares and thought disturbances (Kane and Pokorny, 1975). Respiratory depression is weaker than with morphine and is subject to a 'ceiling' effect (Nagle and Pilcher, 1972).

Trade name: Fortral (Ger, F, UK), Talwin (USA)

The compound has a relevant abuse potential (Reed and Scholl, 1986) and high doses may produce dependence of the morphine type. Pentazocine effects can be antagonized with naloxone and combinations with naloxone are available to discourage parenteral misuse (Baum et al., 1987).

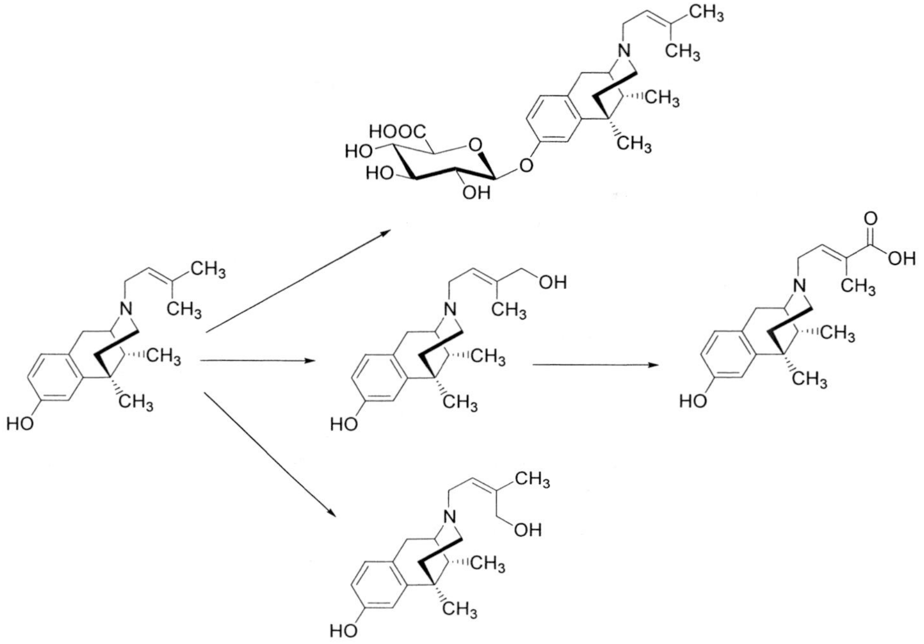

Scheme 42: Metabolic pathway of pentazocine.

Pethidine (Meperidine)

Synthesis (Eisleb (I.G. Farben), 1937, Eisleb (Winthrop), 1939, Smissman and Hite, 1959; Kleemann et al. 1999): the original synthesis involved condensation of benzyl cyanide with *N,N*-bis(2-chloro-ethyl)-*N*-methyl-amine, which is a skin irritant and a carcinogen.

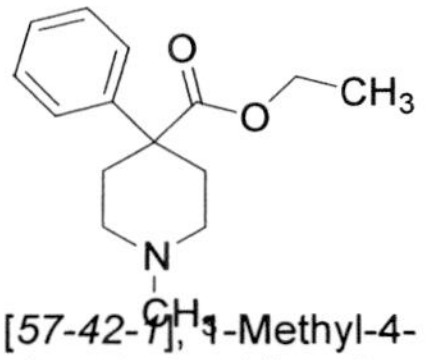

[*57-42-1*], 1-Methyl-4-phenyl-piperidine-4-carboxylic acid ethyl ester, $C_{15}H_{21}NO_2$, M_r 247.33; hydrochloride [*50-13-5*], $C_{15}H_{21}NO_2 \cdot HCl$, M_r 283.80, mp 186-189 °C.

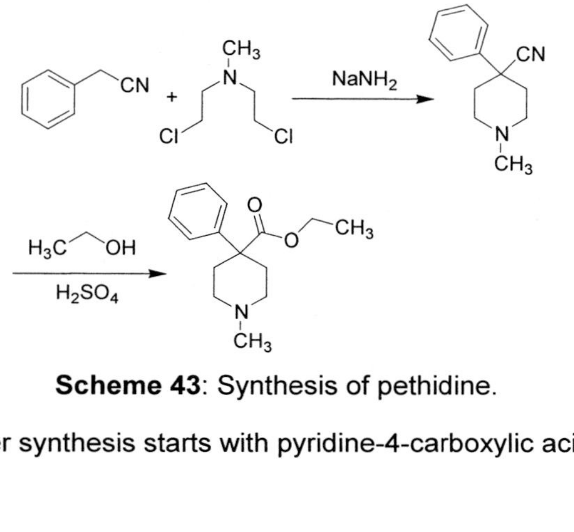

Scheme 43: Synthesis of pethidine.

Another synthesis starts with pyridine-4-carboxylic acid:

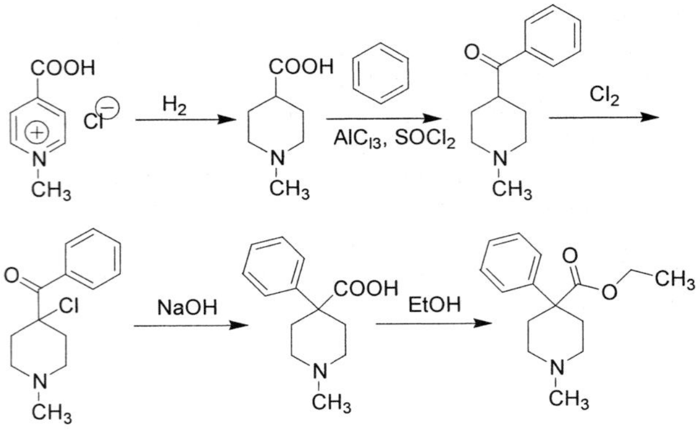

Friderichs and Buschmann

Scheme 44: Synthesis of pethidine.

Pethidine, introduced in 1939, was the first fully synthetic analgesic with morphine-like activity.

Opioid receptor binding: Pethidine is a μ-selective synthetic opioid with an intermediate receptor affinity (Pert and Snyder, 1976).

Analgesic efficacy and clinical use: Pethidine (Clark et al.,1995; Latta et al., 2002) is used for the treatment of moderate to severe pain including labor pain. It is also used as preoperative medication and as an adjunct to anesthesia. Due to its anti-muscarinic properties, it has a weaker muscle stimulant activity than other opioids and does not increase biliary pressure, which makes it suitable for the treatment of pain associated with pancreatitis or biliary colic.

Dosages and routes of administration: For pain inhibition pethidine is used in oral doses of 50-150 mg every 4 hrs, or in subcutaneous, intramuscular or slow intravenous doses of 25-100 mg.

Figure 7 shows the pethidine consumption in different european countries and the United States.

Pharmacokinetic properties: Pethidine (Mather and Meffin, 1978) has a faster onset and a shorter duration of action than morphine. After oral administration about 50% of the drug is eliminated by first-pass metabolism. N-demethylation yields the active metabolite nor-pethidine, and hydrolytic cleavage the inactive metabolites pethidinic and nor-pethidinic acid. The half-life of pethidine is about 3- 6 h. Nor-pethidine has a much slower elimination with a half life of up to 20 h.

Trade name: Dolantin (Ger), Dolosal (F), Demerol (USA)

Side-effects: Pethidine induces morphine-type side-effects with a lower incidence of constipation. Higher doses induce central stimulation and antimuscarinic effects accompanied with pupil dilatation. In even larger doses toxic symptoms including muscular twitching, tremor, mental confusion and convulsions occur, which are partly attributed to the more toxic metabolite nor-pethidine (Jiraki, 1992). Severe side-effects including coma and cyanosis have been observed in combination with MAO inhibitors (Meyer and Halfin, 1981). Pethidine induces morphine type tolerance and dependence and addicts using high doses of pethidine have an increased risk of excitatory side-effects.

Figure 7: Pethidine consumption (1995) in different countries in kg compound /Mio inhabitants (Sohn and Zenz, 1998)

Piritramide

Synthesis: By condensation of 4-piperidinopiperidine-4-carboxamide with 3,3-diphenyl-3-cyano propyl bromide (Janssen, P. (Janssen), 1961; Kleemann et al. 1999).

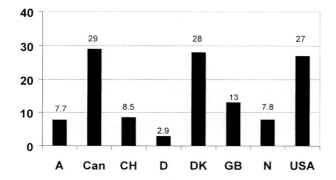

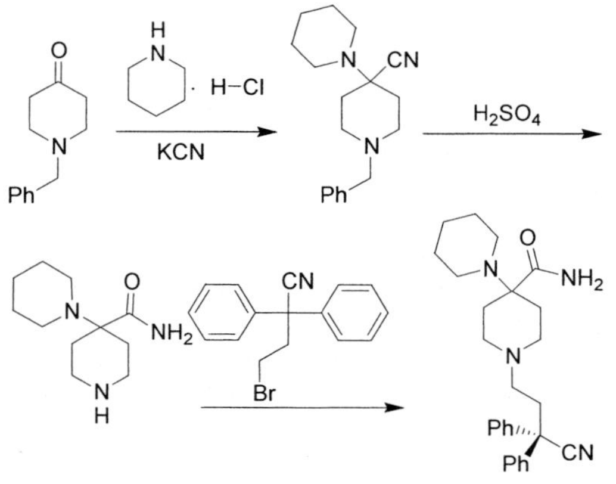

Scheme 45: Synthesis of piritramide.

Piritramide

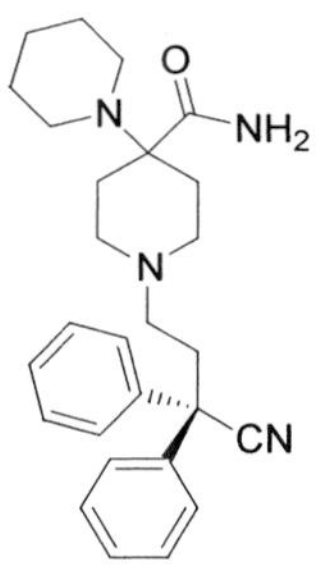

[*302-41-0*], 1'-(3-Cyano-3,3-diphenyl-propyl)-[1,4']bipiperidinyl-4'-carboxylic acid amide, $C_{27}H_{34}N_4O$, M_r 430.59, 149-150 °C

Opioid receptor binding: Piritramide is a synthetic µ-opioid with morphine-like affinity and receptor selectivity.

Analgesic efficacy and clinical use: Piritramide (Gibb and Pikler, 1973; Kumar and Rowbotham, 1999) is used for the treatment of acute, preferentially postoperative pain (Lehmann et al., 1986) and as an adjunct to anesthesia. It is less potent than morphine.

Dosages and routes of administration: Piritramide is used only parenterally by the intravenous, intramuscular or subcutaneous route. The standard dose is 15 mg.

Pharmacokinetic properties: Piritramide is extensively metabolized by first-pass metabolism in the liver and gut (Bouillon et al., 1999). After parenteral administration it is rapidly distributed. The compound is eliminated slowly and has a half-life of about 10 h.

Trade name: Dipidolor (Ger, B, NL), Piridolan (S)

Side-effects: Piritramide has a morphine-like side-effect profile and may induce tolerance and dependence.

Remifentanil

Remifentanil

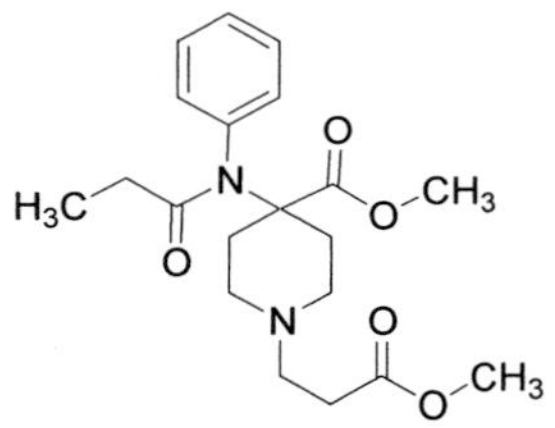

[*132875-61-7*], 1-(2-Methoxycarbonyl-ethyl)-4-(phenyl-propionyl-amino)-piperidine-4-carboxylic acid methyl ester, 4-(methoxycarbonyl)-4-[(1-oxopropyl)phenylamino]-1-piperidinepropanoic acid methyl ester, $C_{20}H_{28}N_2O_5$, M_r 376.45; monohydrochloride [132539-07-2], $C_{20}H_{28}N_2O_5 \cdot$ HCl, M_r 412.91; oxalate (1 : 1) [*132875-62-8*], $C_{20}H_{28}N_2O_5 \cdot C_2H_2O_4$, M_r 466.49

Synthesis: The reaction of 1-benzyl-4-piperidone with aniline and KCN in acetic acid gives the aminonitrile **i**, which is treated with H_2SO_4 at room temperature to yield the carboxamide **ii**. The hydrolysis of **ii** with refluxing aqueous HCl affords the carboxylic acid **iii**, which is esterified with MsOH and methanol to provide the methyl ester **iv**. Acylation of the NH group of **iv** with propionic anhydride gives the propionamide **v**, which is debenzylated with H_2 over Pd/C to yield the piperidine **vi**. Finally condensation of 4-(phenyl-propionyl-amino)-piperidine-4-carboxylic acid methyl ester with acrylic acid methyl ester in hot acetonitrile affords the target compound (Feldman et al. (Glaxo) 1990; Feldmann et al., 1991; Drugs Fut. 1994, Drugs Fut. 1995, Drugs Fut. 1997, Coleman 1999; Kleemann et al. 1999).

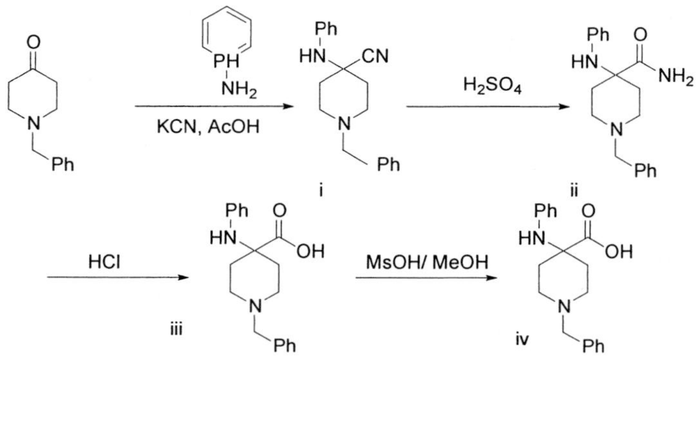

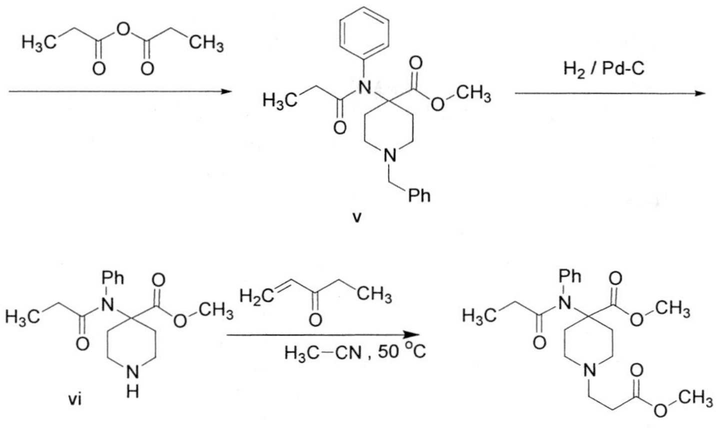

Scheme 46: Synthesis of remifentanil.

Opioid receptor binding: Remifentanil (Patel and Spencer, 1996) is a μ-opioid with a higher receptor affinity than fentanyl.

Analgesic efficacy and clinical use: Remifentanil (Glass,1995) has short-acting strong analgesic and anesthetic properties. It has been developed as an ultra-short anesthetic and can be used for ambulatory surgery (Servin, 1997; Haigh, 2000), general surgery and intensive care. As primary anesthetic or adjunct to other anesthetics it affords potent intra-operative analgesia and has a sparing effect on sedatives and hypnotics (Cohen and Royston, 2001).

Dosages and routes of administration: Remifentanil is given as intravenous short infusion in doses of 0.5-1 µg/kg or as continuous infusions in the range of 0.0025-2 µg/kg/min.

Pharmacokinetic properties: Remifentanil is an ultra-short acting compound (Michelsen and Hug, 1996), rapidly inactivated by plasma and tissue esterases. The terminal elimination half-life is 10-20 min.

Side-effect profile: Remifentanil has a μ-opioid-type side-effect profile with strong CNS and respiratory depressant properties. It has a morphine-like addiction and dependence potential.

Trade name: Ultiva (Ger, UK)

Sufentanil

Synthesis: In the literature several synthetic pathways to sufentanil have been described (Janssen and van Daele

Sufentanil

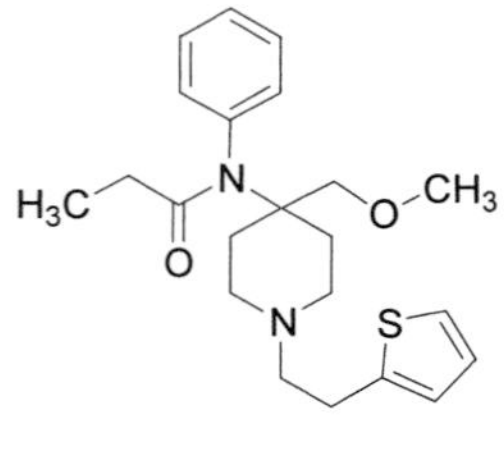

[*56030-54-7*], N-[4-
(Methoxymethyl)-1-[2-(2-
thienyl)ethyl]-4-piperidinyl]-
N-phenylpropanamide, *N*-[4-
Methoxymethyl-1-(2-
thiophen-2-yl-ethyl)-
piperidin-4-yl]-*N*-phenyl-
propionamide, $C_{22}H_{30}N_2O_3S$,
M_r 386.56, *mp* 96.6 °C;
citrate (1 : 1) [*60561-17-3*],
$C_{22}H_{30}N_2O_3S \cdot C_6H_8O_7$, M_r
578.68

(Janssen), 1976, van Daele et al., 1976; Castaner and
Roberts, 1977; Bever et al., 1976; Kleemann et al. 1999).

The esterification of 1-benzyl-4-(phenylamino) piperidine-
4-carboxylic acid with ethanol and H_2SO_4 gives the corresponding ethyl ester, which is reduced with
$LiAlH_2(OCH_2CH_2OCH_3)_2$ in benzene affording 1-benzyl-4-
(phenylamino)piperidine-4-methanol. The methylation of
this compound with methyl iodide and NaH in HMPA
yields 1-benzyl-4-methoxymethyl-4-(phenylamino)-
piperidine, which is refluxed with propionic anhydride to
give N-[4-(methoxymethyl)-1-benzyl-4-piperidyl]propion-
anilide . The following hydrogenolysis of with H_2 over
Raney Ni in methanol yields N-[4-(methoxymethyl)-4-
piperidyl]propionanilide, which is finally condensed with 2-
thiopheneethanol methanesulfonate by means of Na_2CO_3
in methyl isobutyl ketone.

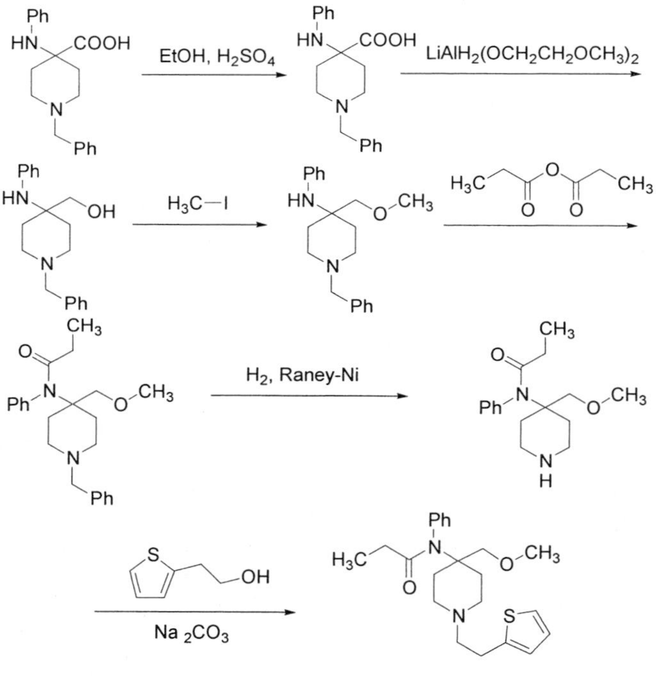

Scheme 47: Synthesis of sufentanil.

Another total synthesis of sufentanil has been described:
the cyclization of 2-(2-thienyl)ethylamine with allyl-
trimethylsilane and formaldehyde gives 4-hydroxy-1-[2-(2-
thienyl)ethyl]piperidine, which is oxidized with oxalyl
chloride in DMSO/dichloromethane to 1-[2-(2-thienyl)
ethyl]piperidin-4-one. The epoxidation of this compound by
means of trimethylsulfonium iodide and the sodium salt of
DMSO yields the spiro-epoxide, which is opened with

aniline and boron trifluoride ethearate giving a 1.8 : 1 mixture of 4-(hydroxymethyl)-4-(phenylamino) piperidine and 4-hydroxy-4-(phenylamino) piperidine which can be conveniently separated. The methylation of the OH group with diazomethane and SiO$_2$ affords the methoxymethyl compound, which is finally acylated with propionic anhydride to provide sufentanil.

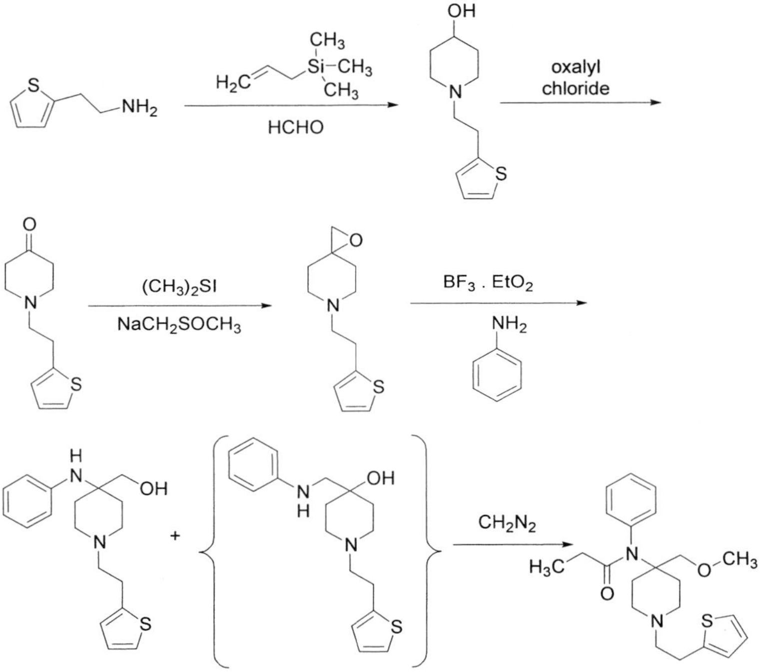

Scheme 48: Synthesis of sufentanil.

The reaction of 4-oxopiperidine-1-carboxylic acid ethyl ester with CHCl$_3$, benzyl triethylammonium chloride and NaOH in THF/water gives the spirooxirane derivative, which is treated with aniline and NaOH to yield the corresponding anilide. The methylation of the amide nitrogen by means of NaH and CH$_3$I in THF affords the methylated anilide. The reaction of methylated anilide with KOH in refluxing isopropanol causes elimination of its ethoxycarbonyl group, providing compound **i**, which is reduced with lithium triethylborohydride in THF to give 4-(hydroxymethyl)-4-(phenylamino)piperidine. The condensation of *N*-(4-methoxymethyl-piperidin-4-yl)-*N*-phenyl-propionamide with 2-(2-thienyl)ethyl mesylate by means of K$_2$CO$_3$ in refluxing acetonitrile yields the adduct **ii**, which is methylated with NaH and CH$_3$I in THF to afford the methoxy derivative sufentanil.

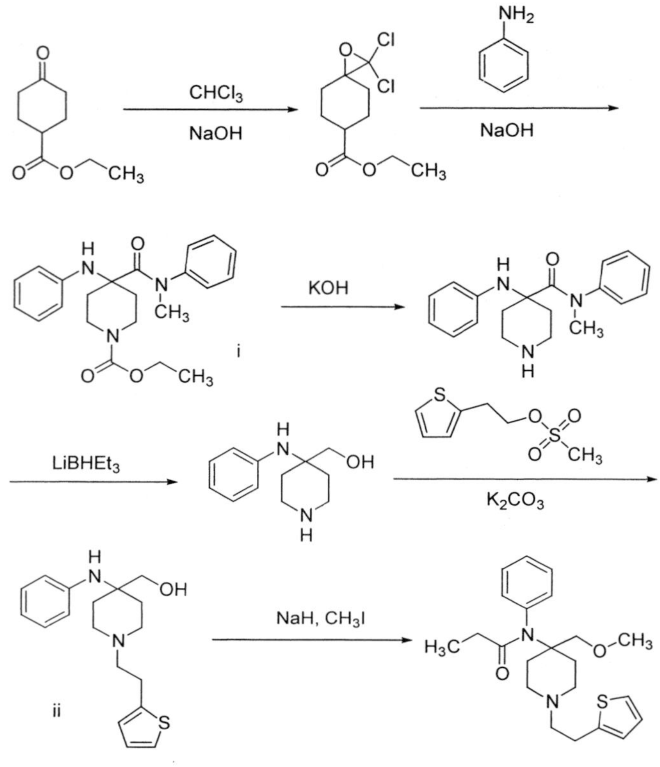

Scheme 49: Synthesis of sufentanil.

Opioid receptor binding: Sufentanil is a μ-selective opioid with an about 10-fold higher receptor affinity than fentanyl (Leysen et al., 1983).

Analgesic efficacy and clinical use: Sufentanil (Rosow, 1984; Monk et al., 1988) is a very potent fentanyl analog with analgesic and anesthetic properties and a more rapid onset and a shorter duration of action. It is used for perioperative analgesia, short duration anesthesia and as an adjunct to various anesthetic procedures including neuroleptanalgesia (Isaacson, 1992).

Dosages and routes of administration: Sufentanil is mostly given parenterally as an intravenous bolus or as brief injection or infusion during anesthesia. For pain treatment, intravenous or epidural on-demand procedures are in use. Doses up to 8 μg/kg are adequate for pain treatment and higher doses up to 30 μg/kg for surgery (Grass, 1992).

Pharmacokinetic properties: Following parenteral administration sufentanil has a rapid onset and a short duration of action. The compound is very lipophilic and is subject to high plasma protein binding of ~ 90%. The short duration of action is more dependent on redistribution than on metabolic inactivation. Redistribution half-life is about 20 min as compared to a elimination half-life of 2-3 h. The compound is metabolized by oxidative N- and O-de-methylation to polar metabolites which are excreted in the urine.

Side-effects: Sufentanil has a morphine-type side-effect profile and induces severe respiratory depression and chest wall rigidity in anesthetic dosages (Goldberg et al., 1985). High dose levels have been associated with seizures. Prolonged use may induce tolerance and dependence.

Trade name: Sufenta (B, Ger, F, N, USA)

Tilidine

Synthesis: The reaction of buta-1,3-dienyl-dimethylamine **3** with ethyl atropate **4** yields tilidine as a *cis/trans* mixture (trans : cis = 2 : 3). Most of the analgesically inactive *cis* isomer is separated as a zinc complex and the trans isomer is isolated as the hydrochloride. The *cis* isomer can be epimerized to the trans form by treating the epimeric mixture with acid (Satzinger (Gödecke), 1965; Sallay (Warner-Lambert), 1969, Satzinger, 1972; Satzinger et al., 1978; Overman et al., 1979; Kleemann et al. 1999).

Tilidine

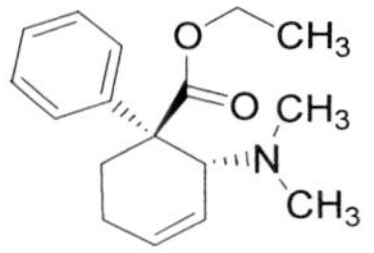

[51931-66-9], *trans*-2-Dimethylamino-1-phenyl-cyclohex-3-enecarboxylic acid ethyl ester, $C_{17}H_{23}NO_2$, M_r 273.17, *mp* 34 °C, *bp* 95.5-96 °C at 0.01 mm pressure; hydrochloride [27107-79-5], $C_{17}H_{23}NO_2$ · HCl, M_r 309.84, *mp* 159 °C; hydrochloride hemihydrate $C_{17}H_{23}NO_2$ · HCl · 1/2 H_2O, M_r 318.80, *mp* 125 °C

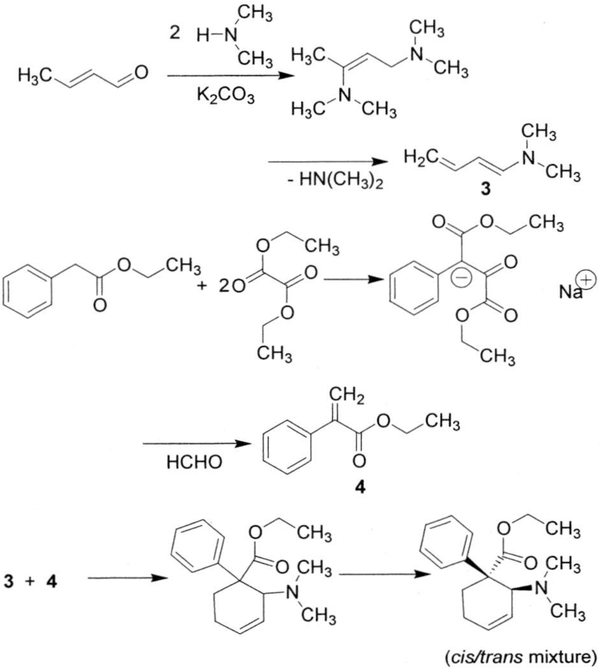

Scheme 50: Synthesis of tilidine.

Opioid receptor binding: Tilidine itself has a low opioid receptor binding affinity, whereas the active metabolites nor-tilidine and bisnor-tilidine have a high affinity and selectivity for the μ-type of opioid receptor (Schulz et al.,1978).

Analgesic efficacy and clinical use: The compound is used for the treatment of acute and chronic moderate to severe pain.

Dosages and routes of administration: Tilidine is most commonly used in oral formulations containing about 10% naloxone to avoid parenteral misuse (Worz and Worz, 1995). Tilidine without naloxone is given rectally and by various parenteral routes including intravenous, intramuscular and subcutaneous routes. Parenteral doses of up to 400 mg/day can be administered; the oral and rectal single doses are 50 and 75 mg, respectively (Martin et al., 1999).

Pharmacokinetic properties: Tilidine is a pro-drug (Vollmer et al., 1989) which is rapidly metabolised in the gut and liver to the analgesically active N-demethyl derivatives nor-tilidine and bisnor-tilidine.

Trade name: Valoron N (Ger), Tilidate (Spain)

Side-effects: Tilidine has a morphine-like side-effect and abuse potential (Trojan and Beil, 1978; Jasinski and Preston, 1986). To inhibit parenteral abuse of oral formulations, a small amount of naloxone is added. Naloxone is completely inactivated after oral administration and does not impede analgesia, whereas after parenteral administration the naloxone component is active and blocks the tilidine effect and can induce withdrawal reactions (Vollmer, 1988). The combination with naloxone, in contrast to pure tildine, is available under normal prescription.

Tramadol

Tramadol

[27203-92-5], cis-2-Dimethylaminomethyl-1-(3-methoxy-phenyl)-cyclohexanol, $C_{16}H_{25}NO_2$, M_r 263.38; hydrochloride [36282-47-0], $C_{16}H_{25}NO_2$. HCl, M_r 299.84, mp 180-181°C

Synthesis: The Grignard reaction of 2-(dimethyl-aminomethyl)cyclohexanone (obtained by Mannich reaction of cyclohexanone, formaldehyde, and dimethyl-amine hydrochloride) and the Grignard reagent of 3-bromoanisole yields tramadol as a *cis/trans* mixture (*cis : trans* = 85 : 15). Tramadol (*cis* isomer) is separated from the reaction mixture via crystallization of the hydrochloride salt. A crystallization of the hydrate or hydrobromide salts has also been described. (Frankus and Flick (Grünenthal) 1964; 1971; Flick et al. 1978; Kleemann et al. 1999).

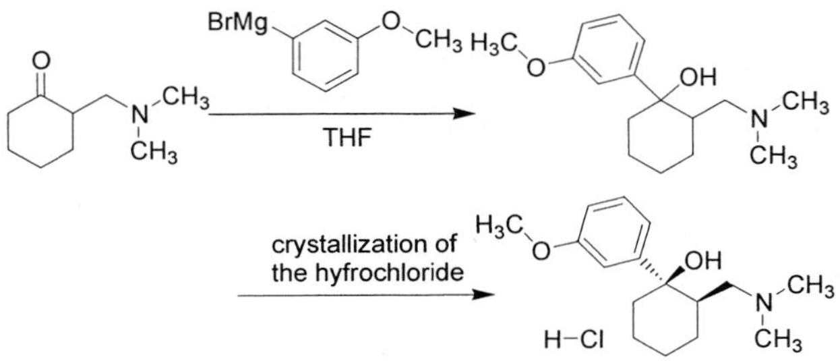

Scheme 51: Synthesis of tramadol.

Opioid receptor affinity: Tramadol (Frink et al., 1996) itself has a weak opioid receptor affinity, the active metabolite O-desmethyl-tramadol has μ-selectivity and μ-affinity about 10 times lower than that of morphine.

Analgesic efficacy and clinical use: Tramadol HCl (Friderichs et al., 1978; Raffa and Friderichs, 1996) is a centrally-acting analgesic with a μ-opioid and non-opioid component of action (Raffa et al., 1992). The non-opioid component induces inhibition of spinal pain transmission via inhibition of noradrenaline (NA) and serotonin (5HT) re-uptake (Driessen and Reimann, 1992; Driessen et al. 1993) Tramadol is a racemate and uptake inhibition and opioid properties are differentially distributed between the enantiomers (Raffa et al., 1993) and the active O-desmethyl metabolite. μ-Opioid receptor binding, NA uptake inhibition and 5HT uptake inhibition are regarded as the relevant (Desmeules et al., 1996; Raffa and Friderichs, 1996) components of the complex analgesic action profile of the compound; (+)-O-desmethyl-tramadol mainly contributes to μ-activity, (-)-tramadol to NA uptake inhibition and (+)-tramadol to 5HT uptake inhibition, respectively.

Tramadol is a potent analgesic (Lee et al., 1993). The compound is marketed worldwide and has become one of the most important centrally-acting analgesics (Bamigbade, 1998; Scott and Perry, 2000) for the treatment of acute and chronic moderate to severe pain.

Dosages and routes of administration: Tramadol is used in single doses of 50-100 mg up to daily doses of 300-400 mg. The compound has high oral bio-availability and can be given by mouth, rectally or by intramuscular, subcutaneous or slow intravenous injection or infusion (Lintz et al. 1981).

Pharmacokinetic properties: Tramadol is extensively metabolized by O- and N-demethylation yielding the active metabolite O-desmethyl-tramadol (M1) and several inactive derivatives like N-desmethyl-tramadol (M2), N-bis-desmethyl-tramadol (M3), O-desmethyl-N-desmethyl-tramadol (M5) and O-desmethyl-N-bis-desmethyl-tramadol (M4).

Trade name: Tramal (Ger, Switzerland, Austr.,Fin.), Zydol (UK), Ultram (USA), Adolonta (Spain), Contramal (F,I, Belg.), Nobligan (N)

Side-effects: Typical side-effects of tramadol are nausea, sweating and dizziness. In rare cases seizures after high i.v. doses are reported, mostly in combination with other proconvulsant componds or in patients with reduced seizure theshold (Gardner et al., 2000). Tramadol shows a reduced level of opioid side-effects, especially respiratory depression and constipation are less frequent and severe than with standard opioids such as morphine. Tramadol has a very limited abuse potential and is not subject to narcotic control (Cossmann et al., 1997).

References

Aasmundstad, T.A., Xu, B.Q., Johansson, I., Ripel, A., Bjorneboe, A., Christophersen, A.S., Bodd, E., Morland, J.: *Biotransformation and pharmacokinetics of ethylmorphine after a single oral dose*, Br. J. Clin. Pharmacol. **1995**, *39*, 611-620.

Akil, H., Watson, S.J., Young, E., Lewis, M. E., Khachaturian, H., Walker, J. M.: *Endogenous opioids: biology and function*, Annu. Rev. Neurosci. **1984**, *7*, 223-55.

Alford, B. T., Burkhart, R. L., Johnson, W. P.: *Etorphine and diprenorphine as immobilizing and reversing agents in captive and free-ranging mammals*, J. Am. Vet. Med. Assoc.: **1974**,*164*, 702-705.

Ameer, B., Salter, F. J.: *Drug therapy reviews: evaluation of butorphanol tartrate*, Am. J. Hosp. Pharm. **1979**, *36*, 1683-1691.

Ammon, S., Hofmann, U., Griese, E. U., Gugeler, N., Mikus, G.: *Pharmacokinetics of dihydrocodeine and its active metabolite after single and multiple oral dosing*, Br. J. Clin. Pharmacol. **1999**, *48*, 317-22.

Aparasu, R., McCoy, R. A., Weber, C., Mair, D., Parasuraman, T. V.: *Opioid-induced emesis among hospitalized nonsurgical patients: effect on pain and quality of life*, J. Pain Symptom. Manage. **1999**, *18*, 280-288.

Archer, S., Albertson, N. F., Harris, L. S., Pierson, A. K., Bird, J. G.: J. Med. Chem. **1964**, *7*, 123-127.

Archer, S.: *State-of-the-art analgesics from the agonist-antagonist concept*, NIDA Res. Monogr. **1992**, *119*, 71-75.

Ashburn, M. A. and Streisand, J. B.: *Oral transmucosal fentanyl. Help or hindrance?* Drug Saf. **1994**, *11*, 295-300.

Atkinson, R.E., Schofield, P., Mellor, P.:*The efficacy in sequential use of buprenorphine and morphine in advanced cancer pain. In: (Ed.:D. Doyle) Opioids in the treatment of cancer pain*, London, Royal Society of Medicine **1990**, 81-87.

Awouters, F., Megens, A., Verlinden, M., Schuurkes, J., Niemegeers, C., Janssen, P.A.: *Loperamide. Survey of studies on mechanism of its antidiarrheal activity*, Dig. Dis. Sci. **1993**, *38*, 977-95.

Bamigbade, T.A. and Langford, R.M.: *Tramadol hydrochloride: an overview of current use*, Hosp. Med. **1998**, *59*, 373-376.

Banbery, J., Wolff, K., Raistrick, D.: *Dihydrocodeine: a useful tool in the detoxification of methadone-maintained patients*, J. Subst. Abuse Treat. **2000**, *19*, 301-305.

Barber, A. and Gottschlich, R.: *Novel developments with selective , non-peptidic kappa-opioid receptor agonists*, Exp. Opin. Invest. Drugs **1997**, *6*, 1354-1368.

Barnes, N.M., Bunce, K.T., Naylor, R.J., Rudd, J.A.: *The actions of fentanyl to inhibit drug-induced emesis*, Neuropharmacology **1991**, *30*, 1073-1083.

Baum, C., Hsu, J.P., Nelson, R.C.: *The impact of the addition of naloxone on the use and abuse of pentazocine*, Public Health Rep. **1987**, *102*, 426-429.

Beaver, W.T.: *Analgesic efficacy of dextropropoxyphene and dextropropoxyphene-containing combinations: a review*, Hum. Toxicol. **1984**, *3*, 191S-220S.

Beckett, A.H. and Casy, A.F.: *Synthetic analgesics: Stereochemical considerations*, J. Pharm. Pharmacol. **1954**, *6*, 986-1000.

Benyhe, S.: *Morphine: new aspects in the study of an ancient compound*, Life Sci. **1994**, 55, 969-979.

Bentley, K.W.: *The Chemistry of the morphine alkaloids*, Oxford, **1954**.

Bentley, K.W., Hardy, D.G.: Proc. Chem. Soc. (London) **1963**, 220.

Bentley, K. W. (Reckitt & Colman): *In 7-Stellung substituierte 6,14-endo-Äthanotetrahydrothebain-, tetrahydronorthebain- und −tetrahydronororipavinverbindungen, Verfahren zu ihrer Herstellung und ihre Verwendung als Arzneimittel*, DE 1620206, **1966**.

Bentley, K. W. (Reckitt & Sons Ltd.): *Endoethano nor oripavines and nor thebains*, US 3 433 791, **1969**.

Bentley, K.W.: *Beta-phenylethylamines and the isoquinoline alkaloids*, Nat. Prod. Rep. **2000**, 17, 247.

Berkowitz, B.: *Pharmacokinetics and neurochemical effects of pentazocine and its optical isomers*, Adv. Biochem. Psychopharmacol. **1973**, *8*, 495-501.

Berkowitz, B.A.: *The relationship of pharmacokinetics to pharmacological activity: morphine, methadone and naloxone*, Clin. Pharmacokinet. **1976**, *1*, 219-230.

Bertorelli, R., Calo, G., Ongini, E., Regoli, D.: *Nociceptin/orpanin FQ and its receptor: a potential target for drug discovery*, Trends Pharmacol. Sci. **2000**, *21*, 233-234.

Bever, van W. F. M., Niemegeers, C. J. E., Schellekens, K. H. L., Janssen, P. A. J.: *N-4-Substituted 1-(2-arylethyl)-4-piperidinyl-N-phenylpropanamides, a novel series of extremely potent analgesics with unusually high safety margin*, Arzneim.-Forsch./Drug Res. **1976**, *26*, 1548-1556.

Blaine, J.D., Renault, P., Levine, G.L., Whysner, J.A.: *Clinical use of LAAM*, Ann. N.Y. Acad. Sci. **1978**, *311*, 214-231.

Blake, A.D., Bot, G., Tallent, M., Law, S.F., Li, S., Freeman, J.C., Reisine, T.: *Molecular regulation of opioid receptors*, Receptors Channels **1997**, *5*, 231-235.

Blancquaert, J.P., Lefebvre, R.A., Willems, J.L.: *Emetic and antiemetic effects of opioids in the dog*, Eur. J. Pharmacol. **1986**, *128*, 143-150.

Blane G.F. and Boura A.L.: *Analgesic and other actions of morphine antagonists*, Naunyn Schmiedebergs Arch. Exp. Pathol. Pharmakol. **1968**, *259*, 154-155.

Blumberg, H., Flushing, I. J. P., Matossian, Z. (Endo Laboratories): *14-Hydroxydihydronormorphinone derivatives*, US 3 332 950, **1967** CH 493522, **1970**, DE1795797, **1973**.

Bockmühl, M. and Ehrhart, G. (Farbw. Hoechst): *Verfahren zur Herstellung von basischen Ketonen*, DBP 865 314, **1941**.

Bockmühl, M. and Ehrhart, G.: Justus Liebigs Ann. Chem. **1948**, *561*, 52-85.

Boehringer, *Verfahren zur Alkylierung von Morphin*, DRP 247 180, **1912**.

Bondesson, U., Arner, S., Anderson, P., Boreus, L.O., Hartvig, P.: *Clinical pharmacokinetics and oral bioavailability of ketobemidone*, Eur. J. Clin. Pharmacol. **1980**; *17*, 45-50.

Bouillon, T., Kietzmann, D., Port, R., Meineke, I., Hoeft, A.: *Population pharmacokinetics of piritramide in surgical patients*, Anesthesiology **1999**, *90*, 7-15.

232   *Friderichs and Buschmann*

Bourke, M., Hayes, A., Doyle, M., McCarroll, M.A.: *Comparison of regularly administered sustained release oral morphine with intramuscular morphine for control of postoperative pain*, Anesth. Analg. **2000**, *90*, 427-430.

Bowdle, T.A.: *Adverse effects of opioid agonists and agonist-antagonists in anaesthesia*, Drug Saf. **1998**, *19*, 173-189.

Brandt, W., Barth, A., Holtje, H.D.: *A new consistent model explaining structure (conformation)-activity relationships of opiates with mu-selectivity*, Drug Des. Discov. **1993**, *10*, 257-283.

Bradley, G., Cavalla, J. F., Edington, T., Shepherd, R. G., White, A. C., Bushell, B. J., Johnson, J. R., Weston, G. O.: *Synthetic studies on meptazinol. Anion chemistry in the synthesis of α-aryl lactams*, Eur. J. Med. Chem. - Chim. Ther. **1980**, *15*, 375-85.

Brogden, R.N., Speight, T.M., Avery, G.S.: *Pentazocine: a review of its pharmacological properties, therapeutic efficacy and dependence liability*, Drugs **1973**, *5*, 6-91.

Brown, R. and Lo, R.: *The physical and psychosocial consequences of opioid addiction: an overview of changes in opioid treatment.* Aust. N.Z. J. Ment. Health Nurs. **2000**, *9*, 65-74.

Brownstein, M.J.: *A brief history of opiates, opioid peptides, and opioid receptors*, Proc. Natl. Acad. Sci. USA **1993**, *90*, 5391-5393.

Buchanan, J.F. and Brown, C.R.: *'Designer drugs'. A problem in clinical toxicology*, Med. Toxicol. Adverse Drug Exp. **1988**, *3*, 1-17.

Cairns, R.: *The use of oxycodone in cancer-related pain: a literature review*, Int. J. Palliat. Nurs. **2001**, *7*, 522-527.

Calo, G., Bigoni, R., Rizzi, A., Guerrini, R., Salvadori, S., Regoli, D.: *Nociceptin/orphanin FQ receptor ligands*, Peptides **2000**, *21*, 935-947.

Campora, E., Merlini, L., Pace, M., Bruzzone, M., Luzzani, M., Gottlieb, A., Rosso, R.: *The incidence of narcotic-induced emesis*, J. Pain Symptom. Manage. **1991**, *6*, 428-430.

Carroll, F.I., Brine, G.A., Chen, T., Kohl, D.W., Welch, C.D.: *Synthesis of (-)-α-acetylmethadol metabolites and related compounds*, J. Org. Chem. **1950**, *41*, 3521-3524.

Castaner, L. and Roberts, P.J.: *Sufentanil*, Drugs Fut. **1977**, *2*, 334-337.

Castaner, L., and Roberts, P.J.: *Nalbuphine*, Drugs Fut. **1977**, *2*, 613-615.

Casy, A.F. and Parfitt, R.T.: *Opioid analgesics*, Plenum Press, New York, **1986**.

Cavalla, J. F. and White, A. C. (Wyeth): *Hexahydroazepine, ihre Herstellung und Verwendung*, DOS 1 941 534, **1969**; GB 1 285 025, **1969**.

Challoner, K.R., McCarron, M.M., Newton, E.J.: *Pentazocine (Talwin) intoxication: report of 57 cases*, J. Emerg. Med. **1990**, *8*, 67-74.

Chen, J.C., Smith, E.R., Cahill, M., Cohen, R., Fishman, J.B.: *The opioid receptor binding of dezocine, morphine, fentanyl, butorphanol and nalbuphine.* Life Sci. **1993**, *52*, 389-396.

Chen, Z.R., Irvine, R.J., Somogyi, A.A., Bochner, F.: *Mu receptor binding of some commonly used opioids and their metabolites.* Life Sci. **1991**, *48*, 2165-2171.

Cherny, N.I.: *Opioid analgesics: comparative features and prescribing guidelines.* Drugs **1996**, *51*, 713-737.

Childers, S.R., Creese, I., Snowman, A.M., Synder, S.H.: *Opiate receptor binding affected differentially by opiates and opioid peptides*, Eur. J. Pharmacol. **1979**, *55*, 11-18.

Childers, S.R.: *Opioid receptor-coupled second messenger systems*, Life Sci. **1991**, *48*, 1991-2003.

Christensen, C.B.: *The opioid receptor binding profiles of ketobemidone and morphine*, Pharmacol. Toxicol. **1993**, *73*, 344-345.

Christoph, T. and Buschmann, H.: *Zwei komplexe Wirkprinzipien in einer Struktur - Gemischte opioide Agonisten/Antagonisten und partielle Agonisten (Two complex action principles in one structure - mixed opioid agonists/antagonists and partial agonists)*, Pharm. i. u. Zeit **2002**, *31*, 40-43.

Christrup, L.L.: *Morphine metabolites*. Acta Anaesthesiol. Scand. **1997**, *41*, 116-122.

Clark, R.F., Wie, E.M., Anderson, P.O.: *Meperidine: therapeutic use and toxicity*, J. Emerg. Med. **1995**, *13*, 797-802.

Cleary, J., Mikus, G., Somogyi, A., Bochner, F.: *The influence of pharmacogenetics on opioid analgesia: studies with codeine and oxycodone in the Sprague-Dawley/Dark Agouti rat model*, J. Pharmacol. Exp. Ther. **1994**, *271*, 1528-1534.

Clotz, M.A., Nahata, M.C.: *Clinical uses of fentanyl, sufentanil, and alfentanil*, Clin. Pharm. **1991**, *10*, 581-593.

Cohen, J. and Royston, D.: *Remifentanil*, Curr. Opin. Crit. Care. **2001**, *7*, 227-231.

Coleman, M.J., Goodyear, M.D., Lathan, D.W.S., Whitehead, A.J.: *A convenient method for the N-acylation and esterification of hindered amino acids: synthesis of ultra short acting opioid agonist, remifentanil*, Synlett **1999**, 1923-1924.

Collins, S.L., Edwards, J.E., Moore, R.A., McQuay, H.J.: *Single dose dextropropoxyphene, alone and with paracetamol (acetaminophen), for postoperative pain*, Cochrane Database Syst. Rev. **2000**, CD001440.

Coluzzi, P.H.: *Cancer pain management: newer perspectives on opioids and episodic pain*, Am. J. Hosp. Palliat. Care **1998**, *15*, 13-22.

Cone, E.J., Darwin, W.D., Buchwald, W.F., Gorodetzky, C.W.: *Oxymorphone metabolism and urinary excretion in human, rat, guinea pig, rabbit, and dog*, Drug Metab. Dispos. **1983**, *11*, 446-450.

Coniam, S.W.: *Withdrawal of levorphanol*, Anaesthesia. **1991**, *46*, 518.

Cookson, R.F., Niemegeers, C.J., Vanden Bussche, G.: *The development of alfentanil*, Br. J. Anaesth. **1983**, *55*, 147S-155S.

Copland, V.S., Haskins, S.C., Patz, J.D.: *Oxymorphone: cardiovascular, pulmonary, and behavioral effects in dogs*, Am. J. Vet. Res. **1987**, *48*, 1626-1630.

Cossmann, M., Kohnen, C., Langford, R., McCartney, C.: *[Tolerance and safety of tramadol use. Results of international studies and data from drug surveillance]*, Drugs **1997**, *53*, Suppl 2, 50-62.

Crabtree, B.L.: *Review of naltrexone, a long-acting opiate antagonist*, Clin. Pharm. **1984**, *3*, 273-280.

Daele, van P.G.H., De Bruyn, M.F.L., Boey, J.M., Sanczuk, S., Agten, J.T.M., Janssen, P.A.J.: *Analgesics: N-(1-(2-arylethyl)-4-substituted 4-piperidinyl)-N-arylalkanamides*, Arzneim.-Forsch./Drug Res. **1976**, *26*, 1521-1531.

Darke, S. and Zador, D.: *Fatal heroin 'overdose': a review*, Addiction 1996, *91*, 1765-1772.

Dashwood, M.R., Sykes, R.M., Thomson, C.S.: *Autoradiographic demonstration of [3H] loperamide binding to opioid receptors in rat and human small intestine*, Prog. Clin. Biol. Res. **1990**, *328*, 165-169.

Davis, M.P. and Walsh, D.: *Methadone for relief of cancer pain: a review of pharmacokinetics, pharmacodynamics, drug interactions and protocols of administration*, Support Care Cancer **2001**, *9*, 73-83.

Davies, S.G., Goodwin, C.J., Pyatt, D., Smith, A.D.: *Palladium catalysed laboration of codeine and morphine*, J. Chem. Soc., Perkin Trans. I **2001**, 1413-1420.

De Luca, A. and Coupar, I.M.: *Insights into opioid action in the intestinal tract*, Pharmacol. Ther. **1996**, *69*, 103-115.

De Souza, E.B., Schmidt, W.K., Kuhar, M.J.: *Nalbuphine: an autoradiographic opioid receptor binding profile in the central nervous system of an agonist/antagonist analgesic*, J. Pharmacol. Exp. Ther. **1988**, *244*, 391-402.

Deamer, R.L., Wilson, D.R., Clark, D.S., Prichard, J.G.: *Torsades de pointes associated with high dose levomethadyl acetate (ORLAAM)*, J. Addict. Dis. **2001**, *20*, 7-14.

Desmeules, J.A., Piguet, V., Collart, L., Dayer, P.: *Contribution of monoaminergic modulation to the analgesic effect of tramadol.* Br. J. Clin. Pharmacol. **1996**, *41*, 7-12.

Dhawan, B.N., Cesselin, F., Raghubir, R., Reisine, T., Bradley, P.B., Portoghese, P.S., Hamon, M.: *International Union of Pharmacology. XII. Classification of opioid receptors*, Pharmacol. Rev. **1996**, *48*, 567-592.

Dixon, R., Crews, T., Inturrisi, C., Foley, K.: *Levorphanol: pharmacokinetics and steady-state plasma concentrations in patients with pain*, Res. Commun. Chem. Pathol. Pharmacol. **1983**, *41*, 3-17.

Dondio, G., Ronzoni, S., Petrillo, P.: *Non-peptide δ opioid agonists and antagonists*, Exp. Opin. Ther. Patents **1997**, *7*, 1075-1098.

Dorner, W.G.: *Opioide - wenn der Schmerz zur Qual wird*, Chem. i. u. Zeit **1986**, *15*, 33-46.

Driessen, B., Reimann, W., Giertz, H.: *Effects of the central analgesic tramadol on the uptake and release of noradrenaline and dopamine in vitro*, Br. J. Pharmacol. **1993**, *108*, 806-811.

Driessen, B. and Reimann, W.: *Interaction of the central analgesic, tramadol, with the uptake and release of 5-hydroxytryptamine in the rat brain in vitro*, Br. J. Pharmacol. **1992**, *105*, 147-151.

Drugs Fut. **1977**, *2*, 45 (*Naltrexone*)

Drugs Fut. **1982**, *11*, 842-843.

Drugs Fut. **1994**, *19*, 1088-1092 (*Remifentanil Hydrochloriude, Ultiva*).

Drugs Fut. **1995**, *20*, 1276-1279 (*Remifentanil Hydrochloriude, Ultiva*).

Drugs Fut. **1997**, *22*, 1388-1390 (*Remifentanil Hydrochloriude, Ultiva*).

Drugs Fut. **2000**, *25*, 93-94 (Naltrexone Hydrochloride)

Easton, N.R., Gardner, J.H., Stevens, J.P.: *A New Synthesis and Confirmation of the Structure of Amidone*, J. Am. Chem. Soc. **1947**, *69*, 2941-2942.

Eccles, R.: *Codeine, cough and upper respiratory infection*. Pulm. Pharmacol. **1996**, *9*, 293-297.

Eckenhoff, J.E., Elder, J.D., King, B.D.: *Effect of N-allylnormorphine in treatment of opiate overdose*, Am. J. Med. Sci. **1951**, *222*, 115-117.

Edwards, J.E., McQuay, H.J., Moore, R.A.: *Single dose dihydrocodeine for acute postoperative pain*, Cochrane Database Syst. Rev. **2000**, CD002760.

Ehrhart, G., Ruschig, H.: *Arzneimittel, Entwicklung, Wirkung, Darstellung*, Verlag Chemie, Weinheim **1972**, Vol. I, 79.

Eisleb, O. (I.G. Farben): *Verfahren zur Darstellung von Piperidinverbindungen*, DE 679 281, **1937**.

Eisleb, O. (Winthrop): *Piperidine compounds and a process of preparing them*, US 2 167 351, **1939**.

Eisleb, O.: *New syntheses with sodium amide*, Chem. Ber. **1941**, *74*, 1433-1450.

Eisleb, O. (I.G. Farben): *Verfahren zur Herstellung von 1-Alkyl-4-(m-oxyphenyl)-piperidinverbindungen*, DRP 752 755, **1942**.

E. Merck AG: *Verfahren zur Herstellung von Morphinäthern*, DRP 131 980, **1902**.

Ericsson, C.D. and Johnson, P.C.: *Safety and efficacy of loperamide*, Am. J. Med. **1990**, *20*, 10S-14S.

Errick, J.K., Heel, R.C.: *Nalbuphine. A preliminary review of its pharmacological properties and therapeutic efficacy*, Drugs **1983**, *26*, 191-211.

Essawi, M.Y.H.: *Fentanyl analogues with a modified propanamido group as potential affinity labels: Synthesis and in vivo activity*, Pharmazie **1999**, *54*, 307-308.

Evans, C.J., Keith, D.E. Jr., Morrison, H., Magendzo, K., Edwards, R.H.: *Cloning of a delta opioid receptor by functional expression*, Science **1992**, *258*, 1952-1955.

Evans, J.M., Hogg, M.I., Lunn, J.N., Rosen, M.: *A comparative study of the narcotic against activity of naloxone and levallorphan*, Anaesthesia **1974**, *29*, 721-727.

Feldman, P. L., James, M. K., Brackeen, M. F., Johnson, M. R., Leighton, H. J. (Glaxo): *N-Phenyl-N-(piperidinyl)amides useful as analgesics*, EP 383 579, **1990**.

Feldmann, P.L., James, M.K., Brackeen, F., Bilotta, J.M., Schuster, S.V., Lahey, A.V., Lutz, M.W., Johnson, M.R., Leighton, H.J.: *Design, synthesis, and pharmacological evaluation of ultrashort- to long-acting opioid analgetics*, J. Med. Chem. **1991**, *34*, 2202-2208.

Flick, K., Frankus, E., Friderichs, E.: *Studies on chemical structure and analgetic activity of phenyl substituted aminomethylcyclohexanoles*, Arzneim.-Forsch./Drug Res. **1978**, *28 (I)*, 107-113.

Foldes, F.F., Duncalf, D., Kuwabara, S.: *The respiratory, circulatory, and narcotic antagonistic effects of nalorphine, levallorphan, and naloxone in anaesthetized subjects*, Can. Anaesth. Soc. J. **1969**, *16*, 151-161.

Foldes, F.F.: *Neuroleptanesthesia for general surgery*, Int. Anesthesiol. Clin. **1973**, *11*, 1-35.

Fowler, C.J. and Fraser, G.L.: *Mu-, delta-, kappa-opioid receptors and their subtypes. A critical review with emphasis on radioligand binding experiments*, Neurochem. Int. **1994**, *24*, 401-426.

Frackenpohl, J.: *Morphin und Opioid-Analgetika*, Chem. i. u. Zeit **2000**, *34*, 99-112.

Franklin, R.A.: *The clinical pharmacokinetics and metabolism of the analgesic meptazinol*, Xenobiotica **1988**, *18*, 105-112.

Frankus, E., and Flick, K. (Grünenthal): *Phenol ethers that contain basic groups*, GB 997 399, **1964**; US 3 564 100, **1971**.

Freed, M. E. and Potoski, J. R. (American Home): *Benzobicycloalkanamine und ihre Zwischeprodukte, Verfahren zu ihrer Herstellung und ihre Verwendung*, DE 2 159 324, **1971**; BE 776 173, **1971.**

Freed, M.E., Potoski, J.R., Freed, E.H., Conklin, G.L.: *Bridged aminotetralins as novel potent analgesic substances*, J. Med. Chem. **1973**, *16*, 595-599.

Friderichs, E., Felgenhauer, F., Jongschaap, P., Osterloh, G.: *[Pharmacological studies on analgesia, dependence on and tolerance of tramadol, a potent analgetic drug (author's transl)]*, Arzneimittelforschung **1978**, *28*, 122-134.

Friedrich, G., Braunstein, P., Friedrich, M., Vach, W.: *[Elimination half life of the opiate etorphine]*, Beitr. Gerichtl. Med. **1991**, *49*, 111-119.

Frink, M.C., Hennies, H.-H., Englberger, W., Haurand, M., Wilffert, B.: *Influence of tramadol on neurotransmitter systems of the rat brain*, Arzneimittelforschung **1996**, *46*, 1029-1036.

Fudala, P.J., Jaffe, J.H., Dax, E.M., Johnson, R.E.: *Use of buprenorphine in the treatment of opioid addiction. II. Physiologic and behavioral effects of daily and alternate-day administration and abrupt withdrawal*, Clin. Pharmacol. Ther. **1990**, *47*, 525-534.

Gal, T.J.: *Naloxone reversal of buprenorphine-induced respiratory depression*, Clin. Pharmacol. Ther. **1989**, *45*, 66-71.

Gardner, J.S., Blough, D., Drinkard, C.R., Shatin, D., Anderson, G., Graham, D., Alderfer, R.: *Tramadol and seizures: a surveillance study in a managed care population*, Pharmacotherapy **2000**, *20*, 1423-1431.

Gates, M. and Tschudi, G.: *Synthesis of morphine*, J. Am. Chem. Soc. **1952**, *72*, 1109.

Gaveriaux-Ruff, G. and Kieffer, B.: *Opioid receptors: Gene structure and function. In: Opioids in pain control. Basic and clinical aspects*, edited by C. Stein, Cambridge University Press, Cambridge, **1999**.

Gibb, D.B. and Pikler, N.: *Piritramide - a new long-acting analgesic*, Anaesth. Intensive Care **1973**, *1*, 308-314.

Ginsburg, C.M.: *Lomotil (diphenoxylate and atropine) intoxication*, Am. J. Dis. Child. **1973**, *125*, 241-242.

Glass, P.S.: *Remifentanil: a new opioid*, J. Clin. Anesth. **1995**, *7*, 558-563.

Goldberg, M., Ishak, S., Garcia, C., McKenna, J.: *Postoperative rigidity following sufentanil administration*, Anesthesiology **1985**, *63*, 199-201.

Goldstein, G.: *Pentazocine*, Drug Alcohol Depend. **1985**, *14*, 313-323.

Gomes, I., Jordan, B.A., Gupta, A., Trapaidze, N., Nagy, V., Devi, L.A.: *Heterodimerization of mu and delta opioid receptors: A role in opiate synergy*, J. Neurosci. **2000**, *20*, RC110.

Gonzalez, J.P. and Brogden, R.N.: *Naltrexone. A review of its pharmacodynamic and pharmacokinetic properties and therapeutic efficacy in the management of opioid dependence*, Drugs **1988**, *35*, 192-213.

Goodrich, P.M.: *Naloxone hydrochloride: a review*. AANA J. **1990**, *58*, 14-16.

Grass, J.A.: *Sufentanil: clinical use as postoperative analgesic - epidural/intrathecal route*, J. Pain Symptom. Manage. **1992**, *7*, 271-286.

Grewe, R.: *Das Problem der Morphin-Synthese*, Naturwissenschaften **1946**, *33*, 333-337.

Grover, H.: *Propoxyphene*, J. Indian Med. Assoc. **1988**, *86*, 21-23.

Hagen, N., Thirlwell, M.P., Dhaliwal, H.S., Babul, N., Harsanyi, Z., Darke, A.C.: *Steady-state pharmacokinetics of hydromorphone and hydromorphone-3-glucuronide in cancer patients after immediate and controlled-release hydromorphone*, J. Clin. Pharmacol. **1995**, *35*, 37-44.

Haigh, C.G.: *Drug development in anaesthesia: the remifentanil*, Minerva Anestesiol. **2000**, *66*, 414-416.

Handal, K.A., Schauben, J.L., Salamone, F.R.: *Naloxone*, Ann. Emerg. Med. **1983**, *12*, 438-445.

Hauser, F.M.: *14-Hydroxycodeinone. An improved synthesis*, J. Med. Chem. **1974**, *17*, 1117.

Heel, R.C., Brogden, R.N., Speight, T.M., Avery, G.S.: *Buprenorphine: a review of its pharmacological properties and therapeutic efficacy*, Drugs **1979**, *17*, 81-110.

Heel, R.C., Brogden, R.N., Speight, T.M., Avery, G.S.: *Butorphanol: a review of its pharmacological properties and therapeutic efficacy*, Drugs **1978**, *16*, 473-505.

Heel, R.C., Brogden, R.N., Speight, T.M., Avery, G.S.: *Loperamide: a review of its pharmacological properties and therapeutic efficacy in diarrhoea*, Drugs **1978**, *15*, 33-52.

Heit, H.A.: *The truth about pain management: the difference between a pain patient and an addicted patient*, Eur. J. Pain **2001**, *5*, Suppl A, 27-29.

Hellerbach, J., Grüssner, A., Schnider, O.: *(-)-3-Hydroxy-N-allyl-morphinan und verwandte Verbindungen*, Helv. Chim. Acta **1956**, *39*, 429-440.

Herbert, R.B., Venter, H., Pos, S.: *Do mammals make their own morphine*, Nat. Prod. Rep. **2000**, *17*, 317-322.

Herz, A.: *Multiple opiate receptors and their functional significance*, J. Neural. Transm. Suppl. **1983**, *18*, 227-233.

Hill, J.L. and Zacny, J.P.: *Comparing the subjective, psychomotor, and physiological effects of intravenous hydromorphone and morphine in healthy volunteers*, Psychopharmacology (Berl). **2000**, *152*, 31-39.

Hörner, L., Rösch, W., Deutschel, K. (Knoll): *Verfahren zur Extraktion von Morphin aus Mohnkapseln*, DOS 2 726 925, **1977**.

Hollt, V. and Herz, A.: *In vivo receptor occupation by opiates and correlation to the pharmacological effect*, Fed. Proc. **1978**, *37*, 158-161.

Holmes, B. and Ward, A.: *Meptazinol. A review of its pharmacodynamic and pharmacokinetic properties and therapeutic efficacy*, Drugs **1985**, *30*, 285-312.

Homan, R.V.: *Transnasal butorphanol*, Am. Fam. Physician. **1994**, *49*, 188-192.

Homsi, J., Walsh, D., Nelson, K.A., LeGrand, S.B., Davis, M.: *Hydrocodone for cough in advanced cancer*, Am. J. Hosp. Palliat. Care. **2000**, *17*, 342-346.

Honig, S. and Murray, K.A.: *An appraisal of codeine as an analgesic: single-dose analysis*, J. Clin. Pharmacol. **1984**, *24*, 96-102.

Hopkins, S.J.: *Alfentanil hydrochloride*, Drugs Fut. **1981**, *6*, 335-337.

Hoskin, P.J. and Hanks, G.W.: *Opioid agonist-antagonist drugs in acute and chronic pain states*, Drugs. **1991**, *41*, 326-344.

Howe, E. E. and Sletzinger, M.: *Resolution of dl-methadone and dl-isomethadone*, J. Am. Chem. Soc. **1949**, *71*, 2935.

Howe, E. E., Brook, B., Tishler, M. (Merck & Co): *Salts of D-amidone with an optically active acid and process for resolving DL-amidone*, US 2 644 010, **1953**.

Huang, P., Kehner, G.B., Cowan, A., Liu-Chen, L.Y.: *Comparison of pharmacological activities of buprenorphine and norbuprenorphine: norbuprenorphine is a potent opioid agonist*, J. Pharmacol. Exp. Ther. **2001**, *297*, 688-695.

Hudlicky, T., Butora, G., Fearnley, S.F., Gum, A.G., Stabile, M.R.: *A historical perspective of morphine synthesis*, in: Studies in natural products chemistry, edited by Atta-ur-Rahman, **1996**, Elsevier, Amsterdam, 43-116.

Hull, C.J.: *The pharmacokinetics of alfentanil in man*, Br. J. Anaesth. **1983**, *55*, Suppl 2, 157S-164S.

Husbands, S.M. and Lewis, J.W.; *Structural determinants of efficacy for κ opioid receptors in the orvinol series: /,/-spiro analogues of buprenorphin*, J. Org. Chem. **2000**, *43*, 139-141.

Inturrisi, C.E., Colburn, W.A., Verebey, K., Dayton, H.E., Woody, G.E., O'Brien, C.P.: *Propoxyphene and norpropoxyphene kinetics after single and repeated doses of propoxyphene*, Clin. Pharmacol. Ther. **1982**, *31*, 157-167.

Inturrisi, C.E., Max, M.B., Foley, K.M., Schultz, M., Shin, S.U., Houde, R.W.: *The pharmacokinetics of heroin in patients with chronic pain*, New Engl. J. Med. **1984**, *310*, 1213-1217.

Inturrisi, C.E., Schultz, M., Shin, S., Umans, J.G., Angel, L., Simon, E.J.: *Evidence from opiate binding studies that heroin acts through its metabolites*, Life Sci. **1983**, *33*, Suppl. 1, 773-776.

Isaacson, I.J.: *Clinical use of sufentanil as an anesthetic*, J. Pain Symptom. Manage. **1992**, *7*, 362-364.

Jackson, F.W.: *Fentanyl and the wooden chest*, Gastroenterology **1994**, *106*, 820-821.

Jacobs, A.M. and Youngblood, F.: *Opioid receptor affinity for agonist-antagonist analgesics*, J. Am. Podiatr. Med. Assoc. **1992**, *82*, 520-524.

Jadad, A.R., and Browman, G.P.: *The WHO analgesic ladder for cancer pain management. Stepping up the quality of its evaluation*, J. Am. Med. Assoc. **1995**, *274*, 1870-1873.

Jamison, R.N., Kauffmann, J., Katz, N.P.: *Characteristics of methadone maintenance patients with chronic pain*, J. Pain Symptom Manage. **2000**, *19*, 53-62.

Janssen, P. and Karel, D. (Janssen): *Verfahren zur Herstellung von analgetisch wirksamen, substituierten 4-[Morpholyl-(4)]-2,2-diphenyl-butyramiden*, DE 1 117 126, **1956**; GB 822 055, **1956**.

Janssens, F. (Janssen): *N-Phenyl-N-(4-piperidinyl)-amide, Verfahren zu deren Herstellung und deren Verwendung als Analgetika*, DOS 2 819 873, **1978**.

Janssen, P. (Janssen): *2,2-Diaryl-ω-(4'-phenyl-1'-piperidino)alkanonitriles*, US 2 898 340, **1959**;

Dryden, H. L. and Erickson, R. A. (Searle): *Process for the preparation of tertiary amines*, US 4 086 234, **1978**.

Janssen, P. (Janssen): *Verfahren zur Herstellung von 1-(ω,ω-Diphenylalkyl)-4-amino-piperidin-4- oder 1-(ω,ω-Diphenylalkyl)-3-amino-pyrrolidin-3-carbonsäureamiden und deren Salze und quarternären Ammoniumverbindungen*, DE 1 238 472, **1961**.

Janssen, P. (Janssen): *1-Arylalkyl-4-(N-aryl-carbonyl amino)-piperidiens and related compounds*, US 3 164 600, **1965;**

Janssen, P. (Janssen): *Method for producing analgesia*, US 3 141 823, **1964**.

Janssen, P. (Janssen): *2,2-Diaryl-4-(4'-aryl-4'-hydroxy-piperidino)-butyramides*, US 3 714 159, **1973**.

Janssen, P., Niemegeers, C. j. E. J., Stokbroekx, R. A. (Janssen): *2,2-Diaryl-4-piperidinbutyramide*, DOS 2 126 559, **1971**.

Janssen, P. and van Daele, H. P.: *N-(4-Piperidinyl)-N-phenylamides and -carbamate*s, US 3 998 834, **1976**.

Janssen, P.A. and Jageneau, A.H.: *A new series of potent analgesics: Dextro 2:2 diphenyl-3-methyl-4-morpholino-butyrylpyrrolidine and related amides*, J. Pharm. Pharmacol. **1957**, *9*, 381-400

Janssen, P.A. and Van der Eycken, C.A.: *The chemical anatomy of potent morphine-like analgesics*, in: Drugs affecting the central nervous system, edited by A. Burger, Marcel Decker, New York, **1968**, 25-60.

Janssens, F., Torremans, J., Janssen, P.A.J.: *Synthetic 1,4-disubstituted 1,4-dihydro-5H-tetrazol-5-one derivatives of fentanyl: alfentanil (R 39209), a potent, extremely short-acting narcotic analgesic*, J. Med. Chem. **1986**, *29*, 2290-2297.

Jasinski, D.R. and Preston, K.L.: *Evaluation of tilidine for morphine-like subjective effects and euphoria*, Drug Alcohol Depend. **1986**, *18*, 273-292.

Jeal, W. and Benfield, P.: *Transdermal fentanyl. A review of its pharmacological properties and therapeutic efficacy in pain control*, Drugs **1997**, *53*, 109-138.

Jiraki, K.: *Lethal effects of normeperidine*, Am. J. Forensic Med. Pathol. **1992**, *13*, 42-43.

Johnson, R.E. and Jasinski, D.R.: *Human pharmacology and abuse potential of meptazinol*, Clin. Pharmacol. Ther., *41*, 426-433.

Jonasson, B., Jonasson, U., Holmgren, P., Saldeen, T.: *Fatal poisonings where ethylmorphine from antitussive medications contributed to death*, Int. J. Legal. Med. **1999**, *112*, 299-302.

Jones, T.E., Morris, R.G., Saccoia, N.C., Thorne, D.: *Dextromoramide pharmacokinetics following sublingual administration*, Palliat. Med. **1996**, *10*, 313-317.

Joseph, H., Stancliff, S., Langrod, J.: *Methadone maintenance treatment (MMT): a review of historical and clinical issues*, Mt. Sinai J. Med. **2000**, *67*, 347-364.

Juby, P.F., Hudyma, T.W., Brown, M.: *Preparation and antininflammatory properties of some 5-(2-anilinophenyl)tetrazoles*, J. Med. Chem. **1968**, *11*, 111-117.

Judd, A.T., Tempest, S.M., Clarke, I.M.: *The anaesthetist and the pain clinic: dextromoramide analgesia*, Br. Med. J. (Clin. Res. Ed.) **1981**, *282*, 75-76.

Kägi, H. and Miescher, K.: *New synthesis of 4-phenyl-4-piperidyl alkyl ketones and related compounds with morphinelike action*, Helv. Chim. Acta **1949**, *32*, 2489-2507.

Kaiko, R.F., Benziger, D.P., Fitzmartin, R.D., Burke, B.E., Reder, R.F., Goldenheim, P.D.: *Pharmacokinetic-pharmacodynamic relationships of controlled-release oxycodone*, Clin. Pharmacol. Ther. **1996**, *59*, 52-61.

Kane, F.J. Jr. and Pokorny, A.: *Mental and emotional disturbance with pentazocine (Talwin) use*, South Med. J. 1975, *68*, 808-811.

Karim, A., Ranney, R.E., Evensen, K.L., Clark, M.L.: *Pharmacokinetics and metabolism of diphenoxylate in man*, Clin. Pharmacol. Ther. **1972**, *13*, 407-419.

Kay, B.: *A study of strong oral analgesics: the relief of postoperative pain using dextromoramide, pentazocine and bezitramide*, Br. J. Anaesth. **1973**, *45*, 623-628.

Kay, B.: *Parenteral meptazinol--international clinical experience*, Postgrad. Med. J. **1985**, *61*, Suppl. 2, 23-26.

Kieffer, B.L., Befort, K., Gaveriaux-Ruff, C., Hirth, C.G.: *The delta-opioid receptor: isolation of a cDNA by expression cloning and pharmacological characterization*, Proc. Natl. Acad. Sci. USA **1992**, *89*, 12048-12052.

Kieffer, B.L.: *Opioids: first lessons from knockout mice*, Trends Pharmacol. Sci. **1999**, *20*, 19-26.

Killinger, J.M., Weintraub, H.S., Fuller, B.L.: *Human pharmacokinetics and comparative bioavailability of loperamide hydrochloride*, J. Clin. Pharmacol. **1979**, *19*, 211-218.

Kleemann, A., Engel, J., Kutscher, B., Reichert, D.: *Pharmaceutical Substances, Synthesis, Patents, Applications*, Thieme, Stuttgart, New York, **1999** (available in print and CD-ROM).

Klinger, W.: *Age dependent acute toxicity of ethylmorphine*, Pharmazie **1976**, *31*, 655-656.

Knapp, R.J., Malatynska, E., Collins, N., Fang, L., Wang, J.Y., Hruby, V.J., Roeske, W.R., Yamamura, H.I.: *Molecular biology and pharmacology of cloned opioid receptors*, FASEB J. **1995**, *9*, 516-525.

Knoll AG, *Verfahren zur Darstellung von Dihydromorphinonen*, DRP 607 931, **1935**.

Krauß, W. (E. Merck AG): *Verfahren zur Herstellung von Oxykodeinon*, DRP 411 530, **1925**.

Kreek, M.J.: *Medical safety and side effects of methadone in tolerant individuals*, J. Am. Med. Assoc. **1973**, *223*, 665-668.

Kromer, W.: *Endogenous opioids, the enteric nervous system and gut motility*, Dig. Dis. **1990**, *8*, 361-373.

Kuhlman, J.J. Jr., Lalani, S., Magluilo, J. Jr., Levine, B., Darwin. W.D.: *Human pharmacokinetics of intravenous, sublingual, and buccal buprenorphine*, J. Anal. Toxicol. **1996**, *20*, 369-378.

Kumar, N. and Rowbotham, D.J.: *Piritramide*, Br. J. Anaesth. **1999**, *82*, 3-5.

Larijani, G.E. and Goldberg, M.E.: *Alfentanil hydrochloride: a new short-acting narcotic analgesic for surgical procedures*, Clin. Pharm. **1987**, *6*, 275-282.

Larsen, A. A., Tullar, B. F., Elpern, B., Buck, J. S.: *Resolution of methadon and related compounds*, J. Am. Chem. Soc. **1948**, *70*, 4195-4196.

Latta, K.S., Ginsberg, B., Barkin, R.L.: *Meperidine: a critical review*, Am. J. Ther. **2002**, *9*, 53-68.

Lattin, D.L.: *Treating narcotic overdose: Nalorphine, levallorphan, or naloxone?*, J. Ark. Med. Soc. **1976**, *72*, 465-467.

Law, P.Y. and Loh, H.H.: *Regulation of opioid receptor activities*, J. Pharmacol. Exp. Ther. **1999**, *289*, 607-624.

Lawson, A.A. and Northridge, D.B.: *Dextropropoxyphene overdose. Epidemiology, clinical presentation and management*, Med. Toxicol. Adverse Drug Exp. **1987**, *2*, 430-444.

Lee, C.R., McTavish, D., Sorkin, E.M.: *Tramadol. A preliminary review of its pharmacodynamic and pharmacokinetic properties, and therapeutic potential in acute and chronic pain states*, Drugs **1993**, *46*, 313-340.

Lee, K.O., Akil, H., Woods, J.H., Traynor, J.R.: *Differential binding properties of oripavines at cloned mu- and delta-opioid receptors*, Eur. J. Pharmacol. **1999**, *378*, 323-330.

Lehmann, K.A., Tenbuhs, B., Hoeckle, W.: *Patient-controlled analgesia with piritramid for the treatment of postoperative pain*, Acta Anaesthesiol. Belg. **1986**, *37*, 247-257.

Leysen, J.E., Gommeren, W., Niemegeers, C.J.: *[3H]Sufentanil, a superior ligand for mu-opiate receptors: binding properties and regional distribution in rat brain and spinal cord*, Eur. J. Pharmacol. **1983**, *87*, 209-225.

Lewenstein, M.J. and Weiss, U.: *Morphine derivative*, US 2 806 033, **1955**.

Lewenstein, M. J. and Fishman, J.: *Morphine derivative*, US 3 254 088, **1966**; DE 1 183 508, **1962**.

Lintz, W., Erlacin, S., Frankus, E., Uragg, H.: *[Biotransformation of tramadol in man and animal (author's transl)]*, Arzneimittelforschung **1981**, *31*, 1932-1943.

Lipp, J.: *Possible mechanisms of morphine analgesia*, Clin. Neuropharmacol. **1991**, *14*, 131-147.

Lloyd, R.S., Costello, F., Eves, M.J., James, I.G., Miller, A.J.: *The efficacy and tolerability of controlled-release dihydrocodeine tablets and combination dextropropoxyphene/paracetamol tablets in patients with severe osteoarthritis of the hips*, Curr. Med. Res. Opin. **1992**, *13*, 37-48.

Lo, M.W., Lee, F.H., Schary, W.L., Whitney, C.C.Jr.: *The pharmacokinetics of intravenous, intramuscular, and subcutaneous nalbuphine in healthy subjects*, Eur. J. Clin. Pharmacol. **1987**, *33*, 297-301.

Lotsch, J. and Geisslinger, G.: *Morphine-6-glucuronide: an analgesic of the future?*, Clin. Pharmacokinet. **2001**, *40*, 485-499.

Lowinson, J., Ruiz, P., Alksne, L., Langrod, J.: *Detoxification from methadone: results and inferences*, Curr. Psychiatr. Ther. **1978**, *18*, 165-172.

Lustman, F., Walters, E.G., Shroff, N.E., Akbar, F.A.: *Diphenoxylate hydrochloride (Lomotil) in the treatment of acute diarrhoea*, Br. J. Clin. Pract. **1987**, *41*, 648-651.

Mancini, I. and Bruera, E.: *Constipation in advanced cancer patients*, Support Care Cancer. **1998**, *6*, 356-364.

Mansour, A., Fox, C.A., Akil, H., Watson, S.J.: *Opioid-receptor mRNA expression in the rat CNS: anatomical and functional implications*. Trends Neurosci. **1995**, *18*, 22-29.

Mansour, A., Watson, S.J., Akil, H.: *Opioid receptors: past, present and future*, Trends Neurosci. **1995**, *18*, 69-70.

Martin, W.R., Eades, C.G., Thompson, J.A., Huppler, R.E., Gilbert, P.E.: *The effects of morphine- and nalorphine- like drugs in the nondependent and morphine-dependent chronic spinal dog*, J. Pharmacol. Exp. Ther. **1976**, *197*, 517-532.

Martin, W.R.: *Pharmacology of opioids*, Pharmacol. Rev. **1983**, *35*, 283-323.

Martin, W., Ring, J., Gaupp, M., Arnold, P., Sennewald, R.: *Bioavailability investigation of a new tilidine/naloxone liquid formulation compared to a reference formulation*, Arzneim.-Forsch./Drug-Res. **1999**, *49*, 599-607.

Mather, L.E. and Meffin, P.J.: *Clinical pharmacokinetics of pethidine*, Clin. Pharmacokinet. **1978**, *3*, 352-368.

Matthes, H.W., Maldonado, R., Simonin, F., Valverde, O., Slowe, S., Kitchen, I., Befort, K., Dierich, A., Le Meur, M., Dolle, P., Tzavara, E., Hanoune, J., Roques, B.P., Kieffer, B.L.: *Loss of morphine-induced analgesia, reward effect and withdrawal symptoms in mice lacking the mu-opioid-receptor gene*, Nature **1996**, *383*, 819-823.

Matthys, H., Erhardt, J., Ruhle, K.H.: *[Objectivation of the effect of antitussive agents using tussometry in patients with chronic cough]*, Schweiz. Med. Wochenschr. **1985**, *115*, 307-311.

McFadzean, I.: *The ionic mechanisms underlying opioid actions,* Neuropeptides **1988**, *11*, 173-180.

Meunier, J.-C., Mollereau, C., Toll, L., Suaudeau, C., Moisand, C., Alvinerie, P., Butour, J.-L., Guillemot, J.-C., Ferrara, P., Monsarrat, B., Mazargil, H., Vassart, G., Parmentier, M., Costentin, J.: *Isolation and structure of the endogenous agonist of the opioid receptor-like ORL1 receptor*, Nature **1995**, *377*, 532-535.

Meuzelaar, G.J., van Vliet, M.C.A., Maat, L., Sheldon, R.A.: *Improvements in the total synthesis of morphine*, Eur. J. Org. Chem. **1999**, 2315-2321.

Meyer, D. and Halfin, V.: *Toxicity secondary to meperidine in patients on monoamine oxidase inhibitors: a case report and critical review*, J. Clin. Psychopharmacol. **1981**, *1*, 319-321.

Michelsen, L.G. and Hug, C.C. Jr.: *The pharmacokinetics of remifentanil*, J. Clin. Anesth. **1996**, *8*, 679-682.

Misra, A.L.: *Current status of preclinical research on disposition, pharmacokinetics, and metabolism of naltrexone*, NIDA Res. Monogr. **1981**, *28*, 132-146.

Mollereau, C. and Mouledous, L.: *Tissue distribution of the opioid receptor-like (ORL1) receptor*, Peptides **2000**, *21*, 907-917.

Monk, J.P., Beresford, R., Ward, A.: *Sufentanil. A review of its pharmacological properties and therapeutic use*, Drugs **1988**, *36*, 286-313.

Monkovic, I. and Conway, T. (Bristol-Myers): *Process for the preparation of 14-hydroxymorphinan derivatives*, US 3 775 414, **1973**.

Monkovic, I., Conway, T. T., Wong, H., Perron, Y. G., Pachter, I. J., Belleau, B.: *Total synthesis and pharmacological activities of N-substituted 3,14-dihydroxymorphinans*, J. Am. Chem. Soc. **1973**, *95*, 7910-7911.

Monkovic, I., Bachand, C., Wong, H.: *A stereoselective total synthesis of 14-hydroxymorphinans. Grewe approach*, J. Am. Chem. Soc. **1978**, *100*, 4609-46.

Moody, D.E., Alburges, M.E., Parker, R.J., Collins, J.M., Strong, J.M.: *The involvement of cytochrome P450 3A4 in the N-demethylation of L-alpha-acetylmethadol (LAAM), norLAAM, and methadone*, Drug Metab. Dispos. **1997**, *25*, 1347-1353.

Morrison, A.B.: *Toxicity and abuse of hydrocodone bitartrate*, Can. Med. Assoc. J. **1979**, *120*, 1338.

Moser, P., Sallmann, A., Wiesenberg, I.: *Synthesis and quantitative structure-activity relationships of diclofenac analogues*, J. Med. Chem. **1990**, *33*, 2358-2368.

Mulroy, M.F.: *Monitoring opioids*, Reg. Anesth. **1996**, *21*, Suppl. 6, 89-93.

Mulzer, J. and Trauner, D.: *Practical synthesis of (-)-morphine*, Chirality **1999**, *11*, 475-482.

Nagata, H., Miyazawa, N., Ogasawara, K.: *A concise route to (-)-morphine*, Chem. Commun. **2001**, 1094-1095.

Nagle, R.E. and Pilcher, J.: *Respiratory and circulatory effects of pentazocine. Review of analgesics used after myocardial infarction*, Br. Heart J. **1972**, *34*, 244-251.

Niemegeers, C.J., Lenaerts, F.M., Janssen, P.A.: *Difenoxine (R 15403), the active metabolite of diphenoxylate (R 1132). 2. Difneozine, a potent, orally active and safe antidiarrheal agent in rats*, Arzneimittelforschung **1972**, *22*, 516-518.

Niemegeers, C. J., Lenaerts, F. M., Janssen, P. A.: *Loperamide, a novel type of antidiarrheal agent*, Arzneim.-Forsch. (Drug Res.) **1974**, *24*, 1633.

Noble, F., Smadja, C., Roques, B.P.: *Role of endogenous cholecystokinin in the facilitation of mu-mediated antinociception by delta-opioid agonists*, J. Pharmacol. Exp. Ther. **1994**, *271*, 1127-1134.

Novak, B.H., Hudlicky, T., Reed, J.W., Mulzer, J., Trauner, D.: *Morphin synthesis and biosynthesis - an update*, Curr. Org. Chem. **2000**, *4*, 343-362.

O'Brien, C.P., Greenstein, R., Ternes, J., Woody, G.E.: *Clinical pharmacology of narcotic antagonists*, Ann. N.Y. Acad. Sci. **1978**, *311*, 232-240.

O'Brien, J.J. and Benfield, P.: *Dezocine. A preliminary review of its pharmacodynamic and pharmacokinetic properties, and therapeutic efficacy*, Drugs **1989**, *38*, 226-248.

Ohqvist, G., Hallin, R., Gelinder, S., Lang, H., Samuelson, S.: *A comparison between morphine, meperidine and ketobemidone in continuous intravenous infusion for postoperative relief*, Acta Anaesthesiol. Scand. **1991**, *35*, 44-48.

Olofson, R.A., Schnur, R.C., Bunes, L., Pepe, J.P.: *Selective N-dealkylation of tertiary amines with vinyl chloroformate - an improved synthesis of naloxone*, Tetrahedron Lett. **1977**, 1567-1571.

Olsen, G.D., Wendel, H.A., Livermore, J.D., Leger, R.M., Lynn, R.K., Gerber, N.: *Clinical effects and pharmacokinetics of racemic methadone and its optical isomers*, Clin. Pharmacol. Ther. **1977**, *21*, 147-157.

O´Siordin, L.; *The role of transdermal fentanyl in palliative care*, Clin. Drug Invest. **1998**, *16*, 71-72.

Osborne, R., Joel, S., Trew, D., Slevin, M.: *Morphine and metabolite behavior after different routes of morphine administration: demonstration of the importance of the active metabolite morphine-6-glucuronide*, Clin. Pharmacol. Ther. **1990**, *47*, 12-19.

Otton, S.V., Schadel, M., Cheung, S.W., Kaplan, H.L., Busto, U.E., Sellers, E.M.: *CYP2D6 phenotype determines the metabolic conversion of hydrocodone to hydromorphone*, Clin. Pharmacol. Ther. **1993**, *54*, 463-472.

Overman, L.E., Petty, C.B., Doedens, R.J.: *Synthetic application of N-(acylamino)-1,3-dienes. Control of endo stereoselectivity by the acyl substituent. stereospecific synthesis of the analgesic tilidine*, J. Org. Chem. **1979**, *44*, 4183-4185.

Palangio, M., Morris, E., Doyle, R.T. Jr., Dornseif, B.E., Valente, T.J.: *Combination hydrocodone and ibuprofen versus combination oxycodone and acetaminophen in the treatment of moderate or severe acute low back pain*, Clin. Ther. **2002**, *24*, 87-99.

Pallenbach, E.: *Die Substitutionstherapie bei opiatabhängigen Patienten*, Pharmazie i. u. Zeit **2002**, *31*, 90-95.

Pasternak, G.W., Adler, B.A., Rodriguez, J.: *Characterization of the opioid receptor binding and animal pharmacology of meptazinol*, Postgrad. Med. J. **1985**, *61*, Suppl. 2, 5-12.

Pasternak, G.W. and Wood, P.J.: *Multiple mu opiate receptors,* Life Sci. **1986**, *38*, 1889-1898.

Patel, S.S. and Spencer, C.M.: *Remifentanil*, Drugs **1996**, *52*, 417-427.

Paton, D.M.: *RO-20,2230*, Drugs Fut. **1979**, *4*, 438-441.

Pearson, R.M.: *Pharmacokinetics of propoxyphene*, Hum. Toxicol. **1984**, *3*, 37S-40S.

Pert, C.B. and Snyder, S.H.: *Correlation of opiate receptor affinity with analgetic effects of meperidine homologues*, J. Med. Chem. **1976**, *19*, 1248-1250.

Pfeiffer, A., Brantl, V., Herz, A., Emrich, H.M.: *Psychotomimesis mediated by kappa opiate receptors*, Science **1986**, *233*, 774-776.

Pfister, K. and Tishler, M. (Merck & Co): Process of preparing dihydrocodeinone, US 2 715 626, **1955**.

Pohland, A., Sullivan, H.R.: *Analgesics esters of 4-dialkylamino-1,2-diphenyl-2-butanols*, J. Am. Chem. Soc. **1953**, *75*, 4458-4461.

Pohland, A., Sullivan, H.R.: *Preparation of α-d- and α-l-dimethylamino-1,2-diphenyl-3-methyl-2-propionyloxybutane*, J. Am. Chem. Soc. **1955**, *77*, 3400-3401.

Pohland, A., Peters, L.R., Sullivan, H.R.: *Analgesics. Stereoselective synthesis of α-(+)- and α-(-)-4-dimethylamino-1,2-diphenyl-3-methyl-2-propionoxybutane*, J. Org. Chem. **1963**, *28*, 2483-2484.

Poklis, A.: *Fentanyl: a review for clinical and analytical toxicologists*, J. Toxicol. Clin. Toxicol. **1995**, *33*, 439-447.

Portoghese, P.S., Alreja, B.D., Larson, D.L.: *Allylprodine analogues as receptor probes. Evidence that phenolic and nonphenolic ligands interact with different subsites on identical opioid receptors*, J. Med. Chem. **1981**, *24*, 782-787.

Poyhia, R., Vainio, A., Kalso, E.: *A review of oxycodone's clinical pharmacokinetics and pharmacodynamics*, J. Pain Symptom. Manage. **1993**, *8*, 63-67.

Pugh, G.C., Brown, D.T., Drummond, G.B.: *Effect of nalbuphine hydrochloride on the ventilatory and occlusion pressure responses to carbon dioxide in volunteers*, Br. J. Anaesth. **1989**, *62*, 601-609.

Quigley, C.: *Hydromorphone for acute and chronic pain (Cochrane Review)*, Cochrane Database Syst. Rev. **2002**, CD003447.

Raffa, R.B., Friderichs, E., Reimann, W., Shank, R.P., Codd, E.E., Vaught, J.L., Jacoby, H.I., Selve, N.: *Complementary and synergistic antinociceptive interaction between the enantiomers of tramadol*, J. Pharmacol. Exp. Ther. **1993**, *267*, 331-340.

Raffa, R.B., Friderichs, E., Reimann, W., Shank, R.P., Codd, E.E., Vaught, J.L.: *Opioid and nonopioid components independently contribute to the mechanism of action of tramadol, an 'atypical' opioid analgesic*, J. Pharmacol. Exp. Ther. **1992**, *260*, 275-285.

Raffa, R.B. and Friderichs, E.: *The basic science aspect of tramadol hydrochloride*, Pain Rev. **1996**, *3*, 249-271.

Rapoport, H., Naumann, R., Bissel, E.R., Bonner, R.M.: *The preparation of some dihydro ketones in the morphine series by Oppenauer oxidation*, J. Org. Chem. **1950**, *15*, 1103-1107.

Reder, R.F.: *Opioid formulations: tailoring to the needs in chronic pain*, Eur. J. Pain **2001**, *5*, Suppl. A, 109-111.

Reed, D.A. and Schnoll, S.H.: *Abuse of pentazocine-naloxone combination*, J. Am. Med. Assoc. **1986**, *256*, 2562-2564.

Reinscheid, R.K., Nothacker, H.P., Bourson, A., Ardati, A., Henningsen, R.A., Bunzow, J.R., Grandy, D.K., Langen, H., Monsma, F.J. Jr., Civelli. O.: *Orphanin FQ: a neuropeptide that activates an opioidlike G protein-coupled receptor*, Science **1995**, *270*, 792-794.

Rosow, C.E.: *Butorphanol in perspective*, Acute Care **1988**, *12*, Suppl. 1, 2-7.

Rosow, C.E.: *Sufentanil citrate: a new opioid analgesic for use in anesthesia*, Pharmacotherapy **1984**, *4*, 11-19.

Sallay, I. S. (Warner-Lambert): *Derivatives of iboga alkaloids*, US 3 557 126, **1969**.

Samuelsson, G.: *Drugs of natural origin - a textbook of pharmacognosy*, **1999**, Swedish Pharmaceutical Press, Stockholm (ISBN 918627 481 3).

Sarhill, N., Walsh, D., Nelson, K.A.: *Hydromorphone: pharmacology and clinical applications in cancer patients*, Support. Care Cancer **2001**, *9*, 84-96.

Satzinger, G. (Gödecke): *Verfahren zur Herstellung von basisch substituierten Cyclohexenen*, DE 1 518 959, **1965**.

Satzinger, G.: *Struktur und Eigenschaften der stereoisomeren 3-Dimethylamino-4-phenyl-4-äthoxycarbonyl-1-cyclohexene*, Justus Liebigs Ann. Chem. **1972**, *758*, 43-64.

Satzinger, G.: *Die absolute Konfiguration von (+)- und (-)-3r-Dimethylamino-4c-phenyl-4t-äthoxycarbonyl-1-cyclohexen*, Justus Liebigs Ann. Chem. **1972**, *758*, 65-71.

Satzinger, G., Herrmann, W., Zimmermann, F.: *Analytisches Profil des Tilidins*, Pharm. Ind. **1978**, *40*, 657-664.

Sawynok, J.: *The therapeutic use of heroin: a review of the pharmacological literature*, Can. J. Physiol. Pharmacol. **1986**, *64*, 1-6.

Scheideler, M.A.: *Evidence for the role of δ opioid agonists in pain signaling*, Curr. Opin. CPNS Invest. Drugs **2000**, *2*, 171-77.

Schmidt, W.K., Tam, S.W., Shotzberger, G.S., Smith, D.H. Jr., Clark, R., Vernier, V.G.: *Nalbuphine*, Drug Alcohol Depend. **1985**, *14*, 339-362.

Schnider, O. and Grüssner, A.: *Oxy-morphinane - Optisch aktive 3-Oxymorphinane*, Helv. Chim. Acta **1951**, *34*, 2211-2217.

Schnider, O. and Hellerbach, J.: *Optisch aktive 3-Oxymorphinane*, Helv. Chim. Acta **1950**, *33*, 1437-1448.

Scholz, J., Steinfath, M., Schulz, M.: *Clinical pharmacokinetics of alfentanil, fentanyl and sufentanil. An update*, Clin. Pharmacokinet. **1996**, *31*, 275-292.

Schultz, E.M., Robb, C.M., Sprague, J.M.: *The reaction of 1-dDimethylamino-2-chloropropane with diphenylacetonitrile. The structure of amidone*. J. Am. Chem. Soc. **1947**, *69*, 2454-2459.

Schulz, R., Blasig, J., Wuster, M., Herz, A.: *The opiate-like action of tilidine is mediated by metabolites*, Naunyn Schmiedebergs Arch. Pharmacol. **1978**, *304*, 89-93.

Schwarzinger, S., Hartmann, M., Kremminger, P., Müller, N.: *Hydrophobic forms of morphine-6-glucuronides*, Bioorg. Med. Chem. Lett. **2001**, *11*, 1455-1459.

Scopes, D.I.: *Recent developments in non-peptide kappa receptor agonists*, Drugs Fut.. **1993**, *18*, 933-947.

Scott, L.J. and Perry, C.M.: *Tramadol: a review of its use in perioperative pain*, Drugs **2000**, *60*, 139-176.

Servin, F.: *Remifentanil: when and how to use it*, Eur. J. Anaesthesiol. Suppl. **1997**, *15*, 41-4.

Shee, C.D. and Pounder, R.E.: *Loperamide, diphenoxylate, and codeine phosphate in chronic diarrhoea*, Br. Med. J. **1980**, *280*, 524.

Shook, J.E., Watkins, W.D., Camporesi, E.M.: *Differential roles of opioid receptors in respiration, respiratory disease, and opiate-induced respiratory depression*, Am. Rev. Respir. Dis. **1990**, *142*, 895-909.

Sim, S.K.: *Methadone*, Can. Med. Assoc. J. **1973**, *109*, 615-619.

Simantov, R. and Snyder, S.H.: *The opiate receptor*, Biochem. Soc. Trans. **1977**, *5*, 62-65.

Simonds, W.F.: *The molecular basis of opioid receptor function*, Endocr. Rev. **1988**, *9*, 200-212.

Sinatra, R.S. and Harrison, D.M.: *Oxymorphone in patient-controlled analgesia*, Clin. Pharm. **1989**, *8*, 541-544.

Sindrup, S.H. and Brosen, K.: *The pharmacogenetics of codeine hypoalgesia*, Pharmacogenetics 1995, 5, 335-346.

Smissman, E.E. and Hite, G.: *The quasi-Favorskii rearrangement. I. The preparation of demerol and b-pethidine*, J. Am. Chem. Soc. **1959**, *81*, 1201-1203.

Stein, A.: *Über Dihydrocodein und Dihydrocodeinon*, Pharmazie **1955**, *10*, 180-186.

Sohn, W. and Zenz, M.: *Morphinverschreibung in Europa*, Berlin **1998**; cited in R. Radziwill, PZ Prisma **2000**, *7*, 145-150.

Solmssen, U.V. and Wenis, E.: *Estrogenic phenylindane derivatives*, J. Am. Chem. Soc. **1948**, *70*, 4195-4194.

Stefano, G.B., Scharrer, B., Smith, E.M., Hughes, T.K. Jr., Magazine, H.I., Bilfinger, T.V., Hartman, A.R., Fricchione, G.L., Liu, Y., Makman, M.H.: *Opioid and opiate immunoregulatory processes*, Crit. Rev. Immunol. **1996**, *16*, 109-144.

Stein, C., Cabot, P.J., Schafer, M.: *Peripheral opioid analgesia: Mechanisms and clinical implications*. In: Opioids in pain control. Basic and clinical aspects, edited by C. Stein, **1999**, Cambridge University Press, Cambridge.

Stein, C.: *Opioids in pain control. Basic and clinical aspects*, **1999**, Cambridge University Press, Cambridge.

Stein, C.: *Peripheral analgesic actions of opioids*, J. Pain Symptom. Manage. 1991, 6, 119-124.

Stokbroekx, R.A., Vandenberk, J., Van Heertum, A.H.M.T., van Laar, G.M.L.W., Van der Aa, M.J.M.C., Van Bever, W.F.M., Janssen, P.A.J.: *Synthetic antidiarrheal agents. 2,2-Diphenyl-4-(4´-aryl-4´-hydroxypiperidino)butyramides*, J. Med. Chem. **1973**, *16*, 782-786.

Subramanian, G., Ferguson, D.M.: *Conformational landscape of selectivity m-opioid agonists in gas phase and in aqueous solution: The Fentanyl Series*, Drug Design and Discovery **2000**, *17*, 53-67.

Sullivan, H.R., Beck, J.R., Pohland, A.: *The absolute configuration of α-(+)-4-dimethylamino-1,2-diphenyl-3-methyl-2-propionoxybutane, d-propoxyphene*, J. Org. Chem. **1963**, *28*, 2381-2385.

Strain, E.C., Preston, K.L., Liebson, I.A., Bigelow, G.E.: *Opioid antagonist effects of dezocine in opioid-dependent humans*, Clin. Pharmacol. Ther. **1996**, *60*, 206-217.

Takemori, A.E., Kupferberg, H.J., Miller, J.W.: *Quantitative studies of the antagonism of morphine by nalorphine and naloxone*, J. Pharmacol. Exp. Ther. **1969**, *169*, 39-45.

Taylor, D.A. and Fleming, W.W.: *Unifying perspectives of the mechanisms underlying the development of tolerance and physical dependence to opioids*, J. Pharmacol. Exp. Ther. **2001**, *297*, 11-18.

Thomas, J.B., Herault, X.M., Rothman, R.B., Atkinson, R.N., Burgess, J.P., Mascarella, S.W., Dersch, C.M., Xu, H., Flippen-Anderson, J.L., George, C.F., Carroll, F.I.: *Factors influencing agonist potency and selectivity for the opioid delta receptor are revealed in structure-activity relationship studies of the 4-[(N-substituted-4-piperidinyl)arylamino]-N,N-diethylbenzamides*, J. Med. Chem. **2001**, *44*, 972-987.

Trauner, D., et al.: Synthesis **1998**, 653-664.

Trauner, D., Porth, S., Opatz, T., Bats, J.W., Giester, G., Mulzer, J.: *New ventures in the construction of complex heterocycles. Synthesis of morphine and hasubanan alkaloids*, Synthesis **1998**, 653-664.

Trojan, A. and Beil, H.W.: *Tilidine abuse and dependence*, Drug Alcohol Depend. **1978**, *3*, 383-391.

Umans, J.G. and Inturrisi, C.E.: *Pharmacodynamics of subcutaneously administered diacetylmorphine, 6-acetylmorphine and morphine in mice*, J. Pharmacol. Exp. Ther. **1981**, *218*, 409-415.

Vachharajani, N.N., Shyu, W.C., Greene, D.S., Barbhaiya, R.H.: *The pharmacokinetics of butorphanol and its metabolites at steady state following nasal administration in humans*, Biopharm. Drug Dispos. **1997**, *18*, 191-202.

Vaught, J.L., Rothman, R.B., Westfall, T.C.: *Mu and delta receptors: their role in analgesia in the differential effects of opioid peptides on analgesia*, Life Sci. **1982**, *30*, 1443-1455.

Vermeire, A. and Remon, J.P.: *Stability and compatibility of morphine*, Int. J. Pharmaceutics **1999**, *187*, 17-51.

Vollmer, K.O., Thomann, P., Hengy, H.: *Pharmacokinetics of tilidine and metabolites in man*, Arzneimittelforschung **1989**, *39*, 1283-1288.

Vollmer, K.O.: *[Pharmacokinetic aspects of the Valoron-N principle. Balanced pharmacokinetics of nortilidine and naloxone]*, Fortschr. Med. 1988, 106, 593-596.

Walczak, S.A., Makman, M.H., Gardner, E.L.: *Acetylmethadol metabolites influence opiate receptors and adenylate cyclase in amygdala*, Eur. J. Pharmacol. 1981, 72, 343-349.

Wallach, J.D.: *Etorphine (M-99), a new analgesic-immobilizing agent, and its antagonists*, Vet. Med. Small Anim. Clin. **1969**, *64*, 53-58.

Watson, C.P.: *The treatment of neuropathic pain: antidepressants and opioids*, Clin. J. Pain **2000**, *16*, S49-S55.

Weijlard, J. and Erickson, A. E. (Merck & Co): *N-Allylnormorphine and processes for its production*, US 2 364 833, **1944**.

Weijlard, J. (Merck & Co): *Process for preparing N-allyl-normorphine*, US 2 891 954, **1959**.

Weiss, U.: *Derivatives of morphine, I. 14-hydroxydihydromorphinone*, J. Am. Chem. Soc. **1955**, *77*, 5891-5892.

WHO, *Cancer pain relief*, World Health Organisation, **1986**, Geneva.

Wheeler, G.D.: *ADL-2-1294 - adolor*, IDrugs **2000**, *3*, 1373-1378.

Wilson, J.M., Cohen, R.I., Kezer, E.A., Schange, S.J., Smith, E.R.: *Single- and multiple-dose pharmacokinetics of dezocine in patients with acute or chronic pain*, J. Clin. Pharmacol. **1995**, *35*, 398-403.

Wolven, A. and Archer, S.: *Toxicology of LAAM*, NIDA Res. Monogr. **1976**, *8*, 29-38.

Wood, P.L.: *Multiple opiate receptors: support for unique mu, delta and kappa sites.* Neuropharmacology 1982, 21,.487-497.

Worz, R. and Worz, E.: *[Long-term treatment of chronic pain with tilidine-naloxone. An analysis of 50 patients with chronic pain conditions of non-malignant origin]*. Fortschr. Med. **1995**, *113*, 388-392.

Yaksh, T.L.: *Pharmacology and mechanisms of opioid analgesic activity*, Acta Anaesthesiol. Scand. **1997**, *41*, 94-111.

Yoshida, K., Nambu, K., Arakawa, S., Miyazaki, H., Hashimoto, M.: *Metabolites of loperamide in rats*, Biomed. Mass. Spectrom. **1979**, *6*, 253-259.

Yue, Q.Y., Alm, C., Svensson, J.O., Sawe, J.: *Quantification of the O- and N-demethylated and the glucuronidated metabolites of codeine relative to the debrisoquine metabolic ratio in urine in ultrarapid, rapid, and poor debrisoquine hydroxylators*, Ther. Drug Monit. **1997**, *19*, 539-542.

Zaugg, H. E. (Abbott): *Resolution of DL-methadone*, US 2 983 757, **1961**.

Zenz, M., Piepenbrock, S., Tryba, M., Glocke, M., Everlien, M., Klauke, W.:*[Long-term therapy of cancer pain. A controlled study on buprenorphine]* Dtsch. Med. Wochenschr. **1985**, *110*, 448-53.

3.5 Drug Delivery Systems for Opioids   *Johannes Bartholomäus*

Introduction

Natural opioids have been used as medicines since ancient times (Seefelder, 1986), when Hippocrates and Galen, for example, obtained them from the juice of the poppy. Throughout the Middle Ages from Avicenna to Paracelsus, the number of extraction forms increased, culminating in Sydenham' entry of opium tincture in the pharmacopoeias. The isolation of the active principles, the synthesis of clearly defined new morphine derivatives, analog active principles, and progress in formulation technology paved the way for classical formulations such as injections, oral solutions, tablets, capsules and suppositories. With regard to 'non-therapeutic' use, in which it is not so much a question of an indication-adequate dosage, alternative administration by means of pulmonary or nasal inhalation (opium pipe or alkaline sniffing) came on the scene at an early stage

The development of modern formulations for opioids was and is still determined by the following trends:

- prolongation of action
- reduction of side-effects
- individual therapy
- patient convenience
- leading to an increase in patient compliance

The trends in parenteral, oral, rectal, transdermal, pulmonary and transmucosal administration will be described with the aid of products that are already on the market or are under development.

PCA

Medico-technical instruments such as infusion pumps can be used in PCA (*patient-controlled analgesia*, Fig. 1) to provide patient-orientated and therapy as required, e.g. with morphine injection solutions. Depending on the patients' perception of pain, they may add small doses of analgesics to the basic infusion by means of an electrically controlled infusion pump. The physician specifies the basic dose, which is infused independent of patient demands, the boluses that can be demanded, an hourly maximum dose and a refractory time that cannot be reduced between two doses. The infusion may be given intravenously, subcutaneously, epidurally or intraspinally.

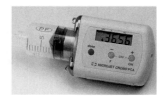

Figure 1: PCA system.

Such technologies focus on acute pain, for example after surgery (Lehmann, 2001).

Oral Prolonged-release Formulations

In (sub)chronic treatment long-acting medicines are mainly used. The breakthrough was the development of oral prolonged-release morphine formulations. The relatively short half-life of morphine (1.7 - 4.5 h) requires a high dosing frequency of 4 - 6 times a day of tablets, capsules or solutions. With the introduction of prolonged-release tablets the frequency of administration was first reduced to twice daily, which was particularly suitable for "'dosing by the clock' in chronic pain instead of symptomatic dosing on the recurrence of pain.

From a technical point of view the challenge of oral morphine prolonged-release was solved by the first preparation MST® Retard/ MS Contin comprising tablets with a matrix of hydrophobic (cetostearyl alcohol) and hydrophilic (hypromellose) elements that release the active substance over a period of 8 - 10 hours (Fig. 2). Various dosage strengths (10, 30, 60, 100 mg and more recently 200 mg) are available to allow for variations in pain intensity and dose adjustment due to the development of tolerance. The different colored tablets of 10 - 100 mg are about 7 mm in diameter and the 10 - 60 mg formulations have virtually the same *in vitro* profile rate (the percentage of the total dose against time, Fig. 2), and the release of the higher 100 mg dose is somewhat more prolonged in order to achieve optimal therapeutic results. This is the aim with the larger 200 mg tablet (approx. 8 mm in diameter), which is bioequivalent despite its somewhat slower *in vitro* release.

Another technical solution for twice-daily morphine treatment are capsules with prolonged-release pellets such as M-long® or Capros®. Release is prolonged by means of diffusion coatings, usually on an ethylcellulose base. The various doses of pellet preparations are obtained by adjusting the number of identical pellets per capsule, and therefore the release profiles of the various 'strengths' are identical. Due to the low dose per pellet and the high solubility of morphine, resulting in the total dissolution of the active substance within the pellets, a first-order release kinetic is achieved after a relatively short time. First-order kinetics and root-t kinetics are quite similar, and therefore M-long® and the above-mentioned matrix tablets are bioequivalent. Using the pellet formulation, in which the dose is distributed over small subunits, the substance can be administered via a stomach tube in patients who have to be fed artificially.

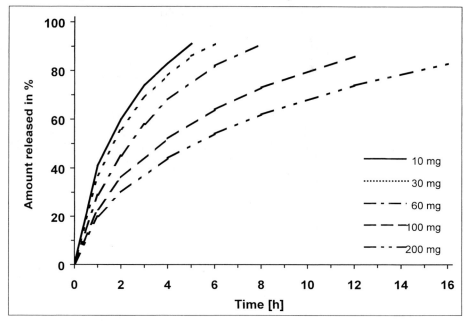

Figure 2: In-vitro release of MST 10 / 30 / 60 / 100 / 200 Mundipharma/MS Contin prolonged-release tablets.

The success of prolonged-release morphine prompted the development of prolonged-release formulations for other opioids, for example the matrix made of hydrophobic and hydrophilic matrix formers, for example on hydrocodeine (DHC retard with cetostearyl alcohol and hydroxyethyl-cellulose), oxycodone (oxygesic with stearyl alcohol and polyacrylate) and tramadol (tramundin with cetostearyl alcohol and ethylcellulose). By virtue of the oblong shape of hydrocodeine and tramadol tablets the prolonged-release tablets can be divided, whereby compared with whole tablets release from the divided tablets is slightly accelerated. The difference with these forms is that with increasing dose the release slows down.

A purely hydrophilic matrix of hypromellose prolongs the release of tramadol from Tramal® long (Fig. 3) developed by Gruenenthal. The tablets have the same dimensions, resulting in an identical release profile for all dosages (100, 150, 200 mg, see Fig. 4). For a titrated effect linear pharmacokinetics on increasing doses produce dose-proportional blood levels at any time. External influences, such as pH value, mechanical stress, surface-active substances and food, have no effect on release (Anonymus, 1995).

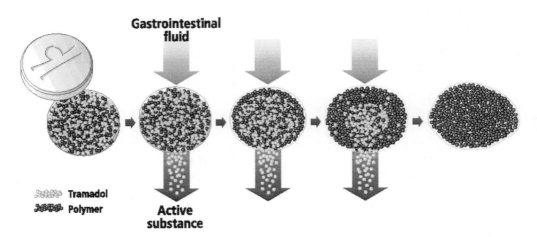

Figure 3: Release from hydrophilic matrices with Tramal®/Contramal®/Adolonta® long of Gruenenthal as an example.

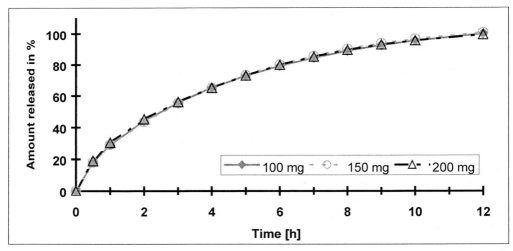

Figure 4: Dose-independent in-vitro release of tramadol hydrochloride from Tramal®/ Contramal®/Adolonta® long 100, 150 and 200 mg (medium up to 0.5 h artificial gastric juice pH 1.2; up to 2 h pH 2.3; up to 3 h pH 6.8; up to 12 h pH 7.4).

Tramadol (Tramadolor® long) is also available as sustained-release pellets with an identical release profile.

Long-acting Oral Formulations

In a number of indications once-daily dosages have proved to be beneficial, and therefore attempts have been made to develop once-daily formulations of opioids. In the case of morphine, a step in this direction was achieved with MST® continus long, which has been approved for once or twice-daily use, by incorporating the active substance in a purely fatty matrix to produce granules with a particle size of about 1 mm, which are then filled into single-dose sachets. Other morphine solutions have been incorporated in prolonged-release pellets with a release rate of about 24 h (e.g. Morphelan developed by Elan).

In Great Britain tramadol is available as once-daily tablets made up of granules in a purely fatty matrix (Zydol® XL), as described above for morphine, which again reduces the release rate compared with the granules.

In other indications such as hypertension, the OROS technology (oral osmotic system developed by ALZA) has already proven its value, and therefore it seemed appropriate to use this technology with its typical, virtually constant, release rate (zero-order kinetics) for once-daily opioid tablets. Such a morphine tablet is already available, but is not yet on the market, and a hydromorphone OROS is currently being clinically developed by Knoll.

Long-acting Enteral Forms

All enteral formulations have one thing in common (at least to date), namely, in view of the gastrointestinal passage times, the dosing frequency must be at least once daily. The only exceptions would be active substances with very long half-lives and having a duration of action of several days. However, these do not include analgesics. Alternative formulations such as Moranex®, which has recently been approved in Great Britain (Fig. 5) and consists of morphine delivered by a rectal xerogel system (Hycore™ Technology developed by CeNeS), still have to gain therapeutic acceptance. The hydrogel formed in the rectum releases the active substance by virtue of the special formulation of the cross-linked gel body via zero-order kinetics, thus producing almost constant blood levels (Fig. 6). However, a new system has to be administered once daily on account of defaecation.

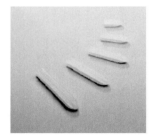

Figure 5: Moraxen™ rectal delivery systems with 35, 50, 75, 100 and 125 mg based on the Hycore™–R technology.

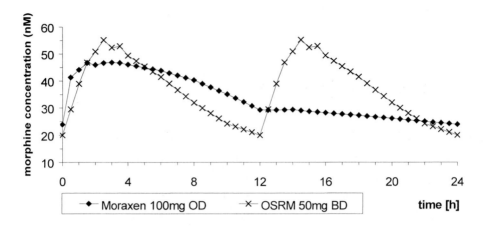

Figure 6: Moraxen™ rectal delivery system. Comparative steady-state simulation of morphine plasma levels after single daily rectal administration of Moraxen™ with 100 mg morphine compared with twice-daily 50 mg morphine (OSRM) in an oral prolonged-release formulation. The simulation is based on the plasma levels from a single-dose study.

Transdermal Patches

A quantum leap in pain therapy with distinct advantages in the form of reduced side-effects and application frequency was achieved with transdermal opioid administration. Transdermal application requires a number of characteristics on the part of the active substance (Fig. 7), the most restrictive being the daily dose, and only very potent opioids which are effective in very low doses, such as fentanyl and buprenorphine, are an option (Sittl and Likar, 2001).

A technical breakthrough was reached by the Drug Delivery System (DDS) developer ALZA with a TTS (Transdermal Therapeutic System) of fentanyl on the basis of a reservoir patch about 0.5 mm thick (Fig. 8). In order to release therapeutically effective amounts of fentanyl from the TTS through the poly(ethylene, vinylacetate) membrane controlling the release of the active substance release and skin penetration, ethanol was used as the solvent and enhancer. The solution in the TTS reservoir is gelated with hydroxyethylcellulose. The 3-day TTS with doses of 25, 50, 75 and 100 μg/h have been clinically developed, approved and marketed by Janssen as Durogesic®. The various dosages that correlate linearly with the corresponding fentanyl blood levels are obtained by proportionally increasing the contents of the reservoir (active substances and excipients) and the contact area

(25 µg/h with 2.5 mg fentanyl citrate and 10 cm² area up to 100 µg/h with 10 mg fentanyl citrate and 40 cm² area).

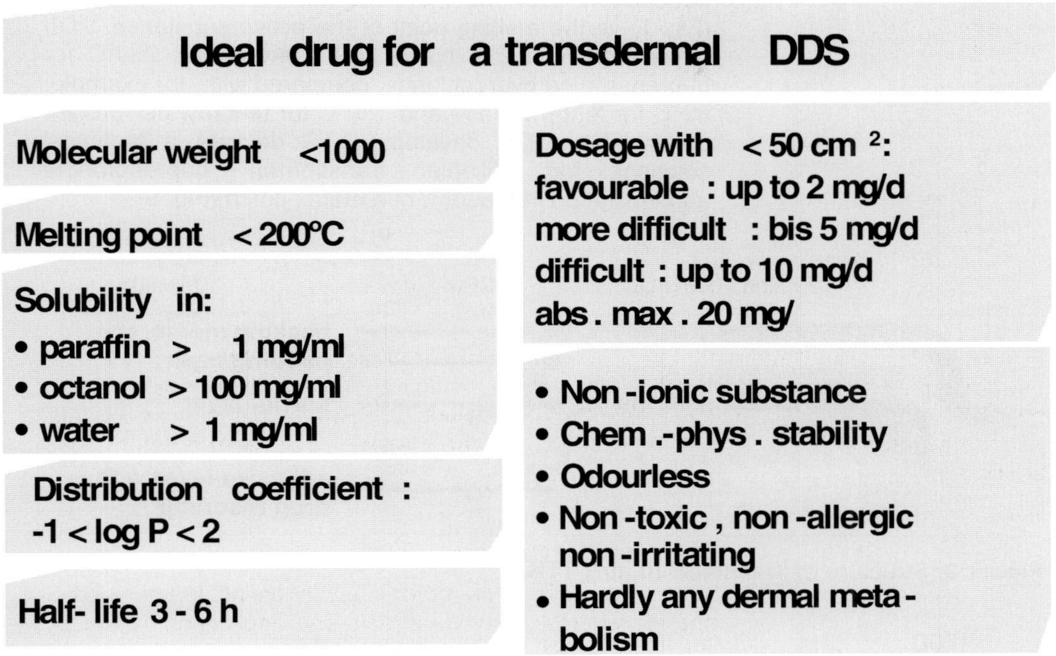

Ideal drug for a transdermal DDS
Molecular weight <1000
Melting point < 200°C
Solubility in:
• paraffin > 1 mg/ml
• octanol > 100 mg/ml
• water > 1 mg/ml
Distribution coefficient :
-1 < log P < 2
Half- life 3 - 6 h
Dosage with < 50 cm ²:
favourable : up to 2 mg/d
more difficult : bis 5 mg/d
difficult : up to 10 mg/d
abs . max . 20 mg/
• Non -ionic substance
• Chem .-phys . stability
• Odourless
• Non -toxic , non -allergic non -irritating
• Hardly any dermal meta - bolism

Figure 7: Requirements for an ideal substance for transdermal administration.

backing membrane
liquid drug reservoir
release controlling membrane
adhesive layer

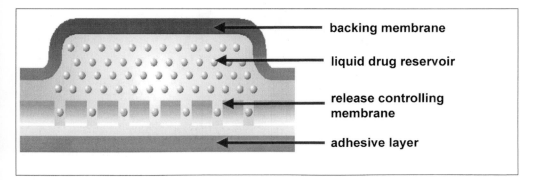

Figure 8: Structure of a reservoir TTS (Durogesic®).

Buprenorphine, the other option for transdermal application on account of its potency, is more difficult to apply dermally in therapeutic doses (Roy et al., 1994; Grond et al., 2000). A surrogate parameter for skin penetration, provided the other prerequisites are fulfilled (Fig. 7), is the melting point of the active substance. With buprenorphine base this is 209°C and about 260°C for buprenorphine hydrochloride, compared with, for example, 83°C for fentanyl base and 150°C for fentanyl dihydrogen citrate. The DDS developer LTS devised a technical solution for reliable transdermal buprenorphine administration in the form of a matrix patch (Fig. 9).

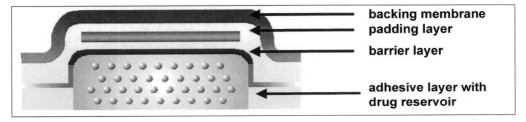

Figure 9: Structure of Transtec® (matrix TTS).

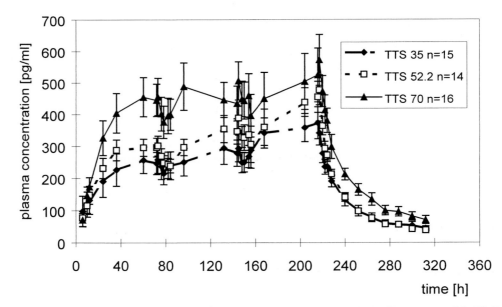

Figure 10: Plasma levels after multiple application of Gruenenthal's Transtec® 35, 52.5 and 70 µg/h for 9 days (three consecutive applications of 3 days each)

In contrast to reservoir patches, there is no risk of dose-dumping a with matrix patch, which releases buprenorphine from a prolonged-release matrix in direct contact with the skin for at least 3 days. The improved solubility necessary to achieve an adequate concentration of dissolved buprenorphine base is obtained by means of well tolerated organic acids that do not form practically insoluble salts with buprenorphine in the undercooled mass in the matrix of the TTS. In Europe transdermal buprenorphine was developed by Grünenthal as Transtec®, which was launched in Germany in 2001 and recently approved in major Europoean markets with dosages of 35, 52.5 and 70 µg/h containing 20, 30 and 40 mg buprenorphine per TDS respectively (Fig. 10; Terlinden et al., 2000).

A typical pharmacokinetic feature of transdermal therapy is a lag-time before measurable concentrations of the active substance circulate in the blood with the first TDS (Grond et al. 2000) from a depot of the active substance in the upper layers of the skin. Therefore when assessing efficacy at least 48 h should elapse before deciding whether the selected patch strength is sufficient or whether a switch should be made to a higher dosage. This depot is also the reason why after removal of the TDS the concentration of the active concentration in the blood only decreases gradually. Mechanical stimulation on removal of the patch also increases perfusion of the skin, producing a small plasma level peak. Steady-state plasma levels are usually reached after a few days and are determined more by the flip-flop kinetics of the delayed absorption of the active substance from the TDS through the skin and the completion of the distribution phase of the relatively lipophilic substances in the various compartments, than by the elimination half-life of the active substance.

In line with the trend towards prolonged application intervals, 3M and Purdue have started developing a fentanyl patch that is effective for 7 days. It will be interesting to see how well long-term application and occlusion at a particular site will be tolerated in comparison with the relatively good dermal tolerance of three days' treatment.

Alternative Transdermal Drug Delivery Systems

An alternative approach to transdermal drug application that differs from patches and classic gels led to the foundation of Acrux, an Australian drug delivery company. The key finding was that certain widely used sunscreens, including C_8- to C_{18}-alkyl substituted-cinnamate,

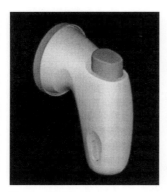

Figure 11: The Acrux MDTS® (Metered Dose Transdermal System) Applicator.

-methoxycinnamate, or -salicylate, caused a significant enhancement of drug absorption through the human skin.

These so-called Across® enhancers are dissolved together with the drug in a volatile solvent for administration. The solution is dosed by means of a volumetric valve combined with a spray nozzle resembling a metered dose inhaler system. Due to its use for transdermal application, the device is called the Metered Dose Transdermal System (MDTS, Fig. 11). The patient positions the unit against the skin and pushes the actuator button to spray a small accurate volume of liquid onto a defined area of skin. The liquid rapidly evaporates leaving an invisible, water resistant depot from which drug is slowly absorbed into the body. This process essentially forms an 'invisible patch' within the upper layer of the skin. One expected advantage of such delivery systems is improved skin tolerability when compared to classical patches. The dosing frequency of these systems would usually be once daily. In addition to formulations containing sex hormones, preliminary results in pigs with fentanyl are available (Klose et al., 2002), exhibiting practically the same absorption rate through human skin as the Duragesic patches (Fig. 12).

Transdermal systems with electrophoretic release of the active substance are under development, e.g. ETRANS® by ALZA with fentanyl for postoperative pain in clinical phase III. By virtue of the electrical field administration of the active substance is faster and on demand, e.g. similar to PCA therapy.

Extremely Long-acting Parenteral Systems

With patches a dosing interval of 1 week may become a possibility in the treatment of pain. Even longer dosing intervals may be achieved by employing implant techniques and formulations that have already become available in the field of hormon treatment including LHRH antagonist formulations. For safety reasons and to remain within the therapeutic window opioids need to be dosed without the 'initial burst' that very often occurs with parenteral microsphere depot formulations based on biodegradable polymers. Very reliable and exact dosing over a long time period has now become available in the form of the DUROS DDS originally developed by ALZA e.g. the once per year Viadur system with leuprolide. This has now been applied to the field of pain control with sufentanyl 3 months depot by DURECT under the brand Chronogesic™, now reaching phase III of clinical development.

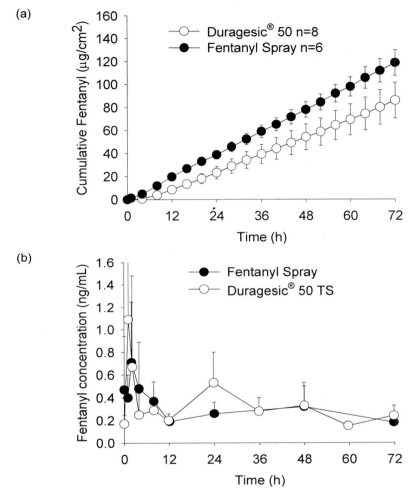

Figure 12: *In vitro* permeation through human skin and *in vivo* animal data after dermal application of fentanyl MDTS. (a) Absorption of fentanyl across human epidermis. Comparison of a fentanyl MDTS® and Duragesic® 50 TS. (b) Mean plasma concentration of fentanyl after a fentanyl MDTS® and Duragesic® 50 TS in male pigs (n = 7).

The DUROS consists of a cylindrical titanium chamber (Fig. 13). The original version was approximately 4 mm in diameter and 4 cm in length; other sizes can be produced (Fisher, 2002). One end of the cylinder is capped with a semipermeable membrane; the other is capped with an orifice designed to permit unidirectional release of the drug. Inside the cylinder, at the membrane end, is a salt tablet, adjacent to which is a piston. The remainder of the cylinder is the reservoir in which the drug is stored.

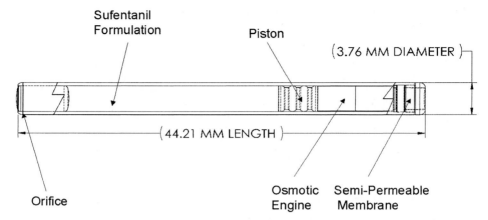

Figure 13: The Durect Chronogesic™ implantable osmotic pump.

During storage in a dry environment, there is no osmotic activity. When the implant is placed in the subcutaneous space or some other body space, there is sufficient relative humidity or water around the implant system to create an osmotic gradient across the membrane. Water is absorbed across the membrane at a zero-order rate that can be controlled to be as low as 0.4 µl (or lower) per day (thereby permitting delivery for 12 months). Water crossing the membrane expands the salt tablet, pushing the piston, and forcing the drug through the orifice into the subcutaneous space from which it is then absorbed.

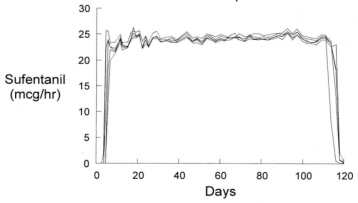

Figure 14: In-vitro release of Sufentanyl from Chronogesic™ DUROS.

Sufentanyl was the selected opioid because it is a very powerful analgesic and could be formulated in a tailor-made high-concentration solution enabling the release of effective doses of drug throughout a 3 months period despite the small capacity of approximately 155 µl filling volume of the Chronogesic™ system. The zero-order *in vitro* release of sufentanyl from the system is shown in Fig. 14.

The Duros implant requires implantation. To date, clinical trials have examined only one implant site, the mesial surface of the upper arm, ~ 10 cm above the antecubital crease. The procedure is performed on an outpatient basis using local anesthesia and requires less than 10 min tocarry out. The polished titanium surface minimizes any adhesions, permitting rapid explant and reimplant (at the same site) once the device is nearly expended.

Fast-acting Transmucosal Formulations

During treatment with long-acting opioid formulations, breakthrough pain (pain peaks) may occur for which basic therapy does not suffice and which requires rapid treatment. In addition to classical formulations such as drops (e.g. Tramal® or morphine solutions), sublingual buprenorphine formulations (Temgesic® sublingual tablets) and FlashTab® dosage forms that rapidly disintegrate in the saliva and are then swallowed, Actiq®, a new transmucosal form in the shape of a fentanyl lozenge on a stick, (Fig. 15), is already on the market in the USA and Europe. The active substance is incorporated into a matrix of sucrose and glucose syrup on a stick in doses of 200, 400, 600, 800, 1200 and 1600 µg. When pain peaks occur the lozenge is moved around in the mouth, especially along the cheeks, twirled often, and actively sucked in about 15 min. About 25% of the active substance is absorbed through the mucous membranes of the mouth, and one-third of the remaining 75% swallowed is said to be absorbed enterally, giving a total bioavailability of about 50% of the fentanyl dose. Plasma level curves are shown in Fig. 16. Any unused remains of the formulation are destroyed as soon as possible by dissolving under running hot water in a wash-basin. Naturally the system must be child-proof. In the USA a 'welcome kit' is also available, with a child-resistant lock, a portable locking pouch, and a child-proof temporary storage bottle for used lozenges.

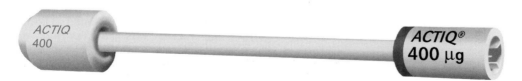

Figure 15: Transmucosal fentanyl drug delivery system Actiq™.

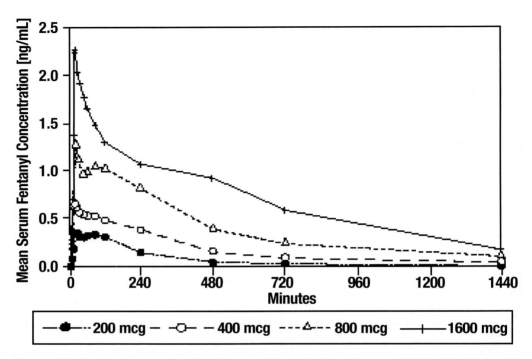

Figure 16: Fentanyl serum levels after sucking Actiq™ at doses of 200, 400, 800 and 1600 µg.

Rapidly Acting Aerosols

In addition to injections, pulmonary administration also allows rapid absorption of analgesics into the blood stream. The AerX® pain management system, which is currently being developed jointly by Aradigm and Glaxo Smith Kline for morphine and fentanyl, produces an aerosol from an active substance solution (Fig. 17).

The active substance is mechanically ejected from a blister through laser-drilled nozzles with a diameter of a few µm and integrated into the blisters by means of punch, to produce a mist consisting of drops measuring 1 - 6 µm. The blister is inserted into an electronically controlled dosing unit that measures the airstream and induces aerosolization in synchrony with inspiration. The bioavailability of morphine sulphate (total dose 8.8 mg) blistered in portions of 1.2 mg was 75% of that on intravenous administration (dose 4 mg), which is much higher than conventional aerosol formulations (Gonda et al., 1999; Otulana et al., 1999).

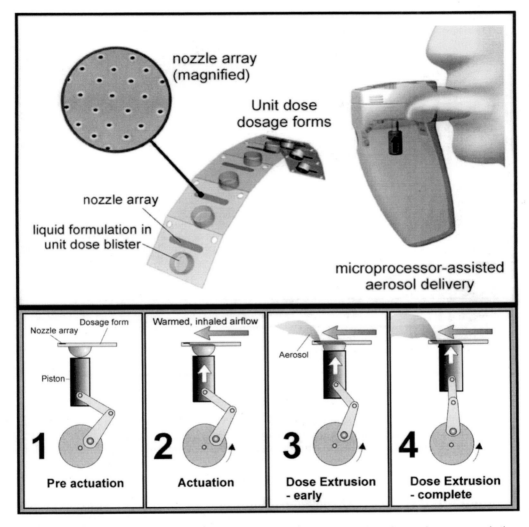

Figure 17: AerX pain management system: the single-dosed active substance solution in the blister is aerosolized by means of a punch through the laser bored nozzles. The blister is inserted into a dosing unit controlled by a microprocessor. Aerosolization is induced by the punch (actuation), when the dosing unit measures a sufficient inspiratory stream and the mist is synchronized with inspiration.

Plasma levels on pulmonary administration corresponded to those resulting from i.v. administration, T_{max} being reached in 2 min (Fig. 18). The electronic control of the AerX system offers interesting opportunities, for example with regard to narcotic safety, such as user identification or lock-out times after a certain number of applications within a certain period to prevent overdosing.

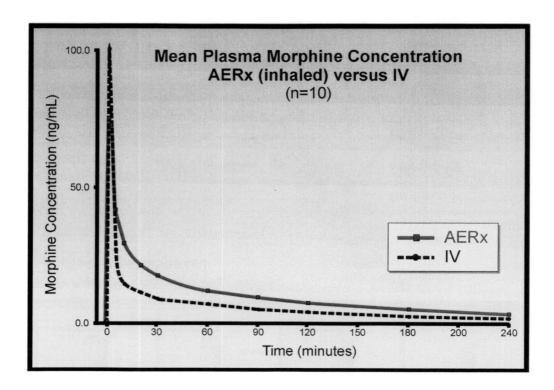

Figure 18: Plasma profiles of inhaled ('AERx') versus intravenous ('IV') morphine. Subjects received four inhalations of morphine sulfate (8.8 mg loaded doses) via the AERx system and 4.0 mg morphine sulfate intravenously on separate days. Both dosages were delivered over a 4 min period.

Conclusions

The development of modern formulations for opioids in the last few years has contributed significantly to pain therapy. New developments will probably optimize pain treatment and thus improve the quality of life of sufferers.

References

Anonymous: *Moderne Galenik erleichtert die Schmerztherapie*, Z. Allg. Med. **1995**, *71* Themenausgabe 3, 1-8.

Fisher, D., DURECT Corporation, Cupertino, CA, USA: *Personal Communication*, **2002**.

Gonda, I., Fiore, M., Johansson, E. T., Liu, R. J., Morishije, R. J., Okikawa, J. K., Otulana, B. A., Rubsamen, R. M.: *Bolus delivery of morphine solutions with the AerX pain management system* (PMS). ISAM Meeting, **1999**, Vienna Austria.*

Grond, S., Radbruch, L., Lehmann, K.A.: *Clinical pharmacokinetics of transdermal opioids*, Clin. Pharmacokinet. **2000**, *38*, 59-89.

Klose, K.T., Humberstone, A.J., Finnin, B.C.: *Comparative transdermal absorption of fentanyl after application of a spray and Duragesic® patch*. PPP Transdermal Conference, April **2002.**

Lehmann, K.A.: *Postoperative Schmerztherapie*, In Lehrbuch der Schmerztherapie, **2001**, edited by Zenz, M. and Jurna, I. WVG Stuttgart.

Otulana, B. A., Morishije, R. J., Beckmann, R. A., Johansson, E. T., Okikawa, J. K., Fiore, M. D., Rubsamen, R. M.: *Oral inhalation system for delivery of morphine produces an iv-like PK profile*. IASP 9th World Congress on Pain, (**1999**).*

Roy, S. D., Hou, S. Y., Witham, S. L., Flynn, G. L.: *Transdermal delivery of narcotic analgesics: comparative metabolism and permeability of human cadaver skin and hairless mouse skin*, J. Pharm. Sci. **1994**, *83*, 1723-1728.

Seefelder, M.: *Opium – Eine Kulturgeschichte*, 3. Auflage, **1996**. Nikol Verlagsgesellschaft, Hamburg.

Sittl, R. and Likar, R.: *Praxis der transdermalen Schmerztherapie*, **2001**. Uni-Med Verlag, Bremen - London - Boston.

Terlinden, R. et al.: *Buprenorphin in einem transdermalen therapeutischen System – Pharmakokinetische Studie bei Mehrfachapplikation*, Der Schmerz **2000**, *14*, Suppl. 1, 80.

*Posters are available on the internet page: www.aradigm.com as a PDF file.

4 NA and 5-HT Reuptake Inhibitors and α_2 agonists

Thomas M. Tzschentke

The discovery that drugs elevating extracellular levels of noradrenaline and/or serotonin have analgesic potential was circumstantial. In 1960, Paoli et al. reported that during an attempt to treat reactive depression in chronic pain patients with the tricyclic antidepressant imipramine they observed an improvement of the patients´ neuralgic pain. Subsequently, it became well established that antidepressant drugs can improve both depression and chronic pain states.

Over the years, antidepressant drugs have become an important treatment option in chronic pain states, in their own right and as adjuncts to opiate treatment. In fact, tricyclic antidepressants are the mainstay of treatment of neuropathic pain conditions such as polyneuropathy, diabetic neuropathy, postherpetic neuralgia and peripheral nerve injury (Sindrup, 1997; Sindrup and Jensen, 1999). Other chronic pain states responsive to antidepressants include osteo- and rheumatoid arthritis, fibromyalgia, and chronic tension headache.

Use of antidepressants against chronic pain

In preclinical tests, antidepressants can also be effective in acute pain models, but in humans the acute analgesic effects are rather small and of no therapeutic relevance. When used as adjunctive treatment, usually doses lower than those required for the treatment of depression are sufficient for improvement of pain, reducing the side-effects arising from this adjunctive treatment. However, antidepressant treatment has clear beneficial effects only in a proportion of patients (McQuay and Moore, 1997) and may not be equally effective in all chronic pain states (Onghena and van Houdenhove, 1992).

One important question to bear in mind when considering the analgesic effectiveness of antidepressant drugs in chronic pain is to what extent this effectiveness is related to a genuine analgesic effect, and to what extent the psychotropic effects of the drugs might contribute to their analgesic effects. It is well known that depressed mood can exacerbate the perception of pain and that chronic pain is often accompanied by depressed mood (´reactive´ depression), thus it appears feasible that drug-induced mood improvement could contribute to a reduction in perceived pain or to an increase in pain tolerance. In the past, a number of possible mechanisms have been proposed to be responsible (at least in part) for the analgesia observed with antidepressants: alleviation of a masked depression, alleviation of a manifest depression, a

It is interesting to note that despite the very widespread use and the generally accepted efficacy of antidepressants in pain therapy, at present not all antidepressant drugs are formally approved for the treatment of pain. Thus, the widespread use of these drugs is, to some extent, off-label, and there does not seem to be much effort in the pharmaceutical industry to market antidepressants explicitley as analgesic drugs.

general sedative effect, or a placebo-like effect (see Onghena and van Houdenhove, 1992). There are several reasons, however, to suggest that antidepressant-induced analgesia is largely independent of their mood-altering effects. Doses of antidepressants needed to produce pain relief are often considerably lower than those that produce antidepressant effects. The onset of analgesia clearly precedes the onset of antidepressant effects; in chronic pain, maximal analgesia is usually achieved within a few days, and in experimental acute pain, antidepressants show an acute analgesic effect, while the antidepressant effects do not become apparent until 2-3 weeks of chronic treatment. Antidepressants that clearly lack sedative effects (e.g. desipramine) show analgesic efficacy, while clearly sedative, benzodiazepines have very little, if any, effect, arguing against the hypothesis that sedative effects contribute to the apparent analgesia (see Onghena and van Houdenhove (1992) for references). This issue is still under discussion, but it seems safe to assume that the main effect is indeed due to a mechanistical pain reduction, although the possibility that in some chronic pain states or in some patients an antidepressant action contributes to the improvement of general well-being and possibly greater pain tolerance cannot be discounted.

Antidepressant-induced analgesia seems to be largely independent of their mood-altering effects

Pharmacological Effects of Antidepressants

The analgesic action of antidepressant drugs is thought to arise mainly from their ability to block the reuptake of the monoamines noradrenaline and/or serotonin, thus increasing the extracellular levels of these transmitters (see Table 1), although other possible mechanisms of action, such as direct interaction with opiate receptors (Sierralta et al., 1995) or histamine receptors (Rumore and Schlichting, 1986), stimulation of adenosine release or blockade of adenosine uptake (Phillips and Wu, 1982; Sawynok et al., 1999), blockade of sodium channels (Song et al., 2000; Sawynok et al., 2001), blockade of calcium channels (Peroutko et al., 1984), blockade of NMDA receptors (Eisenach and Gebhart, 1995), or blockade of substance P (NK1) receptors (Iwashita and Shimizu, 1992) have also been discussed, in particular with regard to tricyclic antidepressants. The latter effect may be important for the antinociceptive effects of antidepressants in pain states involving central sensitization (Eisenach and Gebhart, 1995). The focus of this chapter, however, will be on the monoamine reuptake inhibition produced by these drugs.

Note that there may be a discrepancy between the amount of published data on a particular drug and the actual frequency of clinical use of this drug, since clinical trials are not always well documented in the literature, especially when the trial was unsuccessful

Table 1: Clinical properties of serotonin and noradrenaline reuptake inhibitors (only those drugs are included for which a resonable number of reports on controlled clinical trials are available). For more detailed information see Onghena and van Houdenhove (1992), Philipp and Fickinger (1993), McQuay et al. (1996), and Ansari (2000).

a) TCAs

drug	name/MF/MW/RN	treated symptoms and dosages (examples)	references (examples)
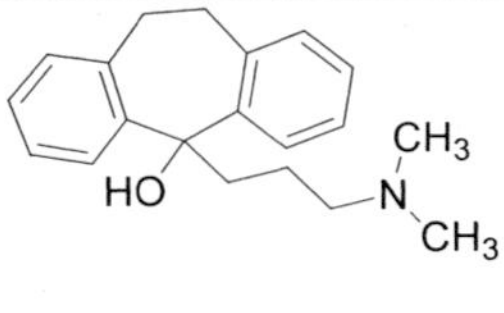 amitriptyline	5-(3-Dimethylamino-propyl)-10,11-dihydro-5H dibenzo[a,d]cyclohepten-5-ol, $C_{20}H_{23}N$, MW 277.41, [50-48-6]	fibromyalgia (20-40 mg/day for 4-32 weeks); diabetic neuropathy (12.5-150 mg/day for 15 weeks)	Goldenberg et al., 1996 Max et al., 1992
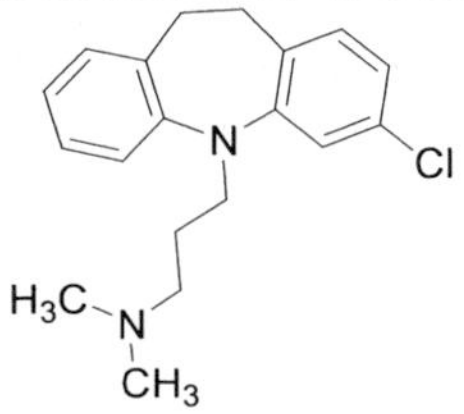 clomipramine	[3-(3-Chloro-10,11-dihydro-dibenzo[b,f]azepin-5-yl)-propyl]-dimethyl-amine, $C_{19}H_{23}ClN_2$, MW 314.86. [303-49-1]	diabetic neuropathy (75-125 mg/day for several weeks)	Sindrup et al., 1990a
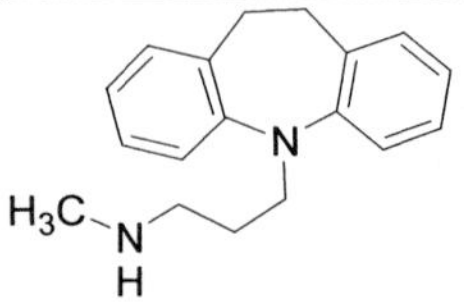 desipramine	[3-(10,11-Dihydro-dibenzo[b,f]azepin-5-yl)-propyl]-methyl-amine, $C_{18}H_{22}N_2$, MW 266.39, [50-47-5]	diabetic neuropathy (12.5-150 mg/day for 15 weeks)	Max et al., 1992 Sindrup et al., 1990a
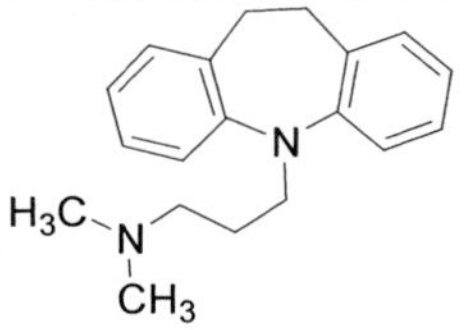 imipramine	[3-(10,11-Dihydro-dibenzo[b,f]azepin-5-yl)-propyl]-dimethyl-amine, $C_{19}H_{24}N_2$, MW 280.42, [50-49-7]	diabetic neuropathy (25-350 mg/day for 7 weeks)	Sindrup et al., 1990b

Prominent side-effects common to the whole drug class (magnitude may vary between drugs): weight gain, drowsiness, dry mouth, constipation, orthostatic hypotension, blurred vision, urinary retention, sedation, dizziness, confusion (especially in the elderly)

Table 1: continued. b) SSRIs, SNRIs

drug	name/MF/MW/RN	treated symptoms and dosages (examples)	references (examples)
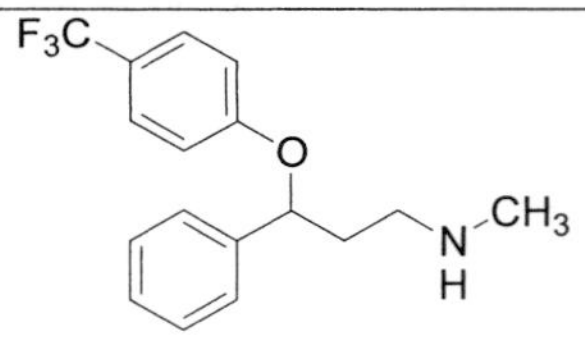 fluoxetine	Methyl-[3-phenyl-3-(4-trifluoromethyl-phenoxy)-propyl]-amine, $C_{17}H_{18}F_3NO$, MW 309.33, [54910-89-3]	headache, migraine (10-80 mg/day for 6-16 weeks); fibromyalgia (20-40 mg/day for 4-32 weeks); *not effective* against diabetic neuropathy (20-40 mg/day for 17 weeks)	Adly et al., 1992 Goldenberg et al., 1996 Max et al., 1992
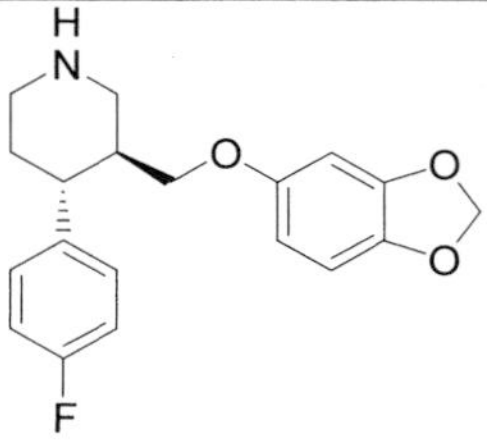 paroxetine	3-(Benzo[1,3]dioxol-5-yloxymethyl)-4-(4-fluoro-phenyl)-piperidine, $C_{19}H_{20}FNO_3$, MW 329.37, [61869-08-7]	headache, migraine (10-50 mg/day for 3-9 months); diabetic neuropathy (40 mg/day for 7 weeks)	Black and Sheline, 1995 Sindrup et al., 1990b
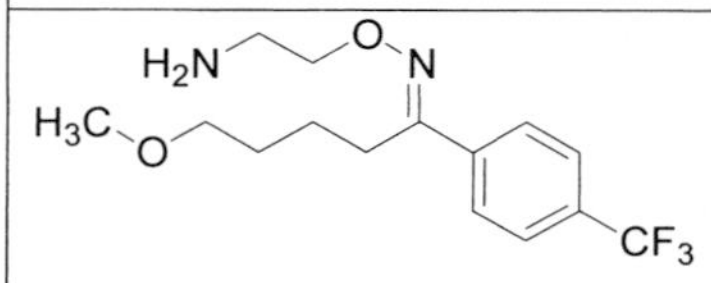 fluvoxamine	5-Methoxy-1-(4-trifluoromethyl-phenyl)-pentan-1-one O-(2-amino-ethyl)-oxime, $C_{15}H_{21}F_3N_2O_2$, MW 318.34, [54739-18-3]	headache, migraine (50-100 mg/day for 8-12 weeks)	Manna et al., 1994
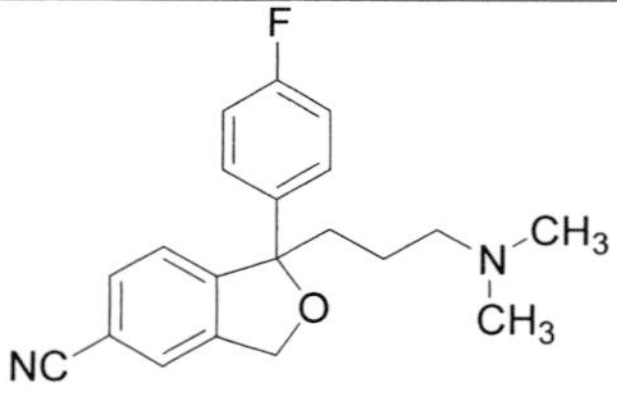 citalopram	1-(3-Dimethylamino-propyl)-1-(4-fluoro-phenyl)-1,3-dihydro-isobenzofuran-5-carbonitrile, $C_{20}H_{21}FN_2O$, MW 324.40, [59729-33-8]	diabetic neuropathy (40 mg/day for 8 weeks); *not effective* against headache and fibromyalgia (20-40 mg/day for 8 -32 weeks)	Sindrup et al., 1992 Norregard et al., 1995
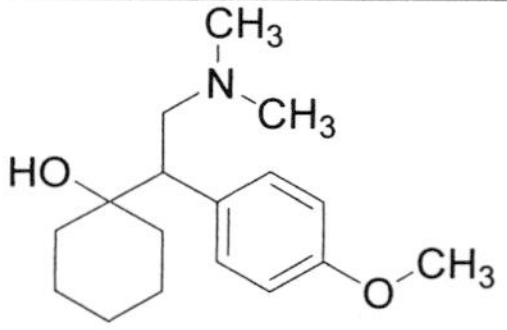 venlafaxine	1-[2-Dimethylamino-1-(4-methoxy-phenyl)-ethyl]-cyclohexanol, $C_{17}H_{27}NO_2$, MW 277.41, [93413-69-5]	various forms of chronic pain (headache, migraine, neuropathies) (37.5-300 mg/day for 4-12 weeks)	Taylor and Rowbotham, 1996

Prominent side-effects common to the whole drug class (magnitude may vary between drugs) agitation: akathisia, insomnia, sexual dysfunction, nausea, gastrointestinal distress/diarrhea, headache, withdrawal effects.

Tricyclic antidepressants (TCAs)

Drugs from this class have multiple pharmacological effects. The most prominent and most important action (for both, antidepressant and analgesic effects) is serotonin and noradrenaline reuptake inhibition. In addition, these drugs act as M1-muscarinic antagonists, α1-adrenergic antagonists, and H1-histaminic antagonists. These actions do not contribute to the therapeutic effectiveness of tricyclic antidepressants but are rather responsible for a number of side-effects. All TCAs block serotonin as well as noradrenaline reuptake, albeit with different potencies. Whereas desipramine and nortriptyline show relative selectivity for noradrenaline, clomipramine shows relative selectivity for serotonin, and imipramine and amitriptyline show about equal affinities for both transporters.

By far the most data on the use of TCAs in the treatment of pain is available on amitriptyline. Because much less data are available on the other drugs, it is difficult to say whether the dominance of this drug in clinical studies reflects a superiority of amitriptyline over other drugs. Results from meta-analyses, however, would suggest that other drugs such as imipramine, doxepine or clomipramine may be equally effective but used less often.

The high efficacy of amitriptyline in chronic pain may be in part related to an antagonistic action at NMDA receptors (Eisenach and Gebhart, 1995) (see Table 2).

In preclinical studies, a number of TCAs (imipramine, amitriptyline, nortriptyline, desipramine) were shown to inhibit pain behavior in the formalin test after systemic as well as after i.t. administration, and this effect did not seem to be related to an antiinflammatory effect of these drugs (Sawynok and Reid, 2001). The effects of TCAs in preclinical acute pain models (involving acute thermal or mechanical stimuli) have been reviewed by Eschalier et al. (1999). TCAs were also active in models of chronic inflammation (Butler et al., 1985) and in models of neuropathic pain involving nerve injury (e.g. Ardid and Guilbaud, 1992; Abdi et al., 1998).

There have been numerous clinical studies examining the analgesic effects of TCAs in chronic pain, and the review of these is beyond the scope of this chapter. There are a number of reviews covering these studies (e.g. Onghena and van Houdenhove, 1992; McQuay et al., 1996; Feuerstein, 1997). In contrast, the effects of TCAs in acute pain have not received much attention in clinical research. There are only a few controlled studies with mixed results, reporting no effect of desipramine or amytriptiline on postoperative dental pain when given alone but enhanced

Nortriptyline

Doxepine

morphine analgesia when combined with desipramine (Levine et al., 1986). In another study, amitriptyline was more effective against acute low back pain than paracetamol (Stein et al., 1996).

Table 2. Pharmacological properties of serotonin and noradrenaline reuptake inhibitors (K_i values [nM]).

	drug	5-HT transporter	NA transporter	5-HT1A receptor	5-HT2A receptor	H1 receptor	M1 receptor	α1 receptor
TCAs	amitriptyline	70	45	>1000	12	2	32	88
	clomipramine	4	48	>1000	64	41	67	88
	desipramine	400	4	>1000	300	200	220	500
	doxepine	230	35	>1000	54	1	110	33
	imipramine	71	31	>1000	130	19	150	190
SSRIs, SNRIs	fluoxetine	11	340	>1000	770	>1000	>1000	>1000
	paroxetine	1	220	>1000	>1000	>1000	280	>1000
	fluvoxamine	7	620	>1000	>1000	>1000	>1000	>1000
	citalopram	2	>1000	>1000	>1000	>1000		
	venlafaxine	77	538					

SSRIs, NSRIs

After a almost 30-year dominance of TCAs in the treatment of depression, selective serotonin reuptake inhibitors (SSRIs) were introduced in the 1980s. Since then, these drugs have also been used in the treatment of chronic pain (Ansari, 2000). SSRIs appear to be less effective in most patients than TCAs. Meta-analyses have shown that, in general, TCAs seem to be more effective than heterocyclic antidepressants or newer generation serotonin- or noradrenaline-selective drugs (Onghena and van Houdenhove, 1992; McQuay et al., 1996; Aigner and Bach, 2000, and references therein) (see Table 2). The same pattern of efficacy also seems to apply to acute pain animal models (Ardid et al., 1992). This pattern may be related to the fact that both serotonin and noradrenaline are involved in pain modulation (see below) and that only a delicately balanced elevation of both transmitters yields the most effective analgesia. On the other hand, SSRIs have an undisputedly better side-effect profile than TCAs. At present, SSRIs are generally viewed as second-choice drugs for patients who do not tolerate TCAs well.

More recently, the selective serotonin and noradrenaline reuptake blocker venlafaxine has been introduced. This drug has a dual action on monoamine reuptake like classical TCAs, yet lacks the side effect-critical affinities for histaminergic, adrenergic and muscarinergic receptors. Venlafaxine has also been used in the treatment of chronic pain, with some success (see Ansari, 2000). It is currently being developed for neuropathic pain. Duloxetine is in clinical development as an antidepressant drug. It has the same mechanisms of action as venlafaxine, but with 10-15-fold higher affinitiy for the NA- and 5-HT transporters. Whether this drug is more effective against chronic pain than venlafaxine remains to be seen.

Duloxetine

Others

Due to their diverse pharmacological actions, and for want of a better categorization, the drugs mentioned below are often referred to as ´atypical antidepressants´, although eventually all of them also act via enhancement of noradrenergic and/or serotonergic neurotransmission.

Mirtazapine, an analog of mianserine (see below), is a drug that combines α2-antagonistic properties (predominantly at inhibitory autoreceptors, thus increasing activity of noradrenergic and serotonergic neurons) with 5-HT2, 5-HT3 and histamine H1 antagonistic properties. 5-HT2 and 5-HT3 antagonism is thought to reduce sexual dysfunction and gastrointestinal problems, respectively, side-effects often observed with SSRIs. We are unaware of any published studies on the use of mitazepine in the treatment of pain.

Mianserine is an α2-antagonist with additional α1, 5-HT2, H1 antagonistic properties. It has been studied extensively for the treatment of chronic pain syndromes, with mixed results (see Ansari, 2000, for references).

Mirtazapine

2-Methyl-1,2,3,4,9,13b-hexahydro-2,4a,5-triaza-tribenzo[a,c,e]cycloheptene, $C_{17}H_{19}N_3$, MW 265.36, [61337-67-5]

Mianserine

2-Methyl-1,2,3,4,9,13b-
hexahydro-2,4a-diaza-
tribenzo[a,c,e]cycloheptene,
$C_{18}H_{20}N_2$, MW 264.37,
[24219-97-4]

Nefazodone

2-{3-[4-(3-Chloro-phenyl)-piperazin-
1-yl]-propyl}-5-ethyl-4-(2-phenoxy-
ethyl)-2,4-dihydro-[1,2,4]triazol-3-one,
$C_{25}H_{32}ClN_5O_2$, MW 506.48,
[82752-99-6]

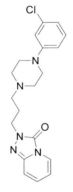

Trazodone

2-{3-[4-(3-Chloro-
phenyl)-piperazin-1-yl]-
propyl}-2H-[1,2,4]
triazolo[4,3-a]pyridin-
3-one, $C_{19}H_{22}ClN_5O$,
MW 371.87, [19794-93-5]

Nefazodone blocks the reuptake of serotonin and noradrenalin and is a 5-HT2 antagonist. This drug is also launched as an analgesic and is being developed for migraine. We are unaware of any published studies in the literature on the use of mitazepine in the treatment of pain.

Trazodone blocks serotonin reuptake and is a 5-HT2, α1, and H1 antagonist. Thus far, the findings on the analgesic efficacy of trazodone are few and inconsistent (Goodkin et al., 1990; Wilson, 1999; see Ansari (2000) for further references).

The Descending Inhibitory Pain System as a Major Target for Noradrenaline and Serotonin Reuptake Inhibitors

The first convincing evidence for a descending inhibitory system came from the discovery of stimulation-induced analgesia: electrical stimulation of the midbrain periaqueductal grey (PAG) produced a highly specific suppression of behavioral responses to noxious stimuli (Reynolds, 1969). Later on, it was discovered that the PAG is part of a CNS circuit that controls the transmission of nociceptive information at the level of the spinal cord. It is in a position to integrate descending information from limbic cortical and diencephalic areas and ascending information from the spinal dorsal horn (Bandler and Keay, 1996). The PAG receives inputs from a number of monoaminergic brainstem nuclei (Herbert and Saper, 1992); in turn, its major descending afferents project to the the rostral ventrolateral medulla (RVM), including the serotonergic nucleus raphe magnus, and to the dorsolateral pons (DLP), including the noradrenergic cells groups A5 (locus coeruleus) and A7 (Cameron et al.,

1995). The RVM and DLP are also reciprocally interconnected (Clark and Proudfit, 1991a), and electrical stimulation of the RVM, like stimulation of the PAG, produces analgesia and inhibits dorsal horn responses to noxious stimuli (Basbaum and Fields, 1984). The analgesic effects of PAG stimulation at the spinal level appear to be relayed in large part via the RVM, since inactivation or inhibition of the RVM largely reduces the spinal effects of PAG stimulation (Behbehani and Fields, 1979). The PAG also projects rostrally to the orbitofrontal cortex and the medial thalamus (Coffield et al., 1992). These projections may underlie a possible ascending control of nociception.

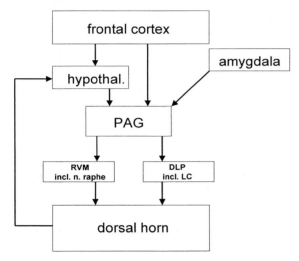

Figure 1: Descending pain modulary pathways: a simplyfied diagram.

Serotonergic and noradrenergic fibers travel from the brain stem through the dorsal lateral funiculus to the spinal cord and terminate in the dorsal horn where they modulate pain signals coming from the periphery (see Fig. 1). These projections have classically been described in terms of descending inhibitory pathways. More recently, evidence has been accumulating that these descending pathways may not only be of inhibitory nature but may modulate spinal pain transmission in a rather complex manner, including facilitatory mechanisms. However, a more detailed consideration of this issue is beyond the scope of this chapter (see Mason (1999) and references therein for details).

Serotonergic and non-serotonergic fibers originating in the RVM terminate predominantly in dorsal horn laminae I, II (substantia gelatinosa), and V, which are the main targets of nociceptive primary afferents (Basbaum et al., 1978). Laminae I and II both contain excitatory and inhibitory interneurons, and both types of interneurons receive input from RVM projections.

The A5 and A7 cell groups are the main source of noradrenergic fibers projecting to the dorsal dorn (Clark and Proudfit, 1991b), and as in the case of PAG and RVM, electrical stimulation of these cell groups inhibits spinal withdrawal reflexes in response to noxious stimulation and the activity of dorsal horn nociceptive neurons (Carstens et al., 1980). In general, the inhibition of nociceptive transmission produced by noradrenaline at the spinal level is mediated via the α2-adrenoceptor (West et al., 1993; Willis and Westlund, 1997). This is consistent with the fact that spinally administered α2-agonists can produce potent analgesia (Curatolo et al., 1997; see below).

Serotonin and noradrenaline probably act both presynaptically on the terminals of nociceptive afferent fibers to reduce the release of excitatory transmitters such as glutamate, CGRP, or substance P (Fürst, 1999) and to increase the release of inhibitory transmitters such as enkephalins and GABA (Feuerstein, 1997; van Schayck et al., 1998), and postsynaptically to activate inhibitory (enkephalinergic or GABAergic) interneurons within the dorsal horn (Alhaider et al., 1991), or to directly inhibit ascending spinothalamic tract neurons (Giesler et al., 1981) (see Fig. 2).

Serotonin and noradrenaline probably act both presynaptically on the terminals of nociceptive afferents and postsynaptically

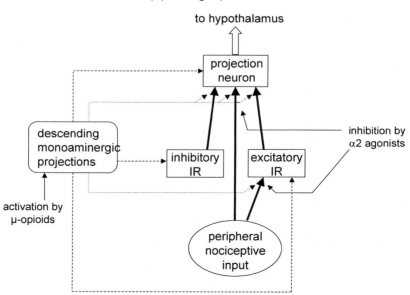

Figure 2: Neuronal circuitry in the dorsal horn of the spinal cord -simplified diagram.

From this anatomical organization it becomes clear that elevation of serotonin and noradrenaline can dampen transmission of nociceptive information at the spinal level via multiple mechanisms.

Possible Supraspinal Sites of Action and Interaction with Endogenous and Exogenous Opioids

Opioid-induced antinociception depends, to some degree, on monoaminergic signaling in the spinal dorsal horn. While opioids can act directly on dorsal horn terminals of primary afferent nociceptive fibers or on excitatory interneurons in lamina II of the dorsal horn to reduce the release of excitatory transmitters (Glaum et al., 1994), the supraspinally mediated analgesic effects of opioids, at least in part, involve interactions with central and spinal serotonergic and noradrenergic transmission.

By acting on monoaminergic brainstem nuclei, either directly or via action in the PAG (Bowker and Dilts, 1988; Budai et al., 1998; see Mason, 1999), opioids may activate descending monoaminergic inhibitory pathways that contribute to the analgesia produced by the activation of non-monoaminergic inhibitory mechanisms (Fitzgerald, 1986; Proudfit, 1988; Borszcz et al., 1996; but see Matos et al., 1992; Gao et al., 1997, 1998) (see Fig. 2). Although the extent of monoamine involvement in opioid action appears to depend on the type of painful stimulus and the test used to assess antinociception, the analgesic effects of intracerebral morphine are attenuated by blockade of serotonergic and α2-adrenergic receptors at the spinal level (Yaksh, 1979; Proudfit, 1988).

Serotonin is also involved in opioid effects on the transmission and processing of nociceptive information at a level rostral to the PAG. Borszcz (1999) and Borszcz and Streltsov (2000) have demonstrated that the antinociceptive effect of morphine administered into the PAG can be attenuated be serotonin antagonism in the central nucleus of the amygdala and the parafascicular nucleus of the thalamus, suggesting that serotonin is also involved in pain processing in higher brain centers.

This discussion shows that the well-documented enhancement of opioid effects by antidepressants ('opioid-sparing effect') is likely to be related to a synergistic effect on monoaminergic transmission, possibly both at the spinal and at the supraspinal level. This synergistic interaction is based on the blockade by antidepressants of the reuptake of serotonin and/or noradrenaline released by the action of an opioid.

Analgesia Produced by α2-Agonists

In contrast to antidepressant drugs, directly-acting α2-agonists such as clonidine or demedetomidine are effective not only in chronic pain states, but also in acute pain. Unfortunately, these agents produce side effects such as cardiovascular depression and sedation when administered systemically; thus, they are most commonly administered by the epidural or intrathecal route, because side-effects are less pronounced following application via these routes. α2-agonists, like antidepressants, besides having analgesic effects, also have opiate-sparing (Motsch et al., 1990), anesthetic-sparing (Bonnet et al., 1990) and anxiolytic effects, making them useful adjuvants in clinical practice.

α2-Agonists Used Clinically

Clonidine has been launched for the treatment of cancer pain (Boehringer Ingelheim). It is effective against malignant and non-malignant pain after spinal administration (Glynn et al., 1988; Eisenach et al., 1995).

Clonidine can also be effective and tolerable when administered by the oral or transdermal route (Zeigler et al., 1992).

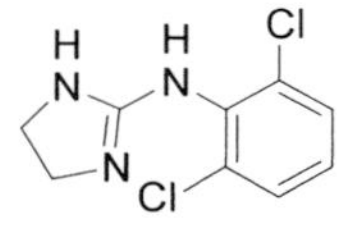

Synthesis (Zeile et al. (Boehringer Ingelheim), 1965; Kleemann et al. 1999):

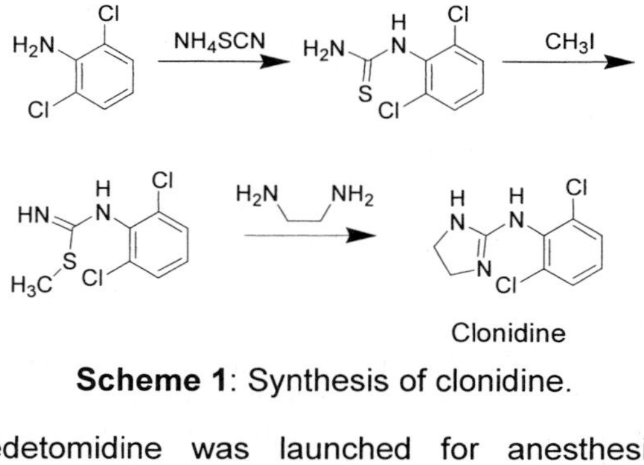

Clonidine

(2,6-Dichloro-phenyl)-(4,5-dihydro-1H-imidazol-2-yl)-amine, $C_9H_9Cl_2N_3$, MW 230.10, [4205-90-7]

Scheme 1: Synthesis of clonidine.

Dexmedetomidine

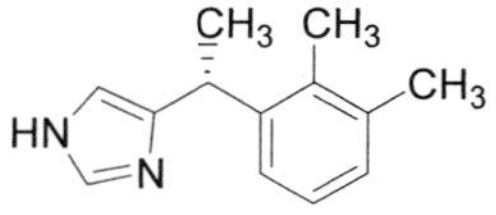

4-[1-(2,3-Dimethyl-phenyl)-ethyl]-1H-imidazole, $C_{13}H_{16}N_2$, MW 200.28, [113775-47-6]

Dexmedetomidine was launched for anesthesia and postoperative pain in the US in 2000 and in Australia in 2001. According to Pharmaprojects, dexmedetomidine alone is effective as an analgesic in 41-44% of patients. Treated patients who require additional analgesics achieve pain relief with half the dose required by those treated with placebo. Dexmedetomidine is generally well tolerated, possible side-effects in the high dose range are nausea, hypotension, decreased heart rate, atrial fibrillation and hypoxia,. The anxiolytic, sedative, analgesic, hemodynamic, stabilizing and anesthetic potentiating effects have been demonstrated in several clinical trials (Orion Pharma; Abbott).

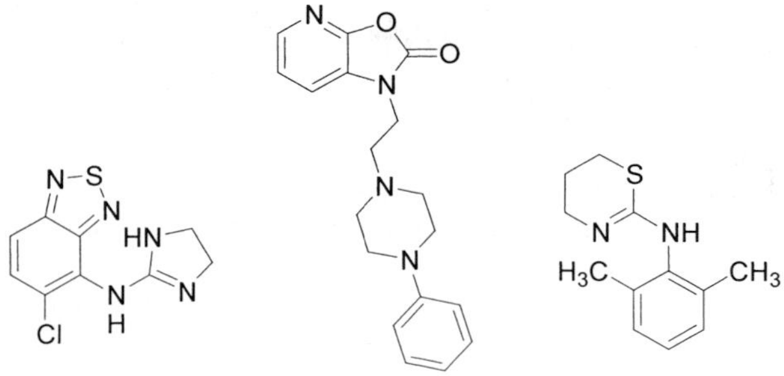

Tizanidine
launched as a muscle relaxant   S-12813-4   Xylazine

Scheme 2: α2-agonists with preclinical effectiveness.

Anatomy and Neuropharmacology of α2-Agonist-Mediated Analgesia

In the spinal cord, α2-agonists act on receptors located on the terminals of primary afferent fibers in the dorsal horn substantia gelatinosa to reduce nociceptive transmission by inhibiting the release of glutamate and substance P (Collin et al., 1994; Hamalainen and Pertovaara, 1995) (see Fig. 2). These receptors appear to be primarily of the α2A subtype which is negatively coupled to adenylate cyclase (Lakhlani et al., 1997; see Millan, 1999; but see Sawamura et al., 2000, and references therein for a discussion of the possible involvement of other α2-receptor subtypes in antinociception). Like activation of µ-opioid receptors, the activation of α2-receptors increases the potassium conductance of the cells bearing these receptors, thus reducing cellular excitability.

In mice with mutations in the α2A-receptor gene it was established that the α2A subtype mediates the analgesic and anesthesia-sparing effects of clonidine and dexmedetomidine, but unfortunately also the sedative and vasodepressor effects of these drugs (Lakhlani et al., 1997). Thus, it seems unlikely that new subtype-selective compounds will lack the major side-effects of the existing drugs.

Chronic constriction injury (CCI) models (Bennett and Xie, 1988; Kim and Chung, 1992; Mosconi and Kruger, 1996) have been used to examine chronic pain states in experimental animals. In these models, intrathecally administered α2-agonists reduced mechanical allodynia and thermal hyperalgesia that developed following nerve constriction (Levy et al., 1994; Yaksh et al., 1995). This action may be partly due to the fact that α2-agonists inhibit the abnormally prolonged response to mechanical stimulation of some mechanoreceptors that develops after nerve ligation (Na et al., 1993). Interestingly, i.t. clonidine can also restore the reduced antinociceptive potency of i.t. morphine in the tail-flick test in nerve-ligated animals (Ossipov et al., 1995), and morphine-tolerant animals remain normally responsive to i.t. serotonin or noradrenaline (Reddy et al., 1980). This is consistent with the observation that in nerve-ligated rats, repeated treatment with desipramine does not result in tolerance to its antihyperalgesic effects (T. Christoph, Grünenthal GmbH, unpublished results). Dexmedetomidine showed antinociceptive actions against carrageenan-induced inflammatory pain and nerve injury pain in the rat (Idanpaan et al., 1994; Poree et al., 1998). It appears to be much more potent than clonidine and does not show an analgesic ceiling effect as is sometimes seen with clonidine (Sullivan et al., 1992).

The 'atypical' opioid drug tramadol has a dual mechanism of action. An important part of its analgesic effects is mediated by the agonistic activity of (+)-tramadol and its O-desmethyl-metabolite at μ-receptors. However, another part of its effects is mediated by noradrenaline and serotonin reuptake inhibition. Noradrenaline reuptake is inhibited primarily by the (-)-enantiomer of tramadol, while the reuptake of serotonin is primarily inhibited by the (+)-enantiomer (Frink et al., 1996), and it has been shown in preclinical models that reuptake inhibition by tramadol contributes to its overall analgesic effects, and that these different mechanisms can yield supra-additive analgesic effects (Kayser et al., 1992; Raffa et al., 1992; Miranda et al., 1999). This augmentation of the opioid effect by monoaminergic mechanisms may be the reason why tramadol can produce very satisfactory analgesia despite its relatively low μ-receptor affinity.

Tramadol

(see chapter 3.4)

Recent Developments

Antidepressants as analgesics are almost a 'closed book' as far as preclinical and clinical development is concerned. TCAs are an old drug class, and because of the rather problematic side-effect profile, interest in developing new drugs from this class is small. BL-1834 (Bioglan Lab.) is an intranasal formulation of doxepine that is in clinical development (phase II) for the treatment of severe pain. In patents on novel monoamine reuptake inhibitors, pain is usually claimed as a possible indication, but depression and anxiety are mentioned as the primary indications in most cases, and we are not aware of novel monoamine reuptake inhibitors that are exclusively developed for pain.

Among the established non-TCA drugs, nefazodone is currently being developed for migraine, and venlafaxine and dexmedetomidine are being developed for neuropathic pain.

Milnacipran (Pierre Fabre), an equipotent serotonin and noradrenaline reuptake inhibitor, was launched in 1997 as an antidepressant and was licensed for development for the treatment of fibromyalgia and related chronic pain disorders in 2001. It is currently in late preclinical development.

The noradrenaline and dopamine reuptake inhibitor bupropion (GlaxoSmithKline) is currently in clinical development (phase II) for neuropathic pain.

Other novel antidepressants in development act on various targets other than noradrenaline or serotonin transporters; thus, the role of these drugs as analgesics is speculative, and its consideration is beyond the scope of this chapter.

VAN-H36 (Vita-Invest) is a serotonin and noradrenaline reuptake inhibitor and μ-receptor agonist (i.e. has a pharmacological profile of action similar to tramadol). It is in early clinical development as an analgesic.

RWJ-37210 (Johnson & Johnson) is the lead structure of a series of α2-receptor agonists in preclinical development for the treatment of pain.

Milnacipran

Bupropion

Outlook

One point for future consideration is that the effects of antidepressants (and drugs like tramadol) may be limited by the activation of somatodendritic 5-HT1A autoreceptors in the raphe nucleus, resulting from the increased extracellular levels of serotonin produced by these drugs. This suggestion is supported by the findings that 5-HT1A-receptor blockade by pindolol accelerates the antidepressant effects of SSRIs (Artigas et al., 1996) and enhances the analgesic potency of tramadol, while the 5-HT1A-receptor agonist 8-OH-DPAT reduces the effects of tramadol (Rojas-Corrales et al., 2000). To our knowledge, it has not been determined whether 5-HT1A-receptor blockade would also enhance the antinociceptive effects of antidepressants, although this strategy would seem promising given the findings outlined above.

Thus, although major breakthroughs in the development of serotonin and noradrenaline reuptake inhibitors as analgesics are unlikely, a refinement of treatment and co-treatment methods may still hold substantial potential in yielding improved therapeutic effectiveness of this drug class.

References

Abdi, S., Lee, D. H., Chung, J. M.: *The anti-allodynic effects of amitryptiline, gabapentin, and lidocaine in a rat model of neuropathic pain*, Anesth. Analg. **1998**, *87*, 1360-1366.

Adly, C., Straumanis, J., Chesson, A.: *Fluoxetine prophylaxis of migraine*, Headache **1992**, *32*, 101-104.

Aigner, M. and Bach, M.: *The antinociceptive effect of antidepressants - noradrenergic versus serotonergic modes of action? / Reply* by Atkinson, J. H., Slater, M. A., Pain **2000**, *88*, 217-218.

Alhaider, A. A., Lei, S. Z., Wilcox, G. L.: *Spinal 5-HT3 receptor-mediated antinociception: possible release of GABA*, J. Neurosci. **1991**, *11*, 1881-1888.

Ansari, A.: *The efficacy of newer antidepressants in the treatment of chronic pain: a review of current literature*, Harv. Rev. Psychiatry **2000**, *7*, 257-277.

Ardid, D. and Guilbaud, G.: *Antinociceptive effects of acute and ´chronic´ injections of tricyclic antidepressant drugs in a new model of mononeuropathy in rats*, Pain **1992**, *49*, 279-287.

Ardid, D., Marty, H., Fialip, J., Privat, A. M., Eschalier, A., Lavarenne, J.: *Comparative effects of different uptake inhibitor antidepressants in two pain tests in mice*, Fundam. Clin. Pharmacol. **1992**, *6*, 75-82.

Artigas, F., Romero, L., de Montigny, C., Blier, P.: *Accelerated effect of selected antidepressant drugs in combination with 5-HT1A antagonists*, Trends Neurosci. **1996**, *19*, 378-383.

Bandler, R. and Keay, K. A.: *Columnar organization in the midbrain periaqueductal gray and the integration of emotional expression*, Prog. Brain Res. **1996**, *107*, 285-300.

Basbaum, A. I. and Fields, H. L.: *Endogenous pain control systems: brainstem spinal pathways and endorphin circuitry*, Annu. Rev. Neurosci. **1984**, *7*, 309-338.

Basbaum, A. I., Clanton, C. H., Fields, H. L.: *Three bulbospinal pathways from the rostral medulla of the cat: an autoradiographic study of pain modulating systems*, J. Comp. Neurol. **1978**, *178*, 209-224.

Behbehani, M. M. and Fields, H. L.: *Evidence that an excitatory connection between the periaqueductal grey and nucleus raphe magnus mediated stimulation produced analgesia*, Brain Res. **1979**, *170*, 85-93.

Bennett, G. J. and Xie, Y. K.: *A peripheral mononeuropathy in rat that produces disorders of pain sensations like those seen in man*, Pain **1988**, *33*, 87-107.

Black, K.J. and Sheline, Y.I.: *Paroxetine as migraine prophylaxis*, J. Clin. Psychiatry **1995**, *56*, 330-331.

Bonnet, F., Buisson, V. B., Francois, Y., Catoire, P., Saada, M.: *Effects of oral and subarachnoid clonidine on spinal anesthesia with bupivacaine*, Reg. Anesth. **1990**, *15*, 211-214.

Borszcz, G. S.: *Differential contributions of medullary, thalamic, and amygdaloid serotonin to the antinociceptive action of morphine administered into the periaqueductal gray: a model of morphine analgesia*, Behav. Neurosci. **1999**, *133*, 612-631.

Borszcz, G. S. and Streltsov, N. G.: *Amygdaloid-thalamic interactions mediate the antinociceptive action of morphine microinjected into the periaqueductal gray*, Behav. Neurosci. **2000**, *114*, 574-584.

Borszcz, G. S., Johnson, C. P., Thorp, M. V.: *The differential contribution of spinopetal projections to increases in vocalization and motor reflex thresholds generated by the microinjection of morphine into the periaqueductal gray*, Behav. Neurosci. **1996**, *110*, 368-388.

Bowker, R. M. and Dilts, R. P.: *Distribution of mu-opioid receptors in the nucleus raphe magnus and nucleus gigantocellularis: a quantitative autoradiographic study*, Neurosci. Lett. **1988**, *88*, 247-252.

Budai, D., Harasawa, I., Fields, H. L.: *Midbrain periaqueductal gray (PAG) inhibits nociceptive inputs to sacral dorsal horn nociceptive neurons through $\alpha2$-adrenergic receptors,* J.Neurophysiol. **1998**, *80*, 2244-2254.

Butler, S. H., Weil-Fugazza, J., Godefroy, F., Besson, J. M.: *Reduction of arthritis and pain behaviour following chronic administration of amitryptiline or imipramine in rats with adjuvant-induced arthritis,* Pain **1985**, *23*, 159-175.

Cameron, A. A., Kahn, I. A., Westlund, K. N., Willis, W. D.: *The efferent projections of the periaqueductal gray in the rat: a Phaseolus vulgaris-leucoagglutinin study. II. Descending projections,* J. Comp. Neurol. **1995**, *351*, 585-601.

Carstens, E., Klumpp, D., Zimmermann, M.: *Differential inhibitory effects of medial and lateral midbrain stimulation on spinal neuronal discharges to noxious skin heating in the cat,* J. Neurophysiol. **1980**, *43*, 332-342.

Clark, F. M. and Proudfit, H. K.: *Projections of neurons in the ventromedial medulla to pontine catecholamine cell groups involved in the modulation of nociception,* Brain Res. **1991a**, *540*, 105-115.

Clark, F. M. and Proudfit, H. K.: *The projection of noradrenergic neurons in the A7 catecholamine cell group to the spinal cord in the rat demonstrated by anterograde tracing combined with immunocytochemistry,* Brain Res. **1991b**, *547*, 279-288.

Coffield, J. A., Bowen, K. K., Miletic, V.: *Retrograde tracing of projections between the nucleus submedius, the ventrolateral orbital cortex, and the midbrain in the rat,* J. Comp. Neurol. **1992**, *321*, 488-499.

Collin, E., Frechilla, D., Pohl, M., Bourgoin, S., Mauborgne, A., Cesselin, F.: *Differential effects of the novel analgesic S12813-4, on the spinal release of substance P and calcitonin gene-related peptide-like materials in the rat,* Naunyn-Schmiedeberg´s Arch. Pharmacol. **1994**, *349*, 387-393.

Curatolo, M., Petersen-Felix, S., Arendt-Nielsen, L., Zbinden, A. M.: *Epidural epinephrine and clonidine: segmental analgesia and effects on different pain modalities,* Anesthesiology **1997**, *87*, 785-794.

Eisenach, J. C. and Gebhart, G. F.: *Intrathecal amitriptyline acts as an N-methyl-D-aspartate receptor antagonist in the presence of inflammatory hyperalgesia in rats,* Anesthesiology **1995**, *83*, 1046-1054.

Eisenach, J. C., DuPen, S., Dubois, M., Miguel, R., Allin, D.: *Epidural clonidine analgesia for intractable cancer pain. The Epidural Clonidine Study Group,* Pain **1995**, *61*, 391-399.

Eschalier, A., Ardid, D., Dubray, C.: *Tricyclic and other antidepressants as analgesics.* In: Sawynok, J., Cowan, A. (eds.) Novel aspects of pain management: opioids and beyond. New York, Wiley-Liss **1999**, 303-319.

Feuerstein, T. J.: *Antidepressiva zur Therapie chronischer Schmerzen,* Der Schmerz **1997**, *11*, 213-226.

Fitzgerald, M.: *Monoamines and descending control of nociception,* Trends Neurosci. **1986**, *9*, 51-52.

Frink, M. C., Hennies, H.-H., Englberger, W., Haurand, M., Wilffert, B.: *Influence of tramadol on neurotransmitter systems of the rat brain,* Arzn.-Forsch./Drug Res. **1996**, *46*, 1029-1036.

Fürst, S.: *Transmitters invloved in antinociception in the spinal cord,* Brain Res. Bull. **1999**, *48*, 129-141.

Gao, K., Kim, Y. H., Mason, P.: *Serotonergic pontomedullary neurons are not activated by antinociceptive stimulation in the periaqueductal gray,* J. Neurosci. **1997**, *17*, 3285-3292.

Gao, K., Chen, D. O., Genzen, J. R., Mason, P.: *Activation of serotonergic neurons in the raphe magnus is not necessary for morphine analgesia,* J. Neurosci. **1998**, *18*, 1860-1868.

Giesler, G. J., Gerhart, K. D., Yezierski, R. P., Wilcox, T. K., Willis, W. D.: *Postsynaptic inhibition of primate spinothalamic neurons by stimulation in nucleus raphe magnus,* Brain Res. **1981**, *204*, 184-188.

Glaum, S. R., Miller, R. J., Hammond, D. L.: *Inhibitory actions of $\delta1$, $\delta2$, and µ-opioid receptor agonists on excitatory transmission in lamina II neurons of adult rat spinal cord,* J. Neurosci. **1994**, *14*, 4965-4971.

Glynn, C., Dawson, D., Sanders, R.: *A double blind comparison between epidural morphine and epidural clonidine in patients with chronic non cancer pain,* Pain **1988**, *34*, 123-128.

Goldenberg, D., Mayskiy, M., Mossey, C., Ruthazer, R., Schmid, C.: *A randomized, double-blind crossover trial of fluoxetine and amitriptyline in the treatment of fibromyalgia*, Arthritis Rheum. **1996**, *39*, 1852-1859.

Goodkin, K., Gullion, C. M., Agras, W. S.: *A randomized, double-blind, placebo-controlled trial of trazodone hydrochloride in chronic low back pain syndrome*, J. Clin. Psychopharmacol. **1990**, *10*, 269-278.

Hamalainen, M. M. and Pertovaara, A.: *The antinociceptive action of an alpha2 adrenoceptor agonist in the spinal horn is due to a direct spinal action and not to activation of descending inhibition*, Brain Res. Bull. **1995**, *37*, 581-587.

Herbert, H. and Saper, C. B.: *Organization of medullary adrenergic and noradrenergic projections to the periaqueductal gray matter in the rat*, J. Comp. Neurol. **1992**, *315*, 34-52.

Idanpaan, J. J., Kalso, E. A., Seppala, T.: *Antinociceptive actions of dexmedetomidine and the κ-opioid agonist U-50488H against noxious thermal, mechanical and inflammatory stimuli*, J. Pharmacol. Exp. Ther. **1994**, *271*, 1306-1313.

Iwashita, T., Shimizu, T.: *Imipramine inhibits intrathecal substance P induced behavior and blocks spinal cord substance P receptors in mice*, Brain Res. **1992**, *581*, 59-66.

Kayser, V., Besson, J. M., Guilbaud, G.: *Evidence for a noradrenergic component in the antinociceptive effect of the analgesic agent tramadol in an animal model of clinical pain, the arthritic rat*, Eur. J. Pharmacol. **1992**, *224*, 83-88.

Kim, S. H. and Chung, J. M.: *An experimental model for peripheral neuropathy produced by segmental spinal nerve ligation in the rat*, Pain **1992**, *50*, 355-363.

Kleemann, A., Engel, J., Reichert, D., Kutscher, B.: *Pharmaceutical Substances*, 3rd edition, Thieme **1999**.

Lakhlani, P. P., MacMIllan, L. B., Guo, T. Z., McCool B. A., Lovinger, D. M., Maze, M., Limbird, L. E.: *Substitution of a mutant α2A-adrenergic receptor via ´hit and run´ gene targeting reveals the role of this subtype in sedative, analgesic, and anesthetic-sparing responses in vivo*, Proc. Natl. Acad. Sci. USA **1997**, *94*, 9950-9955.

Levine, J. D., Gordon, N. C., Smith, R., McBryde, R.: *Desipramine enhances opiate postoperative analgesia*, Pain **1986**, *27*, 45-49.

Levy, R., Leiphart, J., Dills, C.: *Analgesic action of acute and chronic intraspinally administered opiate and α2-adrenergic agonists in chronic neuropathic pain*, Stereotact. Funct. Neurosurg. **1994**, *62*, 279-289.

Manna, V., Bolino, F., Di Cicco, L.: *Chronic tension-type headache, mood depression and serotonin: therapeutic effects of fluvoxamine and mianserine*, Headache **1994**, *34*, 44-49.

Mason, P.: *Central mechanisms of pain modulation*, Curr. Opin. Neurobiol. **1999**, *9*, 436-441.

Matos, F. F., Rollema, H., Brown, J. L., Basbaum, A. I.: *Do opioids evoke the release of serotonin in the spinal cord? An in vivo microdialysis study of the regulation of extracellular serotonin in the rat*, Pain **1992**, *48*, 439-447.

Max, M.B., Lynch, S.A., Muir, J., Shoaf, S.E., Smoller, B., Dubner, R.: *Effects of desipramine, amitriptyline, and fluoxetine on pain in diabetic neuropathy*, N. Engl. J. Med. **1992**, *326*, 1250-1256.

McQuay, H. J., Tramer, M., Nye, B. A., Carroll, D., Wiffen, P. J., Moore, R. A.: *A systematic review of antidepressants in neuropathic pain*, Pain **1996**, *68*, 217-227.

McQuay, H. J. and Moore, R. A.: *Antidepressants and chronic pain - effective analgesia in neuropathic pain and other syndromes*, Br. Med. J. **1997**, *314*, 763-764.

Millan, M. J.: *The induction of pain: an integrative review*, Prog. Neurobiol. **1999**, *57*, 1-164.

Miranda, H. F., Pelissier, T., Pinardi, G.: *Involvement of adrenergic, serotonergic, and opioid mechanisms in tramadol-induced antinociception in mice*, Analgesia **1999**, *4*, 1-7.

Mosconi, T. and Kruger, L.: *Fixed-diameter polyethylene cuffs applied to the rat sciatic nerve induce a painful neuropathy: ultrastructural morphometric analysis of axonal alterations*, Pain **1996**, *64*, 37-57.

Motsch, J., Graber, E., Ludwig, K.: *Addition of clonidine enhances postoperative pain analgesia from epidural morphine: a double blind study*, Anesthesiology **1990**, *73*, 1067-1073.

Na, H. S., Leem, J. W., Chung, J. M.: *Abnormalities of mechanoreceptors in a rat model of neuropathic pain: possible involvement in mediating mechanical allodynia*, J. Neurophysiol. **1993**, *70*, 522-528.

Norregard, J., Volkmann, H., Danneskiold-Samsoe, B.: *A randomized controlled trial of citaloram in the treatment of fibromyalgia*, Pain **1995**, *61*, 445-449.

Onghena, P. and van Houdenhove, B.: *Antidepressant-induced analgesia in chronic non-malignant pain: a meta-analysis of 39 placebo-controlled studies*, Pain **1992**,*49*, 205-219.

Ossipov, M. H., Nichols, M. L., Bian, D., Porreca, F.: *Inhibition by spinal morphine of the tail-flick response is attenuated in rats with nerve ligation injury*, Neurosci. Lett. **1995**, *199*, 83-86.

Paoli, F., Ghaleb, H. A., Cossa, P.: *Note preliminaire sur l'action de l'imipramine das le etats douloureux*, Rev. Neurol. **1960**, *102*, 503-504.

Peroutko, S. J., Banghart, S. B., Allen, G. S.: *Relative potency and selectivity of calcium antagonists used in the treatment of migraine*, Headache **1984**, *24*, 55-58.

Phillipp, M. and Fickinger, M.: *Psychotropic drugs inthe management of chronic pain syndromes*, Pharmacopsychiatry **1993**, *26*, 221-234.

Phillips, J. W. and Wu, P. H.: *The effect of various centrally active drugs on adenosine uptake in the central nervous system*, Comp. Biochem. Physiol. C **1982**, *72*, 179-187.

Poree, L. R., Guo, T. Z., Kingery, W. S., Maze, M.: *The analgesic potency of dexmedetomidine is enhanced after nerve injury: a possible role for peripheral $\alpha2$-adrenoceptors*, Anesth. Analg. **1998**, *87*, 941-948.

Proudfit, H. K.: *Pharmacologic evidence for the modulation of nociception by noradrenergic neurons*, Prog. Brain Res. **1988**, *77*, 357-370.

Raffa, R. B., Friderichs, E., Reimann, W., Shank, R. P., Codd, E. E., Vaught, J. L.: *Opioid and nonopioid components independently contribute to the mechanisms of action of tramadol, an atypical opioid analgesic*, J. Pharmacol. Exp. Ther. **1992**, *260*, 275-285.

Reddy, S. V. R., Maderdrut, J. L., Yaksh, T. L.: *Spial cord pharmacology of adrenergic agonist-mediated antinociception*, J. Pharmacol. Exp. Ther. **1980**, *213*, 525-533.

Reynolds, D. V.: *Surgery in the rat during electrical analgesia by focal brain stimulation*, Science **1969**, *164*, 444-445.

Rojas-Corrales, M. O., Ortega-Alvaro, A., Gibert-Rahola, J., Roca-Vinardell, A., Micó, J. A..: *Pindolol, a beta-adrenoceptor/5-hydroxytryptamine1A/1B antagonist, enhances the analgesic effect of tramadol*, Pain **2000**, *88*, 119-124.

Rumore, M. M. and Schlichting, D. A.: *Clinical efficacy of antihistamines as analgesics*, Pain **1986**, *25*, 7-22.

Sawamura, S., Kingery, W. S., Davies, M. F., Agashe, G. S., Clark, J. D., Kobilka, B. K., Hashimoto, T., Maze, M.: *Antinociceptive action of nitrous oxide is mediated by stimulation of noradrenergic neurons in the brainstem and activation of $\alpha2B$ adrenoceptors*, J. Neurosci. **2000**, *20*, 9242-9251.

Sawynok, J. and Reid, A.: *Antinociception by tricyclic antidepressants in the rat formalin test: differential effects on different behaviours following systemic and spinal administration*, Pain **2001**, *93*, 51-59.

Sawynok, J., Reid, A. R., Esser, M. J.: *Peripheral antinociceptive action of amitriptyline in the rat formalin test: involvement of adenosine*, Pain **1999**, *80*, 45-55.

Sawynok, J., Esser, M. J., Reid, A. R.: *Antidepressants as analgesics: an overview of central and peripheral mechanisms of action*, J. Psychiatry Neurosci. **2001**, *26*, 21-29.

Sierralta, F., Miranda, H. F., Mendez, M., Pinardi, G.: *Interaction of opioids with antidepressant-induced antinociception*, Psychopharmacology **1995**, *122*, 374-378.

Sindrup, S. H.: *Antidepressants as analgesics.* In: Yaksh, T. L., Lynch, C., Zapol, V. M., Maze, M., Biebuyck, J. F., Saidman, L. J. (eds.) Anesthesia. Biologic foundations. Philadelphia: Lippincott-Raven, **1997**, 987-997.

Sindrup, S. H. and Jensen, T. S.: *Efficacy of pharmacological treatments of neuropathic pain: an update and effect related to mechanism of drug action*, Pain **1999**, *83*, 389-400.

Sindrup, S.H., Gram, L.F., Skjold, T., Grodum, E., Brosen, K.: *Clomipramine vs desipramine vs placebo in the treatment of diabetic neuropathy symptoms. A double-blind cross-over study*, Br. J. Pharmacol. **1990b**, *30*, 683-691.

Sindrup, S.H., Gram, L.F., Brosen, K., Eshoj, O., Mogensen, E.F.: *The selective serotonin reuptake inhibitor paroxetine is effective in the treatment of diabetic neuropathy symptoms*, Pain **1990b**, *42*, 135-144.

Sindrup, S.H., Bjerre, U., Deigaard, A., Brosen, K., Aaes-Jorgensen, T., Gram, L.F.: *The selective serotonin reuptake inhibitor citalopram relieves the symptoms of diabetic neuropathy*, Clin. Pharmacol. Ther. **1992**, *52*, 547-552.

Song, J. H., Ham, S. S., Shin, Y. K., Lee, C. S.: *Amitriptyline modulation of Na(+) channels in rat dorsal root ganglion neurons*, Eur. J. Pharmacol. **2000**, *401*, 297-305.

Stein, D., Peri, T., Edelstein, E., Elizur, A., Floman, Y.: *The efficacy of amitryptiline and acetaminophen in the management of acute low back pain*, Psychosomatics **1996**, *37*, 63-70.

Sullivan, A. F., Kalso, E. A., McQuay, H. J., Dickenson, A. H.: *The antinociceptive actions of dexmedetomidine on dorsal horn neuronal responses in the anaesthetized rat*, Eur. J. Pharmacol. **1992**, *215*, 127-133.

Taylor, K. and Rowbotham, M.C.: *Venlafaxine hydrochloride and chronic pain*, West. J. Med. **1996**, *165*, 147-148.

van Schayck, R., Volz, H. P., Meissner, W., Malessa, R.: *Antidepressiva bei chronischen Schmerzen*, Medizin. Monatsschr. f. Pharmazeuten **1998**, *21*, 304-313.

West, W. L., Yeomans, D. C., Proudfit, H. K.: *The function of noradrenergic neurons in mediating antinociception induced by electrical stimulation of the locus coeruleus in two different sources of Sprague-Dawley rats*, Brain Res. **1993**, *626*, 127-135.

Willis, W. D. and Westlund, K. N.: *Neuroanatomy of the pain system and of the pathways that modulate pain*, J. Clin. Neurophysiol. **1997**, *14*, 2-31.

Wilson, R. C.: *The use of low-dose trazodone in the treatment of painful diabetic neuropathy*, J. Am. Pediatr. Med. Assoc. **1999**, *89*, 468-471.

Yaksh, T. L.: *Direct evidence that spinal serotonin and noradrenaline terminals mediate the spinal antinociceptive effects of morphine in the periaqueductal grey*, Brain Res. **1979**, *160*, 180-185.

Yaksh, T. L., Pogrel, J. W., Lee, Y. W., Chaplan, S. R.: *Reversal of nerve ligation-induced allodynia by spinal alpha-2 adrenoceptor agonists*, J. Pharmacol. Exp. Ther. **1995**, *272*, 207-214.

Zeigler, D., Lynch, S. A., Muir, J., Benjamin, J., Max, M. B.: *Transdermal clonidine versus placebo in painful diabetic neuropathy*, Pain **1992**, *48*, 403-408.

Zeile, K., Hauptmann, K.-H., Stahle, H. (Boehringer Ingelheim): *Process for the preparation of 3-aryl-amino-1,3-diazacycloalkenes*, US3202660 (**1965**).

Part III

New Approaches in Pain Therapy

Part III

New Approaches in Pain Therapy

5 Gabapentin and Gabapentinoids

Corinna Maul, Helmut Buschmann and Bernd Sundermann

Introduction

Several antiepileptic drugs like carbamazepine are in use as adjunctive drugs for the treatment of certain symptoms of chronic pain syndromes (Tremonts-Lukats et al., 2000). But, unlike the irreversible GABA transaminase inhibitor vigabatrin and the $GABA_B$ agonist baclofen, gabapentin does not interact directly with $GABA_A$ or $GABA_B$ receptors.

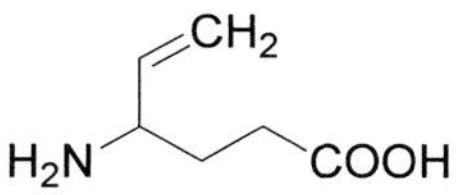

Vigabatrin 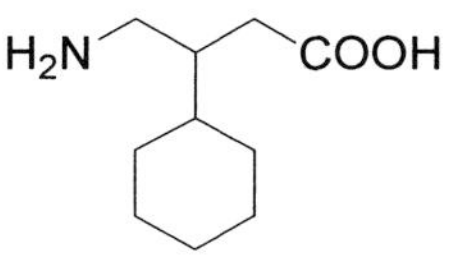   Baclofen 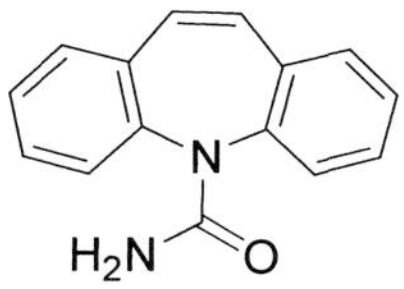   Carbamazepine

Gabapentin

Originally designed as a lipophilic γ-aminobutyric acid (GABA) analog gabapentin was introduced in 1994 as an antiepileptic drug, particularly for the treatment of partial seizures (Mao and Chen, 2000). Although gabapentin is inactive in preclinical pain models designed to assess activity against acute pain – including the p-phenylquinone writhing test in mice and the tail flick test in rats – once gabapentin had been marketed it was recognized to be promising for the treatment of neuropathic pain associated with e.g. postherpetic neuralgia, postpoliomyelitis neuropathy, reflex sympathetic dystrophy, and diabetic peripheral neuropathy. In part this, as well as the clinical potential of gabapentin in the treatment of postoperative pain, has been proven in placebo-controlled clinical trials (Rowbotham et al., 1998; Hemstreet and Lapointe, 2001; Rice and Maton, 2001; Werner et al., 2001). In animal models evidence for the therapeutic usefulness of gabapentin against some trigeminal neuropathic pain

Gabapentin

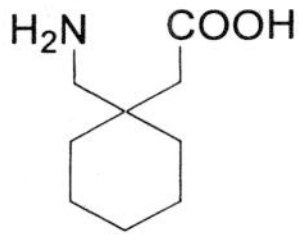

[60142-96-3] (1-Amino-methylcyclohexyl)acetic acid, $C_9H_{17}NO_2$, M_r 171.24

Trade name: Neurontin

disorders has been shown (Christensen et al., 2001, for an overview of gabapentin in neuropathic pain models see Bryans and Wustrow, 1999). Gabapentin is administered in the clinical range between 900 and up to 3600 mg/day in some cases. Because combined therapy of opioids and gabapentin can produce much more effective pain relief in patients, it is used frequently with opioids to treat patients with severe cancer pain. The favorable tolerability and flexibility of the dosage has made gabapentin an important and widely used clinical (adjuvant) analgesic and may make it the first choice drug in the treatment of neuropathic pain (Ripamonti and Dickerson, 2001, Chong et al., 2002; Rose and Kam, 2002). It does, however, possess a relatively short half-life, being excreted unchanged, possibly because it has a very high water solubility and apparent lack of protein binding *in vivo*. Confusion, somnolescence and dizziness are the major adverse events to be expected with gabapentin.

Gabapentin is well absorbed after oral administration and readily crosses the blood-brain barrier via an L-system amino acid transporter when given systemically. Although gabapentin may influence the synthesis and release of GABA, it does not affect the uptake and metabolism of endogenous GABA (Goldlust et al., 1995). Importantly, the antiallodynic effect of gabapentin is not affected by GABA-receptor antagonists. It is thus unlikely that the anti-allodynic effect of gabapentin, as shown in animal studies, is caused by an enhancement of the inhibitory influence via its direct interaction with GABA receptors or its indirect effect via increasing endogenous GABA.

On the other hand, in more recent patents, gabapentin analogs are said to increase newly created GABA at the synaptic junction, therefore acting as GABA agonists which may produce an anticonvulsant or antidepressant effect (Bryans et al., 2000).

A key process of central sensitization is the activation of N-methyl-D-aspartate (NMDA) receptors by glutamate/ aspartate within the central nervous system (see chapter 7.1) and D-serine is an agonist at the NMDA-glycine site. The antihyperalgesic effect of gabapentin has been shown to be reversed by D-serine in models of formalin-induced nociception, substance P and NMDA-induced hyperalgesia, and thermal injury. This data suggests that gabapentin acts as an antagonist at the NMDA-glycine site, and D-serine replaces gabapentin, thereby reversing the gabapentin effect. However, receptor binding studies fail to detect any specific interactions between gabapentin and the NMDA receptor complex. In the absence of specific binding it is unlikely that gabapentin exerts its effect by means of interacting with the NMDA receptor.

Recent results indicate that the effects of gabapentin on NMDA receptors depend on the phosphorylation states of the receptor (or cell). Gabapentin enhances NMDA currents in normal neurons only when protein kinase C (PKC) is added to those cells. The enhancement results from an increase in the affinity of glycine for NMDA receptors by gabapentin. This action of gabapentin can be blocked by the PKC-inhibitor chelerythrine. Since endogenous PKC is elevated in inflamed tissue these results suggest that gabapentin exerts its effects only on cells affected by inflammatory injuries (Gu and Huang, 2001; 2002)

The antinociceptive effect by enhancement of NMDA responses may be exerted through gabapentin's action on inhibitory neurons. An increase in NMDA responses by gabapentin would promote the activity of inhibitory neurons and thus result in a reduction of transmission of nociceptive signals. It was shown that most cells responding to gabapentin were GABA-positive, while those which do not respond to gabapentin are GABA-negative (Gu and Huang, 2001).

A gabapentin-specific binding site was initially identified in the central nervous system. This site was later identified as the $\alpha_2\delta$ subunit of voltage-dependent calcium channels. Besides gabapentin, (*S*)-(+)-3-isobutylgaba (pregabalin, see below), but not (*R*)-(-)-3-isobutylgaba, binds to this calcium channel subunit. Although voltage-dependent calcium channels have been implicated in hyperalgesia, it is difficult to envision that the affinity of gabapentin for voltage-gated calcium channels alone would account for its effects on allodynia and hyperalgesia in animal models: in particular, the average dose of gabapentin used in clinical settings is several hundred-fold larger than that of specific calcium channel blockers. Nevertheless, it was shown recently that 10 μM gabapentin reduces high voltage activated Ca^{2+} current amplitude in DRG cells. This concentration is within the clinically effective range (10-100 μM) found in the serum of human patients. Interestingly, the effect of gabapentin was noticeable only after the membrane was depolarized with either a pre-pulse or a train of stimuli. It was shown that the blockage of high voltage activated Ca^{2+} currents by gabapentin depends on the frequency of stimulation and that it accumulates from pulse to pulse during repetitive stimulation. The decrease of Ca^{2+} currents caused by gabapentin (an average of 25%) is comparable to the

Phenytoin

effect of other anticonvulsant agents that modulate Ca^{2+} influx such as phenytoin and carbamazepine.

These findings may explain the efficacy of gabapentin as an analgesic since DRG neurons are depolarized during pain perception and may implicate the action of the $\alpha_2\delta$ subunit in modulating Ca^{2+} channels with a subsequent reduction in neurotransmitter release (Alden and Garcia, 2001). This hypothesis is supported by the fact that many gabapentin analogs - as shown below – have been identified via binding to the $\alpha_2\delta$ subunit and these compounds were shown to be antinociceptive.

Gabapentin can be synthesized by several methods. The original gabapentin synthesis by Goedecke (Satzinger et al., 1976) and a second generation synthesis are presented below:

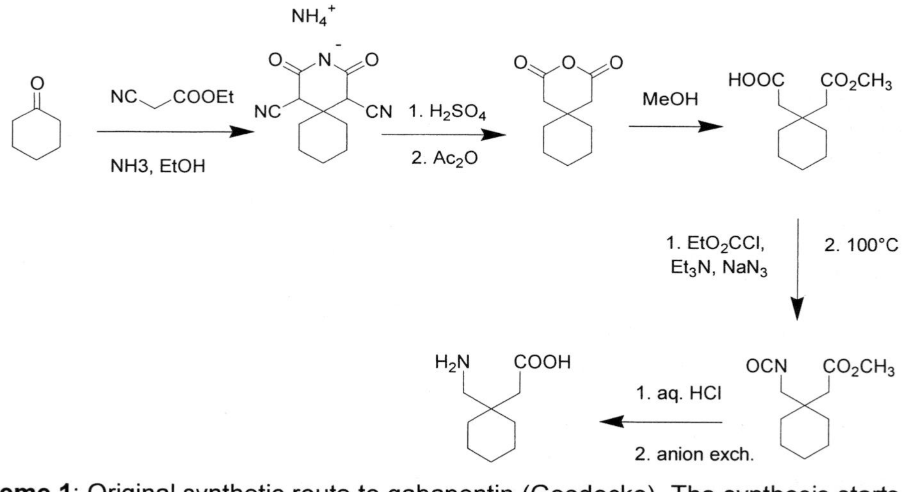

Scheme 1: Original synthetic route to gabapentin (Goedecke). The synthesis starts with the formation of the Guareshi salt and its conversion to the spiro anhydride. The anhydride is then converted to the half ester which is transformed into the isocyanate via a Curtius rearrangement. Acidic hydrolysis followed by ion exchange chromatography yields gabapentin.

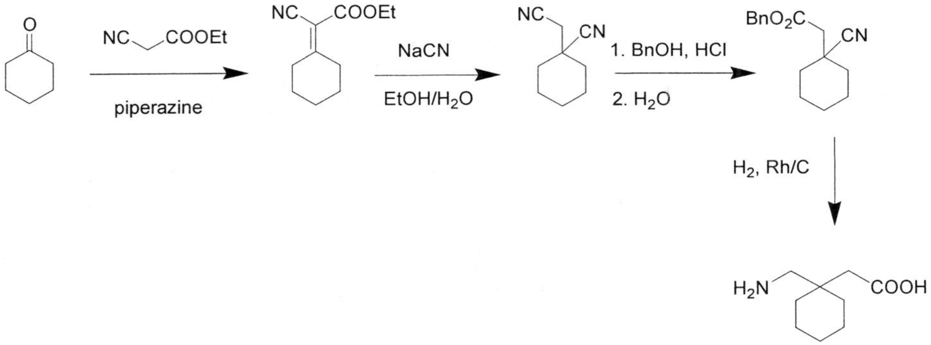

Scheme 2: Alternative route. The synthesis starts with the Knoevenagel condensation of ethyl cyano acetate with cyclohexanone. Ethyl cyano(cyclohexylidine)acetate is then subjected to a Michael addition with cyanide giving the bis-nitrile which is converted to the benzyl ester via the Pinner reaction and finally yields gabapentin by catalytic hydrogenation with rhodium on carbon (Griffiths et al., 1991).

Pregabalin

Pregabalin is the pharmacologically active *S*-enantiomer of 3-aminomethyl-5-methyl hexanoic acid, a 3-alkylated analog of GABA. As with gabapentin, the mechanism of pregabalin is not yet fully understood. It does displace [^{3}H]-gabapentin from its binding site at the $\alpha_2\delta$ subunit of calcium channels. In displacement experiments with [^{3}H]-gabapentin in synaptic plasma membranes from rat neocortex, pregabalin showed an IC_{50} of 37 nm, compared to 80 nm for unlabeled gabapentin (Martin et al., 1999).

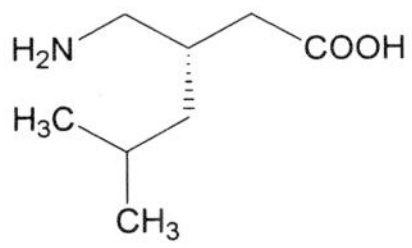

Pregabalin has shown anticonvulsant activity in many animal models. The drug has exhibited a profile similar to that of gabapentin, but active doses have been found to be 3- to 10-fold lower. It has also been found to be effective in rat models of neuropathic pain, including intrathecal substance P- or NMDA-, carrageenan- and formalin-induced pain, thermal injury and postoperative pain. In these models, pregabalin is at least twice as effective as gabapentin against both thermal and mechanical pain. Furthermore, pregabalin does not induce sedation.

Analysis of published phase III trials against epilepsy and diabetic neuropathic pain indicates that pregabalin is more efficacious than gabapentin. In diabetic neuropathic pain, efficacy and tolerability at 300 to 600 mg/day appears to be equivalent to 3600 mg/day of gabapentin.

Following oral administration, pregabalin is absorbed through a large neutral amino acid carrier-mediated intestinal transport mechanism. In a study of healthy

Pregabalin

3-Aminomethyl-5-methyl-hexanoic acid, $C_8H_{17}NO_2$, [148553-50-8]

Clinical efficacy of pregabalin

volunteers, pregabalin had an oral bioavailability of 90%. It is not substantially metabolized (99% unchanged in urine), although the N-methyl derivative of pregabalin is a minor urinary metabolite. It is excreted with a $t_{1/2}$ of 4.6 - 6.8 h, and no drug interactions have been reported yet.

Pregablin can be synthesized by several methods; two methods are described below:

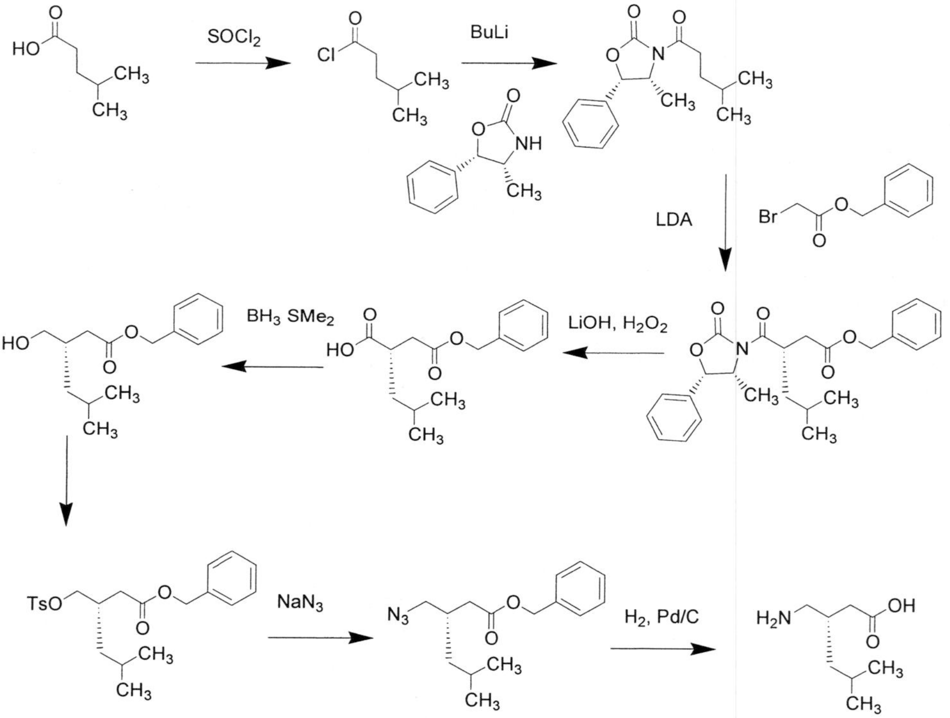

Scheme 3: Synthesis of pregabalin. Condensation of the acyl chloride with a chiral oxazolidinone by means of BuLi in THF yields the corresponding N-acyl derivative. Stereoselective Evans alkylation with benzyl bromoacetate by means of LDA in THF affords the (S)-adduct with 95% ee purity. Elimination of the chiral auxiliary and reduction gives 3-hydroxymethyl-5-methyl-hexanoic acid benzyl ester. The corresponding azide is prepared via the tosylate, and reduction and debenzylation with H_2 over Pd/C yields pregabalin (Hoekstra et al., 1997).

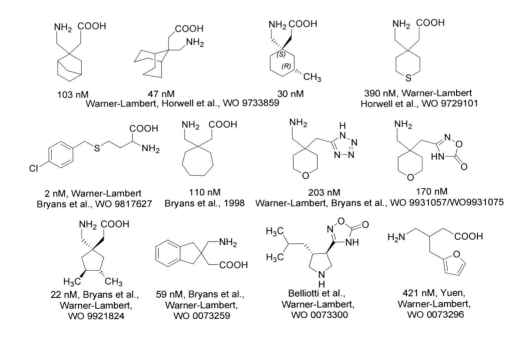

Scheme 4: The reaction of diethyl malonate with 3-methylbutanal by means of dipropylamine in acetic acid gives the corresponding 2-(3-methylbutylidene)malonate derivative, which is treated with KCN to yield 2-(1-cyano-3-methyl-butyl)-malonic acid diethyl ester. Decarboxylative hydrolysis with KOH and reduction with hydrogen over Ni yields racemic pregabalin which is submitted to optical resolution with (*S*)-(+)-mandelic acid (Grote et al. (Warner-Lambert), 1996).

Several series of compounds which are claimed to have the gabapentin mechanism have been published or filed in patent applications, predominantly by Warner-Lambert (now Pfizer):

103 nM

47 nM
Warner-Lambert, Horwell et al., WO 9733859

30 nM

390 nM, Warner-Lambert
Horwell et al., WO 9729101

2 nM, Warner-Lambert
Bryans et al., WO 9817627

110 nM
Bryans et al., 1998

203 nM
Warner-Lambert, Bryans et al., WO 9931057/WO9931075

170 nM

22 nM, Bryans et al.,
Warner-Lambert,
WO 9921824

59 nM, Bryans et al.,
Warner-Lambert,
WO 0073259

Belliotti et al.,
Warner-Lambert,
WO 0073300

421 nM, Yuen,
Warner-Lambert,
WO 0073296

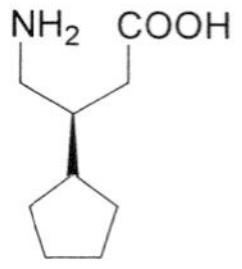

108 nM
Belliotti and Wustrow,
Warner-Lambert,
WO 0031020

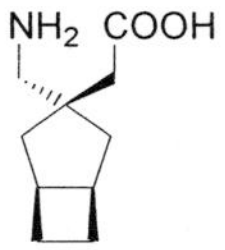

38 nM, Bryans et al.,
Warner-Lambert,
WO 0128978

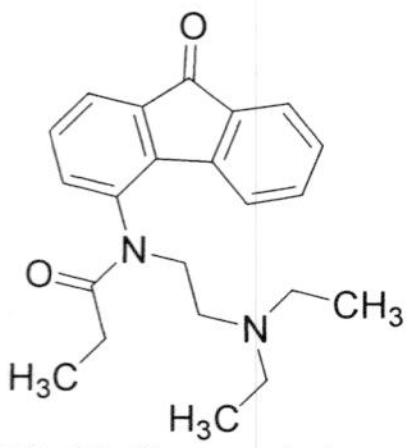

58 nM, Bryans et al.,
Warner-Lambert,
WO 0068184

Scheme 5: Compounds claimed to have the gabapentin mechanism

References

Alden, K. J. and Garcia, J.: *Differential effect of gabapentin on neurnal and muscle calcium currents*, J. Pharmacol. Exp. Ther. **2001**, *297*, 727-735.

Belliotti, T. R. and Wustrow, D. J. (Warner-Lambert): *Improved gamma amino butyric acid analogs*, WO 0031020.

Belliotti, T. R., Thorpe, A. J., Wustrow, D. J. (Warner-Lambert): *Amino heterocycles useful as pharmaceutical agents*, WO 0073300.

Bryans, J. S., Horwell, D. C., Kneen, C. O., Wustrow, D. J., Thorpe, A. J. (Warner-Lambert): *Substituted gamma aminobutyric acids as pharmaceutical agents*, WO 9817627.

Bryans, J. S., Capiris, T., Horwell, D. C., Kneen, C. O., Wustrow, D. J. (Warner-Lambert): *1-Substituted-1-aminomethyl-cycloalkane derivatives (= gabapentin analogues), their preparations and their use in the treatment of neurological disorders*, WO 9931075.

Bryans, J. S., Davies, N., Gee, N. S., Dissanayake, U. K., Ratcliffe, G. S., Horwell, D. C., Kneen, C. O., Morrell, A. I., Oles, R. J., O'Toole, J. C., Perkins, G. M., Sigh, L., Suman-Chauhan, N., O'Neill, J. A.: *Identification of novel ligands for the gabapentin binding site on the $\alpha_2\delta$ subunit of a calcium channel and their evaluation as anticonvulsant agents,* J. Med. Chem. **1998**, *41*, 1838-1845.

Bryans, J. S., Horwell, D. C., Kneen, C. O., Wustrow, D. J. (Warner-Lambert): *4(3)Substituted – 4(3)-aminomethyl-(thio)pyran or –piperidine derivatives (= gabapentin analogues), their preparation and their use in the treatment of neurological disorders*, WO 9931057.

Bryans, J. S., Horwell, D. C., Osborne, S. (Warner-Lambert): *Fused polycyclic amino acids as pharmaceutical agents*, WO 0073259.

Bryans, J. S., Horwell, D. C., Thorpe, A. J., Wustrow, D. J., Yuen, P.-W. (Warner-Lambert): *Cyclic amino acids and derivatives thereof useful as pharmaceutical agents*, WO 9921824.

Bryans, J. S., Blakemore, D. C., Osborne, S., Receveur, J.-M. (Warner-Lambert): *Bicyclic amino acids as pharmaceutical agents*, WO 0128978.

Bryans, J. S., O'Toole, J. C., Horwell, D. C. (Warner-Lambert): *Aromatic amides*, WO 0068184.

Chong, M. S., Smith, T. E., Hanna, M.: Case reports - reversal of sensory deficit associated with pain relief after treatment with gabapentin, Pain **2002**, *96*, 329-333.

Christensen, D., Gautron, M., Guilbaud, G., Kayser, V.: *Effect of gabapentin and lamotrigine on mechanical allodynia-like behaviour in a rat model of trigeminal neuropathic pain*, Pain **2001**, *93*, 147-153.

Goldlust, A., Su, T. Z., Welty, D. F. et al.: *Effects of anticonvulsant drug gabapentin on the enzymes in metabolic pathways of glutamate and GABA*, Epilepsy research **1995**, *22*, 1-11.

Griffiths, G., Mettler, H., Mills, L. S., Previdoli, F.: *Novel syntheses of gabapentin via addition of hydrocyanic acid to cyclohexylidenemalonate or cyano(cyclohexylidene)acetate*, Helv. Chim. Acta **1991**, *74*, 309-414.

Grote, T. M., Huckabee, B. K., Mulhern, T., Sobieray, D. M., Titus, R. D. (Warner-Lambert*): Method of making (S)-3-(aminomethyl)-5-methylhexanoic acid*, WO 9640617.

Gu, Y.and Huang, L.-Y. M.: *Gabapentin actions on N-methyl-D-aspartate receptor channels are protein kinase C dependent*, Pain **2001**, *93*, 85-92.

Gu, Y. and Huang, L.-Y. M.: *Gabapentin potentiates N-methyl-d-aspartate receptor mediated currents in rat GABAergic dorsal horn neurons*, Neuroscience Letters **2002**, *324*, 177-180.

Hemstreet, B. and Lapointe, M.: *Evidence for the use of gabapentin in the treatment of diabetic peripheral neuropathy*, Clin. Ther. **2001**, *23*, 520-531.

Hoekstra, M. S., Sobieray, D. M., Schwindt, M. A., Mulhern, T. A., Grote, T. M., Huckabee, B. K., Hendrickson, V. S., Francklin, L. C., Granger, E. J., Karrick, G. L.: *Chemical development of CI-1008, an enantiomerically pure anticonvulsant*, Org. Proc. Res. Dev. **1997**, *1*, 26-38.

Horwell, D. C., Bryans, J. S., Kneen, C. O., Ratcliffe, G. S. (Warner-Lambert): *Novel cyclic amino acids as pharmaceutical agents*, WO 9729101.

Horwell, D. C., Bryans, J. S., Kneen, C. O., Morrell, A. I., Ratcliffe, G. S.: *Novel briged cyclic amino acids as pharmaceutical agents*, WO 9733859.

Horwell, D. C., Bryans, J. S., Kneen, C. O., Morrell, A. I., Ratcliffe, G. S., Hartenstein, J. (Warner-Lambert): *Novel substituted cyclic amino acids as pharmaceutical agents,* WO 9733858.

Mao, J. and Chen, L.: *Gabapentin in pain management*, Anesth. Analg. **2000**, *91*, 680-687.

Martin, L., Rabasseda, X., Leeson, J., Castaner, J.: *Pregabalin*, Drugs of the Future **1999**, *24*, 862-870.

Rice, A. S. C. and Maton, S.: *Gabapentin in postherpetic neuralgia: a randomised, double blind, placebo controlled study*, Pain **2001**, *94*, 215-224.

Ripermonti, C. and Dickerson, E. D.: *Strategies for the treatment of cancer pain in the new millenium,* Drugs **2001**, *61*, 955-977.

Rose, M. A. and Kam, P. C. A.,: *Gabapentin: pharmacology and its use in pain management*, Anaesthesia **2002**, *57*, 451-462.

Rowbotham, M., Harden, N., Stacey, B. et al.: *For the Gabapentin postherpetic neuralgia study group. Gabapentin for the treatment of postherpetic neuralgia. A randomized controlled trial*, JAMA **1998**, *280*, 1837-1842.

Satzinger, G., Hartenstein, J., Herrmann, M., Heldt, W. (Goedecke A.-G.): *Cyclic amino acids*, Ger. Offen. **1976**, DE 2460891.

Tremont-Lukats, I. W., Megeff, C., Backonja, M.-M.: *Anticonvulsants for neuropathic pain syndromes*, Drugs **2000**, *60*, 1029-1052.

Werner, M. U., Perkins, F. M., Holte, K., Pedersen, J. L., Kehlet, H.: *Effects of gabapentin in acute inflammatory pain in humans*, Reg. Anesth. Pain Med. **2001**, *26*, 322-328.

Yuen, P.W. (Warner-Lambert): *3-Heteroalkyl substituted GABA analogs*, WO 0073296.

6 Voltage-gated Ion Channels

6.1 Sodium Channels

Petra Bloms-Funke

Voltage-dependent sodium channels have long been recognized as potential drug targets for the treatment of pain. In fact, even before the mechanism of sodium channel blockade had been elucidated, Carl Koller had introduced in 1884, the use of the naturally-occurring alkaloid cocaine in clinical surgery, taking advantage of its local anesthetic properties (Vandam, 1987). Today sodium channel blockers, including local anesthetic, anticonvulsant and antiarrhythmic agents, are clinically used for local anesthesia and chronic pain management. As sodium channels are ubiquitously responsible for rapid excitatory transmission, the therapeutic window for the use of systemic sodium channel blockers is limited due to toxic side-effects especially on the cardiovascular and the central nervous system. The application of molecular biological techniques has led to the identification of sodium channel subtypes preferentially expressed in primary sensory neurons, thus opening promising approaches to find effective and well-tolerated sodium channel blockers in particular for their use in chronic pain (for review see Waxman et al., 2000; Anger et al., 2001; Wood et al., 2002).

The natural alkaloid **cocaine** was introduced as the first local anesthetic drug in clinical surgery

Voltage-gated Sodium Channels: Structure and Function

Voltage-gated sodium channels are large glycoproteins that form voltage-dependent, Na^+-selective pores through the plasma membrane of electrically excitable cells (i.e. neurons, cardiac cells, muscle cells). Their primary function is to generate the rapid regenerative upstroke of action potentials as first described by Hodgkin and Huxley (1952). They play a central role in modulation of the firing activity of excitable cells and in the transmission of depolarizing impulses through the neuronal network including pain pathways.

Sodium channels are densely expressed in axons, somata and dendrites of neurons. In the rat brain and spinal sensory neurons, sodium channels are heterotrimeric integral membrane proteins consisting of one major pore-forming α-subunit which associates with two smaller auxiliary β-subunits (one β1 or β3 assembled with one β2 subunit; Black et al., 1996; Morgan et al., 2000; for review see Catterall, 1992; Denac et al., 2000). The deduced

Voltage-gated sodium channels generate the rapid regenerative upstroke of action potentials and hence play a central role in modulation of the firing activity of excitable cells. They form heterotrimeric transmembrane Na^+-conducting pores

primary structure of the α-subunit indicates four homologous domains (DI - DIV) each of which built up with six potential α-helical transmembrane segments (S1 - S6). There are several phosphorylation and glycosylation consensus sequences allowing differential modulation of channel function (Bennett et al., 1997; Fitzgerald et al., 1999; Tyrrell et al., 2001). Although the α-subunit alone is capable of establishing functional channels, the β1-subunit is crucial for rapid rates of channel activation and inactivation (Patton et al., 1994). Recently a β3-subunit, a β1-like member of the family, was cloned which shows largely a complemantary distribution to β1 and inactivates the sodium current more slowly when expressed in oocytes of the South African clawed frog, *Xenopus laevis* (Morgan et al., 2000). The β2-subunit is proposed to be an important regulator of channel expression and localization in neurons (Isom et al., 1995).

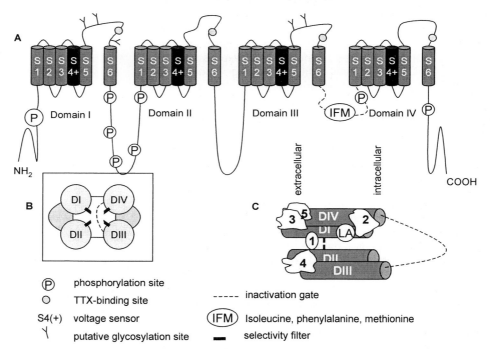

Figure 1: Topology of the α-subunit of voltage-gated sodium channels. (**A**) The α-subunit is built up of four homologous transmembrane domains (DI - DIV) each containing six transmembrane segments (S1 - S6). The extracellular and intracellular loops contain putative glycosylation and phosphorylation sites, as indicated. The IFM-motif is probalby crucial for channel inactivation. (**B**) Transmembrane arrangement of DI - DIV domains around the channel pore. (**C**). Binding sites (1 - 5) of the α-subunit. LA: putative local anesthetic binding site. TTX, tetrodotoxin. (Adapted from Denac et al., 2000).

On depolarization of the plasma membrane, sodium channels are rapidly activated leading to a dramatic increase in Na$^+$ permeability and thus to an inward current of Na$^+$ ions into the cell. The fourth transmembrane segment, S4, of the α-subunit is believed to be the voltage sensor: According to the sliding helix model (Caterall, 1986), depolarization induces a spiral-shaped motion of the positively charged transmembrane α-helix with an outward displacement by 5 Å finally leading to channel activation. The open channel closes rapidly within a range of 0.5 to several milliseconds transforming to an 'inactivated', refractory state. The isoleucine, phenylalanine, methionine (IFM) motif within the intracellular loop between domains DIII and DIV is proposed to function as an inactivation gate (for review see Denac et al. (2000)). In addition to fast inactivation, sodium channels show a slow component of inactivation which lasts for several seconds. Repriming or reactivation of sodium channels requires repolarization of the plasma membrane leading to the so-called 'resting' state, which is non-conducting, but activatable.

Taking into account the fast gating properties of voltage-gated sodium channels, a simplified three-state model has been developed to understand voltage- and frequency-dependent properties which are characteristic for many sodium channel blockers including local anesthetic, anticonvulsant, and antiarrhythmic drugs (Caterall, 1987; Ragsdale et al., 1996; Marban et al., 1998). Voltage-dependency is attributed to a high binding affinity of the drug to the channel in the inactivated state (k_3/k_{-3} » k_1/k_{-1}, k_2/k_{-2}; Fig. 2). Thereby, the channel is stabilized in this state and the inactivation curve is shifted to more negative potentials, thus the extent of channels in the inactivated state is increased at the resting membrane potential . For example, the anticonvulsant drugs carbamazepine, phenytoin and lamotrigine have been shown to shift the voltage of half-maximal inactivation from -67 mV under control conditions to -74, -79 and -82 mV, respectively, at drug concentrations of 100 µM each as shown in a comprehensive study by Lang et al. (1993). Frequency dependency is explained by a faster rate of drug binding to the activated state (k_2 » k_1, k_3). If the drug detaches after a repeated stimulus, the amount of bound drug and thus channel block increases with repeated stimuli until the rates of association and dissociation are equal. This accumulated block during trains of stimulation is called use-dependency or also phasic block. The antagonistic potencies of the piperidine-derived local anesthetic drugs mepivacaine, ropivacaine, and bupivacaine, for instance, were increased 2-5 - fold by the 10th pulse of a stimulus

Sodium channel blockers including local anesthetic, anticonvulsant and antiarrhythmic drugs exhibit voltage- and frequency-dependent blockade which makes them useful drugs for blocking hyperexcitable neurons

train at a frequency of 2 Hz as compared to the block by the first pulse (i.e. tonic block; Bräu et al., 2000). Voltage- and frequency-dependent blocking mechanisms give rise to a preferred block of highly active cells and comparatively less interference with normal physiological sensory and motor function. With regard to chronic pain conditions these properties of many sodium channel blockers make them useful for blocking pain pathways with hyperexcitable neurons.

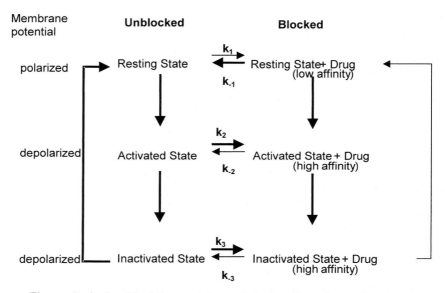

Figure 2: A simplified three-state model of sodium channel gating.

A variety of toxins that modulate voltage-gated sodium channels have been used to probe channel function. They can be classified on the basis of five discrete binding sites (Table 1). These binding sites are commonly found on all α-subunits and are being characterized at the molecular level. The sensitivity to the puffer fish poison tetrodotoxin (TTX) has been used to subdivide voltage-gated sodium channels (Table 3).

The puffer fish poison tetrodotoxin (TTX).

(4R,4aR,5R,7S,9S,10S,10aR,11S,12S)-Octahydro-12-(hydroxymethyl)-2-imino-5,9:7,10a-dimethano-10aH-[1,3]dioxocino[6,5-d]pyrimidine-4,7,10,11,12-pentol, $C_{11}H_{17}N_3O_8$, MW 319.27, [4368-28-9]

Table 1: Toxin and drug binding sites on α-subunits of voltage-gated sodium channels (Catterall, 1992).

Site	Modulators	Effect
1	Tetrodotoxin Saxitoxin	Inhibition of ion conductance
2	Batrachotoxin Veratridine	Persistent activation
3	α-Scorpion toxin Sea anemone toxins	Delay of inactivation, enhancement of persistent activation
4	β-Scorpion toxin	Shift of voltage-dependency of activation
5	Brevetoxin	Repetitive firing; enhancement of activation and block of inactivation
	Local anesthetics, antiarrhythmic, anticonvulsant drugs	Voltage- and use-dependent block

It has been found that six distinct α-subunits are expressed and often co-expressed in the primary sensory neurons, which play an important role in pain transmission. They are activated by nociceptive stimuli on the body surface, skeletal muscle and viscera and encode this information in the form of a series of action potentials which are conveyed to the spinal cord and brain (Black et al., 1996; Goldin et al., 2000; for review see Waxman et al., 2000; Wood et al., 2002). Among the heterogeneous sodium channel subtypes in the primary sensory neurons, $Na_v1.8$ and $Na_v1.9$ are characterized by their resistance to tetrodotoxin (TTX) with IC_{50} values in a micromolar range compared to low nanomolar ranges for TTX-sensitive (TTX-S) subtypes (Table 2).

Channel	Previous name	Gene symbol	Primary tissue
$Na_v1.1$	Type I	SCN1A	CNS, PNS
$Na_v1.2$	Type II	SCN2A	CNS, PNS
$Na_v1.3$	Type III	SCN3A	CNS, (PNS after axotomy)
$Na_v1.4$	SkM1	SCN4A	Skeletal muscle
$Na_v1.5$	SkM2	SCN5A	Heart
$Na_v1.6$	NaCh6	SCNA8A	CNS, PNS
$Na_v1.7$	PN1 / NaS	SCN9A	CNS, PNS
$Na_v1.8$	PN3 / SNS / NaNG	SCN10A	PNS
$Na_v1.9$	NaN / SNS II	SCN11A	PNS
Na_x	$Na_v2.1$ / NaG	SCN6A / SCN7A	heart, uterus, CNS, PNS (glia-specific)

Table 2: Subtypes of voltage-gated sodium channel α-subunits: nomenclature and distribution (Goldin et al., 2000)

CNS / PNS: central / peripheral nervous system.

In neuropathic pain conditions, TTX-resistant channels are downregulated and hyperexcitability of the injured primary sensory neurons is predominantly due to TTX-sensitive channels

Following nerve injury or inflammation of innervated peripheral tissue, primary sensory neurons become hyperexcitable showing spontaneous firing or abnormal high-frequency activity characteristic for chronic pain situations (Nordin et al., 1984; Zhang et al., 1997; Amir et al., 1999). At the same time, the sodium channel subtypes $Na_V1.3$, $Na_V1.7$, $Na_V1.8$ and $Na_V1.9$ are distinguished by preferential distribution in primary sensory neurons and by temporally- and regionally-specific regulation of gene expression, respectively, which qualifies them as potential drug targets for selective treatment of chronic pain. The mRNA of $Na_V1.3$, which is expressed in embryonic, but not adult spinal sensory neurons, is re-expressed in animal models following injury of peripheral nerves either by axotomy or by chronic constriction injury (Waxman et al., 1994; Dib-Hajj et al., 1999; Kim et al., 2001). Since $Na_V1.3$ sodium channels are rapidly repriming, their upregulation might give rise to abnormal high-frequency activity which is recorded in dorsal root ganglions (DRGs) after nerve injury (Amir et al., 1999; Cummins et al., 2001). The $Na_V1.7$ channel, which is highly expressed in DRGs under normal conditions, shows a unique ability to activate upon slow membrane depolarization and has the ability to amplify small excitatory inputs like sensory generator potentials close to resting potential (Cummins et al., 1998). Therefore, the $Na_V1.7$ channel might play a crucial role in modulation of spontaneous activity of DRG neurons. Additionally, two distinct TTX-resistant (TTX-R) sodium channels $Na_V1.8$ and $Na_V1.9$ are densely expressed within a subpopulation of small- and medium-diameter, unmyelinated DRG neurons referred to as nociceptors (Akopian et al., 1996; Tate et al., 1998). Strong evidence for the important role of $Na_V1.8$ in chronic pain situations was revealed by Porreca et al. (1999) showing that intrathecal application of antisense oligo-deoxynucleotide (ODN) to $Na_V1.8$ prevented tactile allodynia as well as thermal hyperalgesia in rat models for neuropathic pain (spinal nerve injury model) and for chronic inflammatory pain (Complete Freund's adjuvant injection). Administration of antisense ODN to $Na_V1.9$, however, did not change pain behavior in neuropathic rats. On the other hand, mRNA for both TTX-R sodium channels are downregulated in the ipsilateral DRG, but are aggregated at the distal tip of injured neurons and upregulated in adjacent, uninjured DRG neurons after axotomy and chronic constriction injury (Dib-Hajj et al., 1996, 1998, 1999; Tzoumaka et al., 1997; Novakovic et al., 1998; Wood et al., 2002). As in animal models, $Na_V1.8$ and $Na_V1.9$ are also highly expressed in human DRGs and, several days after peripheral sensory nerve injury, they are downregulated in the DRG and accumulate at the site of injury (Coward et al., 2000). The nerve damage-induced regulation of gene expression indicates that hyperexcitability in the respective DRG is predominantly due to TTX-S, and not to TTX-R channels. In fact, in animal models for neuropathic pain, increased firing rates of sensory neurons as well as the pain behavior is sensitive to low doses of TTX (Amir et al., 1999; Lyu et al., 2000). The role of TTX-R sodium channels upregulated at the site of injury and in the uninjured adjacent DRG remains to be elucidated (Waxman et al., 2000).

In contrast to neuropathic pain conditions, the mRNAs for $Na_v1.8$ and $Na_v1.9$ are upregulated in DRGs in chronic inflammatory pain models (Tanaka et al., 1998; Tate et al., 1998). Furthermore, a potentiation of sodium currents through $Na_v1.8$ channels by inflammatory mediators (e.g. prostaglandins, serotonin) probably via PKA-dependent phosphorylation has been shown (England et al., 1996; Gold et al., 1996; Fitzgerald et al., 1999). The inactivation kinetics of TTX-R sodium currents is about 10-fold slower than for TTX-S (about 5 ms versus 0.5 ms; Cummins and Waxman, 1997) thus giving rise to persistent TTX-R sodium currents. At the resting membrane potential of DRG neurons which is usually in the range of -55 to -60 mV (Zhang et al., 1997), more TTX-R Na_v 1.8 channels than TTX-S channels are in the resting state and can be activated by depolarizing stimuli as indicated by their relatively high voltage of half-maximal inactivation (Table 3). As a result of their functional properties together with their upregulation and potentiation by inflammatory mediators, TTX-R channels induce increased, persistent sodium conductance and hence might play an important role in generation of hyperexcitability in inflammatory pain conditions.

In inflammatory pain conditions, TTX-resistant channels are upregulated and play an improtant role in generation of hyperexcitability of primary sensory neurons

Table 3: Subtypes of voltage-gated sodium channel α-subunits: biophysical properties and TTX-sensitivity. V½: potential of 50 % activation or inactivation, respectively.

Channel	Activation V½	Inactivation V½	TTX-Block, IC_{50}
$Na_v1.3$	-26 mV [1]	-64.9 mV [1]	0.0018 µM [2]
$Na_v1.7$	-31 mV [3]	-78 mV [3]	0.0043 µM [3]
$Na_v1.8$	+ 13 mV [4]	-54 mV [4]	>100 µM [5]
$Na_v1.9$	-45 mV [6]	-44 mV [7]	1 µM [6]

[1]Cummins et al., 2001; [2] Joho et al., 1990, [3]Sangameswaran et al., 1997; [4]Koch et al., 1997; [5]Sangameswaran, 1996; [6] Tate et al., 1998; [7] Cummins et al., 1999.

Despite considerable efforts to develop subtype-specific sodium channel blockers, there are no specific compounds available as yet

The diversity of sodium channels indicates a complex interaction in modulation of the sensory neuronal activity which might be severely disturbed after dysregulation in neuropathic and inflammatory pain conditions. TTX-R and TTX-S sodium channels in primary sensory neurons can be blocked by several drugs with anti-neuropathic properties such as lidocaine, carbamazepine, lamotrigine and mexilitine in animal models and in patients (Roy and Narahashi, 1992; Xie et al., 1996; Bräu et al., 2001). However, these compounds are not selective for pain-relevant subtypes of sodium channels and despite considerable chemical efforts, there are no specific compounds available as yet. The development of new technologies for functional high-throughput screens (e.g. fluorescence resonance energy transfer (FRET); Gonzalez et al., 1999) should facilitate selective sodium channel drug discovery.

Sodium Channel Blockers in Clinical Use

Local Anesthetic drugs (LAs)

LAs block nerve conduction when applied locally to nervous tissue by a voltage- and frequency-dependent inhibition of sodium currents (see 'Voltage-gated Sodium Channels: Structure and Function'). Due to this mechanism, they preferentially block hyperexcitable cells and interfere comparatively less with normal physiological sensory and motor function. However, they are not selective for pain-relevant sodium channel subtypes so that they have a relatively high risk of adverse effects associated with the central nervous and cardiovascular systems when administered systemically. Known LAs are not active when administered orally.

Local anesthetic drugs block sodium channels in a voltage- and frequency-dependent manner. They are not selective for pain-relevant subtypes of sodium channels

LAs are reported to bind in a charged form within the pore of sodium channels near the cytoplasmic surface of the plasma membrane (for review see Butterworth and Strichartz, 1990; Tetzlaff, 2000). Before binding LAs have to cross the lipid layer of the plasma membrane probably in an uncharged form. The common structure of LAs is a hydrophilic moiety (usually a tertiary amine) linked by a short alkyl chain and an ester or amide group to a hydrophobic moiety (usually an aromatic residue). The linkage is enzymatically degraded in the plasma.

Local anesthetic drugs probably bind to sodium channels in a charged form after they have penetrated the lipid plasma membrane in an uncharged form which explains why physico-chemical porperties largely determine their clinical properties including potency, onset and duration of action, and toxicitiy

The pharmacological activity of LAs is determined by several physicochemical properties including lipophilicity, protein binding, and pKa which can be explained by their mechanism of action. A general structure - activity relationship was described by Courtney and Strichartz (1987), according to which an increase in the hydrophobicity leads to a parallel increase in anesthetic potency and duration of action, but also an increase in toxicity which results from an improved access to the binding site within the membrane, leading to reduced degradation by plasma enzymes. These effects are further enhanced by high plasma protein binding. The pKa determines the onset of action: the lower the pKa value, the higher the percentage of the neutral form which can penetrate the plasma membrane.

Following plasma uptake by the vasculature of the tissue or after unintentional intravascular injection, LAs interfere with the function of all organs in which transmission of impulses occur due to their non-selective block of sodium currents, thus giving rise to adverse effects especially in the central nervous, cardiac and vascular systems. In fact, with high plasma concentrations LAs can induce tonic-clonic convulsions and cardiovascular depression possibly leading to severe ventricular arrhythmias. Therefore, it is essential that the main dose of LAs is injected incrementally until satisfactory anesthesia is achieved and with sufficient pauses between each bolus to allow observation of any systemic consequences. Furthermore, with application of a LA with a relatively high risk of systemic side-effects or for treatment in children or pregnant patients, the upper drug concentration of the preparation is limited. Allergic reactions to local anaesthetics are rare and are usually related to the presence of an ester function.

Table 4. Local anesthetic drugs: Physicochemical properties and plasma protein binding.

Drug	LogP	Protein binding	pKa
Benzocaine	1.86 [4]	-	3.5 [2]
Bupivacaine	3.41 [3]	95.5 % [1]	8.2 [1]
Cocaine	2.45 [4]	91 % [4]	8.8 [4]
Etidocaine	3.69 [3]	94 % [5]	7.7 [2]
Lidocaine	2.48 [3]	64 % [1]	7.8 [1]
Levobupivacaine	*	93.4 % [1]	8.2 [1]
Mepivacaine	1.95 [3]	77 % [1]	7.8 [1]
Prilocaine	8.0 [5]	55 % [1]	7.8 [1]
Procaine	1.91 [3]	6 % [5]	8.9 [2]
Ropivacaine	2.90 [3]	94 % [1]	8.2 [1]
Tetracaine	3.56 [3]	76 % [5]	8.6 [2]

[1]Whiteside and Wildsmith, 2001; [2]Tetzlaff, 2000; [3]Strichartz et al., 1990; [4] Dr. K. Fuchte, Grünenthal GmbH, personal communication; [5] Büch and Rummel, 1996, * (S)-enantiomer of bupivacaine.

When tolerability of the compound is sufficient to allow systemic administration, local anesthetic drugs can be employed for relief of neuropathic pain and acute treatment of migraine headache in addition to the broad application for local anesthesia as proven for lidocaine

In clinical practice, LAs are applied for topical anesthesia using solutions, creams or patches, for infiltration anesthesia (injection directly into the wound), for field block anesthesia (parallel margin infiltration), for nerve block anesthesia (injection into or around a peripheral nerve), for intravenous regional anesthesia and for spinal anesthesia with intrathecal and epidural injection. Aiming at a prolongation of action and a reduction in plasma uptake, clinical preparations of LAs often contain a vasoconstrictor like adrenaline (1 : 200,000) to reduce local tissue perfusion. However, care must be taken to avoid tissue ischemia in areas without collateral blood supply such as nose, penis, fingers, or ears. In addition to these traditional applications of LAs to provide surgical anesthesia and analgesia for acute pain, LAs are also found to be effective in chronic pain conditions including neuropathic pain syndromes and acute migraine headache when administered systemically (for review see Backonja, 1994).

The chemical search for synthetic substitutes started in 1892 and gave rise to several compounds with improved properties which largely replaced the naturally occurring cocaine.

The natural substance cocaine was already beeing employed for local anesthesia in ophthalmological surgery in 1884 (Vandam, 1987). However, the clinical use of cocaine is limited because of its abuse potential, its intense vasoconstriction and eventual arrhythmias due to its reuptake-inhibition of catecholamines, and instability upon sterilization. The chemical search for synthetic substitutes started in 1892 and gave rise to several compounds without abuse potential and with improved onset and duration of action, tolerability and stability of the preparation.

Benzocaine

Benzocaine

4-Amino-benzoic acid ethyl ester, $C_9H_{11}NO_2$, MW 165.19, [94-07-7}

Anaesthesine® (Germany), Auralgan® , Tympagesic® (USA)

Benzocaine is an ester local anesthetic with a moderate onset of action and short duration. It is minimally absorbed and therfore relatively free from systemic adverse effects (toxic range of total dose: 200 to 300 mg; Tetzlaff, 2000).

Clinical use: Due to the low lipophilicity and therefore the low ability to penetrate neuronal membranes, the clinical use of benzocaine is limited to topical anesthesia such as mucous membrane anesthesia prior to endoscopic examination or for temporary relief of oral or dental pain. With higher doses, oxidation of the ferric form of hemoglobin to the ferrous form can occur; the resulting methemoglobinemia is usually benign and can be reversed with methylene blue. Benzocaine is more likely to cause contact sensitization than amide-type LAs.

Bupivacaine

Synthesis (Kleemann et al., 1999):

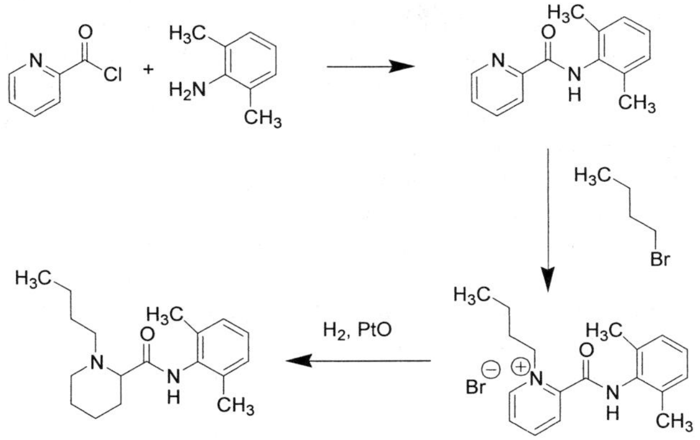

Bupivacaine

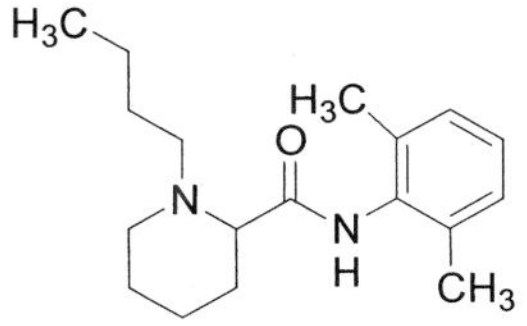

1-Butyl-piperidine-2-carboxylic acid (2,6-dimethyl-phenyl)-amide, $C_{18}H_{28}N_2O$, MW 288.44, [2180-92-9]

Trade names: Marcaine® (F, GB), Sensorcaine® (USA), Bupivacain® (D)

Bupivacaine

Alternative synthesis (Ekenstam and Egner, 1957; Kleemann et al., 1999):

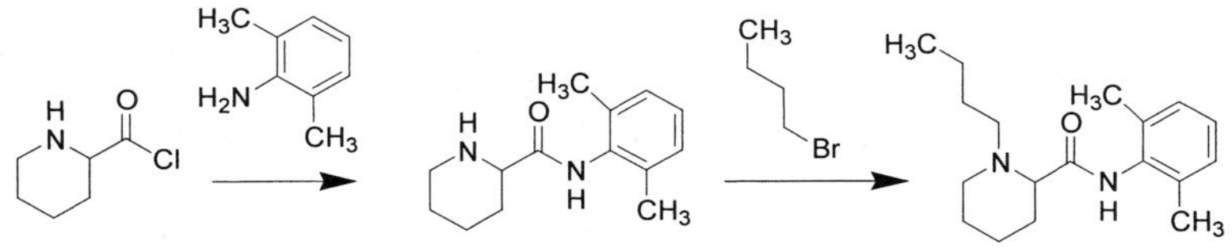

Scheme 1: Synthesis of bupivacaine.

The racemic compound bupivacaine, which was first synthesized by Ekenstam et al. in 1957, is an amide-type LA with a high lipophilicity, protein binding and pKa giving rise to an intermediate onset and a long duration of action. At the same time, bupivacaine has a high toxicity potential relatively often associated with convulsions and life-threatening cardivascular collapse (Moore et al., 1978). Levobupivacaine, the (*S*)-enantiomer of bupivacaine, has recently been developed for clinical use addressing the enantioselectivity of side-effects of bupivacaine (see below).

Clinical use: Because of its long duration of action, bupivacaine is indicated for long surgical anesthesia where a considerable amount of postoperative pain is expected such as dental and oral surgeries. Infiltration using a 0.25 % solution of bupivacaine produces sensory anesthesia with an onset of 2 to 5 min and a duration of 2 to 4 h or greater (Tetzlaff, 2000). A nerve conduction block with a duration of between 4 to 8 h and occasionally up to 24 h is achieved with injection of 0.5 to 0.75 %

Bupivacaine is a long-acting local anesthetic drug and has a high risk of side-effects which are enantio-selective and mainly associated with the (*R*)-enantiomer

bupivacaine often combined with adrenaline as an vasoconstrictor to decrease plasma uptake. For epidural analgesia employed in perioperative settings, bupivacaine is infused at a concentration of 0.1 or 0.25 % to an upper dose of 150 mg for surgery and 60 mg for labour (Singh and Erwin, 1998; Mandabach, 1999). Careful monitoring of the patient is necessary to avoid motor block and hypotension. A combination with opioids, e.g. 0.1 % bupivacaine with 10 µg/ml fentanyl, is infused epidurally for postoperative analgesia with satisfactory results. Bupivacaine with dextrose is used for spinal analgesia.

With local infiltration, toxic side-effects like convulsions and cardiovascular collaps occur in the dose range of 2.5 to 3 mg/kg body weight. Because of its systemic toxicity, bupivacaine is contraindicated for intravenous regional anesthesia.

Etidocaine

Etidocaine

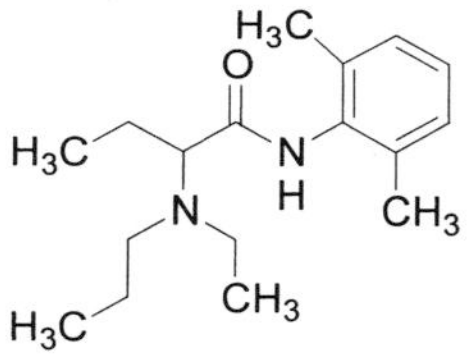

N-(2,6-Dimethyl-phenyl)-2-
(ethyl-propyl-amino)-
butyramide, $C_{17}H_{28}N_2O$, MW
276.43, [36637-18-0]

Duranest®

Etidocaine is a long-acting amide LA with a physicochemical and clinical profile similar to bupivacaine. Toxic side-effects occur at total doses of 300 to 400 mg. It is clinically available in combination with the vasoconstrictor adrenaline.

Synthesis (Adams et al., 1974; Kleemann et al., 1999):

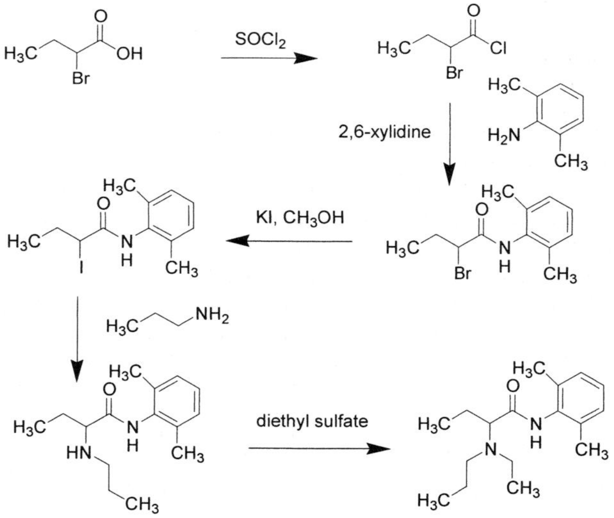

Scheme 2: Synthesis of etidocaine.

Clinical use: Etidocaine in combination with adrenaline is employed for infiltration anesthesia using solutions of 0.5% and peripheral nerve block at 0.5 and 1.0 % with a duration of 3 to 12 h (Tetzlaff, 2000). Epidural anesthesia is achieved with 1.0 to 1.5 % solutions with a duration of 3 to 5 h. Due to a profound motor block sometimes associated with unsatisfactory sensory block etidocaine is disadvantegous compared to bupivacaine.

Levobupivacaine

When the enantioselectivity of the cardiotoxicity of bupivacaine became apparent in preclinical models and in healthy human volunteers (Aberg, 1972; Bardsley et al., 1998), its (*S*)-enantiomer levobupivacaine was developed and finally approved as an alternative long-acting LA in 1999. The majority of preclinical and clinical studies indicate a similar potency, but lower risk of cardiovascular and, at least in preclinical investigations, fewer central side-effects. Levobupivacaine is vasoconstrictive in lower doses (up to 0.1 ml of 0.125 % solutions; Aps and Reynolds, 1978), which explains its longer duration of conduction block than that of bupivacaine, and vasodilatory at higher doses upon intradermal infiltration in healthy human volunteers. In adults, the recommended maximum single dose for surgical anesthesia is 150 mg. As for bupivacaine, the onset of action of levobupivacaine is slow (up to 15 min) with different methods of administration (for review see Foster and Markham, 2000; Whiteside and Wildsmith, 2001).

Clinical use: The indications for levobupivacaine include wound infiltration (0.25 % solution), nerve conduction block (0.25 - 0.5 %), spinal analgesia (0.5 %) and epidural anesthesia (0.5 to 0.75 %). For labour analgesia, lower concentrations of levobupivacaine are recommended when administered as epidural injection (0.125 to 0.25 % up to 25 mg) or infusion (0.25 %). The maximum dose for ilioinguinal or iliohypogastric block in children is 1.25 mg/kg/side (0.25 to 0.5 % solutions). For postoperative pain management, levobupivacaine can be applied epidurally in combination with the opioids fentanyl or morphine or with the α_2-agonist clonidine.

The most common side-effect of levobupivacaine is hypotension. Therefore, levobupivacaine is contra-indicated for in intravenous regional block and patients with severe hypotension.

Levobupivacaine

(S)-(-)-Bupivacaine

(S)-1-Butyl-piperidine-2-carboxylic acid (2,6-dimethyl-phenyl)-amide, $C_{18}H_{28}N_2O$, MW 288.44, [27262-47-1]

Chirocaine®

Synthesis: cp. Bupivacaine

Levobupivacaine, the (S)-enantiomer of bupivacaine, was developed as an alternative long-lasting local anesthetic compound with a similar potency, but improved tolerability.

Lidocaine

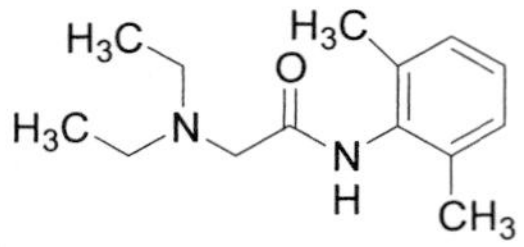

2-Diethylamino-N-(2,6-
dimethyl-phenyl)-acetamide,
$C_{14}H_{22}N_2O$, MW 234.34,
[137-58-6]

Xylocaine®, Gelicain®,
Lidocaine®

Emla®

Lidoderm®

Lidocaine (Lignocaine)

Lidocaine (synonyme: lignocaine) was introduced as the first amide in 1944 and is the most commonly used LA today. It has a rapid onset of action with intermediate duration and an intermediate toxicity. The maximum tolerated dose with infiltration or injection is 200 mg (500 mg when combined with adrenaline). Lidocaine is dealkylated in the liver to monoethylglycine xylidide and glycine xylidide which retain local anesthetic activity. It is available in a variety of preparations including creams, gels, patches and solutions, often in combination with adrenaline.

Synthesis (Löfgren and Lundquist, 1948; Kleemann et al., 1999):

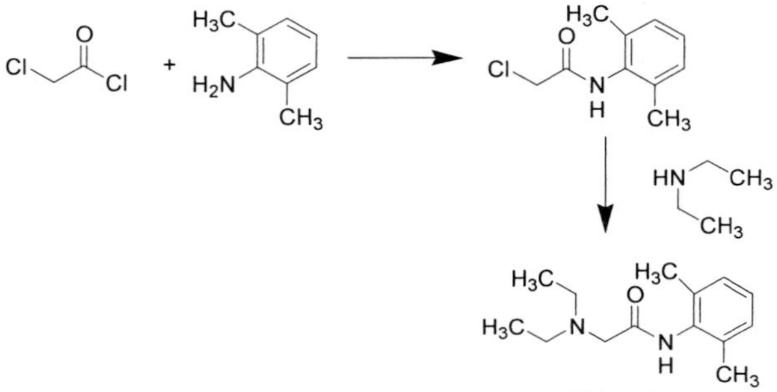

Scheme 3: Synthesis of lidocaine.

Lidocaine is the most commonly used local anesthetic drug. In addition to its effectiveness for local anesthesia, it provides relief of neuropathic pain and acute migraine headache

Clinical use: Topical anesthesia is easiliy performed using 1 to 2 g/10 cm² skin of an eutectic mixture of the LAs (EMLA) lidocaine and prilocaine. Onset of action is achieved between 15 to 120 min depending on the tissue vascularization. Since EMLA is as effective as infiltration anesthesia, but avoids puncture pain and is usually well tolerated due to low risk of systemic absorption, it is widley used for procedures such as superficial skin surgery or lumbar puncture, especially in children. Effective relief of neuropathic pain was achieved with topical administration of lidocaine using a 5% gel or patch formulation (Rowbotham et al., 1995; Devers and Galer, 2000).

When used for infiltration anesthesia, a 1% solution is used which produces anesthesia within 2-3 min lasting for 2 to 4 h. On injection of 1.0 to 1.5 % lidocaine a peripheral nerve conduction block can be achieved with an onset of action of 4 to 10 min and a duration of 1 to 3 h, which can be prolonged with co-administration of adrenaline (Tetzlaff, 2000). Lidocaine is used for intravenous regional anesthesia at a concentration of 0.5 % with a duration of 45 to 60 min. For epidural anesthesia, lidocaine is administered at a concentration of 1.5 to 2.0 % in combination with adrenaline and also with an opioid, e.g. fentanyl (Mandabach, 1999). Injection of lidocaine in a concentration of 5 % in a hyperbaric solution containing 7.5 % glucose is used for spinal anesthesia with a duration of 45 to 90 min.

Systemic injection of lidocaine was also shown to be effective and well tolerated in patients suffering from several neuropathic pain syndromes. Significant relief was reported in patients with neuropathic pain after peripheral nerve damage (Wallace et al., 1996) and after spinal cord injuries and stroke (Attal et al., 2000) and in patients with diabetic neuropathic pain (Kastrup et al., 1987), with postherpetic neuralgia (Rowbotham et al., 1991) and with fibromyalgia (Ellemann et al., 1989). Clinical data concerning cancer-related pain are inconsitent. While Brose and Cousins (1991) found an improvement after systemic lidocaine, there are other clinical trials showing no difference between lidocaine and placebo (Ellemann et al., 1989; Bruera et al., 1992).

Preclinical and clinical data indicate that lidocaine administered by intravenous injection or intranasally is effective in acute treatment of migraine (Bell et al., 1990; Kaube et al., 1994; Maizels, et al., 1996).

In addition to its use for anesthesia and analgesia, lidocaine is also used for acute treatment of ventricular arrhythmias.

Mepivacaine

Mepivacaine is an amide-type LA with a rapid onset, intermediate duration and intermediate toxicity. It has a slight vasoconstrictor action and produces less vasodilatation compared with lidocaine. The daily dose of mepivacaine should not exeed 400 mg.

Clinical use: Mepivacaine has been employed for all types of infiltration and conduction nerve block anesthesia using solutions of 1.0 and 1.5 % lasting for 1.5 to 3 h. Epidural anesthesia with 2.0 % mepivacaine has a rapid onset with a dense motor block. Hyperbaric solutions of mepivacaine have also been used for spinal anesthesia (Tetzlaff, 2000). Mepivacaine has been used for topical applications, but other LA such as lidocaine are more effective.

Mepivacaine

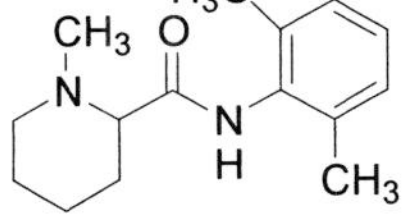

1-Methyl-piperidine-2-carboxylic acid (2,6-dimethyl-phenyl)-amide, $C_{15}H_{22}N_2O$, MW 246.35, [22801-44-1]

Carbocaine[®], Polocaine[®], Isocaine[®], Scandicaine[®]

Bloms-Funke

Synthesis (Ekenstam and Egner, 1957; Kleemann et al., 1999)

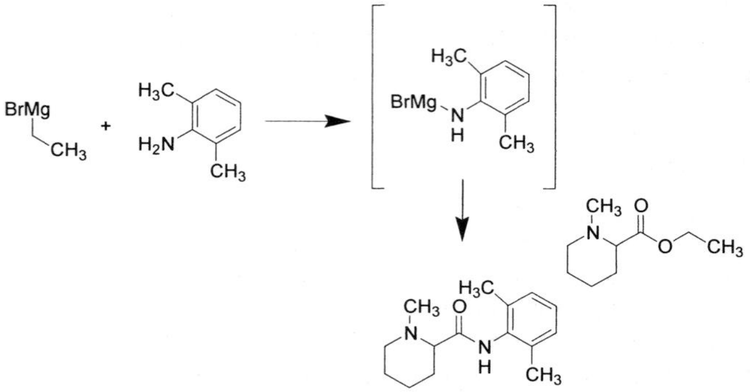

Mepivacaine

Scheme 4: Synthesis of mepivacaine.

Prilocaine

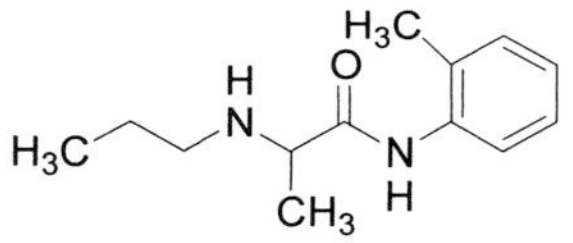

Prilocaine

2-Propylamino-N-o-tolyl-propionamide, $C_{13}H_{20}N_2O$, MW 220.32, [721-50-6]

Citanest $^{®}$, Xylonest $^{®}$ (G)

EMLA Creme$^{®}$ (G), Emlapatch$^{®}$ (GB), Emla$^{®}$ (USA)

Prilocaine is an amide-type LA with a rapid onset and an intermediate duration of action associated with a low toxicity. However, metabolism to ortho-toluidine can cause oxidation of the ferric form of hemoglobin to the ferrous form, creating methemoglobin. In most cases the methemoglobuniemia is benign, but sometimes tissue hypoxia is observed (Eriksson, 1966).

Synthesis (Löfgren et al., 1958; Kleemann et al., 1999):

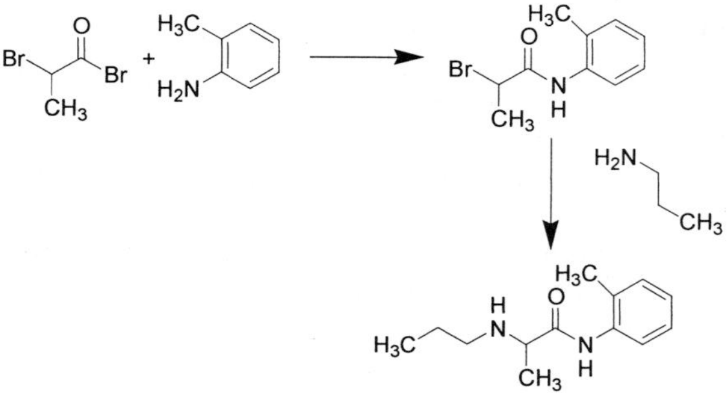

Prilocaine

Scheme 5: Synthesis of prilocaine.

Clinical use: Topical anesthesia is easily achieved using an eutectic mixture of the LAs prilocaine and lidocaine (EMLA, see Lidocaine).

With infiltration of 0.5 to 1.0% prilocaine local anesthesia with a duration of 1 to 2 h is established. Peripheral nerve block is achieved with 1.5 to 2.0 % with a duration of 2 to 3

h. Upon peripheral application, the toxic dose is in the range of 600 mg (Teztlaff, 2000). Because of its low toxicity, prilocaine is also used for intravenous regional anesthesia. Epidural anesthesia with 2 to 3 % prilocaine gives satisfactory results for 1 to 3 h.

Procaine

Procaine, a para-aminobenzoic acid ester, was the first synthetic LA synthesized in 1904. It has a slow onset of action and a short duration and hence low toxicity. Due to its extremely low binding to plasma proteins (only 6 %) procaine is rapidly hydrolyzed by plasma cholinesterases to diethylaminoethanol and para-aminobenzoic acid, which inhibit the actions of salicylates and sulfonamides (Tetzlaff, 2000).

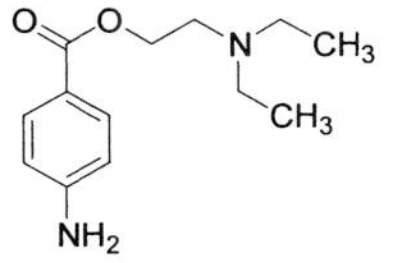

Synthesis (Kleemann and al., 1999):

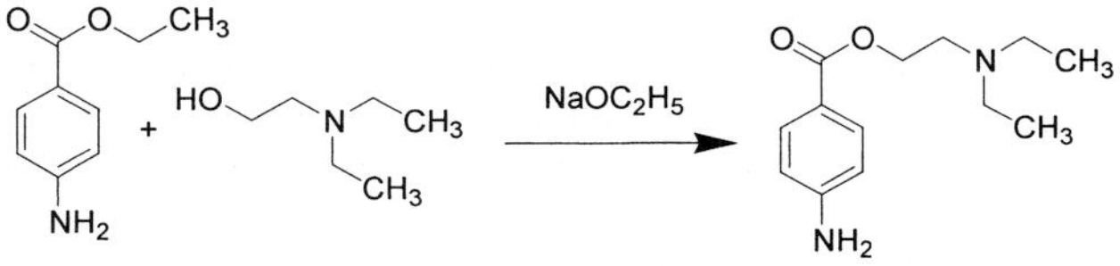

Procaine

4-Amino-benzoic acid 2-diethylamino-ethyl ester, $C_{13}H_{20}N_2O_2$, MW 236.32, [59-46-1]

Novocaine[®]

Scheme 6: Synthesis of procaine.

Clinical use: Because of its poor penetration of intact mucous membranes, procaine is largely ineffective for topical applications and has been mainly used in injection in combination with adrenaline, although in general it has been replaced by other LAs such as lidocaine. For infiltration anesthesia, 0.25 to 0.5 % solutions of procaine have been used in doses up to 600 mg. For peripheral nerve block, a common dose of 500 mg of procaine has been given as a 0.5 to 2.0 % solution.

Ropivacaine

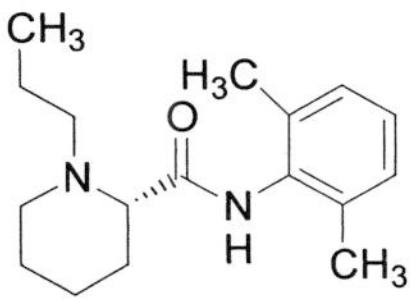

In addition to levobupivacaine, ropivacaine is a new long-lasting amide-type LA that has been produced in order to address the enantioselectivity of the cardiotoxicity of bupivacaine. Ropivacaine, which is an (S)-enantiomer containing an n-propyl instead of the butyl moiety of bupivacaine, was launched in 2000. Clinical data indicate a late onset and long duration of action and the anesthetic potency of ropivacaine is comparable to that of bupivacaine (for review see McClellan and Faulds, 2000; Whiteside and Wildsmith, 2001). In animal models, the

1-Propyl-piperidine-2-carboxylic acid (2,6-dimethyl-phenyl)-amide, $C_{17}H_{26}N_2O$, MW 310.87, [98717-15-8]

cardiotoxic side-effects of ropivacaine are intermediate between that of mepivacaine and bupivacaine. The maximum recommended single dose of ropivacaine is 300 mg. Ropivacaine has slight vasoconstrictor effects in lower doses in healthy human volunteers (Cederholm et al., 1994).

Naropin®, Naropeine®

Synthesis (Thuresson et al., 1985; Kleemann et al., 1999):

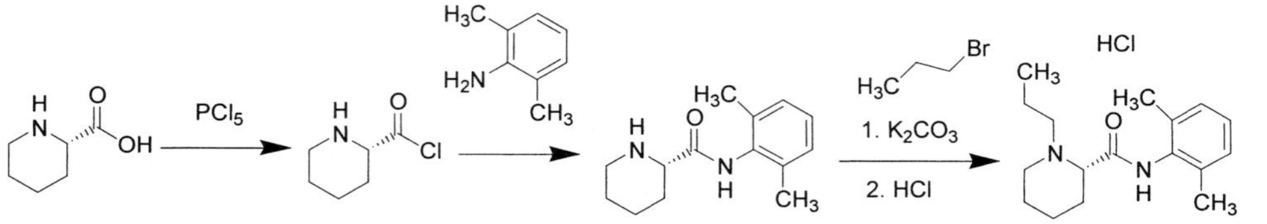

Ropivacaine hydrochloride

Scheme 7: Synthesis of ropivacaine..

Ropivacaine, which is an (*S*)-enantiomer, is a new long-lasting amide local anesthetic drug that has been produced in order to address the enantioselectivity of the cardiotoxicity of bupivacaine.

Clinical use: Ropivacaine is used for local infiltrations such as field block (0.75 % solution) and for nerve block (0.75 %) up to 300 mg and for epidural anesthesia (0.75 and 1.0 %) up to 200 mg. When used for labour analgesia, epidural doses up to 40 mg are recommended. A combination of opioids is often administered via the epidural route for postoperative analgesia.

Hypotension was the most commomly reported side-effect. Co-administration with opioids may raise the incidence of hypotension, nausea, and pruritus (Scott et al., 1999).

Tetracaine

Tetracaine

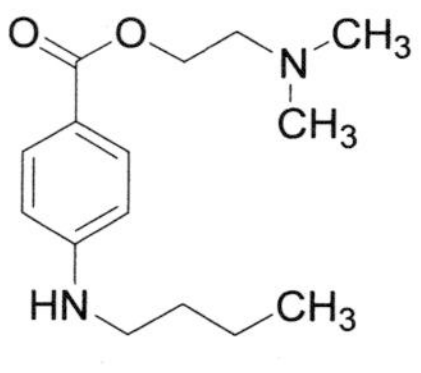

4-Butylamino-benzoic acid 2-dimethylamino-ethyl ester, $C_{15}H_{24}N_2O_2$, MW 264.37, [94-24-6]

Pontocaine®

Tetracaine, an ester of para-aminobenzoic acid, has a slow onset, very short plasma half-life of 2.5 to 4 min and a long duration of action. Toxic effects are rare and only in the case of vascular absorbance from mucous membranes.

Clinical use: Tetracaine is employed by ophthalmologists for surface anesthesia as a 0.5 % solution and by endoscopists for anesthesia of mucous membranes including airways as a 2.0 % solution. For topical anesthesia, a 4.0 % cream of tetracaine can also be used, which is, however, less effective than a lidocaine/prilocaine cream in preventing venipuncture-induced pain in children (van Kan et al., 1997). A combination of tetracaine with adrenaline and cocaine (TAC) is widely used for repair of lacerations to the face or scalp in children (Singh and Erwin, 1998). Tetracaine is commonly used for spinal analgesia at a total dose of 5 to 20 mg often in combination with other LAs with shorter duration in order to prolong anesthesia (Tetzlaff, 2000).

Synthesis (Kleemann et al., 1999; Eisleb, 1932):

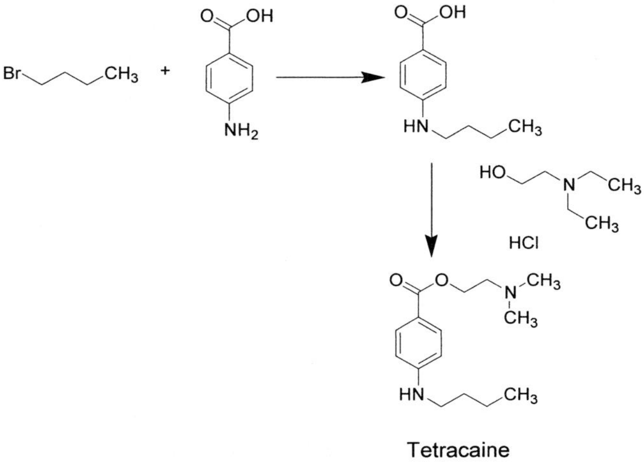

Tetracaine

Scheme 8: Synthesis of tetracaine.

Anticonvulsant Drugs

Over the past few years, it has become increasingly apparent that anticonvulsant drugs are effective in neuropathic pain conditions in animal models and in patients (for review see McQuay, et al., 1995; Tremont-Lukats et al., 2000). Among the large number of anticonvulsant drugs this review will focus on carbamazepine, oxcarbazepine, lamotrigine, and phenytoin whose main mechanism is a voltage- and frequency-dependent block of sodium channels (see 'Voltage-gated Sodium Channels: Structure and Function'). As a result, they preferentially block highly active cells in pain pathways. However, they are not selective for pain-relevant sodium channel subtypes so that adverse effects associated with the central nervous and the cardiovascular systems occur. One of the advantages of the anticonvulsant sodium channel blockers over the local anesthetic lidocaine is that they are orally active.

Anticonvulsant drugs, which block voltage-gated sodium channels in a voltage- and frequency-dependent manner, are used to relief neuropathic pain and for migraine prophylaxis. They appear to have particular utility when there is a paroxysmal, lancinating component as in trigeminal neuralgia. The anticonvulsant drugs are not selective for pain-relevant sodium channel subtypes.

Carbamazepine

Carbamazepine

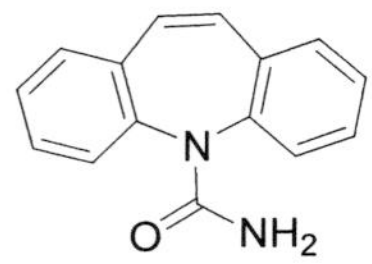

Dibenzo[b,f]azepine-5-
carboxylic acid amide,
$C_{15}H_{12}N_2O$, MW 236.27,
[298-46-4]

Tegretal®, Tegretol®

Carbamazepine is
recommended as the drug
of first choice in the
treatment of trigeminal
neuralgia

In 1962, Blom was the first to report the analgesic properties of carbamazepine in neuropathic pain conditions. In clinical studies in patients suffering from trigeminal neuralgia, oral doses of up to 2400 mg/day for 5 to 14 days produced moderate to excellent results (Campbell et al., 1966; Killian and Fromm, 1968; Nicol, 1969). In fact, carbamazepine is recommended as the drug of first choice in the treatment of trigeminal neuralgia. Results from clinical trials have been positive in the treatment of painful diabetic neuropathy (Rull et al., 1969; Wilton, 1974; Gomez-Perez et al., 1996). After 4 weeks treatment with carbamazepine, central pain after stroke was improved only in five out of 14 patients (Leijon and Boivie, 1989). Carbamazepine was found to be effective for migraine prophylaxis (Rompel and Bauermeister, 1970).

Synthesis (Kleemann et al., 1999):

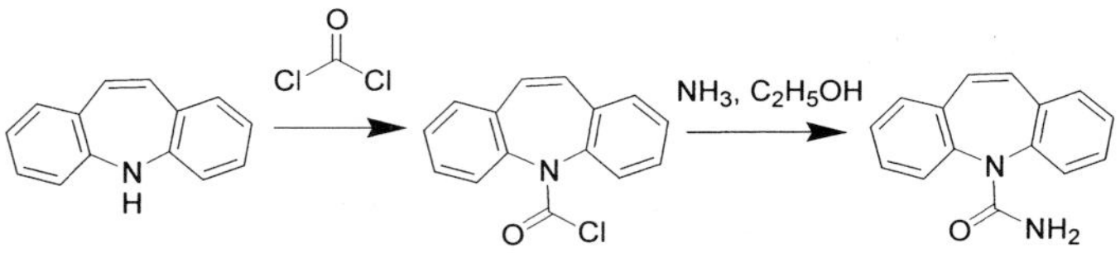

Carbamazepine

Scheme 9: Synthesis of carbamazepine.

The most common side-effects in clinical trials among pain patients were moderate and largely associated with the central nervous system (i.e. sedation, tremor and incoordination). From its broad application as an anticonvulsant since the early 1960s, however, additional rare, but severe adverse effects are known including hematological changes such as aplastic anemia, hepatotoxicity and teratogenicity (for review see Perucca et al., 2000). The 10,11- double bond of carbamazepine is oxidized to an active epoxide metabolite and due to a remarkable induction of drug-metabolizing enzymes in the liver, carbamazepine is associated with intense drug interactions.

In addition to its use for the management of epilepsy and neuropathic pain, carbamazepine is employed for the treatment of manic depression (for review see Elphick,1989).

Lamotrigine

In patients with trigeminal neuralgia, some of whom may be resistant to carbamazepine, lamotrigine in oral doses up to 400 mg/day affords considerable and in some cases complete pain relief. Thus, lamotrigine offers an alternative approach for the management of trigeminal neuralgia (Canavero and Bonicalzi, 1997; Lunardi et al., 1997; Zakrzewska et al., 1997). Lamotrigine in daily doses up to 400 mg is effective in a dose-dependent manner in modulating and controlling diabetic neuropathic pain, as shown in one open and one randomized, placebo-controlled clinical trial (Eisenberg et al., 1988; Luria et al., 2000). In the treatment of painful human immuno-deficiency virus (HIV) -associated peripheral neuropathy, lamotrigine in doses up to 300 mg/day produced effective pain relief versus placebo (Simpson et al., 2000). A clinical study in patients with central post-stroke pain indicates significant improvements with lamotrigine treatment for 8 weeks (200 mg/day).

Lamotrigine

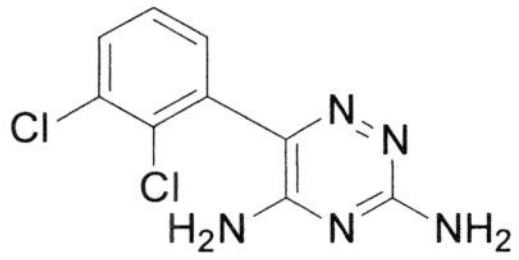

6-(2,3-Dichloro-phenyl)-[1,2,4]triazine-3,5-diamine, $C_9H_7Cl_2N_5$, MW 256.10, [84057-84-1]

Lamictal®

Lamotrigine, which has been shown to be effective in several neuropathic pain conditions, offers an alternative approach to carbamazepine for the management of trigeminal neuralgia

Synthesis (Kleemann et al., 1999):

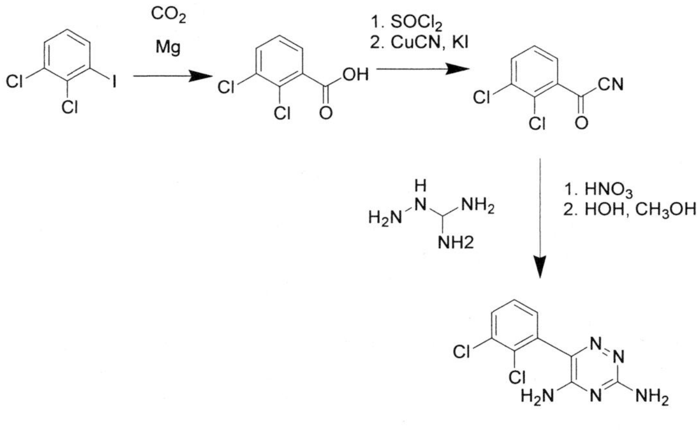

Scheme 10: Synthesis of lamotrigine.

Lamotrigine in doses up to 100 mg/kg/day was successful in migraine prophylaxis as shown in two clinical studies (D'Andrea et al., 1999; Lampl et al., 1999); however, a third study did not show significant effects versus placebo (Steiner et al., 1997). Further controlled trials are warranted to further validate the effectiveness of lamotrigine in prophylactic migraine treatment.

Side-effects are rare and include gastrointestinal adverse effects, skin rashes and headache.

Oxcarbazepine

Oxcarbazepine

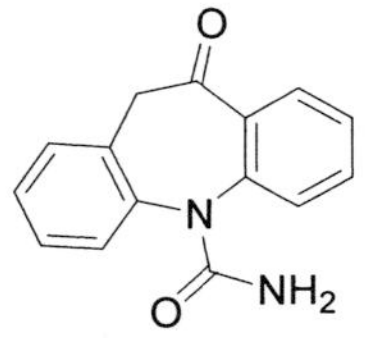

10-Oxo-10,11-dihydro-
dibenzo[b,f]azepine-5-
carboxylic acid amide,
$C_{15}H_{12}N_2O_2$, MW 252.27,
[28721-07-5]

Trileptal®

Oxcarbazepine is a sodium channel blocker which is structurally related to carbamazepine (McLean et al., 1994), but which has the advantage of a lower risk of drug interactions: In humans, it is rapidly and completely degraded to the active 10-monohydroxy metabolite and does not induce drug-metabolizing enzymes in the liver, so that comparatively few drug interactions are associated with this therapy (Feldmann et al., 1978). Administered orally, oxcarbazepine has been shown to be clinically as effective as carbamazepine against partial and generalized tonic-clonic seizures and has better tolerability (Reinikainen et al., 1987; Dam et al., 1989).

Synthesis:

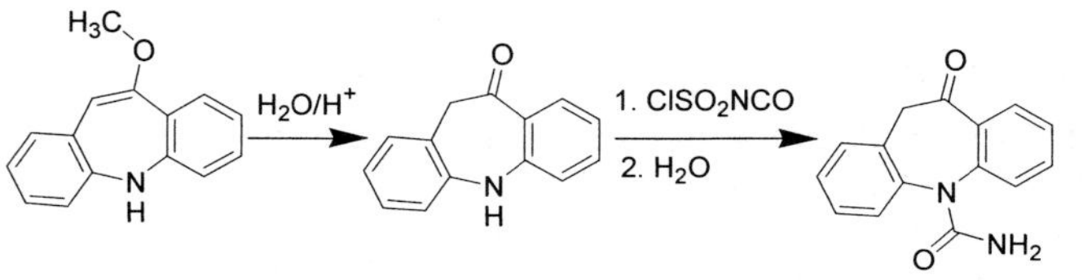

Scheme 11: Synthesis of oxcarbazepine.

In a clinical trial in trigeminal neuralgia patients, Lindström (1987) reported significant pain relief after treatment with 900-2100 mg/day oxcarbazepine which was comparable to the effects of carbamazepine (400-1200 mg/day).

Phenytoin

Phenytoin

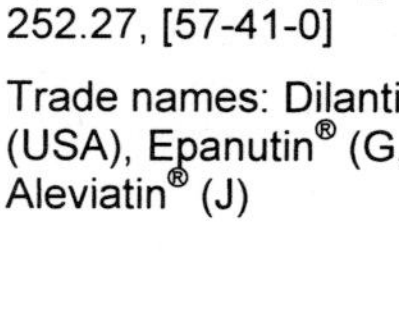

5,5-Diphenyl-imidazolidine-
2,4-dione, $C_{15}H_{12}N_2O_2$, MW
252.27, [57-41-0]

Trade names: Dilantin®
(USA), Epanutin® (G, GB),
Aleviatin® (J)

Phenytoin was the first anticonvulsant to be tested in neuropathic pain patients (Bergouignan, 1942). In two following clinical studies with phenytoin in daily doses of up to 300 mg p.o. or 15 mg/kg i.v. clear reductions of diabetic neuropathic pain were observed (Chadda and Mathur, 1978; McCleane, 1999); however no effect was revealed in a third study using 300 mg/day p.o. (Saudek et al., 1977). Yajnik et al. (1992) found mild to moderate relief of cancer-related pain by phenytoin on its own and a significant enhancement of buprenorphine-induced analgesia.

The side-effect profile of phenytoin is quite similar to that of carbamazepine (see above).

Synthesis (Kleemann et al., 1999):

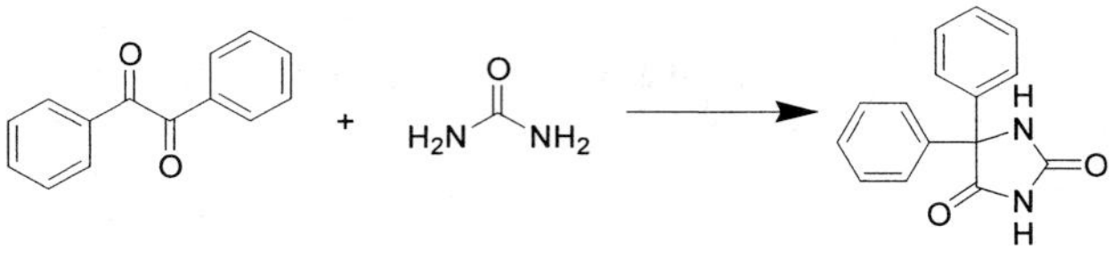

Phenytoin

Scheme 12: Synthesis of phenytoin.

Antiarrhythmic Drugs

As in the previous section, only drugs with sodium channel blocking activities are considered.

Mexilitine

The class Ib antiarrhythmic drug mexilitine is structurally related to the local anesthetic agent lidocaine and also shows a voltage- and frequency-dependent block of sodium channels. Mexilitine is not selective for any pain-relevant subtype of sodium channel. As an advantage over lidocaine, mexilitine can be given orally.

Mexilitine

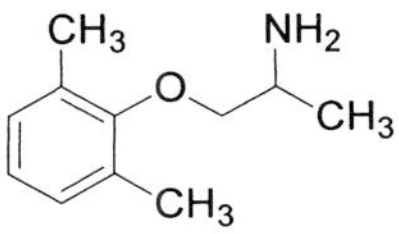

2-(2,6-Dimethyl-phenoxy)-1-methyl-ethylamine,
$C_{11}H_{17}NO$, MW 179.26,
[31828-71-4]

Mexitil ®

Synthesis (Köppe et al., 1972; Kleemann et al., 1999):

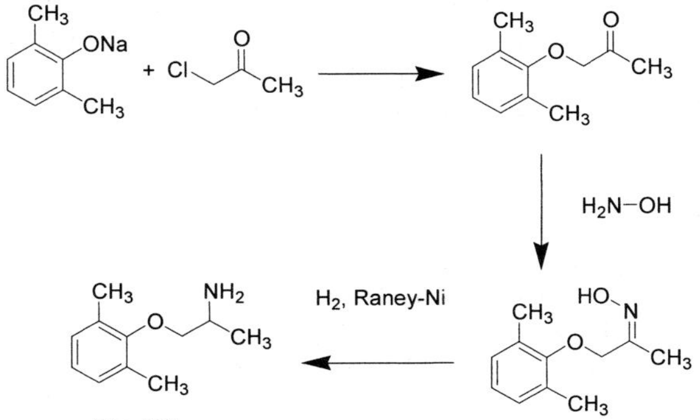

Mexilitine

Scheme 13: Synthesis of mexilitine.

Several clinical trials indicate that mexilitine has analgesic properties in several neuropathic pain syndromes. Mexilitine was first shown to be effective for the treatment of diabetic neuopathic pain at oral doses of 10 mg/kg/day by Dejgard et al. (1988). However, in a large multi-center study by Stracke et al. (1992), the improvement in diabetic neuropathic pain resulting from the administration of mexilitine in daily doses up to 675 mg, was confined to certain subgroups of patients suffering from burning,

Mexilitine has analgesic properties in several neuropathic pain syndromes and is an alternative agent for treatment of patients who fail to respond to tricyclic antidepressants or who cannot tolerate them

stabbing, and heat sensation. In a double-blind placebo-controlled study, Chabal et al. (1992) found a significant improvement in neuropathic pain after peripheral nerve injury following oral administration of mexilitine in daily doses up to 750 mg. Furthermore, mexilitine at a dose of 10 mg/kg/day was used for treatment of a centrally-mediated pain syndrome and led to an improvement of neuropathic pain in eight out of nine patients (Awerbuch, 1990). Sloan et al. (1999) reported three cases of neuropathic cancer pain in which mexilitine was used as an adjuvant to opioids led to further relief of pain.

The most common side-effects in patients receiving mexilitine are gastrointestinal complaints, especially nausea (Jarvis and Coukell, 1998). Neurological side-effects such as tremor, headache, dizziness, and sleep disorders are rare. Although serious cardiac arrhythmias were not reported in neuropathic pain patients, transient tachicardia and palpitations occurred.

Mexilitine is an alternative for treatment of neuropathic pain in patients who fail to respond to tricyclic antidepressants or who cannot tolerate them (Chapter 4 this book; Jarvis and Coukell, 1998).

Sodium channel blockers in development

At present, a multitude of novel sodium channel blockers are in preclinical and clinical development. However, most compounds have been applied to many indications, especially epilepsy and stroke. This review includes only those substances for which activities in pain models have been reported.

In spite of remarkable efforts to develop sodium channel blockers which are selective for subtypes preferentially expressed in primary sensory neurons, no such pain-selective compound has as yet been found.

Co102862

Co102862, a semicarbazone, is a novel chemical entity structurally unrelated to other sodium channel blockers.

(Purdue Pharma)

The semicarbazone Co102862 is a novel chemical entity structurally unrelated to other sodium channel blockers and is currently being investigated preclinically for epilepsy and pain. When studied in an HEK-293 cell line, stably expressing $Na_v1.4$ channels, Co102862 induced a concentration-dependent shift of the voltage of half-maximal inactivation from -77.6 to -95.4 mV at a concentration of 6 µM, thus indicating a preferential block of the sodium channel in the inactivated state (Illyin, 1999). Furthermore, channel repriming was significantly delayed. At steady-state, Co102862 was more potent than the local anesthetic drugs lidocaine and bupivacaine. In addition to its anticonvulsant activities (Carter et al., 1997), Co102862 reduced pain behavior with ED_{50} values in the range of 5 to 10 mg/kg i.p. and p.o. in the formalin test in mice, a model for chronic, peristent pain (Tran et al., 1997). After spinal nerve injury in rats, reduction of tactile allodynia and mechanical hyperalgesia were marked and only moderate, respectively, in a dose range of 1.25 to 20 mg/kg p.o. (Carter et al., 1999).

In recent preclinical saftey studies, formation of bone lesions in the rat, probably mediated by the semicarbazide metabolite, have been reported (Srinivasan et al., 2001).

Crobenetine (BIII 890 CL)

Crobenetine, in phase II clinical studies for stroke, is characterized as a voltage- and frequency-dependent sodium channel blocker (Carter et al., 2000). Crobenetine shifted the half-maximal voltage of inactivation of $Na_v1.2$ channels by up to -27 mV in concentrations up to 10 μM. With trains of stimuli at 5 Hz, crobenetine at a concentration of 1.85 μM induces a pronounced use-dependent inhibition. The analgesic potential of the compound was investigated in a model for chronic inflammatory pain after induction of monoarthritis with intraatricular injection of Complete's Freund adjuvant into the right ankle (Laird et al., 2001). Following treatment for 5 days, crobenetine as well as mexilitine dose-dependently reduced mechanical joint hyperalgesia and impaired mobility with ED_{50} values of 15.5 and 18.1 mg/kg/day s.c., respectively. No effects on the edema and stiffness of the ankle were observed.

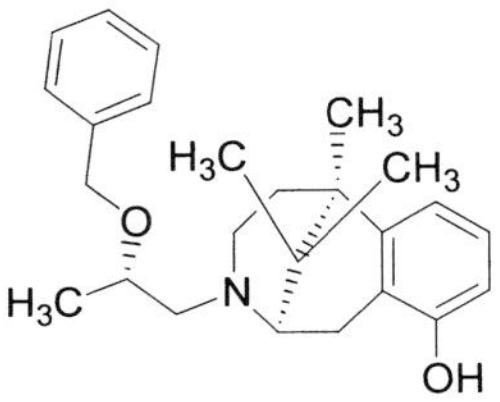

Crobenetine, a neuroprotectant compound, induces anti-hyperalgesia in an animal model for chronic inflammatory pain

(Boehringer Inglheim Pharma KG)

GW4030W92

Since lamotrigine has been shown to inhibit TTX-R channels (Xie et al., 1996), a systematic search for more potent analgesics from the lamotrigine series has led to the new compound GW4030W92. Due to steric loading and the restricted rotation around the two aromatic ring systems, GW4030W92 possesses a stereocenter with the R-(−)-confirmation being preferred (Nobbs and Rodgers, 1996).

GW4030W92

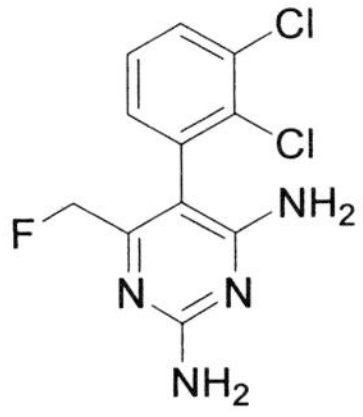

Derived from lamotrigine (Glaxo Wellcome), The compound is a potent voltage- and frequency-dependent blocker of TTX-resitant and TTX-sensitive sodium channels. The compound induces anti-hyperalgesic and anti-allodynic effects in animal models of chronic neuropathic and inflammatory pain

GW4030W92 has been shown to block TTX-R as well as TTX-S sodium channels in a voltage- and use-dependent manner (Trezise et al., 1998). TTX-R currents, induced by test pulses from -60 to 0 mV, were reduced with an IC_{50} value of 22 µM. GW4030W92 leads to a shift of the voltage of half-maximal inactivation only with long-lasting prepulses (i.e. 4 s), but not with pulse width in the range of milliseconds. (see above: 'Voltage-gated Sodium Channels: Structure and Function'). Furthermore, use-dependency is obvious using trains of relatively long-lasting pulses (20 ms), but absent with application of short pulses (3.5 ms). These properties indicate a unique preferential effect of GW4030W92 on TTX-R channels in the slow inactivation state. TTX-S, currents induced from -70 to 0 mV, are inhibited with an IC_{50} value of 5 µM and the steady-state inactivation curve is shifted to more negative potentials.

In a chronic constriction injury model for neuropathic pain in rats, GW4030W92 induces total relief of mechanical hyperalgesia and a significant reduction of mechanical allodynia after subchronic treatment with an oral dose of 10 mg/kg b.i.d. (Collins et al., 1998). In animal models for chronic, persistent and inflammatory hyperalgesia (Formalin test, Carrageenan and Complete Freund's adjuvant tests), GW4030W92 showed significant anti-hyperalgesic effects with ED_{50} values between 4 and 19 mg/kg p.o. (Clayton et al., 1998.). In addition, an anti-edemic property was found to be associated with GW4030W92 .

Development of GW4030W92 has been discontinued in phase II clinical trials.

Safinamide

Safinamide (NW1015, PNU 151774E)

(Newron Pharmaceuticals)

Safinamide is a mixed Na^+ and Ca^{2+} channel blocker with anticonvulsant, neuroprotective and anti-parkinsonian properties and is currently in phase II clincical trials for the indications epilepsy and Morbus parkinson (for review see Chazot, 2001). Additionally, analgesic activity has been shown in acute pain models (hot plate, tail flick) and more pronounced in a chronic, persistent pain model (formalin test) in mice in a dose range of 7.5 to 120 mg/kg p.o. (Salvati et al., 1999).

RGH-5002

RGH-5002 is a tolperisone-type centrally acting muscle relaxant. In isolated DRG neurons, RGH-5002 inhibited both TTX-R and TTX-S sodium currents. RGH-5002 shifted the voltage of half-maximal inactivation towards the hyperpolarizing direction for both channel types, thus indicating voltage-dependent channel block (Bielik et al., 1997). There was also a moderate fequency-dependency with trains of stimuli of 1 to 33 Hz. When investigated in hemisected spinal cord preparations excised form 6-day-old rats, RG-5002 inhibited ventral root potentials evoked by supramaximal stimulation of the dorsal root with a higher potency than the local anesthetic drug lidocaine (Farkas et al., 1997).

Development of RG-5002 has been discontinued in phase I clinical trials.

RGH-5002 (Silperisone)

(Gedeon Richter Ltd.)

Conclusion and prospects

The therapeutic potential of voltage-gated sodium channels for pain management has been established by the efficacy of several sodium channel blockers including local anesthetic, anticonvulsant and antiarrhythmic drugs. In several preclinical and clinical studies, these drugs have been found to be useful for the treatment of various types of neuropathic pain. Further clinical trials are necessary to assess the risk - benefit ratio and hence the place of sodium channel blockers in the management of neuropathic pain especially in comparison with tricyclic antidepressant drugs (for review see McQuay et al., 1995, Chapter 4 this book).

The common mechanism of voltage- and frequency-dependent block of sodium channels gives rise to a preferred block of hyperexcitable neurons within pain pathways and comparatively less interference with normal physiological sensory and motor function. In clinical studies, adverse effects are usually reported as mild or moderate; however, there are also rare, but life-threatening incidents associated with the central nervous and cardiovascular systems.

The discovery of several subtypes of sodium channel with an outstanding relevance for pain has provided a rational basis to develop more selective and disease-specific compounds with an improved side-effect profile. Thus, there is a challenge to develop compounds combining the properties of voltage- and use-dependent block of sodium channels with subtype selectivity. However, despite considerable efforts, there are no such compounds available as yet. Developments of new technologies for functional high-throughput should facilitate selective sodium channel drug discovery.

References

Adams, H. J. F., Kronberg, G. H., Takman, B. H. (Astra Pharmaceutical Products): *Acylxylidide local anaesthetics,* US 3812147 (**1974**).

Åberg, G.: *Toxicological and local anesthetic effects of optically acitve isomers of two local anesthetic compounds,* Acta Pharmacol. Toxicol. **1972**, *31*, 444-450.

Akopian, A. N., Sivilotty, L., Wood, J. N.: *A tetrodotoxin-resistant voltage-gated sodium channel expressed by sensory neurons,* Nature **1996**, *379*, 257-262.Amir, R. , Michaelis, M., Devor, M.: *Membrane oscillations in dorsal root ganglion neurons: role in normal electrogenesis and neuropathic pain,* J. Neurosci. **1999** *19*, 8589-8596.

D'Andrea, G., Granella, F., Cadaldini, M., Manzoni, G. C.: *Effectiveness of lamotrigine in the prophylaxis of migraine with aura: an open pilot study,* Cephalalgia **1999** *19*, 64-66.

Anger, T., Madge, D. J., Mulla, M., Riddal, D.: *Medicinal chemistry of neuronal voltage-gated sodium channel blockers,* J. Med. Chem. **2001**, *44*, 115-137.

Aps, C. and Reynolds, F.: *An intradermal study of the local anaesthetic and vascular effects of the isomers of bupivacaine,* Br. J. Clin. Pharmacol. **1978**, *6*, 63-68.

Attal, N., Brasseur, L., Guirimand, M. D., Parker, F., Gaude, V., Bouhassira, D.: *Effects of intravenous lidocaine of spontaneous and evoked pains in patients with CNS injury,* in: Proceedings of the 9th World congress on Pain. Progress on pain research and management **2000**, *16*, edited by M. Devor, M. C. Rowbotham, Z., Wiesenfeld-Hallin, 863-874, IASP Press.

Awerbuch, G. I.: *Mexilitine for thalamic pain syndrome,* Int. J. Neurosci. **1990**, *55*, 129-133.

Backonja, M.-M.: *Local anesthetics as adjuvant analgesics,* J. Pain Symptom. Manage. **1994**, *9*, 491-499.

Bardsley, H., Gristwood, R., Baker, H., Watson, N., Nimmo, W.: *A comparison of the cardiovascular effects of levobupivacaine and rac-bupivacaine following intravenous administration to healthy volunteers,* Br. J. Clin. Pharm. **1998**, *46*, 245-249.

Bell, R., Montoya, S., Shuaib, A., Lee, M. A.: *A comparative trial of three agents in the treatment of acute migraine headache,* Ann. Emerg. Med. **1990** *19*, 1079-1082.

Bennett, E., Urcan, M., Tinkle, S., Koszowski, A., Levinson, S.: *Contribution of sialic acid to the voltage dependence of sodium channel gating. A possible electrostatic mechanism,* J. Gen. Physiol. **1997**, *109*, 327-343.

Bergouignan, M.: Cures heureuses de nevralgies faciales essentielles par diphenyl-hidantoinate de soude, Rev. Laryngol. Otol. Rhinol. **1942**, *63*, 34-41.

Bielik, N., Kocsis, P., Farkas, S.: *Whole-cell patch-clamp analysis of the effect of RGH-5002, a novel centrally acting muscle relaxant drug on voltage-gated sodium channels of dorsal root ganglion neurons,* Naunyn Schmiedeberg's Arch. **1997**, *356*, Suppl 1, R25.

Black, J. A:, Dib-Hajj, S., McNabola, K., Jeste, S., Rizzo, M. A., Kocsis, J. D., Waxman, S. G.: *Spinal sensory neurons express multiple sodium channel α-subunit mRNAs,* Mol. Brain Res. **1996**, *43*, 117-131.

Blom, S.: *Trigeminal neuralgia: its treatment with a new anticonvulsant drug,* Lancet **1962**, I, 839-840.

Bräu, M. E., Branitzki, P., Olschewski, A., Vogel, W., Hempelmann, G.: *Block of neuronal tetrodotoxin-resistant Na+ currents by stereoisomers of piperidine local anesthetics,* Anest. Analg. **2000**, *91*, 1499-1505.

Bräu, M. E., Dreimann, M., Olschewski, A., Vogel, W., Hempelmann, G.: *Effect of drugs used for neuropathic pain management on tetrodotoxin-resistent Na+ currents in rat sensory neurons.* Anesthesiology **2001**, *94*, 137-144.

Brose, W. G. and Cousins, M. J.: *Subcutaneous lidocaine for treatment of neuropathic cancer pain.* Pain **1991**, 501-505.

Bruera, E., Ripamonti, C., Brennis, C., Macmillan, K., Hanson, J.: *A randomized double-blind crossover trial of intravenous lidocaine in the treatment of neuropathic cancer pain,* J. Pain Symptom Manage. **1992**, 7, 138-141.

Büch, H. P. and Rummel, W.: *Lokalanästhetika,* in: Allgemeine und spezielle Pharmakologie und Toxikologie **1996**, edited by W. Forth, D., Henschler, W., Rummel, K., Starke, Spektrum Akademischer Verlag, Heidelberg, Berlin, Oxford, 227-233.

Butterworth J. F. and Strichartz, G. R.: *Molecular mechanisms of local anesthesia: A review.* Anesthesiology **1990**, 72, 711-734.

Campbell, F. G., Graham, J. G., Zilkha, K. J.: *Clinicl trial for carbamazepine (Tegretol) in trigeminal neuralgia,* J. Neurol. Neurosurg. Psychiatry **1966**, 29, 265-267.

Canavero, S. and Bonicalzi, V.: *Lamotrigine control of trigeminal neuralgia: an expanded study,* J. Neurol. **1997**, 244, 527.

Carter, R. B., Lam, G., Vanover, K. E., Illyin, V. I., White, H. S., Wolf, H. H., Puthucode, R. N., Dimmock, J. R., Nakamura, L., Monaghan, E. P., Ramu, K.: *Characterization of the anticonvulsant and pharmacokinetic properties of Co102862, a novel blocker of voltage-gated sodium channels,* Epilepsia **1997**, 28, suppl 8, 1038.

Carter, R. B., Vanover, K. E., Wilent, W., Xu, Z., Woodward, R. M., Illyin, V. I.: *Anti-allodynic and anti-hyperalgesic effects of the novel voltage-dependent sodium channel blocker Co102862 in a rat model of peripheral neuropathy,* Adv. Ion Channel Res., San Francisco **1999,** Abstract book, P-19.

Carter, A. J., Grauert, M., Pschorn,U., Bechtel, W. D., Bartmann-Lindholm, Qu, Y., Scheuer, T., Catterall., W. A., Weiser, T.: *Potent blockade of sodium channels and protection of brain tissue from ischemia by BIII 890 CL,* Proc. Natl. Acad. Sci. USA **2000**, 97, 4944-4949.

Caterall, W. A.: *Voltage-dependent gating of sodium channels: correlating structure and function.* Trends Neurosci. **1986**, 9, 7-10.

Caterall, W. A.: *Common modes of drug action on Na$^+$ channels: local anesthetics, antiarrhythmics and anticonvulsants,* Trends Pharmacol. Sci. **1987**, 8, 57-65.

Catterall, W. A.: *Cellular and molecular biology of valtage-gated sodium channels,* Physiol. Rev. **1992**, 72, 15-48.

Cederholm, I, Åckerman, B., Evers, H.: *Local analgesic and vascular effects of intradermal ropivacaine and bupivacaine in various concentrations with and without adrenaline in man,* Acta Anaesthesiol. Scand. **1994**, 38, 322-327.

Chabal, C., Jacobson, L., Mariano, A., Chaney, E., Britell, C. W.: *The use of oral mexilitine for the treatment of pain after peripheral nerve injury,* Anesthesiology **1992**, 76, 513-517.

Chadda, V. S. and Mathur, M.S.: *Double blind study of the effects of diphenylhydantoin sodium on diabetic neuropathy,* J. Assoc. Physicians India **1978**, 26, 403-406.

Chapman, P. J.: Review: *Bupivacaine – a long acting local anesthetic,* Aust. Dent. J. **1987**, 32, 288-291.

Chazot, P. L.: *Safinamide,* Curr. Opin. Invest. Drugs **2001**, 2, 809-813.

Clayton, N. M., Collins, S. D., Sargent, R., Brown, T., Nobbs, M., Bountra, C., Trezise, D. J.: *The effect of the novel sodium cahnnel blocker 4030W92 in models of acute and chronic inflammatory pain in the rat,* Br. J. Pharmacol. **1998**, 124, 953-963.

Collins, S. D., Clayton, N. M., Nobbs, M., Bountra, C.: *The effect of 4030W, a novel sodium channel blocker, on the treatment of neuropathic pain in the rat,* Br. J. Pharmacol. **1998**, 123, 16 P.

Courtney, K. R., Strichartz, G. R.: *Structural elements which determine local anesthetic activity,* in: Local Anesthetics. Handbook of Experimental Pharmacology **1987**, 81, edited by G. R. Strichartz, 53-94, Springer Verlag, Berlin.

Coward, K., Saldanha, G., Birch, R., Carlstedt, T.: Anand, P. *SNS/PN3 and NaN/SNS2 sodium channel immunoreactivity in human pain states,* in: Proceedings of the 9th World congress on Pain.

Progress on pain research and management **2000**, *16,* edited by M. Devor, M. C., Rowbotham, Z. Wiesenfeld-Hallin, 711-716, IASP Press, Seattle.

Cummins, T. R. and Waxman, S. G.: *Downregulation of tetrodotoxin- resistant sodium currents and up-regulation of a rapidly repriming tetrodotoxin-sensitive sodium current in small spinal sensory neruons after nerve injury,* J. Neurosci. **1997**, *17,* 3503-3514.

Cummins, T. R., Howe, J. R., Waxman, S. G.: *Slow closed-state inactivation: a novel mechanism underlying ramp currents in cells expressing the hNE/PN1 sodium channel,* J. Neurosci. **1998**, *18,* 9607-9619.

Cummins, T. R., Dib-Hajj, S. D., Black, J. A., Akopian, A. N., Wood, J. N., Waxman, S. G.: *A novel persistent tetrodotoxin-resistant sodium current in SNS-null and wild-type smal primary sensory neurons,* J. Neurosci. **1999** 19, RC43, 1-6.

Cummins, T. R., Aglieco, F., Renganathan, M., Herzog, R. I., Dib-Hajj, S. D., Waxman, S. G. :*Nav1.3 sodium channels: Rapid repriming and slow closed-state inactivation display quantitative differences after expression in a mammalian cell line and in spinal sensory neurons,* J. Neurosci. **2001**, *21,* 5952-5961.

Dam, M., Ekberg, R., Løyning, Y., Waltimo, O., Jacobsen, K.: *A double-blind study comparing oxcarbazepineamazepine and carbamazepine in patients with newly diagnosed, previously untreated epilepsy,* Epilepsy Res. **1989**, *3,* 70-76.

Dejgard, A., Petersen, P., Kastrup, J: *Mexilitine for treatment of chronic painful diabetic neuropathy,* Lancet **1988**, *1,* 9-11.

Denac, H., Mevissen, M., Scholtysik, G.: *Strucure, function and pharmacology of voltage-gated sodium channels,* Naunyn-Schmiedeberg's Arch. Pharmacol. **2000**, *362,* 453-479.

Devers, A. and Galer, B. S.: *Topical lidocaine patch relieves a variety of neuropathic pain conditions: An open-label study,* Clin. J. Pain **2000**, *16,* 205-208.

Dib-Hajj, S. D., Black, J. A., Felts, P., Waxman, S. G.: *Down-regulation of transcripts of Na channel α-SNS in spinal sensory neurons following axotomy,* Proc. Natl. Acad. Sci. USA **1996**, *93,* 14950-14954.

Dib-Hajj, S. D. , Tyrell, L., Black, J. A., Waxman, S. G.: *NaN, a novel voltage-gated Na channel, is expressed preferentially in peripheral sensory neurons and down-regulated after axotomy,* Proc. Natl. Acad. Sci. USA **1998**, *95,* 8963-8968.

Dib-Hajj, S. D., Fjell, J., Cummins, T. R., Zheng, Z., Fried, K., LaMotte, R.: *Plasticity of sodium channel expression in DRG neurons in the chronic constriction injury model of neuropathic pain,* Pain **1999**, *83,* 591-600.

Eisenberg, E., Alon, N., Daoud, D., Yarnitsky, D.: *Lamotrigine in the treatment of painful diabetic neuropathy.* Eur. J. Neurol. **1998**, *5,* 167-173.

Eisleb, O. (Winthrop): Beta-Dimethylaminoethyl ester of para-butylamino-benzoic acid, US 1889645 (**1932**).

Ekenstam, B. T. and Egner, B. P. H. (Bofors): *Anilides of heterocyclic compounds,* US 2792399 (**1957**).

Ekenstam, B., Enger, B., Petterson, G.: *N-alkyl prolidine and N-alkyl peperidine carboxylic acid amines,* Acta Chem. Scand. **1957**, *11,* 183-195.

Ellemann, K., Sjøgren, P., Banning, A. M., Jensen, T. S., Smith, T., Geertsen, P.: *Trial of intravenous lidocaine on painful neuropathy in cancer patients,* Clin. J. Pain **1989**, *5,* 291-294.

Elphick, M.: *Clinical issues in the use of carbamazepine in psychiatry: A review,* Psychol. Med. **1989**, *19,* 591-604.

England, S., Bevan, S., Docherty, R.: *PGE$_2$ modulates the tetrodotoxin-resistant sodium current in neonatal rat dorsal root ganglion neurons via the cyclic AMP-protein kinase A cascade.* J Physiol **1996**, *495,* 429-440.

Eriksson, E.: *Review of the properties of two new local anesthetics, pripocaine and lidocaine,* Acta Anesthesiol. Scand. **1966**, *25,* 54-58.

Farkas, S., Kocsis, P., Bielik, N.: *Comparative characterisation of the centrally acting muscle relaxant RGH-5002 and tolperisone and of lidocaine based on their effects on rat spinal cord in vitro,* Neurobiology **1997**, *5*, 57-58.

Feldmann, K. F., Brechbühler, S., Faigle, J. W., Imhof, P.: *Pharmacokinetics and metabolism of GP 47 680, a compound related to carbamazepine, in animals and man,* in: Advances in epileptology **1978**, edited by H. Meinardi, A. J. Rowan, 290-294, Amsterdam: Swets & Zeitlingerr BV.

Fitzgerald, E. M., Okuse, K., Wood, J. N., Dolphin, A. C., Moss, S. J.: *cAMP-dependent phosphorylation of the tetrodotoxin-resistant voltage-dependent sodium channel SNS,* J. Physiol. **1999**, *516*, 433-446.

Foster, R. H. and Markham, A.: *Levobupivacaine: A review of its pharmacology and use as a local anesthetic.* Drugs **2000**, *59*, 551-579.

Gold, M. S., Riechling, D. B., Shuster, M. J., Levine, J. D.: *Hyperalgesic agents increase tetrodotoxin-resitant Na^+ current in nociceptors,* Proc. Nat. Acad. Sci. USA **1996**, *93*, 1108-1112.

Goldin, A. L., Barchi, R. L., Caldwell, J. H., Hofmann, F., Howe, J. R., Hunter, J. C., Kallen, R. G., Mandel, G., Meisler, M. H., Netter, Y. B., Noda, M., Tamkun, M. M., Waxman, S. G., Wood, J. N., Catterall, W. A.: *Nomenclature of voltage-gated sodium channels,* Neuron **2000**, *28*, 365-368.

Gomez-Perez, F. J., Choza, R., Rios, J. M., Reza, A., Huerta, E., Aguilar, C. A.: *Nortriptyline-fluphenazine vs. carbamazepine in the symptomatic treatment of diabetic neuropathy,* Arch. Med. Res. **1996**, *27*, 525-529.

Gonzalez, J. E., Oades, K., Leychkis, Y., Harootunian, A., Negulescu, P. A.: *Cell-based assays and instrumentation for screening ion-channel targets,* Drug Discovery Today **1999**, *4*, 431-439.

Hodgkin, A. L. and Huxley, A.F.: *A quantitative description of memebrane current and its application to conduction and excitation in the nerve,* J. Physiol. (Lond.) **1952**, *117*, 500-544.

Illyin, V.I.: *Comparative study of inhibition of hSkM1 sodium channels by Co102862, lidocaine and bupivacaine,* Biophysical. J. **1999**, *76*, A82.

Isom, L. L., Ragsdale, D. S., deJongh, K. S., Westenbroek, R. E., Reber, B. F. X., Scheuer, T., Catterall, W. A.: *Structure and function of the β2 subunit of brain sodium channels, a transmembrane glycoprotein with a CAM motif,* Cell **1995**, *83*, 433-442.

Jarvis, B. and Coukell, A. J.: *Mexilitine. A review of its therapeutic use in painful diabetic neuropathy.* Drugs **1998**, *56*, 691-707.

Joho, R. H., Moorman, J.R., Vandongen, A. M. J., Kirsch, G. E., Silberberg, H., Schuster, G., Brown, A. M.: *Toxin and kinetic profile of rat brain type III sodium channels expressed in Xenopus oocytes,* Mol. Brain Res. **1990**, *7*, 105-113.

Kan, van, H. J., Egberts, A. C., Rijnvos, W. P., Pelkwijk, ter, N. J., Lenderink, A. W.: *Tetracaine versus lidocaine-prilocaine for preventing venipuncture-induced pain in children,* Am. J. Health Syst. Pharm. **1997**, *54*, 388-392.

Kastrup, J., Petersen, P., Dejgard, A., Angelo, H., Hilsted, J.: *Intravenous lidocaine infusion – a new treatment of chronic painful diabetic neuropathy?* Pain **1987**, *28*, 69-75.

Kaube, H., Hoshkin, K. L., Goadsby, P. J.: *Lignocaine and headache: an electrophysiological study in the cat with supporting clinical observations in man,* J. Neurol. **1994**, *241*, 415-420.

Killian, J. M., Fromm, G. H.: *Carbamazepine in the treatment of neuralgia. Use of side effects,* Arch. Neurol. **1968** *19*, 129-136.

Kim, C..H., Oh, Y., Chung, J. M., Chung, K.: *The changes in expression of three subtypes of TTX sensitive sodium channels in sensory neurons after spinal nerve ligation,* Brain Res Mol **2001**, *95*, 153-161.

Kleemann, A., Engel, J., Kuscher, B., Reichert, D.: *Pharmaceutical substances,* **1999**, Georg Thieme Verlag, Stuttgart.

Koch, B. D., Sangameswaran, L., Dietrich, P., Delgado, S. G., Fish, L. M., Herman, R. C., Hunter, J. C.: *Electrophysiological properties of rat homologs of SCN9A and SCN10A sodium channels expressed in Xenopus oocytes,* Biophysical. J. **1997**, *72*, A116.

Köppe, H., Zeile, K., Kummer, W., Stähle, H. (Boehinger Ingelheim): 1-(2',6'-Dimethyl-phenoxy)-2-amino-alkanes and salts thereof, US 3954872 (**1972**).

Laird, J. M. A., Carter, A. J., Grauert, M., Cervero, F.: *Analgesic activity of a novel use-dependent sodium channel blocker, crobenetine, in mono-arthritic rats,* Br. J. Pharmacol. **2001**, *134*, 1742-1748.

Lampl, C., Buzath, A., Klinger, D., Neuman, K.: *Lamotrigine in the prophylactic treatment of migraine aura: a pilot study,* Cephalalgia **1999**, *19*, 58-63.

Lang, D. G., Wang, C. M., Cooper, B. R.: *Lamotrigine, phenytoin and carbamezepine interactions on the sodium current present in N4TG1 mouse neuroblastoma cells,* J. Pharmacol. Exp. Therap. **1993**, *266*, 829-835.

Laijon, G. and Boivie, J.: *Central post-stroke pain – a controlled trial of amitriptyline and carbamazepine,* Pain **1989**, *36*, 27-36.

Löfgren, N. M. and Lundquist, B. J. (Astra): *Alkyl glycinanilides,* US 2441498 (**1948**).

Löfgren, N. M. (Astra): *Substituted toluidides and compositions containing them,* GB 839943 (**1958**).

Lindström, P.: *The analgesic effect of carbamazepine in trigeminal neuralgia,* Pain **1987**, *4*, S85.

Lunardi, G., Leandri, M., Albano, C., Cultreara, S., Fracassi, M., Rubino, V.: *Clinical effectiveness of Lamotrigine and plasma levels in essential and symptomatic trigeminal neuralgia.* Neurology **1997**, *48*, 1714-1717.

Luria, Y., Brecker, C., Daoud, D., Ishay, A., Eisenberg, E.: *Lamotrigine in the treatment of painful diabetic neuropathy: a ramdomized, placebo-controlled study,* in: Proceedings of the 9th World congress on Pain. Progress on pain research and management **2000**, edited by M. Devor, M. C. Rowbotham, Z. Wiesenfeld-Hallin, 16, IASP Press, Seattle.

Lyu, Y. S., Park, S. K., Chung, K., Chung, J. M.: *Low doses of tetrodotoxin reduce neuropathic pain behaviors in an animal model,* Brain Res. **2000**, *871*, 98-103.

Maizels, M., Scott, B., Cohen, W., Chen, W.: *Intranasal lidocaine for treatment of migraine: a randomized, double-blind, controlled trial,* JAMA **1996**, *276*, 319-321.

Mandabach, M. G.: *Intrathecal and epidural analgesia.* Crit. Care Clin. **1999**, *15*, 105-118.

Marban, E., Yamagishi, T., Tomaselli, G.: *Structure and function of voltage-gated sodium channels,* J. Physiol. **1998**, *3*, 647-657.

McClellan, K. J. and Faulds, D.: *Ropivacaine: An update of its use in regional anesthesia,* Drugs **2000**, *60*, 1065-1093.

McLean, M. J., Schmutz, M., Wamil, A. W., Olpe, H.-R., Portet, C., Feldmann, F.: *Oxcarbazepine: mechanisms of action,* Epilepsia **1994**, *35*, 5-9.

McQuay, H., Dawn, C., Jadad, A. R., Wiffen, P.: *Anticonvulsant drugs for management of pain: a systematic review,* BMJ **1995**, *311*, 1047-1052.

McCleane, G. J.: *A prospective audit of the use of lamotrigine in 300 chronic pain patients,* The Pain Clinic **1998**, *11*, 97-102.

McCleane, G.J.: *Intravenous infusion of phenytoin relieves neuropathic pain: a randomized, double-blinded, placebo-controlled, crossover study,* Anesth. Analg. **1999**, *89*, 985-988.

Moore, D. C., Bridenbaugh, L. D., Thompson, G. E., Balfour, R.I., Horton, W. G.: *Bupivacaine: A review of 11,080 cases,* Anest. Analg. **1978,** *57*, 42-53.

Morgan, K., Stevens, E. B., Shah, B., Cox, P. J., Dixon, A. K., Lee, K., Pinnock, R. D., Hughes, J., Richardson, P. J., Mizuguchi, K., Jackson, A. P.: *Beta3: an additional auxiliary subunit of the voltage-sensitive sodium channel that modulates channels gating with distinct kinetics,* Proc. Natl. Acad. Sci. USA **2000**, *97*, 2308-2313.

Nicol, C.F.: *A four year double blind study of tegretol in facial pain,* Headache **1969**, *9*, 54-57.

Nobbs., M. S. and Rodgers, S. J. (Glaxo Group Ltd): *Preparation of (R)-2,4-Diamino-5-(2,3-dichlorophenyl)-6-fluoromethylpyrimidine as a drug,* WO 97095317

Nordin, M., Nyström, B., Wallin, U., Hagbarth, K.-E.: *Ectopic sensory discharges and paresthesiae in patients with disorders of peripheral nerves, dorsal roots and dorsal columns,* Pain **1984** 20, 231-245.

Novakovic, S. D., Tzoumaka, E., McGivern, J. G., Haraguchi, M. Sangameswaran, L., Gogas, K. R.: *Distribution of the tetrodotoxin-resistant sodium channel PN3 in rat sensory neurons in normal and neuropathic conditions,* J. Neurosci. **1998**, *18*, 2174-2187.

Patton, D. E., Isom, L. L., Catterall, W. A., Goldin, A. L.: *The adult rat brain β1 subunit modifies activation and inactivation gating of multiple sodium channel α subunits,* J Biol Chem **1994**, *269*, 17649-17655.

Perucca, E., Beghi, E., Dulac, O., Shorvon, S., Tomson, T.: *Assessing risk benefit ratio in antiepileptic drug therapy,* Epilepsy Res **2000**, *41*, 107-139.

Porreca, F., Lai, J., Bian, D., Wegert, S., Ossipov, M. H., Eglen, R. M., Kassotakis, L., Novakovic, S., Rabert, D. K., Sangameswaran, L., Hunter, J. C.: *A comparison of the potential role of the tetrodotoxin-insensitive sodium channels, PN3/SNS and NaN/SNS2, in rat models of chronic pain,* Proc. Natl. Acad. Sci. USA **1999**, *96*, 7640-7644.

Ragsdale, D. S., McPhee, J. C., Scheuer, T., Catterall, W. A.: *Common molecular determinants of local anesthetics, antiarrhythmic, and anticonvulsant block of voltage-gated Na^+ channels,* Proc. Natl. Acad. Sci. USA **1996**, 9270-9275.

Reinikainen, K. J., Keränen, T., Halonen, T., Komulainen, H., Riekinen, P. *J.: Comparison of oxcarbazepine and carbamazepine: a double-blind study,* Epilepsy Res **1987**, 1, 284-289.

Rompel, H., Bauermeister, P. W. *Aetiology of migraine and prevention with carbamazepine (tegretol): results of a double-blind, cross-over study,* S. Afr. Med. **1970**, *44*, 75-78.

Rowbotham, M. C., Reisner-Keller, L. A., Fields, H. L.: *Both intravenous lidocaine and morphine reduce the pain of postherpetic neuralgia,* Neurology **1991**, *41*, 1024-1028.

Rowbotham, M. C., Davies, P. S., Fileds, H. L.: *Topical lidocaine gel relieves postherpetic neuralgia,* Ann. Neurol. **1995**, *37*, 246-253.

Roy, M. L. and Narahashi, T.: *Differential properties of tetrodotoxin-sensitive and tetrodotoxin-resistant sodium channels in rat dorsal root ganglion neurons,* J. Neurosci. **1992**, *12*, 2104-2111.

Rull, J., Quibrera, R., Gonzalez-Millan, H., Lozano Castaneda, O.: *Symptomatic treatment of peripheral diabetic neuropathy with carbamazepine: doubleblind crossover study,* Diabetologia **1969**, *5*, 215-220.

Salvati, P., Maj, R., McArthur, R. A., Cervini, M. A., Kozak, W., Benatti, L., Fariello, R. G.: *PNU-151774E, a novel Na+ channel blocker, shows analgesic effects in some animal models,* Soc. Neurosci. Abstr. **1999**, *25,* 1947.

Sangameswaran, L., Delgado, S. G., Fish, L. M., Koch, B. D., Jakeman, L. B., Stewart, G. R., Sze, P. Hunter, J. C., Eglen, R. M. Herman, R. C.: *Structure and function of a novel voltage-gated, tetrodotoxin-resistant sodium channel specific to sensory neurons,* J. Biol. Chem. **1996**, *271*, 5953-5956.

Sangameswaran, L., Fish, L. M., Koch, B. D., Rabert, D. K., Delgado, S. G., Ilnicka, M., Jakeman, L.B., Novakovic, S., Wong, K., Sze, P., Tzoumaka, E., Stewart, G. R., Herman, R. C., Chan, H., Eglen, R. M., Hunter, J. C.: *A novel tetrodotoxin-sensitive, voltage-gated sodium channel expressed in rat and human dorsal root ganglia,* J. Biol. Chem. **1997**, *271*, 14805-14809.

Saudek, C. D., Werns, S., Reidenberg, M. M.: *Phenytoin in the treatment of diabetic symmetrical polyneuropathy,* Clin. Pharmacol. Ther. **1977**, *22*, 196-199.

Scott, D. A., Blake, D., Buckland, M, Etches, R., Halliwell, R., Marsland, C., Merridew, G., Murphy, D., Paech, M., Schug, S. A., Turner, G., Walker, S., Huizar, K., Gustafsson, U.: *A comparison of epidural ropivacaine infusion alone and in combination with 1.2 and 4 µg/mL fentanyl for seventy-two hours of postoperative analgesia after major abdominal surgery,* Anesth. Analg. **1999**, *88*, 857-864.

Simpson, D. M, Olney, R. K., McArthur, J. C., Khan, A., Godbold, J., Ebel-Frommer, K.: *A placebo-controlled trial of lamotrigine for painful HIV-associated neuropathy,* Neurology **2000**, *54,* 2115-2119.

Singh, R. and Erwin, D.: *Local anesthetics: an overview of current drugs,* Hosp. Med. **1998**, *59,* 880-883.

Sloan, P., Basta, M., Storey, P., Gunten, von, C.: *Mexilitine as an adjuvant analgesic for the management of neuropathic pain,* Anesth. Analg. **1999**, *89,* 760-761.

Srinivasan, V., Chow, C.P., Leyshon, A., Smith, S., Castelli, M.C., Subrahmanyan, V., Sullivan, T.: *Semicarbazide-mediated bone toxicity of V102862 in Sprague-Dawley rats.* Drug Metab. Rev. **2001**, *33,* 235.

Steiner, T. J., Findley, L. J., Yuen, A. W.: *Lamotrigine versus placebo in the prophylaxis of migraine with and without aura,* Cephalalgia **1997**, *17,* 1009-112.

Stracke, H., Meyer, U., Schumacher, H., Federlin, K.: *Mexilitine in the treatment of diabetic neuropathy,* Diabetes Care **1992**, *15,* 1550-1555.

Strichartz, G. R., Sanchez, V., Arthur, G.R., Chafetz, R., Martin, D.: *Fundamental properties off local anesthetics. II. Measured octanol:buffer partition coefficients and pKa values of clinically used drugs,* Anesth. Analg. **1990**, *71,* 158-170.

Tanaka, M. Cummins, T. R., Ishikawa, K., Dib-Hajj, S. D. , Black, J. A., Waxman, S. G.: *SNS Na$^+$ channel expression increases in dorsal root ganglion neurons in the carrageenan inflammatory pain model,* Neuroreport **1998**, *9,* 967-972.

Tate, S., Benn, S., Hick, C., Trezise, D., John, V., Mannion, R. J., Costigan, M., Plumpton, C., Grose, D., Gladwell, Z., Kendall, G., Dale, K., Bountra, C., Woolf, C. J.: *Two sodium channels contribute to the TTX-R sodium current in primary sensory neurons,* Nature **1998**, *1,* 653-655.

Tetzlaff, J. E.: *The pharmacology of local anesthetics,* Anesthesiol. Clin. North Am. **2000**, *18,* 217-233.

Thuresson, A. F., Ekenstam, B., Bovin, C., Kaggs, N. (Apothekernes Lab., Astra): L-N-n-Propylpipecolic acid-2-6-xylidide and method for preparing the same, WO 8500599.

Tran, M., Lufty, K., Xu, Z., Puthucode, R.N., Dimmock, J.R., Woodward, R.M.: *Antinocieceptive effects of Co102862, a novel anticonvulsant in tail flick and formalin tests in mice,* Soc. Neurosci. Abstr. **1997**, *23,* 840.7.

Trezise, D. J., John, V. H., Xie, X. M.: *Voltage- and use-dependent inhibition of Na+ channels in rat sensory neurons by 4030W92, a new hyperalgesic agent,* Br. J. Pharmacol. **1998**, *124,* 953-963.

Tremont-Lukats, I. W., Megeff, C., Backonja, M. M.: *Anticonvulsants for neuropathic pain syndromes: mechanisms of action and place in therapy,* Drugs **2000**, *60,* 1029-1059.

Tyrrell, L., Renganathan, M., Dib-Hajj, S. D., Waxman, S. G.: *Glycolization alters steady-state inactivation of sodium channel Na$_v$1.9 / NaN in dorsal root ganglion neurons and is developmentally regulated,* J. Neurosci. **2001**, *21,* 9629-9637.

Tzoumaka, E., Novakovic, S. D., Haraguchi, M., Sangameswaran, L., Wong, K., Gogas, K. R., Hunter, J. C.: *PN3 sodium channel distribution in the dorsal ganglia of normal and neuropathic rats,* Proc. West. Pharmacol. Soc. **1997**, *40,* 69-72.

Vandam, L. D.: *Some aspects of the history of local anesthesia,* in: Local anesthetics 1987, edited by G. R. Strichartz, 1-19, Handbook of Experimental Pharmacology, 81, Springer-Verlag, Berlin.

Wallace, M.S., Dyck, J.B., Rossi, S.S., Yaksh, T.L.: *Computer-controlled lidocaine infusion for evaluation of neuropathic pain after peripheral nerve injury,* Pain **1996**, *66,* 69-77.

Waxman, S. G., Kocsis, J. D., Black, J. A.: *Type III sodium channel mRNA is expressed in embryonic but not adult spinal sensory neurons, and is reexpressed following axotomy,* J. Neurophysiol. **1994**, *72,* 466-470.

Waxman, S. G., Cummins, T. R., Dib-Hajj, S. D., Black, J. A.: *Voltage-gated sodium channels and the molecular pathogenesis of pain: A review,* J. Rehabil. Res. Dev. **2000,** *37,* 517-528.

Whiteside, J. B. and Wildsmith, J. A. W.: *Developments in local anesthetic drugs,* Brit. J. Anesth. **2001**, *87,* 27-35.

Wilton, T.: *Tegretol in the treatment of diabetic neuropathy*, S. Afr. Med. J. **1974**, *27*, 869-872.

Wood, J. N., Akopian, A. N., Baker, M., Ding, Y., Geoghegan, F., Nassar, M., Malik-Hall, M., Okuse, K., Poon, L., Ravenall, S., Sukumaran, M., Souslova, V.: *Sodium channels in primary sensory neurons: relationship to pain states,* Novartis Found. Symp. **2002**, *241*, 159-168.

Woolf, C. J., Safieh-Garabedian, B., Ma, Q.-P., Crilly, P., Winters, J.: *Nerve growth factor contributes to the generation of inflammatory sensory hypersensitivity,* Neuroscience **1994**, *62*, 327-331.

Xie, X. M., Dale, T. J., Trezise, D. J.: *Voltage-dependent inhibition of tetrodotoxin-resistant Na+ currents in rat sensory neurons by lamotrigine.* Soc. Neurosci. Abstr. **1996**, *22*, 33.3.

Yajnik, S., Singh, G. P., Singh, G., Kumar, M.: *Phenythoin as a coanalgesic in cancer pain,* J. Pain Symptom. Manage. **1992**, *7,* 209-213.

Zakrzewska, J. M, Chaudhry, Z., Nurmikko, T. J., Patton, D. W., Mullens, E. L.: *Lamotrigine (lamictal) in refractory trigeminal neuralgia: results from a double-blind placebo controlled crossover trial,* Pain **1997**, *73*, 223-230.

Zhang, J.-M, Donnelly, D. F., Song, X.-J., LaMotte, R. H.: *Axotomy increases the excitability of dorsal root ganglion cells with unmyelinated axons*, J. Neurophysiol. **1997**, *78*, 2790-2794.

6.2 Potassium Channels

Wolfgang Schröder

Structure, Function and Distribution of K⁺ Channels

Based on their functional properties as well as the degree of amino acid sequence homology, potassium (K^+) channels are grouped into several families and subfamilies with voltage-gated K^+ channels (Kv), Ca^{2+}-activated K^+ channels, inward rectifier K^+ (Kir) channels (including the ATP-dependent K_{ATP} channels) and two-pore-domain K^+ channels constituting the main classes. Over 80 mammalian genes for K^+ channel subunits have been cloned to date. In the case of Kv channels each subunit consists of six transmembrane (TM) segments. The fourth segment (S4) contains the voltage sensor. A pore-forming loop is located between S5 and S6. The subunits of Kir channels only possess two TM domains connected by the pore-forming loop. Unlike K_v channels they lack an intrinsic voltage sensor. Both functional Kv and Kir channels form homo- or heteromeric tetramers composed of four identical or related subunits, often with associated auxiliary β–subunits. K_{ATP} channels form octameric complexes of Kir6.x and regulatory sulphonylurea receptor (SUR) subunits with a 4:4 stochiometry. Three different SUR subunits have been identified so far (SUR1, SUR2A, SUR2B). They are expressed in a cell type-specific manner and confer different pharmacological sensitivities to the functional channel complexes. Subunits of the two-pore-domain K^+ channels may be regarded as composed of two connected Kir subunits. Hence, they possess 4 TM domains and two pore-forming loops. They probably dimerize to yield the functional channel.

Different K^+ channels can be distinguished by their characteristic electrophysiological properties as well as differential sensitivities to pharmacological modulation. For example, Kv channels are blocked by 4-aminopyridine (4-AP), tetraethylammonium (TEA) and millimolar concentrations of Ba^{2+}. In contrast, Kir channels are also blocked by TEA but show selective sensitivity to sub-millimolar concentrations of Ba^{2+}. Furthermore, certain peptide toxins (e.g. dendrotoxins, tertiapin) can sometimes discriminate between K^+ channels belonging to the same family. The K^+ channel openers diazoxide, pinacidil and cromakalim (see below) act on the three SUR subunits with a differential order of potency thereby affecting K_{ATP} channels in a cell type-specific manner (Yokoshiki et al., 1998).

The activation of K^+ channels leads to membrane hyperpolarization which exerts an inhibitory influence on

4-aminopyridine

tetraethylammonium

Glx-Pro-Arg-Arg-Lys-Leu-Cys-
Ile-Leu-His-Arg-Asn-Pro-Gly-
Arg-Cys-Tyr-Asp-Lys-Ile-Pro-
Ala-Phe-Tyr-Tyr-Asn-Gln-Lys-
Lys-Lys-Gln-Cys-Glu-Arg-Phe-
Asp-Trp-Ser-Gly-Cys-Gly-Gly-
Asn-Ser-Asn-Arg-Phe-Lys-
Thr-Ile-Glu-Glu-Cys-Arg-Arg-
Thr-Cys-Ile-Gly

α-Dendrotoxin

H-Ala-Leu-Cys-Asn-Cys-
Asn-Arg-Ile-Ile-Ile-Pro-His-
Met-Cys-Trp-Lys-Lys-Cys-
Gly-Lys-Lys-NH$_2$

Tertiapin

Activated K$^+$ channels in the neuronal circuitry of pain processing areas may either directly or indirectly interfere with the transmission of nociceptive signals

cell excitability. According to their electrophysiological properties the different types of potassium channels fulfill specialized functions in that they shape individual action potentials, determine the frequency of action potential firing, contribute to the afterhyperpolarization following an action potential or stabilize the membrane potential near the K$^+$ equilibrium potential. Common to all these actions is that they dampen excitability. An excellent introductory overview of the field of K$^+$ channel biology is provided by Hille (2001).

Depending on the location of a specific type of K$^+$ channel in the neuronal circuitry of pain processing areas they may either directly or indirectly interfere with the transmission of nociceptive signals when activated. For example, opening of K$_{ATP}$ channels seems to mediate peripheral morphine analgesia by directly hyperpolarizing peripheral terminals of primary afferent fibers preventing action potential discharge and hence leading to antinociception. The activation of a K$^+$ conductance can also indirectly modulate pain processing via disinhibitory processes as will be discussed in detail for the supraspinal action of morphine (see below).

However, due to the ubiquitous expression of K$^+$ channels in virtually all excitable cells the general question arises how can they be exploited as targets for drug therapy of painful states? To put it in other words, what is required to ascertain a specific antinociceptive action when modulating K$^+$ channel functioning?

First, a considerable body of evidence for the involvement of K$^+$ channels in antinociceptive signaling that has been accumulated from both *in vitro* and *in vivo* studies of acute pain will be reviewed.

Second, the mechanisms by which altered K$^+$ channels contribute to the development of chronic pain states and what needs must be met by the channels in order to constitute attractive drug targets with respect to the problem of ensuring a specific antinociceptive action will be discussed. Corresponding examples for this will be given.

K$^+$ channels and supraspinal analgesia

In 1956 it was recognized that insulin pretreatment enhanced morphine-induced analgesia (Davis et al., 1956). It was further suggested that this potentiation was due to a reduced level of intracellular ATP (Singh et al., 1983).

K$_{ATP}$ channels

The identification of ATP-sensitive K$^+$ (K$_{ATP}$) channels in brain tissue (Bernardi et al., 1988) provoked a series of *in vivo* studies which demonstrated that these channels are involved in morphine-induced supraspinal analgesia (Table 1). Intracerebroventricular (i.c.v.) injection of K$_{ATP}$ channel blockers antagonized morphine-induced antinociception in a dose-dependent manner (Ocana et al., 1990; Narita et al., 1992; Ocana et al., 1993). Interestingly, the order of potency of these blockers responsible for antagonizing the effect of morphine was the same as for blocking K$_{ATP}$ channels in neurones, i.e. gliquidone > glipizide > glibenclamide > tolbutamide (Ocana et al., 1993). On the other hand, intracerebroventricularly administered K$_{ATP}$ channel openers (KCOs) such as pinacidil (Vergoni et al., 1992), cromakalim (Ocana et al., 1996) as well as diazoxide and levcromakalim (Lohmann and Welch, 1999b) potentiated morphine-induced analgesia in a dose-dependent manner.

glipizide

glibenclamide (glyburide)

tolbutamide

gliquidone

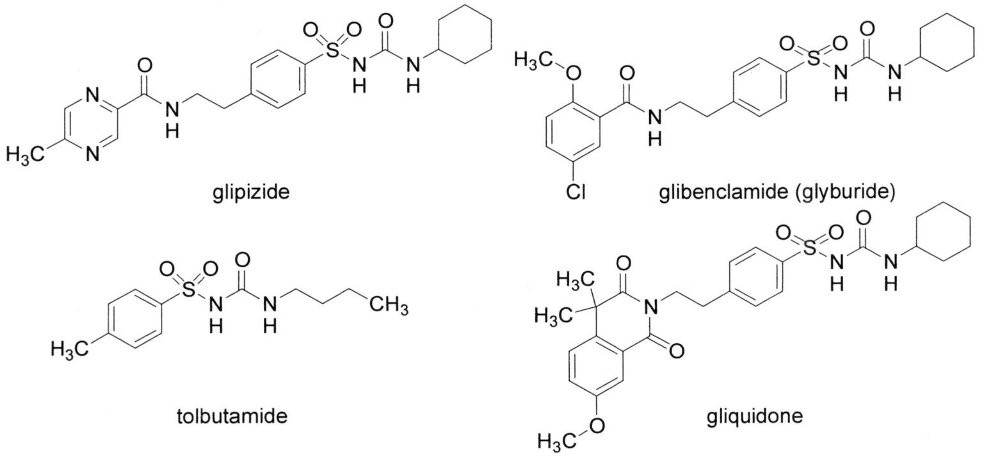

Scheme 1: K$_{ATP}$ channel blockers.

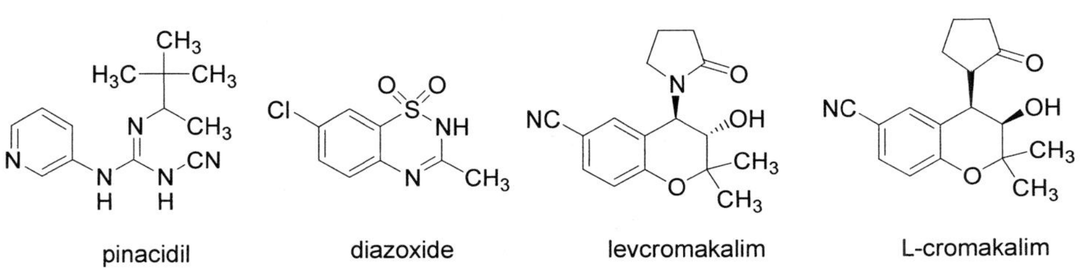

pinacidil

diazoxide

levcromakalim

L-cromakalim

Scheme 2: K$_{ATP}$ channel openers.

Table 1: Involvement of K$^+$ channels in supraspinal analgesia.

Analgesics	Supraspinal K$^+$ channels		
	K$_{ATP}$ channels	TEA, 4- AP sensitive K$^+$ channels	Ca^{2+} - activated K$^+$ channels
μ-opioid receptor agonists	+ (1, 2, 3, 4, 5, 6)	- [1, 7] + [8] (Kv1.1)	n.d.
κ-opioid receptor agonists	- [2, 5, 9]	- [9]	n.d.
GABA$_B$ receptor agonists	- [5, 9]	+ [8, 9] (Kv1.1)	n.d.
α$_2$ adrenoceptor agonists	+ (5, 9, 10, 11)	+ [11] (Kv1.1)	- [11]
Tricyclic antidepressants	+ [12]	+ [12, 13] (Kv1.1)	+ [12]
5-HT$_{1A}$ receptor agonists	+ [14]	- [14]	n.d.
H1 histamine receptor antagonists	+ [15]	- [15] (Kv1.1)	+ [15]
A1 adenosine receptor agonists	+ [16]	- [16]	n.d.

(1) Ocana et al., 1990; (2) Narita et al., 1992; (3) Vergoni et al., 1992; (4) Ocana et al., 1993; (5) Ocana et al., 1996; (6) Lohmann and Welch, 1999a, b; (7) Ocana et al., 1995; (8) Galeotti et al., 1997a; (9) Ocana and Baeyens, 1993; (10) Raffa and Martinez, 1995; (11) Galeotti et al., 1999a; (12) Galeotti et al., 2001; (13) Galeotti et al., 1997b; (14) Robles et al., 1996; (15) Galeotti et al., 1999b; (16) Ocana and Baeyens, 1994

n.d. = not determined

The disinhibition of PAG output neurones mediates the supraspinal analgesia of morphine and serotonin

Morphine exerts its supraspinal analgesia by presynaptically blocking GABA release from tonically active inhibitory interneurones projecting to output neurones of the caudal ventrolateral periaqueductal grey matter (PAG) (Yaksh et al., 1976; Vaughan et al., 1997). This disinhibition of PAG output neurones stimulates serotoninergic and noradrenergic descending analgesic pathways which originate in the rostro-ventral medulla and terminate in the spinal cord where they modulate spinal nociceptive transmission (A detailed description of the PAG's functional anatomy can be found in Bandler and Shipley; 1994 and in Beitz, 1995).

Opioids including morphine acting on metabotrobic μ–opioid receptors produce their inhibitory effect on cellular excitability in part by activation of G$_{i/o}$-protein-coupled K$^+$ channels thereby hyperpolarizing the membrane potential (Williams et al., 1982; Han et al.,

1999; Ikeda et al., 2000; Narita et al., 2000). K_{ATP} channels have been shown to be opened by $G_{i/o}$-proteins (Edwards and Weston, 1993) and could thus mediate the inhibitory effect of morphine at the cellular level. Furthermore, such an interaction would also explain the antagonism and potentiation of morphine analgesia by K_{ATP} channel blockers and openers, respectively (see above). However, a recent electrophysiological study demonstrated that K_{ATP} channels do not mediate the effect of morphine in ventrolateral PAG neurones (Chiou and How, 2001).

The disinhibition of PAG output neurones described above presumably also mediates supraspinal analgesia produced by serotonin which by acting on 5-HT_{1A} receptors stimulates a G-protein-gated inward rectifier K^+ current (Jeong et al., 2001). As with morphine, this leads to presynaptic inhibition of GABA release from inhibitory interneurones. Indeed, stimulation of 5-HT_{1A} and μ–opioid receptors synergistically modulate GABA release in PAG neurones since combining subthreshold concentrations of agonists of both receptors produces significant inhibitory effects (Kishimoto et al., 2001).

Currently, an alternative view of K_{ATP} channel involvement in supraspinal morphine analgesia is gradually emerging. Based on experiments which show that KCO-mediated antinociception is attenuated both by antisense oligonucleotides to opioid receptors and opioid antagonists, Lohmann and Welch (1999a, b) hypothesize that K_{ATP} channel openers stimulate the release of endogenous opioids which in turn may act on opioid receptors in the PAG. Most interestingly, when combining inactive doses of both KCOs and opioid receptor agonists a significant antinociception could be achieved. One important practical implication of this might be that morphine doses could be decreased when KCOs are concomitantly applied thereby reducing the side-effects of opioid therapy such as constipation, respiratory depression and abuse liability.

K_{ATP} channel openers seem to stimulate the release of endogenous opioids

However, currently available KCOs do not cross the blood-brain barrier and therefore had to be administered intracerebroventricularly for experimental purposes.

Novel classes of K_{ATP} channel openers have been claimed to be useful in the management of pain and migraine (Mogensen et al. (Novo Nordisk), 1999; Carroll et al., (Abbott), 2000-2001).

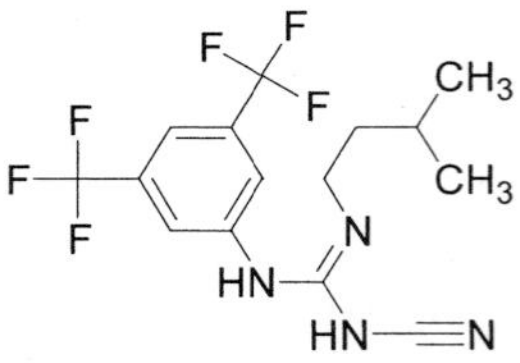

Mogensen et al. (Novo Nordisk),
WO9958497

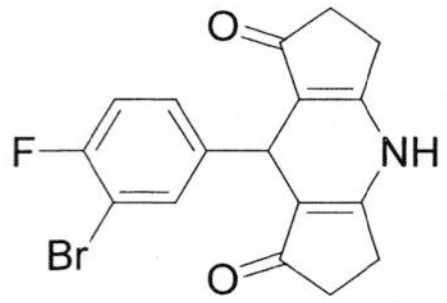

Carroll et al. (Abbott)
WO0051986

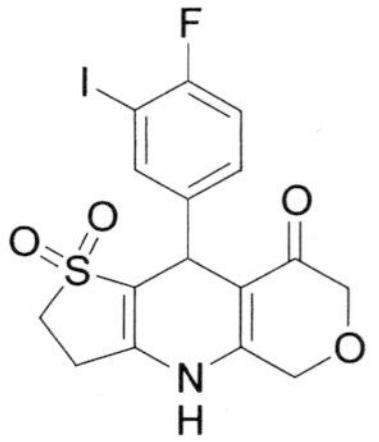

Carroll et al. (Abbott),
WO0183484

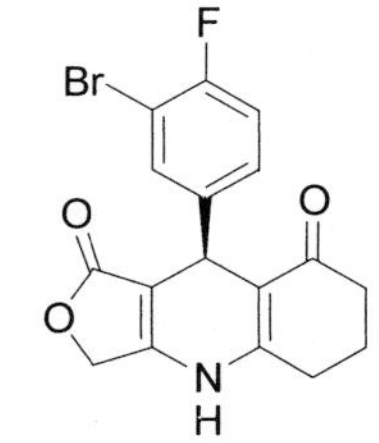

Carroll et al. (Abbott),
WO0183480

Scheme 3: K_{ATP} channel openers.

Morphine interacts with the endogenous opioid system

The systemic administration of morphine has been shown to elevate endogenous opioid peptide levels in plasma and cerebrospinal fluid (Höllt et al., 1978; Natsuki and Dewey, 1993). Hence, K_{ATP} channel openers and blockers could interfere with this positive feedback loop to modulate supraspinal morphine analgesia by altering an additional antinociceptive component which is mediated by the morphine-induced release of endogenous opioids. Two findings may support this assumption. First, K_{ATP} channel blockers alone do not produce any effect on nociceptive thresholds (see below). Second, the antagonism of morphine-induced supraspinal analgesia by K_{ATP} channel blockers is not complete even with the highest doses tested. It is noteworthy that no cross-tolerance develops between KCOs and morphine, hence KCOs produce antinociception in morphine tolerant mice (Welch and Dunlow, 1993) possibly indicating that K_{ATP} channels interact with other transmitter systems involved in nociceptive processing.

Indeed, using the same experimental approach (i.e. i.c.v. administration of K_{ATP} channel openers and blockers) it was shown that supraspinal K_{ATP} channels are also involved in producing antinociceptive effects of several other classes of analgesic substances (Table 1). The K_{ATP} channels involved in supraspinal antinociception are not tonically activated since none of the K_{ATP} channel blockers exerted any effect when given alone.

Kv1.1 channel

Likewise, by intracerebroventricular administration of antisense oligonucleotides to the voltage-gated K^+ channel Kv1.1 Galeotti and her colleagues (1997a) demonstrated that this K^+ channel is also associated with morphine-induced supraspinal analgesia. This finding is supported by electrophysiological experiments performed in the PAG demonstrating opioid-induced inhibition of inhibitory postsynaptic currents (due to reduced GABA release) by activating a 4-aminopyridine- and dendrotoxin-sensitive K^+ conductance (Vaughan et al., 1997). Again, supraspinal Kv1.1 channels have been implicated in antinociception produced by other classes of analgesic substances (Table 1). The fact that Kv1.1 knockout mice exhibit pronounced hyperalgesia and reduced responsiveness to morphine further underlines the important role played by this channel in nociceptive signaling (Clark and Tempel, 1998).

Ca^{2+}-activated K^+ channels

The i.c.v. injection of apamin or charybdotoxin, specific blockers of the SK and BK type of Ca^{2+}-activated K^+ channels, respectively, prevented the antinociception mediated by tricyclic antidepressants and H1 histamine receptor antagonists whereas α_2 adrenoceptor-mediated supraspinal analgesia did not depend on the activation of these K^+ channels (Table 1).

Immunoreactivities of the SK1 and IK1 type of Ca^{2+}-activated K^+ channels were demonstrated to be down-regulated by chronic nerve injury thereby probably contributing to increased excitability in neuropathic states (Boettger et al., 2002). SK, IK (Jensen et al. (Neurosearch), 2000) and BK channel opening compounds (Sit and Meanwell (BMS), 1998; Hewawasam et al. (BMS), 1999; Hewawasam and Starrett (BMS), 2000) were claimed to be suitable for the treatment of migraine.

Jensen et al.
(Neurosearch),
WO0033834

Cys-Asn-Cys-Lys-Ala-Pro-Glu-Thr-Ala-Leu-
Cys-Ala-Arg-Arg-Cys-Gln-Gln-His-NH$_2$

Apamin

pGlu-Phe-Thr-Asn-Val-Ser-Cys-Thr-Thr-Ser-
Lys-Glu-Cys-Trp-Ser-Val-Cys-Gln-Arg-Leu-
His-Asn-Thr-Ser-Arg-Gly-Lys-Cys-Met-Asn-
Lys-Lys-Cys-Arg-Cys-Tyr-Ser

Charybdotoxin

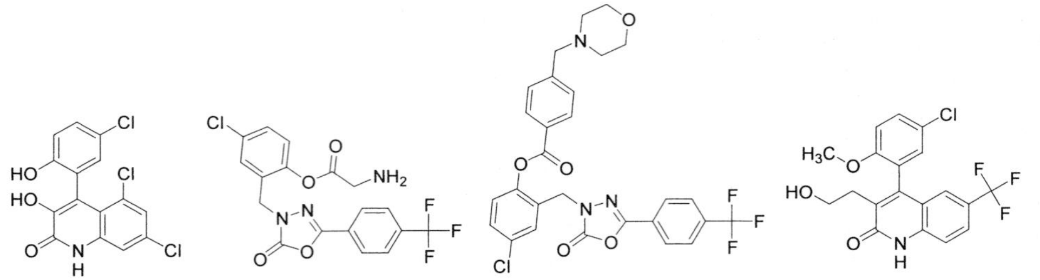

| Sit and Meanwell (BMS), WO9823273 | Hewawasam et al. (BMS), WO9938853 | Hewawasam et al. (BMS), WO9938854 | Hewawasam and Starrett (BMS), WO0034244 |

Scheme 4: BK channel openers.

K$^+$ channels and spinal analgesia

Spinal K_{ATP} channels were shown to be involved in the antinociception produced by intrathecally (i.t.) administered morphine, norepinephrine, apomorphine and carbachol as deduced from the dose-dependent inhibition by i.t. glibenclamide.

Table 2: Involvement of K$^+$ channels in spinal and peripheral analgesia

Analgesics	Spinal K$^+$ channels		
	K_{ATP} channels	TEA, 4- AP sensitive K$^+$ channels	Ca^{2+} -activated K$^+$ channels
μ-opioid receptor agonists	+ (1, 2, 3, 4, 5, 6)	n.d.	+ [1]
α$_2$ adrenoceptor agonists	+ [2, 3, 5]	n.d.	n.d.
5-HT receptor agonists	- [3]	n.d.	n.d.
adenosine receptor agonists	- [2, 3]	n.d.	n.d.
dopamine D1/D2 receptor agonists	+ [4]	n.d.	n.d.
muscarinic receptor agonists	+ [7]	n.d.	n.d.
	Peripheral K$^+$ channels		
μ-opioid receptor agonists	+ [8]	- [8]	- [8]

(1) Welch and Dunlow, 1993; (2) Yang et al., 1998; (3) Kang et al., 1998a; (4) Kang et al., 1998b; (5) Asano et al., 2000; (6) Campbell and Welch, 2001; (7) Kang et al., 1997; (8) Rodrigues and Duarte, 2000

Interestingly, apart from their glibenclamide-sensitivity all these antinociceptive effects were also inhibited by i.t. naloxone suggesting a requirement for spinal opioid receptor activation. Kang et al. (1998b) proposed that norepinephrine, apomorphine and carbachol exert their spinal antinociception by releasing endogenous opioids which in turn act on opioid receptors that possibly coexist with K_{ATP} channels in neuronal membranes postsynaptic to opioidergic local interneurones. Morphine analgesia in the spinal cord is partly mediated by the release of adenosine from central terminals of capsaicin-sensitive primary afferent fibers (Sawynok et al., 1989). Accordingly, analgesia produced by i.t. norepinephrine could be blocked by both i.t. naloxone and the adenosine receptor antagonist aminophylline (Zhang et al., 1994). However, K_{ATP} channels do not participate in the analgesic effects elicited by adenosine agonists (Table 2).

Again, as is the case for K_{ATP} channels involved in supraspinal analgesia those participating in spinal antinociception are not tonically activated since none of the K_{ATP} channel blockers exerted any effect per se.

Activation of spinal opioid receptors appears to be central for antinociception elicited by several classes of analgesics

K⁺ channels and peripheral analgesia

Peripheral endogenous opioid analgesia occurring under inflammatory conditions has been of much interest in the last few years (reviewed in Stein et al., 2001). Opioid receptors were shown to be expressed on the peripheral terminals of primary afferent fibers. Inflammation not only upregulates these receptors but also attracts immunocytes to the inflamed tissue to secrete endogenous opioid peptides thereby eliciting local analgesia. Rodrigues and Duarte (2000) showed that activation of K_{ATP} channels is involved in this process since peripherally applied blockers of those channels were able to reverse the antinociceptive effects of peripherally administered morphine. The hyperpolarization of primary afferent fibers due to K⁺ channel activation leads to diminished action potential discharge and is thus thought to enhance the threshold for pain perception.

The action of several anesthetics has also been associated with a modulation of K⁺ channels. In addition to blocking Na⁺ currents in spinal neurones of the superficial dorsal horn the local anesthetics bupivacaine, lidocaine and mepivacaine reduce transient, A-type K⁺ currents in these cells whereas delayed rectifier K⁺ currents proved to be resistant (Olschewski et al., 1998). Since the A-type K⁺ current determines the frequency pattern of repetitively firing neurones (Hille, 2001) their suppression in dorsal

K⁺ channels are affected by anesthetics

horn neurones might contribute to the modulation of pain perception. However, a reduced A-type K^+ current would increase the firing frequency of the respective neurone. How this might be related to the analgesic action is at present unknown. Bupivacaine also inhibits G-protein gated inward rectifier K^+ channels (Zhou et al., 2001).

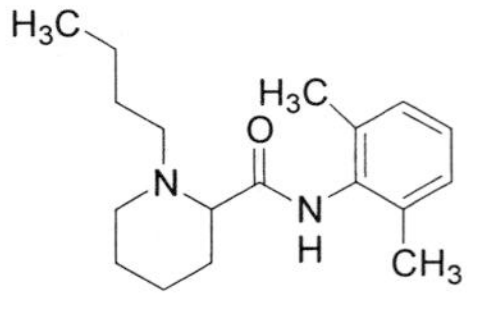

Bupivacaine

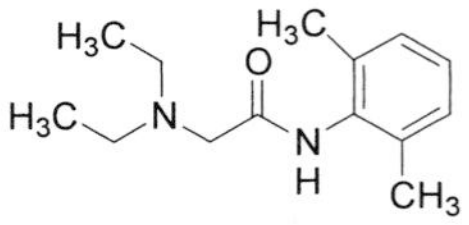

Lidocaine

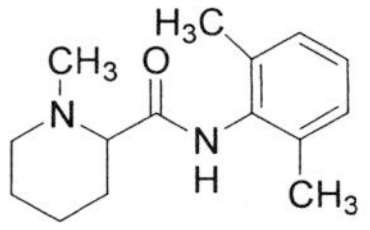

Mepivacaine

Scheme 5: Anesthetics modulating K^+ channels.

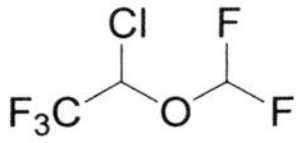

Isoflurane 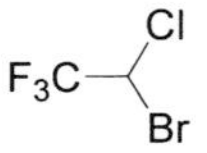   Halothane

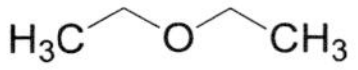

Diethylether

CHCl$_3$

Chloroform

In contrast, currents through the two-pore-domain K^+ channels TREK-1, TASK-1 and TASK-2 are activated by the volatile general anesthetics halothane, isoflurane chloroform and diethyl ether (Patel et al., 1999; Sirois et al., 2000; Gray et al., 2000). The resulting hyperpolarization in cortical, hippocampal and cerebellar neurones where these channels are abundantly expressed may explain how anesthesia is produced by volatile anesthetics. Moreover, halothane also enhanced background currents through heteromeric Kir3.1/3.4 and homomeric Kir3.1 G-protein gated inward rectifier K^+ channels whereas homomeric Kir3.2-mediated currents were inhibited (Weigl and Schreibmayer, 2001; Yamakura et al., 2001). In addition, volatile anesthetics reduce neuronal excitability by stimulating GABA$_A$ and glycine receptors (Mihic et al., 1997) as well as by reducing AMPA and NMDA receptor functioning (Cheng and Kendig, 2000). The mechanisms of action of general anesthetics have been reviewed comprehensively by Thompson and Wafford (2001).

K^+ channels and chronic pain

So far, a role in mediating acute antinociceptive responses has been ascribed to different types of K^+ channels using *in vivo* pain models such as the tail-flick or the hot-plate test.

However, finding new drugs to combat chronic pain with negligible deleterious side-effects is a major challenge for pharmaceutical research. Side-effects generally arise when the drug's cellular target shows a broad tissue distribution and also becomes activated outside the area of interest.

For instance, cardiac expression of TASK and TREK (both in the myocardium and conductive tissue) is compatible with bradycardia and the negative inotropic effect observed with volatile anesthetics (Terrenoire et al., 2001).

In the CNS, K_{ATP} channels show an ubiquitous neuronal expression (Dunn-Meynell et al., 1998). Moreover, they have been detected in astroglial cells of the cortex, hippocampus and cerebellum (Zawar et al., 1999; Thomzig et al., 2001). Outside the nervous system K_{ATP} channels are well known to occur in heart (Kir6.2/SUR2A) pancreas (Kir6.2/SUR1) and vascular smooth muscle (Kir6.1/SUR2B) cells where they are involved in the phenomenon of ischemic cardiac preconditioning as well as in regulating insulin release and blood pressure (reviewed in Yokoshiki et al., 1998). Hence, interfering with K_{ATP} channel function may potentially provoke a series of effects apart from the intended modulation of pain perception mentioned above. To ensure a rather specific antinociceptive action an expression pattern of the target largely confined to areas involved in pain processing such as the PAG, dorsal root ganglion (DRG) cells or the spinal cord dorsal horn would be highly desirable.

Among K^+ channels, two candidates that meet these requirements (i.e. involvement in chronic pain as well as restricted expression) are now emerging: the KCNQ2/3 heteromere and the Kv1.4 homomere.

KCNQ2/3 K^+ channel

The heteromeric KCNQ2/3 K^+ channel is exclusively expressed in the nervous system with high abundance in neurones of the cortex, hippocampus, sympathetic ganglia and the DRG. This channel underlies a current referred to as the M-current since it is blocked by muscarinic agonists as was initially shown in sympathetic ganglion neurones (Brown and Adams, 1980; Wang et al., 1998). Due to its activity in the subthreshold voltage range the M-current critically determines cellular excitability and responsiveness to synaptic inputs. Most recently, the KCNQ2 protein was shown to be expressed in regions particularly prone to seizure generation namely in thalamo-cortical and septo-hippocampal neuronal circuits that are crucial determinants of synchronized activity in the brain (Cooper et al., 2001). Indeed, mutations in the channel protein resulting in a reduced current density have been associated with a special form of epilepsy (reviewed by Rogwaski, 2000). Hence, the potent and selective KCNQ2/3 agonist retigabine which is bioavailable after

Activating KCNQ2/3 channels produces both anticonvulsant and analgesic effects

systemic administration proved to be effective as an anticonvulsant both *in vitro* and *in vivo* (Hetka et al., 1999; De Sarro et al., 2001; Straub et al., 2001).

Retigabine

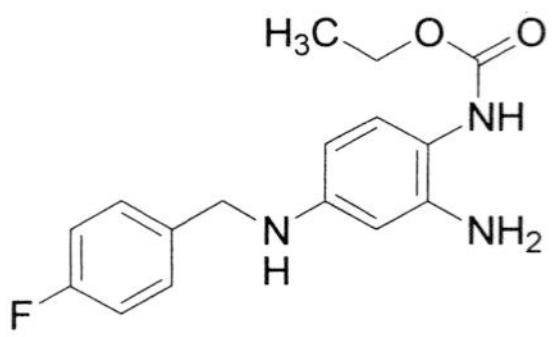

[2-Amino-4-(4-fluoro-benzylamino)-phenyl]-carbamic acid ethyl ester, $C_{16}H_{18}FN_3O_2$, MW 303.33, [150812-12-7]

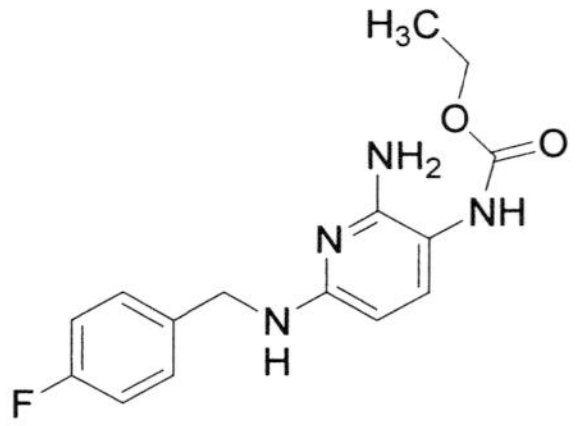

Retigabine opens KCNQ2/3 channels by shifting the voltage of activation to more hyperpolarized potentials as well as by accelerating the rate of activation and slowing deactivation (Main et al., 2000; Rundfeldt and Netzer, 2000; Wickenden et al., 2000; Tatulian et al., 2001). An overview of pathophysiological conditions associated with KCNQ channels is given by Robbins (2001).

Retigabine which is in phase II clinical trials for epilepsy, is a derivative of the analgesic flupirtine which also has anticonvulsant activity. The anticonvulsant action of retigabine is greater than that of flupirtine, however retigabine is not effective in models of acute pain.

Flupirtine

Therefore, it was surprising to find that retigabine had remarkable antihyperalgesic properties (as demonstrated by the dose-dependent inhibition of the second phase of the formalin test). Furthermore, it exerted a robust anti-allodynic effect in the chronic sciatic nerve constriction model of neuropathic pain (Rostock et al., 2000; Rundfeldt et al., 2001). The usefulness of retigabine and KCNQ2/3 channel openers in general for the treatment or prevention of chronic inflammatory and neuropathic pain has also been stressed by Burbidge et al. (2001).

Synthesis (Dieter et al. (Asta Medica), 1993):

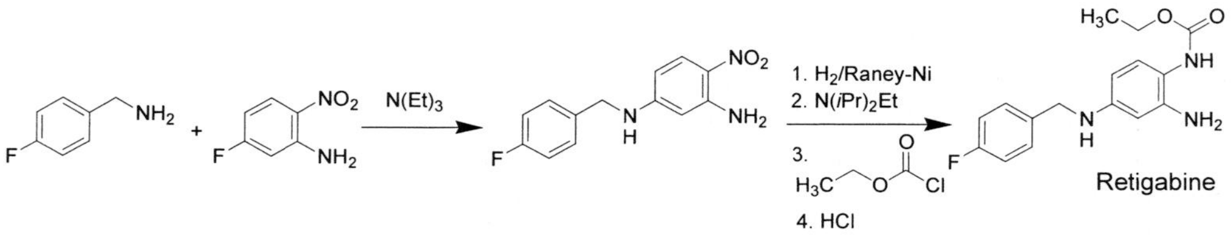

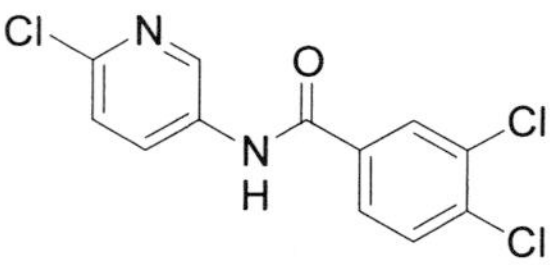

McNaughton-Smith et al. (Icagen), KCNQ2/3 channel opener WO0110380

The newly discovered KCNQ2/3 channel openers of the benzanilide class including those with a previously undescribed 2-substituted-5-aminopyridine substructure have been also demonstrated to be effective against inflammatory pain after systemic administration (McNaughton-Smith et al. (Icagen), 2001; Wickenden et al. (Icagen), 2001).

Kv1.4

Sciatic nerve injury causes a reduction of transient and delayed rectifier Kv currents in large-diameter DRG neurones that leads to hyperexcitability (Everill and Kocsis, 2000). Recently, Rasband et al. (2001) showed a dramatic down-regulation of Kv1.1, Kv1.2 and Kv1.4 channels in DRG neurones in the same model of neuropathic pain. Most interestingly, homomeric Kv1.4 channels appear to critically determine C fiber excitability since no other Kv subunits are expressed by small-diameter DRG neurones. Consistent with this a dendrotoxin-insensitive transient A-type K^+ current with properties corresponding to homotetrameric Kv1.4 channels is found in these cells (Pearce and Duchen, 1994). Moreover, chronic bladder inflammation is also characterized by a suppression of a Kv1.4-like A-type K^+ current in C fiber bladder afferents resulting in enhanced excitability (Yoshimura and de Groat, 1999).

In most neurones Kv1.4 forms part of the heteromultimeric channels. Hence, the development of openers specific for homotetrameric Kv1.4 channels may prove an attractive alternative to Na^+ channel antagonists in selectively reducing excitability of nociceptive C fibers as was suggested by Rasband and colleagues.

Summary

In vivo studies employing tests of acute pain unequivocally showed the involvement of K_{ATP}, Kv1.1 and Ca^{2+}-activated K^+ channels in supraspinal, spinal and peripheral analgesia produced by different classes of analgesics. Furthermore, two-pore-domain and G-protein gated inward rectifier (Kir3.x) K^+ channels are affected by volatile anesthetics. The latter also contribute to μ– and κ-opioid receptor-mediated analgesia (Ikeda et al., 2000).

Synergistic effects as described for the supraspinal interaction of opioids with either KCOs or serotonin are interesting in terms of providing a rationale for reducing opioid doses by using co-administration regimes, e.g. with tricyclic antidepressants which are known to increase serotonin levels in the synaptic cleft.

Keeping in mind the large number of known K^+ channels, our current knowledge on their involvement in analgesia is undoubtedly very limited. This is mainly due to methodological reasons such as the relative paucity of modulators specific for individual K^+ channels. Consequently, it cannot be ruled out that other K^+ channels might also participate in mediating antinociceptive effects.

However, the ubiquitous expression of the vast majority of them does not allow the intended antinociceptive effects to be dissociated from a plethora of side-effects when they are modulated. This will probably prevent common K^+ channel openers to be used as analgesics to a large extent. On the other hand, due to their segregated expression pattern KCNQ2/3 and homomeric Kv1.4 channels have proven promising targets for treating chronic pain states.

References

Abdulla, F. A. and Smith, P. A.: *Axotomy- and autotomy-induced changes in Ca^{2+} and K^+ channel currents of rat dorsal root ganglion neurons*, Journal of Neurophysiology **2001**, *85*, 644-658.

Asano, T., Dohi, S., Iida, H.: *Antinociceptive action of epidural K_{ATP} channel openers via interaction with morphine and an α_2-adrenergic agonist in rats*, Anesthesia and Analgesia **2000**, *90*, 1146-1151.

Bandler, R. and Shipley, M. T.; *Columnar organization in the midbrain periaqueductal gray: modules for emotional expression?*, Trends in Neuroscience **1994**, *17*, 379-389.

Beitz, A. J., *Periaqueductal gray* in: The rat nervous system, 2nd edition **1995**, edited by G. Paxinos, 173-182.

Bernardi, H., Fosset, M. Lazdunski, M.: *Characterization, purification and affinity labeling of the brain [^{3}H]glibenclamide-binding protein, a putative neuronal ATP-regulated K^+ channel*: Proceedings of the National Academy of Science **1988**, *85*, 9816-9820.

Boettger, M. K., Till, S., Chen, M. X., Anand, U., Otto, W. R., Plumpton, C., Trezise, D. J., Tate, S. N., Bountra, C., Coward, K., Birch, R., Anand, P.: *Calcium-activated potassium channel SK1-and IK1-like immunoreactivity in injured human sensory neurones and its regulation by neurotrophic factors*, Brain **2002**, *125*, 252-260.

Brown, D. A. and Adams, P. R.: *Muscarinic suppression of a novel voltage-sensitive K^+ current in a vertebrate neurone*: Nature **1980**, *283*, 673-676.

Burbidge, S. A., Clare, J. F., Cox, B., Dupere, J., Hagan, R. M., Xie, X., (Glaxo Group Ltd.): *New uses for potassium channel openers*, WO0101970.

Campbell, V. C. and Welch, S. P.: *The role of minoxidil on endogenous opioid peptides in the spinal cord: a putative co-agonist relationship between K_{ATP} openers and opioids*, European Journal of Pharmacology **2001**, *417*, 91-99.

Carroll, W. A., Chen, Y., Drizin, I., Kerwin, J. F., Moore, J. L.; (Abbott Laboratories): *Cyclopentanone dihydropyridine compounds useful as potassium channel openers*, WO0051986.

Carroll, W. A., Agrios, K., Basha, F. Z., Chen, Y., Kort, M. E., Kym, P. R., Tang, R., Turner, S., Yi, L., (Abbott Laboratories): *Dihydropyridine compounds and methods of use*, WO0183480.

Carroll, W. A., Agrios, K., Altenbach, R. J., Drizin, I., Kort, M. E., (Abbott Laboratories): *Pyrano, piperidino, and thiopyrano compounds and methods of use*, WO0183484.

Cheng, G. and Kendig, J. J.: *Enflurane directly depresses glutamate, AMPA and NMDA currents in mouse spinal cord motor neurons independent of actions on $GABA_A$ or glycine receptors*, Anesthesiology **2000**, *93*, 1075-1084.

Chiou, L.-C. and How, C.-H.: *ATP-sensitive K^+ channels and cellular actions of morphine in periaqueductal gray slices of neonatal and adult rats*, The Journal of Pharmacology and Experimental Therapeutics **2001**, *298*, 493-500.

Clark, J. D. and Tempel, B. L.: *Hyperalgesia in mice lacking the Kv1.1 potassium channel gene*, Neuroscience Letters **1998**, *251*, 121-124.

Cooper, E. C., Harrington, E., Jan, Y. N., Jan, L. Y.: *M channel KCNQ2 subunits are localized to key sites for the control of neuronal network oscillations and synchronization in mouse brain*, The Journal of Neuroscience **2001**, *21*, 9529-9540.

Davis, W. M., Miya, T. S., Edwards L. D.: *The influence of glucose and insulin pretreatment upon morphine analgesia in the rat*, Journal of the American Pharmacological Association **1956**, *45*, 60-62.

De Sarro, G., Di Paola, E. D., Conte, G., Pasculli, M. P., De Sarro, A.: *Influence of retigabine on the anticonvulsant activity of some antiepileptic drugs against audiogenic seizures in DBA/2 mice*, Naunyn-Schmiedeberg's Archiv of Pharmacology **2001**, *363*, 330-336.

Dieter, H.-R., Engel, J., Kutscher, B., Polymeropoulos, E., Szelenyi, S., Nickel, B. (Asta Medica): *Neue 1,2,4-Triaminobenzol-Derivate und Verfahren zu deren Herstellung (New 1,2,4-triaminobenzene-derivatives and synthesis procedures)*, EP0554543 (**1993**).

Dunn-Meynell, A. A., Rawson, N. E., Levin, B. E.: *Distribution and phenotype of neurons containing the ATP-sensitive K$^+$ channel in rat brain*, Brain Research **1998**, *814*, 41-54.

Edwards, G. and Weston, A. H.: *The pharmacology of ATP-sensitive potassium channels*, Annual Reviews Pharmacology Toxicology **1993**, *33*, 597-637.

Everill, B. and Kocsis, J. D.: *Nerve growth factor maintains potassium conductance after nerve injury in adult cutaneous afferent dorsal root ganglion neurons*, Neuroscience **2000**, *100*, 417-422.

Galeotti, N., Ghelardini, C., Papucci, L., Capaccioli, S., Quattrone, Bartolini, A.: *An antisense oligonucleotide on the mouse Shaker-like potassium channel Kv1.1 gene prevents antinociception induced by morphine and baclofen*, The Journal of Pharmacology and Experimental Therapeutics **1997a**, *281*, 941-949.

Galeotti, N., Ghelardini, C., Capaccioli, S., Quattrone, A., Nicolin, A., Bartolini, A.: *Blockade of clomipramine and amitriptyline analgesia by an antisense oligonucleotide to mKv1.1, a mouse Shaker-like K$^+$ channel,* European Journal of Pharmacology **1997b**, *330*, 15-25.

Galeotti, N., Ghelardini, C., Vinci, M. C., Bartolini, A.: *Role of potassium channels in the antinociception induced by agonists of α_2- adrenoceptors*, British Journal of Pharmacology **1999a**, *126*, 1214-1220.

Galeotti, N., Ghelardini, C., Bartolini, A.: *The role of potassium channels in antihistamine analgesia*, Neuropharmacology **1999b**, *38*, 1893-1901.

Galeotti, N., Ghelardini, C., Bartolini, A.: *Involvement of potassium channels in amitriptyline and clomipramine analgesia*, Neuropharmacology **2001**, *40*, 75-84.

Gray, A. T., Zhao, B. B., Kindler, C. H., Winegar, B. D., Mazurek, M. J., Xu, J., Chavez, R. A., Forsayeth, J. R., Yost, C. S.: *Volatile anesthetics activate the human tandem pore domain baseline K$^+$ channel KCNK5*, Anesthesiology **2000**, *92*, 1722-1730.

Han, S. H., Cho, Y. W., Kim, C. J., Min, B., I., Rhee, I. S., Akaike, N.: *μ-opioids agonist-induced activation of G-protein-coupled inwardly rectifying potassium current in rat periaqueductal gray neurons*, Neuroscience **1999**, *90*, 209-219

Hetka, R., Rundfeldt, C., Heinemann, U., Schmitz, D.: *Retigabine strongly reduces repetitive firing in rat entorhinal cortex*, European Journal of Pharmacology **1999**, *386*, 165-171.

Hewawasam, P., Chen, X., Starrett, J. E., (Bristol-Myers Squibb): *Amino acid derivatives of diaryl 1,3,4-oxadiazolone*, WO9938853.

Hewawasam, P., Chen, X., Ding, M., Starrett, J. E., (Bristol-Myers Squibb): *Benzoate derivatives of diaryl 1,3,4-oxadiazolone*, WO9938854.

Hewawasam, P. and Starrett, J. E. (Bristol-Myers Squibb): *3-Substituted-4-arylquinolin-2-one derivatives as potassium channel modulators*, WO0034244.

Hille, B.: *Ion channels of excitable membranes*, 3rd edition **2001**, Sinauer Associates Inc..

Höllt, V., Przewlocki, R., Herz, A.: *β-Endorphine-like immunoreactivity in plasma, pituitaries and hypothalamus of rats following treatment with opiates*, Life Sciences **1978**, *23*, 1057-1066.

Hohman, T. C., Cotter, M. A., Cameron, N. E.: *ATP-sensitive K$^+$ channel effects on nerve function, Na$^+$, K$^+$ ATPase, and glutathione in diabetic rats*, European Journal of Pharmacology **2000**, *397*, 335-341.

Ikeda, K., Kobayashi, T., Kumanishi, T., Niki, H., Yano, R.: *Involvement of G-protein-activated inwardly rectifying K^+ (GIRK) channels in opioid-induced analgesia*, Neuroscience Research **2000**, *38*, 113-116.

Jensen, B. S., Jorgensen, T. D., Ahring, P. K., Christophersen, P., Strobaek, D., Teuber, L., Olesen, S. P., (Neurosearch A/S): *Use of isatin derivatives as ion channel activating agents*, WO0033834.

Jeong, H.-J., Han, S.-H., Min, B.-I., Cho, Y.-W.: *5-HT$_{1A}$ receptor-mediated activation of G-protein-gated inwardly rectifying K^+ current in rat periaqueductal gray neurons*, Neuropharmacology **2001**, *41*, 175-185.

Kang, Y., Zhang, C., Qiao, J.: *Involvement of endogenous opioids and ATP-sensitive potassium channels in the mediation of carbachol-induced antinociception at the spinal level: a behavioral study in rats*, Brain Research **1997**, *761*, 342-346.

Kang, Y.-M., Zhang, Z.-H., Yang, S.-W., Qiao, J.-T., Dafny, N.: *ATP-sensitive K^+ channels are involved in the mediation of intrathecal norepinephrine- or morphine-induced antinociception at the spinal level: a study using EMG planimetry of flexor reflex in rats*, Brain Research Bulletin **1998a**, *45*, 269-273.

Kang, Y.-M., Hu, W.-M., Qiao, J.-T.: *Endogenous opioids and ATP-sensitive potassium channels are involved in the mediation of apomorphine-induced antinociception at the spinal level: a behavioral study in rats*, Brain Research Bulletin **1998b**, *46*, 225-228.

Kishimoto, K., Koyama, S., Akaike, N.: *Synergistic μ-opioid and 5-HT$_{1A}$ presynaptic inhibition of GABA release in rat periaqueductal gray neurons*, Neuropharmacology **2001**, *41*, 529-538.

Lohmann, A. B. and Welch, S. P.: *Antisenses to opioid receptors attenuate ATP-gated K^+ channel opener-induced antinociception*, European Journal of Pharmacology **1999a**, *384*, 147-152.

Lohmann, A. B. and Welch, S. P.: *ATP-gated K^+ channel openers enhance opioid antinociception: indirect evidence for the release of endogenous opioid peptides*, European Journal of Pharmacology **1999b**, *385*, 119-127.

Main, M. J., Cryan, J. E., Dupere, J. R. B., Cox, B., Clare, J. J., Burbidge, S. A.: *Modulation of KCNQ2/3 potassium channels by the novel anticonvulsant retigabine*, Molecular Pharmacology **2000**, *58*, 253-262.

McNaughton-Smith, G. A., Gross, M. F., Wickenden, A. D., (Icagen Inc.): *Benzanilides as potassium channel openers*, WO0110380.

Mihic, S. J., Ye, Q., Wick, M. J., Koltchine, V. V., Krasowski, M. D., Finn, S. E., Mascia, M. P., Valenzuela, C. F., Hanson, K. K., Greenblatt, E. P., Harris, R. A., Harrison, N. L.: *Sites of alcohol and volatile anaesthetic action on GABA$_A$ and glycine receptors*, Nature **1997**, *389*, 385-389.

Mogensen, J. P., Hansen, J. B., Tagmose, T. M., (Novo Nordisk A/S): *Substituted guanidines and diaminonitroethenes, their preparation and use*, WO9958497.

Narita, M., Suzuki, T., Misawa, M., Nagase, H., Nabeshima, A., Ashizawa, T., Ozawa, H., Saito, T., Takahata, N.: *Role of central ATP-sensitive potassium channels in the analgesic effect and spinal noradrenaline turnover-enhancing effect of intracerebroventricularly injected morphine in mice*, Brain Research **1992**, *596*, 209-214.

Narita, M., Mizoguchi, H., Narita, M., Dun, N. J., Hwang, B. H., Endoh, T., Suzuki, T., Nagase, H., Suzuki, T., Tseng, L. F.: *G protein activation by endomorphins in the mouse periaqueductal gray matter*, Journal of Biomedical Science **2000**, *7*, 221-225.

Natsuki, R. and Dewey, W. L.: *Changes in the levels of several endogenous opioid peptides in dog cerebrospinal fluid following morphine administration*, Japanese Journal of Alcohol and Drug Dependence **1993**, *28*, 379-394.

Ocana, M., Del Pozo, E., Barrios, M., Robles, L. I., Baeyens, J. M.: *An ATP-dependent potassium channel blocker antagonizes morphine analgesia*, European Journal of Pharmacology **1990**, *186*, 377-378.

Ocana, M., Del Pozo, E., Baeyens, J. M.: *ATP-dependent K^+ channel blockers antagonize morphine- but not U-504,88H-induced antinociception*, European Journal of Pharmacology **1993**, *230*, 203-207.

Ocana, M. and Baeyens, J. M.: *Differential effects of K^+ channel blockers on antinociception induced by α_2-adrenoceptor, $GABA_B$ and κ-opioid receptor agonists*, British Journal of Pharmacology **1993**, *110*,1049-1054.

Ocana, M. and Baeyens, J. M.: *Role of ATP-sensitive K^+ channels in antinociception induced by R-PIA, an adenosine A1 receptor agonist*, Naunyn-Schmiedeberg's Archiv of Pharmacology **1994**, *350*, 57-62.

Ocana, M., Del Pozo, E., Barrios, M., Baeyens, J. M.: *Subgroups among μ-opioid receptor agonists distinguished by ATP-sensitive K^+ channel-acting drugs*, British Journal of Pharmacology **1995**, *114*, 1296-1302.

Ocana, M., Barrios, M., Baeyens, J. M.: *Cromakalim differentially enhances antinociception induced by agonists of α_2 adrenoceptors, γ-aminobutyric acid$_B$, μ and κ opioid receptors*, The Journal of Pharmacology and Experimental Therapeutics **1996**, *276*, 1136-1142.

Olschewski, A., Hempelmann, G., Vogel, W., Safronov, B.: *Blockade of Na^+ and K^+ currents by local anesthetics in the dorsal horn neurons of the spinal cord*, Anesthesiology **1998**, *88*, 172-179.

Patel, A. J., Honoré, E., Lesage, F., Fink, M., Romey, G., Lazdunski, M.: *Inhalational anesthetics activate two-pore-domain background K^+ channels*, Nature Neuroscience **1999**, *2*, 422-426.

Pearce, R. J. and Duchen, M. R.: *Differential expression of membrane currents in dissociated mouse primary sensory neurons*, Neuroscience **1994**, *63*, 1041-1056.

Raffa, R. B. and Martinez, R. P.: *The glibenclamide-shift of centrally-acting antinociceptive agents in mice*, Brain Research **1995**, *677*, 277-282.

Rasband, M. N., Park, E. W., Vanderah, T. W., Lai, J., Porecca, F., Trimmer, J. S.: *Distinct potassium channels on pain-sensing neurons*, Proceedings of the National Academy of Science **2001**, *98*, 13373-13378.

Robbins, J., *KCNQ potassium channels: physiology, pathophysiology, and pharmacology*, Pharmacology and Therapeutics **2001**, *90*, 1-19.

Robles, L.-I., Barrios, M., Del Pozo, E., Dordal, A., Baeyens, J. M.: *Effects of K^+ channels blockers and openers on antinociception induced by agonists of $5\text{-}HT_{1A}$ receptors*, European Journal of Pharmacology **1996**, *295*, 181-188.

Rodrigues, A. R. A. and Duarte, I. D. G.: *The peripheral antinociceptive effect induced by morphine is associated with ATP-sensitive K^+ channels*, British Journal of Pharmacology **2000**, *129*, 110-114.

Rogawski, M. A.: *KCNQ2/KCNQ3 K^+ channels and the molecular pathogenesis of epilepsy: implications for therapy*, Trends in Neuroscience **2000**, *23*, 393-398.

Rostock, A., Rundfeldt, C., Bartsch, R.: *Effects of the anticonvulsant retigabine in neuropathic pain models in rats* Poster presentation, 41st Annual Meeting of the German Society of Pharmacology and Toxicology **2000**

Rundfeldt, C., Bartsch, R., Rostock, A., Tober, C., Dost, R., (Asta Medica AG): *Use of retigabine for treating neuropathic pain,* WO0122953.

Rundfeldt, C. and Netzer, R.: *The novel anticonvulsant retigabine activates M-current in Chinese hamster ovary-cells transfected with human KCNQ2/3 subunits*, Neuroscience Letters **2000**, *282*, 73-76.

Sawynok, J., Sweeney, M. I., White, T. D.: *Adenosine release may mediate spinal analgesia by morphine*, Trends in Pharmacological Sciences **1989**, *10*, 186-189.

Singh, I. S., Chatterjee, T. K., Ghosh, J. J.: *Modification of morphine antinociceptive response by blood glucose status: possible involvement of cellullar energetics*, European Journal of Pharmacology **1983**, *90*, 437-439.

Sirois, J. E., Lei, Q., Talley, E. M., Lynch III, C., Bayliss, D. A.: *The TASK-1 two-pore domain K^+ channel is a molecular substrate for neuronal effects of inhalational anesthetics*, The Journal of Neuroscience **2000**, *20*, 6347-6354.

Sit, S.-Y. and Meanwell, N. A., (Bristol-Myers Squibb): *4-Aryl-3-hydroxyquinolin-2-one derivatives as ion channel modulators*, WO9823273.

Stein, C., Machelska, H., Binder, W., Schäfer, M.: *Peripheral opioid analgesia*, Current Opinion in Pharmacology **2001**, *1*, 62-65.

Straub, H., Köhling, R., Höhling, J.-M., Rundfeldt, C., Tuxhorn, I., Ebner, A., Wolf, P., Pannek, H., Speckmann, E.-J.: *Effects of retigabine on rhythmic synchronous activity of human neocortical slices*, Epilepsy Research **2001**, *44*, 155-165.

Tatulian, L., Delmas, P., Abogadie, F. C., Brown, D. A.: *Activation of expressed KCNQ potassium currents and native neuronal M-type potassium currents by the anti-convulsant drug retigabine*, The Journal of Neuroscience **2001**, *21*, 5535-5545.

Terrenoire, C., Lauritzen, I., Lesage, F., Romey, G., Lazdunski, M.: *A TREK-1-like potassium channel in atrial cells inhibited by beta-adrenergic stimulation and activated by volatile anesthetics*, Circulation Research **2001**, *89*, 336-342.

Thompson, S.-A. and Wafford, K.: *Mechanism of action of general anaesthetics – new information from molecular pharmacology*, Current Opinion in Pharmacology **2001**, *1*, 78-83.

Thomzig, A., Wenzel, M., Karschin, C., Eaton, M. J., Skatchkov, S. N., Karschin, A., Veh, R. W.: *Kir6.1 is the principal pore-forming subunit of astrocyte but not neuronal plasma membrane K-ATP channels*, Molecular and Cellular Neuroscience **2001**, *18*, 671-690.

Vaughan, C. W., Ingram, S. L., Connor, M. A., Christie, M. J.: *How opioids inhibit GABA-mediated neurotransmission*, Nature **1997**, *390*, 611-614.

Vergoni, A. V., Scarano, A., Bertolini, A.: *Pinacidil potentiates morphine analgesia*, Life Sciences **1992**, *50*, 135-138.

Wang, H.-S., Pan, Z., Shi, W., Brown, B. S., Wymore, R. S., Cohen, I. S., Dixon, J. E., McKinnon, D.: *KCNQ2 and KCNQ3 potassium channel subunits: molecular correlates of the M-channel*, Science **1998**, *282*, 1890-1893.

Weigl, L. G. and Schreibmayer, W.: *G protein-gated inwardly rectifying potassium channels are targets for volatile anesthetics*, Molecular Pharmacology **2001**, *60*, 282-289.

Welch, S. P. and Dunlow, L. D.: *Antinociceptive activity of intrathecally administered potassium channel openers and opioid agonists: a common mechanism of action?*, The Journal of Pharmacology and Experimental Therapeutics **1993**, *267*, 390-399.

Wickenden, A. D., Yu, W., Zou, A., Jegla, T., Wagoner, P. K.: *Retigabine, a novel anti-convulsant, enhances activation of KCNQ2/Q3 potassium channels*, Molecular Pharmacology **2000**, *58*, 591-600.

Wickenden, A. D., Rigdon, G. C., McNaughton-Smith, G. A., Gross, M. F., (Icagen Inc.): *Methods for treating or preventing pain and anxiety*, WO0110381.

Williams, J. T., Eagan, T. M., North, R. A.: *Enkephalin opens potassium channels in mammalian central neurons*, Nature **1982**, *299*, 74-77.

Yaksh, T. L., Yeung, J. C., Rudy, T. A.: *Systematic examination in the rat of brain sites sensitive to the direct application of morphine: observation of differential effects within the periaqueductal gray*, Brain Research **1976**, *114*, 83-103.

Yamakura, T., Lewohl, J. M.; Harris, R. A.: *Differential effects of general anesthetics on G protein-coupled inwardly rectifying and other potassium channels*, Anesthesiology **2001**, *95*, 144-153.

Yang, S.-W., Kang, Y.-M., Guo, Y.-Q., Qiao J.-T.: *ATP-sensitive potassium channels mediate norepinephrine- and morphine-induced antinociception at the spinal cord level*, International Journal Neuroscience **1998**, *93*, 217-223.

Yokoshiki, H., Sunagawa, M., Seki, T., Sperelakis, N.: *ATP-sensitive K^+ channels in pancreatic, cardiac, and vascular smooth muscle cells*, American Journal of Physiology **1998**, *274*, 25-37.

Yoshimura, N. and de Groat, W. C.: *Increased excitability of afferent neurones innervating rat urinary bladder after chronic bladder inflammation*, The Journal of Neuroscience **1999**, *19*, 4644-4653.

Zawar, C., Plant, T. D., Schirra, C., Konnerth, A., Neumcke, B.: *Cell-type specific expression of ATP-sensitive potassium channels in the rat hippocampus*, Journal of Physiology **1999**, *514*, 327-341.

Zhang, Z. H., Yang, S. W., Xie, Y. F., Qiao, J. T.: *Effects of naloxone and aminophylline on the antinociception induced by serotonin and norepinephrine at the spinal level*, Chinese Journal of Physiological Sciences **1994**, *10*, 139-145.

Zhou, W., Arrabit, C., Choe, S., Slesinger, P. A.: *Mechanism underlying bupivacaine inhibition of G protein-gated inwardly rectifying K$^+$ channels*, Proceedings of the National Academy of Science **2001**, *98*, 6482-6487.

6.3   Calcium Channels

Hagen-Heinrich Hennies and Bernd Sundermann

Introduction

Calcium channel antagonists - also known as Ca^{2+} channel inhibitors or Ca^{2+} entry blockers - have now played a pivotal role in the treatment of hypertension for more than 20 years. Nifedipine, diltiazem and verapamil, the three prototype drugs of the L-type Ca^{2+} channel, were introduced in the late 1970s and early 1980s. But in addition to the interaction with the cardiovascular system, voltage-dependent ion channels also are attractive drug targets for analgesia and neuroprotection (Cox and Denyer, 1998; Williams et al., 1999). Voltage-dependent calcium channels (VDCC) are involved in the regulation of many physiological functions of excitable cells such as neurite outgrowth, enzyme regulation, neurotransmitter release, hormone release and gene expression in cell bodies (Kater et al., 1988; Tsien et al., 1988; Cox and Denyer, 1998). Molecular cloning, biochemical and pharmacological studies have shown that there are several subtypes of VDCC.

VDCC form hetero-oligomeric complexes. The α 1-subunit is pore-forming and provides the extracellular binding site(s) for virtually all agonists and antagonists. The α 1-subunit belongs to a heterogeneous family. Ten cloned α-subunits of 1610 - 2424 amino acids in length are known (α 1S, α 1A, α 1B, α 1C, α 1D, α 1E, α 1F, α 1G, α 1H and α 1I). From these 10 α 1-subunits three families emerge:

VDCC subtypes can be categorised by α 1-subunit families

1. L-type channels (high-voltage activated dihydropyridine- (DHP) sensitive channels): α 1C, α 1D, α 1S, α 1F.

2. N-, P/Q-, R-type channels (high-voltage and moderate-voltage activated DHP-insensitive channels): α 1B, α 1A, α 1E.

3. T-type channels (low-voltage activated channels): α 1G, α 1H, α 1I.

Each subunit has four homologous repeats (I - IV), each having six transmembrane domains (see Fig. 1). Gating is thought to be associated with the membrane-spanning S4 segment, which contains highly conserved positive charges. Many of the α 1-subunit genes give rise to alternatively spliced products. When expressed alone many α 1-subunits produce functional Ca^{2+} channels. However, at least for high-voltage activated channels, it is likely that native channels comprise co-assemblies of α 1-,

The structure of VDCCs

β-, α 2-, δ- and possibly γ-subunits (reviews: Tsien et al., 1991; Catterall and Striessnig, 1992; Catterall, 1993; Isom et al., 1994; Striessnig et al., 1998; Alexander and Peters, 2000).

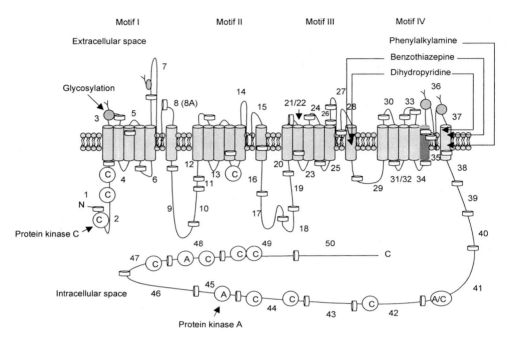

Figure 1: Proposed arrangement of the polypeptide chain of the channel-forming α1c subunit of the L-type calcium channel in humans.

The four repetitive motifs (I, II, III, IV) each consist of six putative transmembrane segments. Both the N terminal and C terminal point into the cytoplasm. White rings separate the segments encoded by numbered exons. The transmembrane segments encoded by alternative exons 8 or 8A, 21 or 22, and 31 or 32 are shown. Sequences encoded by invariant exons which are subject to constitutive splicing are 7, 33, and 45. Exons 40, 41, and 42 are subject to alternative splicing. Putative sites of glycosylation and of phosphorylation involving protein kinase C (C) and protein kinase A (A) are shown, as are the discrete binding areas of the three types of calcium antagonists – phenylalkylamine (verapamil-like), benzothiazepine (diltiazem-like), and dihydropyridine (nifedipine-like) (adapted from Abernethy and Schwartz, 1999).

Activation and localization of calcium channels

Arrival of the nerve impulse at a nerve terminal leads to the opening of voltage-gated Ca^{2+} channels and rapid influx of Ca^{2+}. The increase in Ca^{2+} concentration at the active zone from a basal level of 100 nM to more than 200 µM results in an appropriate neurotransmitter release within 200 µs (Barrett and Stevens, 1972; Linas et al., 1981; 1992; Augustine and Neher, 1992; Zucker, 1993; Heidelberger et al., 1994).

N-type Ca^{2+} channels for instance are located at presynaptic termini of neurons where they are directly involved in the regulation of neurotransmitter release. Staining of the dorsal laminae of the rat spinal cord revealed a complementary distribution of class A and class B Ca^{2+} channels in nerve terminals in the deeper versus the superficial laminae. Many of the nerve terminals immunoreactive for class B N-type Ca^{2+} channels also contain substance P, an important neuropeptide in pain pathways, suggesting the N-type Ca^{2+} channels are predominant at synapses that carry nociceptive information to the spinal cord (Westernbroek et al., 1998).

L-type Ca^{2+} channels can be detected in peripheral neurons, central neurons, synaptosomes as well as in non-neuronal cells (review: Tsien et al., 1988). In general the following gene products were found to be expressed, at least in part, in the central nervous system (CNS) (Birnbaumer et al., 1994; Alexander and Peters, 2000):

α 1A (P/Q-type Ca^{2+} channel)
α 1B (N-type Ca^{2+} channel)
α 1C (L-type Ca^{2+} channel)
α 1D (L-type Ca^{2+} channel)
α 1E (R-type Ca^{2+} channel)

Predominant distribution of the α 1-subunit of the L-type channel:

α 1S: skeletal muscle

α 1C: cardiac and smooth muscle, brain

α 1D: endocrine, kidney and brain

α 1F: appears to be confined to the retina

Preclinical Data

Antinociceptive Effects of L-type Ca^{2+} Channel Antagonists

There are several reports in the literature showing that L-type blockers are more or less active in pharmacological testing systems such as the formalin, writhing, hot plate and tail flick assays (see Table 1). In addition to this data there are further publications reporting an enhancement of opioid-mediated antinociception by L-type Ca^{2+} channel antagonists. All scientific groups listed in Table 2 report that L-type Ca^{2+} channel blockers enhance the antinociceptive effect of µ-opioid agonists without exception. Positive results were reported with all three types of L-type Ca^{2+} channel inhibitors in combination with several µ-opioid receptor agonists such as morphine, DAMGO ((D-Ala^2,N-Me-Phe^4,Gly-ol^5)-enkephalin), fentanyl or sufentanyl. These pharmacological pain models employed mice as well as rats. In general the combination of µ-opioid agonists with an L-type Ca^{2+} entry blocker leads to an enhancement or potentiation of the antinociceptive effect. The dose - response curve of the opioid is shifted to the left. At the spinal level this is also

Enhancement of opioid mediated antinociception by L-type Ca^{2+} channel antagonists

true for μ-agonists, but an enhancement of δ- or κ-opioid agonist-induced antinociception by an L-type VDCC inhibitor was not detectable (Table 2, Dogrul et al., 2001).

Table 1: Antinociceptive activity of L-type Ca^{2+} channel antagonists in specified pharmacological assays.

Model	Species	Compound	Application	Effect	References
Formalin test	Rat	Nifedipine, Nimodipine, Verapamil, Diltiazem	1 – 30 mg/kg i.p.	all drugs are active	Miranda et al. (1992)
Formalin test	Rat	Nifedipine	5 and 15 mg/kg i.p.	active at 15 mg/kg i.p.	Bustamante et al. (1989)
Formalin test	Rat	Nicardipine, Nitrendipine, Diltiazem, Verapamil	10-40 mg/kg i.p.	all drugs are active	Gürdal et al. (1992)
Writhing (acetic acid)	Mouse	Verapamil, Nimodipine, Nifedipine, Diltiazem	0.5 – 400 µg/kg i.c.v. depending on the substance	V > Nim. > D > Nif.	Miranda et al. (1993)
Writhing (phenyl-quinone)	Mouse	Diltiazem Verapamil Nifedipine	10 mg/kg s.c. 5 mg/kg s.c. 10 mg/kg s.c.	all comps. are active	Al-Humayyd (1991)
Writhing (acetic acid)	Mouse	Nifedipine, Nimodipine, Verapamil, Diltiazem	1-30 mg/kg i.p.	Nim. and Nif. are more active than V and D	Miranda et al. (1992)
Hot plate (55°C)	Mouse	Verapamil Diltiazem	15 – 120 µg 60 – 120 µg i.c.v.	significant antinocic. effects	Del Pozo et al. (1990)
Hot plate (63°C)	Mouse	Nifedipine Nimodipine Verapamil Diltiazem	1 – 30 mg/kg i.p.	only Nim. is active	Miranda et al. (1992)
Hot plate (55° C)	Rat	Nifedipine	2.5 – 20 µM epidurally	active at 20 µM, but short duration of action	Wong et al. (1994)
Tail flick	Rat	Nifedipine	2.5 – 20 µM epidurally	active at 5-20 µM	Wong et al. (1994)

Table 1 continued:

Model	Species	Compound	Application	Effect	References
Tail flick	Mouse	Nifedipine	2.5 and 5 mg/kg i.p.	N has no effect on TF-latencies	Pavone et al. (1992)

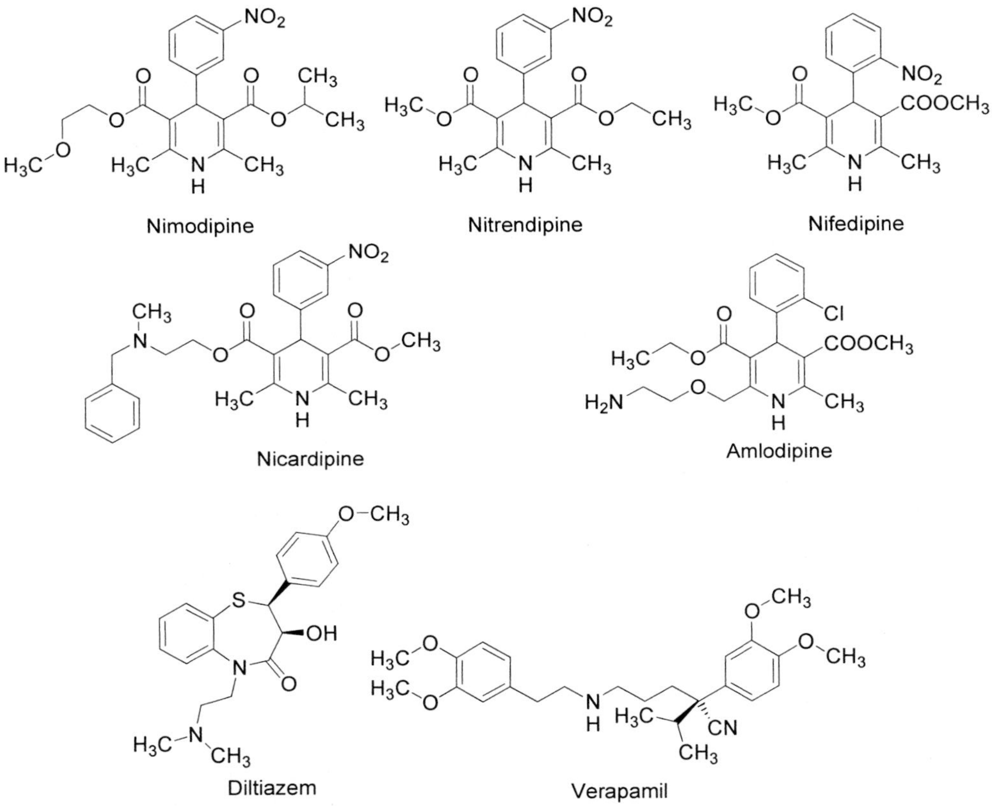

Nimodipine

Nitrendipine

Nifedipine

Nicardipine

Amlodipine

Diltiazem

Verapamil

Scheme 1: Structures of several clinically relevant L-type Ca^{2+} channel antagonists.

In contrast, a low dose of the Ca^{2+} channel <u>agonist</u> BAY K 8644, a dihydropyridine derivative, antagonizes the antinociceptive effect of μ-opioids. This is in agreement with results from Smith and Stevens (1995), who reported that Ca^{2+}, when administered i.c.v., antagonizes morphine-induced antinociception in the mouse tail flick assay. The dose - response curve of morphine is shifted to the right by i.c.v. administration of calcium ions.

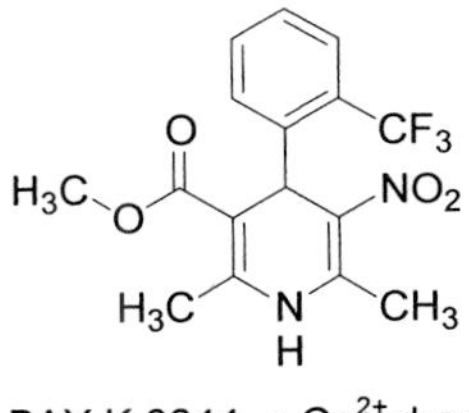

BAY K 8644, a Ca^{2+} channel <u>agonistic</u> dihydropyridine

Table 2: Enhancement of opioid antinociception by L-type Ca^{2+} channel antagonist.

Model	Species	Opioid	L-type Ca^{2+} channel antagonist	Application	Effect	References
Hot plate (55°C)	Mouse	Morphine	Diltiazem or Verapamil	M: 1 mg/kg s.c.; D and V: 30-120 µg/kg i.c.v.	Both Ca^{2+} antag. lead to an enhancement of the M effect $\geq$ 30 µg/kg	Del Pozo et al. (1990)
Hot plate (55°C)	Mouse	Morphine	Diltiazem or Verapamil	M: 1-8 mg/kg s.c.; D and V: 40 µg/kg s.c.	The dose - response curve of M is shifted to the left by an additional application of D or V	Del Pozo et al. (1990)
Tail flick	Rat	Morphine	Verapamil or Nicardipine or Diltiazem	M: 2 µg i.t. plus: V: 50 µg i.t. or N: 20 µg i.t. or D: 100 µg i.t.	M alone and the Ca^{2+} antag. alone have no effect. In combination there is a very pronounced enhancement of the tail flick latencies	Omote et al. (1993)
Tail flick	Rat	Morphine	Verapamil or Nicardipine or Diltiazem	i.t.	The dose - response curve of M is shifted to the left by V, N or D	Omote et al. (1993)
Tail flick	Rat	DAMGO	Verapamil	D: 0.4 nmol i.c.v. V: 20 nmol i.c.v.	Large enhancement of the AUC of D by additional V application	Spampinato et al. (1994)
Hot plate (53.5°C)	Rat	Morphine	Diltiazem	M: 4, 6 and 8 mg/kg s.c.; D: 20 mg/kg s.c.	Potentiation and prolongation of the M effect by additional application of D	Beredek and Szikszay (1984)
Tail flick	Mouse	Morphine	Nifedipine	M: 5 mg/kg i.p.; N: 2.5 and 5 mg/kg i.p.	N prolongs M induced TF latencies	Pavone, et al. (1992)
Tail flick	Mouse	Morphine DAMGO DPDPE U-50,488H	Amlodipine	i.t.	I.t. administration of A potentiated M- and DAMGO -induced antinoc. by shifting their dose response curves to the left. However i.t. admin. of A did not effect DPDPE and U-induced tail flick latencies. These data indicate that L-type VDCC blockers potentiate the analgesic effects of µ-opioid receptor agonists, but not δ an κ receptor agonists, at the spinal level	Dogrul et al. (2001)

Table 2 continued:

Model	Species	Opioid	L-type Ca^{2+} channel antagonist	Application	Effect	References
Tail flick	Rat	Sufentanil	Nimodipine	S: 0.26 µg/kg s.c. (~ED$_{50}$); N: 200 µg/kg i.p.	N potentiated the antinociceptive effect of S by reducing the ED$_{50}$ from 0.26 to 0.08 µg/kg s.c.	Dierssen et al. (1990)
Tail flick	Rat	Sufentanil	BAY K 8644 (Agonist)	S: 0.26 µg/kg s.c. (~ED$_{50}$); BAY K 8644: 20 µg/kg i.p.	BAY K 8644 in this low dose behaves as a calcium agonist and antagonized the effect of S (ED$_{50}$ = 0.26 → 0.58 µg/kg s.c.), whereas at a high dose (200 µg/kg i.p.) it potentiated this action (ED$_{50}$ = 0.26 → 0.15 µg/kg s.c.)	Dierssen et al. (1990)
Hot plate	Mouse	Fentanyl	Dihydro-pyridines (DHPs)	F: i.v.; DHPs: i.v.	F antinociceptive effects are potentiated by simultaneous i.v. administration of the Ca^{2+} antagonists	Hoffmeister and Tettenborn (1986)
Hot plate	Mouse	Fentanyl	BAY K 8644 (Agonist)		BAY K 8644 increases reaction time in the hot plate test dose-dependently (1-10 mg/kg p.o.)	Hoffmeister and Tettenborn (1986)
several	Rat	Fentanyl	BAY K 8644 (Agonist)		The influence on F antinociception in the rat of the Ca^{2+} agonist BAY K 8644 is biphasic: low doses attenuate, high doses potentiate F antinociception. It is concluded that calcium antagonism potentiates µ-receptor agonist antinociceptive effects, whereas calcium agonism antagonizes µ-receptor agonist antinociception	Hoffmeister and Tettenborn (1986)

Due to the crosstalk between G-proteins of metabotropic receptors and the α1 subunit of Ca^{2+} channels a highly regulated and dynamic control of neurotransmitter release results (Herlitze et al., 1996; Zamponi et al., 1997). This crosstalk has also been documented with respect to opioid receptors and Ca^{2+} channels (Moises et al., 1994; Bourinet et al., 1996). There are several publications

Crosstalk between opioid receptors and Ca^{2+} channels

claiming that co-administration of L-type Ca^{2+} channel blockers has a positive result with respect to opioid-induced tolerance and/or withdrawal symptoms (Bongianni et al., 1985; 1986; Baeyens et al., 1987; Barrios and Baeyens, 1988; Contreras et al., 1988; Alfaro et al., 1990; Antkiewicz-Michaluk et al., 1990; 1993; Welch and Olson, 1991; Ruiz et al., 1993; Diaz et al., 1995; Garaulet et al., 1996; Tokuyama and Ho, 1996; Michaluk et al., 1998).

Evidence suggesting a fundamental role for VDCCs in the development of opioid tolerance and dependence

In morphine-tolerant mice an increased number of $[^3H]$-nitrendipine binding sites (B_{max}) was determined while the dissociation constant was unchanged (K_d; Ramkumar and El-Fakahany, 1984). In rats an increased DHP binding induced by prolonged opioid treatment was localized to the cortex, hippocampus and brainstem but not to the cerebellum and striatum (Ramkumar and El-Fakahany, 1988). These data were confirmed by Zharkovsky et al. (1993), who reported that in rats concurrent nimodipine treatment prevented the rise in the density of central DHP binding sites which occurred during chronic treatment. The authors suggest that chronic nimodipine treatment attenuates the development of withdrawal symptoms which occur on termination of chronic morphine treatment by preventing the upregulation of central DHP-sensitive binding sites. These pharmacological effects still have to be confirmed clinically.

Low antinociceptive strength of L-type Ca^{2+} channel antagonists for the treatment of pain

We reevaluated these experiments to determine the relationship between antinociceptive efficacy and possible side-effects which were only poorly reported in the literature. The first approach - application of L-type Ca^{2+} channel antagonists alone - was not convincing. The antinociceptive effect was rather poor and, since L-type Ca^{2+} channel antagonists have been used for the treatment of hypertension for many years, side-effects like hypotension are to be expected.

Potent antinociception and reduced side-effects through the combination of µ-opioid agonists with L-type Ca^{2+} channel antagonists

The second approach however - enhancement of opioid antinociception by L-type Ca^{2+} channel antagonists - offers the possibility for very effective antinociception with a reduced spectrum of side effects due to the opioid-sparing effect (Reimann (Grünenthal GmbH), 1998).

The rationale of this concept is:

- Ca^{2+}-antagonists are able to enhance the antinociceptive effect of opioids

- for this reason the µ-component can be reduced by an additional Ca^{2+} antagonistic component to achieve equipotent analgesia

- lowering the opioid component has the advantage that opioid mediated side-effects are no longer prominent

The aim of this concept was to synthesize drugs which combine both activities in one molecule. Before *in vitro* screening was started, excellent correlation between pharmacological effects and L-type channel as well as μ opioid binding affinity was ensured (data not shown).

The biochemical screening procedure consisted of a μ-opioid-, DHP-, PAA-, BTZ- and BTX- (Batrachotoxinin A 20-α-benzoate - binding site 2 of the Na^+ channel) radio-ligand binding assay essentially according to Frink et al. (1996), Murphy and Snyder (1982), Reynolds et al. (1983), Schoemaker and Langer (1985) and Pauwels et al. (1986). In contrast to DHPs, compounds binding to the PAA- and BTZ-site of the L-type Ca^{2+} channel exhibit a more or less pronounced interaction with the BTX-binding site of the Na^+ channel. For structural reasons we nevertheless decided to combine an agonistic μ-opioid affinity with an L-type Ca^{2+} channel blocking affinity mediated by the PAA and/or BTZ site(s).

During the drug discovery campaign we found that all compounds with a very high affinity for the BTX-site of the sodium channel had an insufficient safety index - the LD_{50}/ED_{50} ratio was too narrow. In this respect the BTX-assay was used as an early safety indicator.

Selected orally active compounds (Graudums et al. (Grünenthal GmbH), 1997; Sundermann et al. (Grünenthal GmbH), 2000) exhibited a wide range of μ-opioid affinity (Ki 0.1 to 0.0001 μM) but affinities to the PAA and/or BTZ site were always quite constant (Ki 1 to 0.1 μM). Compounds with very pronounced μ-affinities are at least 10 times more potent than morphine *in vivo*, have an excellent safety index and a relatively mild effect on respiration in comparison to other very strong opioids, e.g. fentanyl.

Compounds with moderate μ-affinities are very potent in a variety of pain models in mice and rats. In addition to anti-nociceptive efficacy in models of acute pain (tail flick, writhing) these compounds inhibit acute and persistent inflammatory pain (Randall Selitto, formalin test). Furthermore, they show strong inhibition of acute visceral pain (colorectal distension) and of tactile and cold allodynia in models of neuropathic pain (spinal nerve ligation (Chung), chronic constriction injury (Bennett)). The data suggest these compounds to be potential candidates for the management of clinical pain indications. Somatic and visceral pain with and without inflammatory conditions as well as neuropathic pain might be addressed with this approach.

Combining μ-opioid agonism and L-type Ca^{2+} channel antagonism in one molecule

L-type Ca^{2+} channels are the only VDCC which have three different drug binding sites, the

- Dihydropyridine (DHP)
- Phenylalkylamine (PAA)
- Benzothiazepine (BTZ)

sites (Glossmann and Striessnig, 1990; Catterall and Striessnig, 1992; Varadi et al., 1995; Striessnig et al., 1998).

Pronounced interaction with binding site 2 of the Na^+ channel leads to an insufficient safety index

Compounds with dual mode of action (Ki/μM):

μ-opioid affinity	affinty to PAA / BTZ site
0.1 - 0.0001	1 - 0.1

Antinociceptive Effects of N- and P/Q- type Ca²⁺ Channel Antagonists

Peptides from cone snails and spiders – molecular probes for N- and P/Q- type Ca^{2+} channels

Unlike DHP-sensitive L-type channels ω-conotoxin-sensitive N-type Ca^{2+} channels are exclusively expressed in the CNS. L-type channels inactivate very slowly whereas N-type channels inactivate more rapidly and are blocked by ω-conotoxin GVIA. ω-[^{125}I]conotoxin GVIA is an ideal ligand for binding experiments. The dissociation constant (K_D) for this toxin in rat brain membranes is 60 pM (Wagner et al., 1988).

P-type channels inactivate extremely slowly and are insensitive to both DHPs and ω-conotoxin GVIA, but are blocked by the spider venom peptide ω-agatoxin IVA, a peptide consisting of 48 amino acids isolated from the American funnel-web spider *Agelenopsis aperta*.

The inactivation kinetics of the Q-type channel are similar to the N-type channel but are resistant to DHPs and ω-conotoxin GVIA. Q-type channels are inhibited by ω-agatoxin IVA but less effectively than ω-agatoxin IVA blocks P-type channels (review: Miljanich and Ramachandran, 1995).

Table 3: Sequences of naturally-occurring ω-conopeptides.
(from Miljanich and Ramachandran, 1995)

Name	Sequence (I)	Species
SNX-124 (GVIA)	C K S X G S S C S X T S Y N C C R - S C N X Y T K R C Y	*Conus geographus*
SNX-178 (GVIIA)	C K S X G T X C S R G M R D C C T - S C L L Y S N K C R R Y	*C. geographus*
SNX-111 (MVIIA)	C K G K G A K C S R L M Y D C C T G S C - R - S G K C	*Conus magus*
SNX-159 (MVIIB)	C K G K G A S C H R T S Y D C C T G S C N R - - G K C	*C. magus*
SNX-230 (MVIIC)	C K G K G A P C R K T M Y D C C S G S C G R - R G K C	*C. magus*
SNX-238 (MVIID)	C Q G R G A S C R K T M Y N C C S G S C N R - - G R C	*C. magus*
SNX-157 (SVIA)	C R S S G S X C G V T S I - C C - G R C - - Y R G K C T	*Conus striatus*
SNX-183 (SVIB)	C K L K G Q S C R K T S Y D C C S G S C G R - S G K C	*C. striatus*
SNX-185 (TVIA)	C L S X G S S C S X T S Y N C C R - S C N X Y S R K C	*Conus tulipa*

(I) All synthetic peptides are amidated at the carboxy terminus. Dashes indicate gaps. X: Hydroxyproline.

Cone snails are found in tropical waters, often in the neighborhood of coral reefs. These molluscs produce a complex venom delivered through a specialized radular tooth that serves as a harpoon to immobilize their prey (Olivera et al., 1990; 1991). Complete immobilisation of the prey takes only a few seconds (Terlau et al., 1996). The venom from a single cone snail can contain up to 200 different biologically-active components (review: Shen et al., 2000). The primary structure of the naturally-occurring ω-conopeptides derived from several species of Conus are shown in Table 3 (taken from Miljanich and Ramachandran, 1995). The ω-conopeptides are simple peptides built from 24 to 29 amino acids. All contain six cysteine residues linked to form three disulfide bridges. The SNX numbers refer to synthetically prepared peptides.

Table 4 summarizes the antinociceptive effects of several ω-conotoxins and ω-agatoxin IVA in different animal models. The peptides are administered by the i.t. or i.c.v. route.

ω-conotoxins and -agatoxins

Concerning the ω-conopeptides, SNX-111 (Ziconotide) seems to be one of the proteins with the highest intrinsic antinociceptive activity in the formalin test (Table 4, Malmberg and Yaksh, 1994). This may be the main reason why most of the papers cited deal with this special synthetic peptide.

SNX-111 (Ziconotide)

SNX-111, when given alone, is active in the Chung model (spinal nerve ligation), tactile allodynia test (hindpaw UV burn) and paw pressure test. In the hot plate assay there is only a small but significant effect of about 20% increase in response latency (Table 4, Malmberg and Yaksh, 1994).

ω-agatoxin IVA has been reported to be active in the formalin test whereas it is inactive in the hot plate assay (Table 4, Malmberg and Yaksh, 1994).

ω-agatoxin IVA

SNX-111 combined with morphine in the hot plate assay results in response latencies greatly exceeding those produced by either compound alone (Table 4, Bowersox et al., 1998). In the formalin test a combination of both drugs leads to an additive effect (Table 4, Wang et al., 2000). In the tail immersion test the effect of both compounds together is higher than those produced by each drug alone. Morphine, when administered for 7 days leads to rapid tolerance. SNX-111 in combination with this μ-opioid agonist did not prevent tolerance to morphine analgesia (Table 4, Wang et al., 2000). In contrast to opioids only minimal development of tolerance was observed in the formalin test after chronic administration of SNX-111 over 7 days (Malmberg and Yaksh, 1995).

Combination of SNX-111 with morphine - additive to synergistic antinociception

In the tail flick assay ω-conotoxin GVIA in combination with morphine leads to an additive effect similar to the combination of morphine with SNX-111 in the formalin test. But when ω-conotoxin GVIA was applied 24 h before morphine, antinociception was greatly reduced. In morphine-dependent rats, ω-conotoxin GVIA given i.c.v. 15 min before naloxone challenge (2 mg/kg i.p.), significantly attenuated the withdrawal symptoms (Table 4, Basilico et al., 1992).

Table 4: Antinociceptive activity of N-, P- and/or Q-type VDCC inhibitors <u>in rats</u>.

Model	Opioid	Compound	Application	Effect	References
Formalin test	-	N-type blocker SNX-111 SNX-159 SNX-183 SNX-199 SNX-239 P- and/or Q-type blocker ω-Agat.-IVA SNX-231	i.t.	ED_{50} (nmol) Phase 1 Phase 2 0.003 0,003 >0.26 0.12 0.010 0.009 >0.30 0.23 0.54 0.052 >0.006 0.001 >0.24 >0.24	Malmberg and Yaksh (1994)
Hot plate (52.5°C)	- -	SNX-111 ω-Agat.-IVA	0.008 nmol i.t. 0.006 nmol i.t.	Small, but sign. effect Very small insign. effect	Malmberg and Yaksh (1994)
Paw pressure	-	SNX-111	0.1, 0.3 and 1.0 µg i.t.	Sign. antinoc. effect at 0.3 and 1.0 µg	Bowersox et al. (1998)
Tactile allodynia (UV burn, hindpaw)	-	SNX-111	0.3 µg i.t.	≈ 4-fold increase in the hindpaw withdrawal threshold to mechan.stim.	Bowersox et al. (1998)
Formalin test (2nd phase)	-	SNX-111	0.1 µg i.t.	Suppression of nociceptive responses (flinch behavior)	Bowersox et al. (1998)
Chung model (spinal nerve ligation)	-	SNX-111	0.03, 0.1 and 0.3 µg i.t.	Dose-dependent blockade of mechan. allodynia in neuropathy rats	Bowersox et al. (1998)
Hot plate	Morphine	SNX-111 (Ziconotide)	M: 15 µg/hr S: 30 ng/hr; continuous spinal infusion for 7 days	Both drugs alone at this dose = little effect; in combination = response latencies greatly exceed those produced by either compound alone	Bowersox et al. (1998)
Chung model	-	SNX-111 SNX-159 SNX-239	3.0 µg i.t. 1.0 µg i.t. 3.3 µg i.t.	Significant suppression of allodynia	Chaplan et al. (1994)
Extracellular recording of dorsal horn neurones after s.c. formalin injection	-	ω-Con.-GVIA w-Agat.-IVA	0.1 and 0.4 µg i.t. 0.125 and 0.5 µg i.t.	Both phases of the formalin response were inhibited by ω-Con-GVIA, ω-Agat-IVA blocks only the second phase	Diaz and Dickenson (1997)

Table 4 continued:

Model	Opioid	Compound	Application	Effect	References
Formalin test	Morphine	SNX-111 (Ziconotide)	dose-response curves alone and in combination i.t.	Isobolographical analysis: combination of both drugs results in an additive effect	Wang et al. (2000)
Tail immersion test	Morphine	SNX-111 (Ziconotide)	M: 15 µg/h S: 30 ng/h; continuous spinal infusion for 7 days	The effect of both compounds together exceed those produced by either compound alone. Morphine alone leads to rapid tolerance. SNX-111 in combination with M did not prevent tolerance to M analgesia	Wang et al. (2000)
Tail flick	Morphine	ω-Con.-GVIA	M: 1.5 µg/rat ω-C.: 20 ng/rat i.c.v.; M: 3.0 µg/rat ω-C.: 20 ng/rat i.c.v.	When ω-C. was given immediately before M, analgesic effect was additive. But, when the toxin was given 24 h before M, M analgesia was greatly reduced	Basilico et al. (1992)
Morphine-dependent rats	Morphine	ω-Con.-GVIA	two M. pellets (75mg each) implanted s.c. for 72 h; ω-C.: 20 ng/rat i.c.v.	ω-C injected in M dependent rats 15 min before naloxone challenge (2 mg/kg i.p.) signif. attenuated the abstinence syndrome	Basilico et al. (1992)

High doses of the N-type VDCC inhibitors produce characteristic shaking behavior, serpent-like tail movements, and impaired coordination. At antinociceptive doses however there is no significant motor effect although some of the N-type Ca^{2+} channel antagonists produce tail movements (Malmberg and Yaksh, 1994).

Side-effects of N-type VDCC inhibitors

ω-Conotoxins (as well as ω-agatoxin) cannot be applied orally but the intrathecal route is, at any rate, far from ideal. To overcome the disadvantages of intrathecal administration the pharmaceutical industry has endeavored to develop orally-active small molecule inhibitors of the N-type VDCC. There is a large list of small molecules having a pronounced affinity for the N-type VDCC (review: Cox and Denyer, 1998). The majority of these compounds are not really selective and interact with other targets like the dopamine D_2 receptor (neuroleptics

Small molecule N-type VDCC inhibitors

like fluspirilene and pimozide), the NMDA receptor (eliprodil) and others.

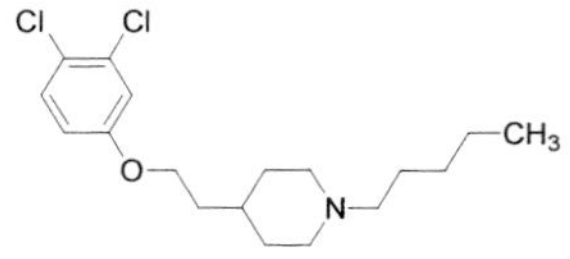

Since 1992 SmithKlineBeecham have published more than 20 patents on a range of piperidine and cycloalkylamine derivatives such as SB-201823 which are claimed to be non-DHP-like VDCC modulators. The main indication for these compounds is stroke (review including structures: Cox and Denyer, 1998) but no compound has yet been reported to be in clinical trials for the treatment of stroke or any other indication.

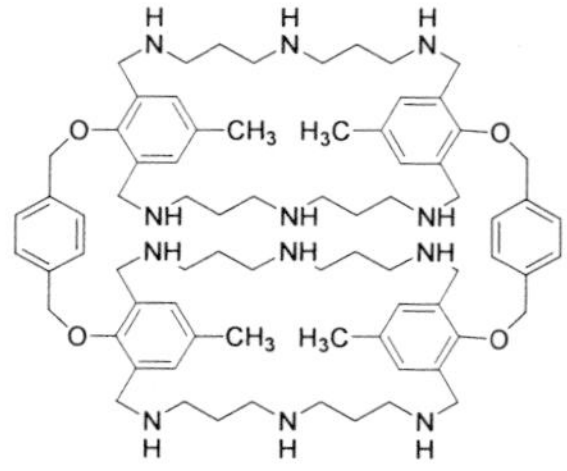

SB-201823

McNaughton et al. (1999) published data on LY310315, a synthetic macrocyclic polyamine. Effects of this compound were investigated on recombinant human N-type Ca^{2+} channels expressed in HEK293 cells. The electro-physiological characterization revealed that LY310315 is a potent and reversible N-type Ca^{2+} channel antagonist with an IC_{50} of approximately 0.4 μM at pH 7.35. Although most effective on N-type Ca^{2+} channels LY310315 also inhibits P-type and L-type Ca^{2+} channels.

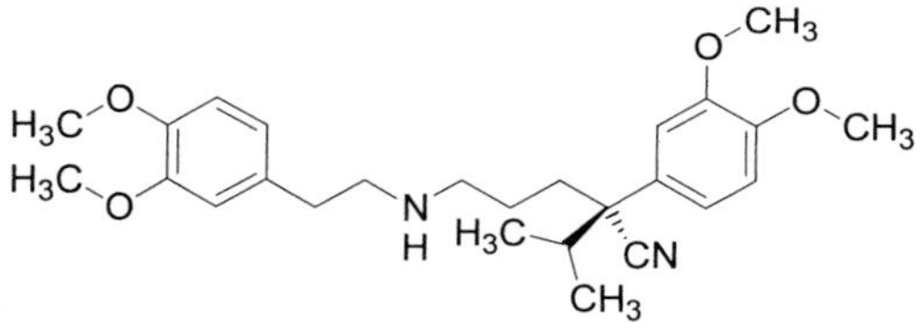

LY310315

Verapamil

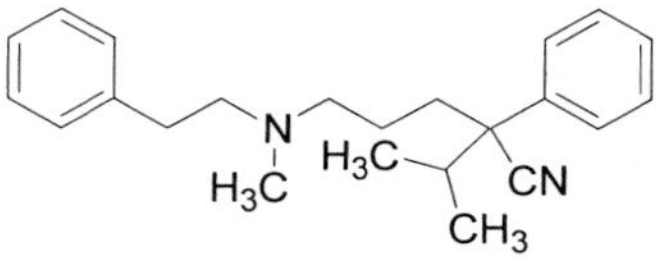

Emopamil

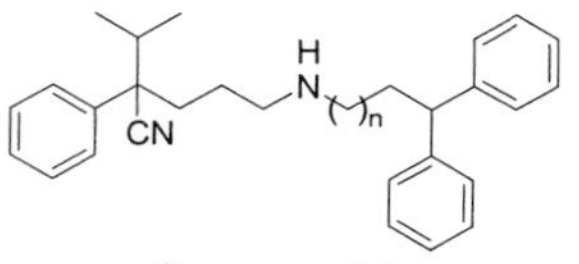

Compound 1

Through the modification of the known L-type VDCC inhibitors verapamil and its desmethoxy analog emopanil, Eli Lilly identified a novel series of amino acid containing phenylalkylamines which demonstrate submicromolar inhibition of neuronal non-L-type VDCC while showing markedly decreased activity on L-type channels. They initially investigated the modification of the phenethylamine moiety and found that chain elongation and incorporation of a second phenyl substituent (compound 1) markedly shifted activity away from L-towards non-L-type inhibition.

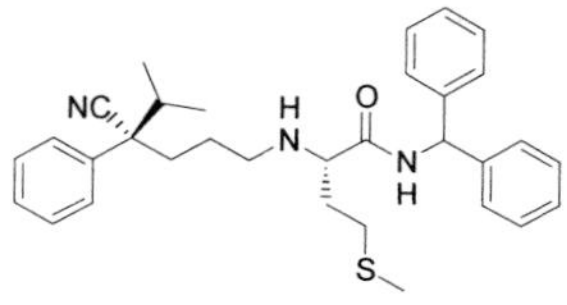

One of the best compounds of this series is the methionine-derived compound 2. It shows preferential inhibition of human α 1B construct (N-channel) with respect to α 1A (P/Q-channel) and α 1E (R-channel) (Ambler et al., 1997).

Compound 2

Warner-Lambert/ParkeDavis have published data on several N-type compounds for the treatment of stroke and pain (review: Cox and Denyer, 1998). PD157667, although potent at the N-type Ca^{2+} channel, was found to have significant Na^+ and K^+ channel blocking activity at 10 µM. PD158143 however is selective with respect to sodium channel, potassium channel or L-type calcium channel activities.

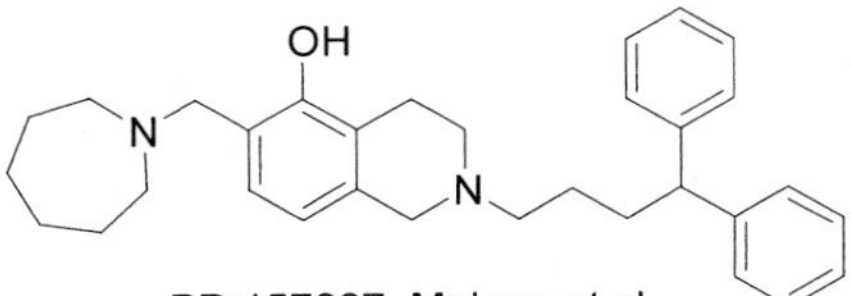

PD 157667, Malone et al.,
Warner-Lambert, WO9705125

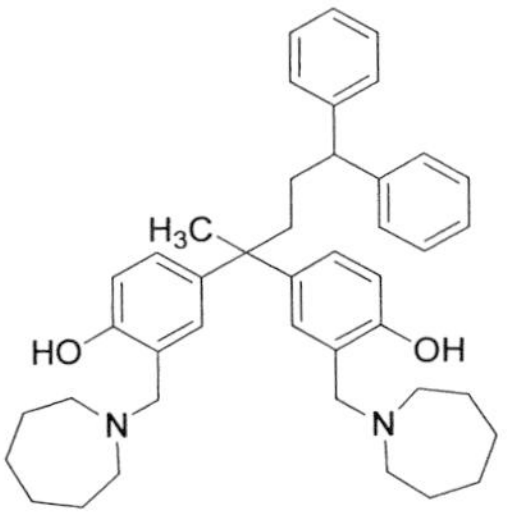

PD158143,
Yuen, Warner-Lambert,
US5767129, 1998

Neurex/Warner-Lambert and Elan/Warner-Lambert have published additional data on PD-151307 and PD-175069 and analogs thereof (Drug Data Report **1999**, *21*, 403, 576, 589):

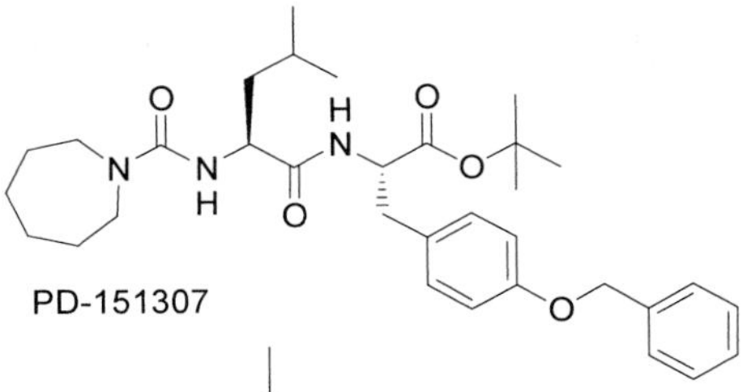

PD-151307

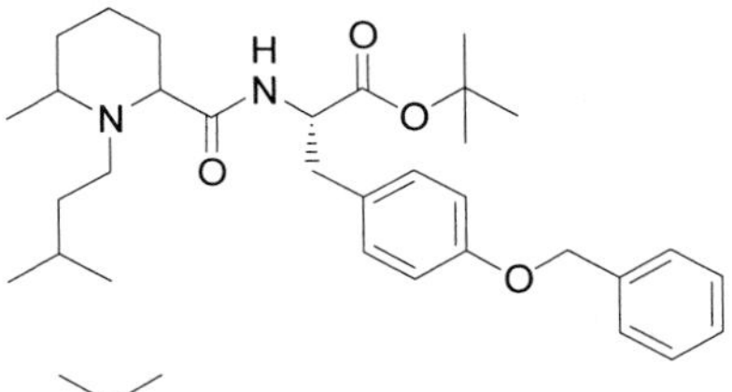

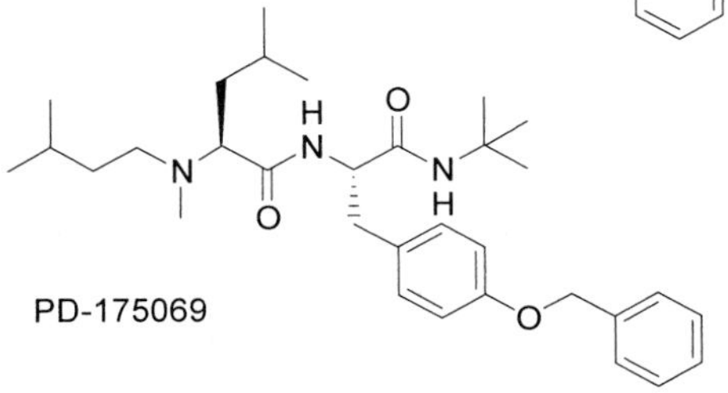

PD-175069

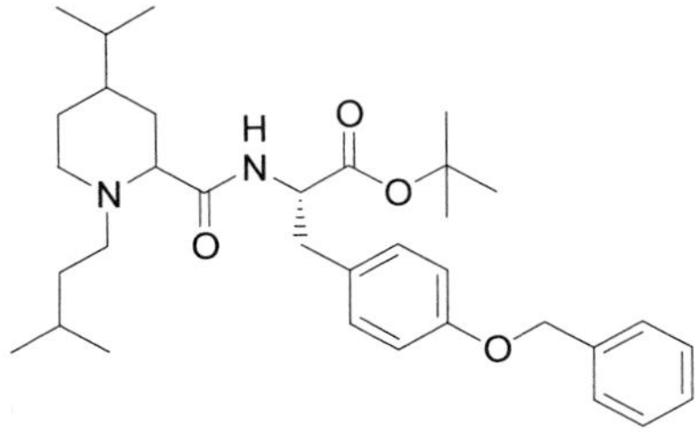

These compounds block N-type calcium channels in human neuroblastoma IMR-32 cells. PD-151307 (IC_{50} = 0.22 µM) shows about 40-fold selectivity for N- over L-type calcium channels (IC_{50} = 9.1 µM in GH3 cells). These compounds may also be potentially useful in the treatment of cerebral ischemia and chronic intractable pain.

Pfizer reported on a small-molecule calcium channel antagonist (compound 3) with potential for the treatment of pain (Song et al., 2000). Its antagonistic activity toward neuronal N-type calcium channels was confirmed by electrophysiology studies. It has an IC_{50} value of 1.3 µM against N-type calcium channels in superior cervical ganglion neurons. But it is also active, although to a lesser extent, against Na^+ channels (IC_{50} = 5.1 µM) and K^+

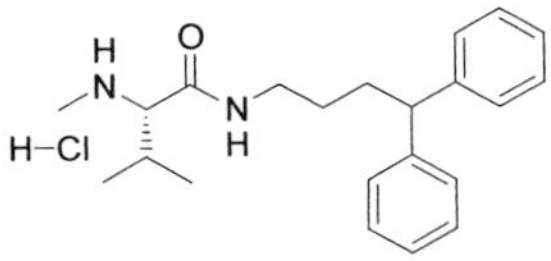

Compound 3

Compound 4,
Kazuyuki et al., Shionogi &
Co., WO9801121

Compound 5

	R_1	R_2	n
A-53930A	$CONH_2$	H	4
A-53930B	$CONH_2$	H	5
A-53930C	H	$CONH_2$	5

channels (IC_{50} = 9.9 μM). Furthermore this compound inhibits the activity of L-type calcium channels in smooth muscles. Fluorescence measurements, using Oregon Greens 488 Bapta-1 dye in the A10 smooth muscle cell line (FLIPR-assay) revealed an IC_{50} value of 0.4 μM. This compound penetrates into the CNS after i.v. and p.o. administration.

Shinogi and Co. has filed a patent application on P/Q-type calcium channel antagonists such as compound 4. Suppression of Ca^{2+} ion influx was evaluated using rat cerebellar synaptosomes. An IC_{50} value of 1.0 μM was obtained. Compounds in this series are claimed to be useful as antiischemic nerve cell disorder agents, anticonvulsants, migraine agents and analgesics and for the treatment of diseases caused by excessive release of neurotransmitters in the CNS.

Cypros Pharm. Corp. describes the use of polyguanidino derivatives as presynaptic N- and P/Q-type calcium channel blockers for i.v. (or i.c.v.) administration (Marangos et al. (Cypros Pharmaceutical Corp.), WO9836743). Compound 5 was administered to gerbils (7.5 mg/kg i.v.) prior to bilateral carotid occlusion. After 72 h the animals were sacrificed. Brains were perfusion-fixed and sections were stained to enable quantitative cell counts of live and dead neurons. The number of damaged neurons in the subiculum was 91.5 compared to 214 for a control treated with saline. It has been claimed that this compound can be used for the treatment of neuropathic pain and for the protection of neurons from excitatory damage under conditions of cerebral hypoxia.

The Sankyo compounds A-53930A, B and C are natural products and were isolated from the culture broth of *Streptomyces vinaceusdrappus*. A-53930A and B are new compounds (JP08208690), whereas A-53930C is identical to streptothricin B. A-53930A, B and C inhibit [^{125}I]ω-conotoxin MVIIA binding to N-type Ca^{2+} channels (IC_{50} = 0.17, 0.091 and 0.071 μM respectively). There is no interaction with the DHP binding site of the L-type Ca^{2+} channel. It was also revealed that although A-53930C has antimicrobial activity against Gram-negative and -positive bacteria and fungi, A-53930A and B only show weak activity against Gram-negative bacteria (Hisamoto et al., 1998).

Clinical Data

L-type VDCC Inhibitors in Combination with a μ-Opioid Agonist

To demonstrate the enhancement of μ-opioid-mediated antinociception by L-type VDCC a nearly ineffective dose (threshold dose) of an opioid agonist can be used. All three types of L-type VDCC inhibitors enhance the opioid-mediated effect in an additive or synergistic manner, depending upon the pharmacological model used. For clinical investigations, however, such a study design may not be approved by the ethics commission. From this point of view clinical investigations are not as easy to carry out as the pharmacological investigations described in the section 'Antinociceptive effects of L-type Ca^{2+} channel antagonists'. By and large the following clinical trials reflect the results described in 'Preclinical data'. Nevertheless there are some reports with insignificant effects.

To the best of our knowledge the first clinical study in this field was carried out at the universities of Giessen and Marburg (Germany) and reported by Bormann et al. in 1985. Twenty patients undergoing cardiovascular surgery were investigated in two groups. The 10 patients in the first group received high-dose fentanyl anesthesia (mean: 2.45 mg/patient), whereas the 10 patients in the second group were treated with only 0.1 mg fentanyl/patient in addition to nimodipine 1.0 μg/kg/min. Although the patients in the second group received only ≈ 1/25 of the μ-opioid dose compared to the first group, there were no differences with respect to perioperative course and postoperative demand for analgesics. So nimodipine can be used very effectively to reduce the necessary dose of fentanyl in cardiovascular surgery.

Fentanyl and nimodipine in cardiovascular surgery

In a second paper, published 2 years later, the same group confirmed the data concerning the positive interaction of fentanyl with nimodipine. Forty-five men scheduled for aorto-coronary bypass operation received fentanyl according to their individual demands. Nimodipine at infusion rate of 1.0 μg/kg/min reduced the demand for fentanyl significantly. Astonishingly, nifedipine at infusion rate of 0.7 μg/kg/min failed to reduce the need for fentanyl during surgical procedures without influencing the quality of anesthesia (Boldt et al., 1987).

Fentanyl and nimodipine in aorto-coronary bypass operations

A randomized double-blind study including 40 patients undergoing elective hysterectomy under standardized balanced anesthesia were reported by Lehmann et al. in 1989. In a recovery room patients were allowed to self-administer fentanyl by means of the On-Demand Analgesia Computer. Demand dose was 34.5 μg, infusion rate 4 μg/h, lockout time 1 min, hourly max. dose = 250 μg. The patients were randomly and double-blindly assigned to have an additional infusion of either placebo

Fentanyl and nimodipine in elective hysterectomy

or nimodipine(N) (N = 15 µg/kg/h during the first 2 h, 30 µg/kg/h from the third to the 12th hour). Fentanyl consumption, pain scores, blood pressure, heart rate, respiratory rate and side-effects were monitored. At each time interval (4 h) when the fentanyl consumption was calculated, the nimodipine group had a lower consumption rate in comparison with the placebo group. Nevertheless, none of these differences were statistically significant. Further studies are necessary to evaluate this potential drug interaction at different dose ranges.

Morphine and nifedipine in orthopedic surgery and hysterectomy

Additional data concerning the influence of nifedipine on morphine analgesia was reported by Carta et al. (1990). In a double-blind, placebo-controlled experimental design, slow-release 20 mg tablets of nifedipine or identical placebo control tablets were used. The half-life of slow-release nifedipine is 15.2 ± 4.3 h (standard nifedipine tablets = 3.9 ± 2.3 h). Per randomization, persons were divided into a placebo (P) and a verum (V) group. Nifedipine significantly increased the analgesic effect of morphine (orthopedic surgery: P = 5; V = 5; hysterectomy: P = 8; V = 8). Respiratory and cardiovascular functions were not significantly changed by this L-type VDCC inhibitor.

Epidural morphine and sublingual nifedipine

Pereira et al. (1993) evaluated postoperative pain relief and incidence of side-effects of the combination of epidural morphine (0.5 mg) and sublingual nifedipine (10 mg). In this double-blind, placebo-controlled study 36 women were submitted to elective operations (hysterectomy and colpoperineoplasty). The nifedipine-treated group showed a significant drop in blood pressure which was controlled by rehydration. The results indicate that epidural morphine-induced postoperative pain relief may be enhanced by systemic administration of nifedipine with easily controlled side-effects.

Morphine and diltiazem, verapamil or nimodipine

Negative results were reported by Hasegawa and Zacny (1997). They examined the effects of three L-type VDCC inhibitors (diltiazem 30 mg p.o.; nimodipine 60 mg p.o. and verapamil 80 mg p.o.) on morphine (10 mg/70 kg i.v.) in a cold-pressor test with nine healthy volunteers. Subjects first ingested the oral drugs or placebo and 120 min later were injected with morphine or saline. Morphine alone and in combination with the VDCC inhibitors reduced pain ratings. No statistically significant differences in the pain measures between the morphine and the L-type VDCC blockers/morphine conditions were observed. Other conditions e.g. altered dose or time regimes of the p.o. and i.v. drug administration were not tested.

Another negative result was reported by Roca et al. (1996). They assessed the ability of nimodipine to increase the analgesic effect of morphine in 32 patients suffering from cancer pain. In this double-blind, placebo-controlled cross-over study morphine administration began a few days before the start of the study. The analgesic effects of two combinations were compared: morphine plus placebo and morphine plus 90 mg/24 h nimodipine. The study spanned 8 days, including the wash-out period. No significant statistical differences were found in analgesic effect between the two groups. Higher doses of the L-type VDCC inhibitor were not tested.

In contrast to this study Santillán et al. (1994) used a higher dose of nimodipine and reported positive results for nimodipine - morphine association in a non-placebo controlled trial with cancer patients. Nimodipine succeeded in reducing the daily dose of morphine in 16 of 23 patients (p.o. n = 13; i.t.: n = 3), and failed to modify it in two patients. Total oral daily dose of morphine was significantly reduced by nimodipine (120 mg/day) from 283 to 159 mg. Intrathecal morphine was also reduced. This data was confirmed by a randomized, double-blind, placebo-controlled study which was published 4 years later (Santillán et al., 1998). The study started with 54 cancer patients. A total of 30 patients completed the study (14 in the nimodipine group and 16 in the placebo group). The dose of morphine was reduced from 313 to 174 mg/day (p < 0.001) in the nimodipine group (120 mg/day), and non-significantly from 254 to 218 mg/day in the placebo group. The authors conclude that the introduction of nimodipine in patients chronically treated with morphine may be a safe alternative to reducing the daily requirement of the µ-opioid agonist. It is further suggested that interference with Ca^{2+}-related events may attenuate the development and/or expression of tolerance to morphine in a clinically relevant way.

Morphine and nimodipine in cancer pain

N-type VDCC Inhibitors

Clinical studies of N-type VDCC inhibitors are limited to SNX-111 (Ziconotide), a synthetic peptide related to the naturally-occurring ω-conopeptide MVIIA (see Table 3; for clinical reviews see Hunter, 1999 and Prado, 2001).

In 1997 Brose et al. published the result of a single case study. SNX-111, administered i.t. by continuous, constant-rate infusion, produced dose-dependent pain relief in a 43-year-old male patient with a 23-year history of intractable deafferentation and phantom limb pain secondary to brachial plexus avulsion and subsequent amputation. Dizziness, blurred vision, and lateral-gaze nystagmus

Clinical trials with SNX-111 (Ziconotide)

were dose-dependent side-effects that resolved with decreasing dose levels. Complete pain relief was achieved in this patient without side-effects after dose adjustment.

A second report was published by Atanassoff et al. (2000). This was a randomized, double-blind, placebo-controlled study including patients undergoing elective total abdominal hysterectomy, radical prostatectomy, or total hip replacement. Ziconotide was administered as a continuous i.t. infusion at a rate of 0.7 µg/h or 7.0 µg/h. Thirty patients received the study drug, 26 were evaluable for efficacy. Mean daily morphine consumption was less in patients receiving Ziconotide than in placebo-treated patients (p = 0.040). Four of six patients who received the high dose of Ziconotide (7.0 µg/h) developed adverse events such as dizziness, blurred vision, nystagmus and sedation. The conclusion of the report was that an i.t. infusion of Ziconotide results in a significant morphine-sparing effect. The dose of 0.7 µg/h may be closer to the ideal dose than 7.0 µg/h.

Adverse effects of SNX-111 (Ziconotide)

The first study dealing with the adverse effects after i.t. administration of Ziconotide was published by Penn and Paice (2000). This clinical report described the experiences of three patients suffering from chronic pain, who developed very serious side-effects after continuous i.t. infusion of the drug. In addition to the side-effects described in previous papers, nasal congestion, urinary retention, bradycardia, orthostatic hypotension, nausea and vomiting, coma, ataxia, dysmetria, agitation, hallucination, rash, hypoglycemia and diarrhoea were reported by the authors. Penn and Paice (2000) point out that these complications occurred within a highly monitored environment. Widespread use in general clinical conditions are likely to lead to an even greater prevalence of adverse effects, with potentially more serious outcomes.

Conclusions

L-type VDCC inhibitors

In pharmacological experiments L-type VDCC inhibitors are not convincingly effective for the treatment of pain. In combination with a µ-opioid agonist, however, all three classes of L-type inhibitors lead to an enhancement of opioid-induced antinociception. This enhancement may be additive or even over-additive (synergistic), depending on the species and pain model under investigation. To achieve equipotent antinociception the µ-component can be reduced. This opioid-sparing effect has also been documented in double-blind, placebo-controlled clinical studies without drastic changes to respiratory and cardiovascular function. Observed side-effects can be easily controlled. A large body of evidence points to the possibility that L-type VDCC blockers may prevent the development of opioid tolerance. Thus, a new generation of drugs which exhibit a μ-agonistic and an L-type VDCC antagonistic activity in the same molecule is of great interest.

N - and/or P/Q - type VDCC inhibitors (ω-conotoxins and ω-agatoxin IVA) are active in a variety of pharmacological pain models. In contrast to opioids, only minimal development of tolerance was observed when SNX-111 (Ziconotide), a synthetic peptide related to the naturally-occurring ω-conopeptide MVIIA, was administered chronically over 7 days. Ziconotide and related peptides can only be administered i.t. or i.c.v. An opioid-sparing effect is also evident. The enhancement of opioid antinociception with N-type VDCC blockers was reported to be additive. Clinical studies with N-type VDCC inhibitors are limited to SNX-111 (Ziconotide). Although positive results have been reported in patients suffering from chronic pain after continuous constant i.t. infusion of Ziconotide, severe side-effects seem to limit the usefulness of this peptide. To overcome the disadvantages of intrathecal administration, small molecule N -, or P/Q - type VDCC blockers for i.v. and/or p.o. application are under investigation.

N - and/or P/Q - type VDCC inhibitors

Clinical trials with new L- type and especially N - or P/Q - type VDCC inhibitors are eagerly awaited.

References

Abernethy, D.R. and Schwartz, J.B.: *Calcium-Antagonist Drugs,* Drug Therapy **1999**, *341,* 1447-1457.

Alexander, S.P.H. and Peters, J.A.: *Receptor and ion channel nomenclature,* Trends Pharmacol. Sci. **2000** (Suppl.), 98-99.

Alfaro, M.J., Colado, M.I., Lopez, F. and Martin, M.I.: *Effect of clonidine, nimodipine and diltiazem on the* in vitro *opioid withdrawal response in the guinea-pig ileum,* Br. J. Pharmacol. **1990**, *101,* 958-960.

Al-Humayyd, M.S.: *Effect of diltiazem, nifedipine and verapamil on the antinociceptive action of acetylsalicylic acid in mice,* Gen. Pharmac.**1991**, *22,* 121-125.

Ambler, S.J., Bleakman, D., Boot, J.R., Bowman, D., Gilmore, J., Harris, J.R., Harvey, J., Hotten, T.M., O'Brien, A.J., Timms, G.H., Tupper, D.E., Wedley, S.: *Novel antagonists of neuronal (non L-type) voltage-dependent calcium channels,* 27th Annual Society for Neuroscience Meeting, New Orleans, USA: **1997**, 472.1.

Antkiewicz-Michaluk, L., Michaluk, J., Romanska, I., Vetulani, J.: *Cortical dihydropyridine binding sites and a behavioral syndrome in morphine-abstinent rats,* Eur. J. Pharmacol. **1990**, *180,* 129-135.

Antkiewicz-Michaluk, L., Michaluk, J., Romanska, I., Vetulani, J.: *Reduction of morphine dependence and potentiation of analgesia by chronic co-administration of nifedipine,* Psychopharmacology **1993**, *111,* 457-464.

Atanassoff, P.G., Hartmannsgruber, M.W.B., Thrasher, J., Wermeling, D., Longton, W., Gaeta, R., Singh, T., Mayo, M., McGuire, D., Luther, R.R.: *Ziconotide, a new N-type calcium channel blocker, administered intrathecally for acute postoperative pain,* Reg. Anesth. Pain Med. **2000**, *25,* 274-278.

Augustine, G.J. and Neher, E.: *Neuronal Ca^{2+} signalling takes the local route,* Curr. Opin. Neurobiol. **1992**, *2*, 302-307.

Baeyens, J.M., Esposito, E., Ossowska, G., Samanin, R.: *Effects of peripheral and central administration of calcium channel blockers in the naloxone-precipitated abstinence syndrome in morphine-dependent rats,* Eur. J. Pharmacol. **1987**, *137*, 9-13.

Barrett, E.F. and Stevens, C.F.: *The kinetics of transmitter release of the frog neuromuscular junction,* J. Physiol. (Lond.) **1972**, *227*, 691-708.

Barrios, M. and Bayens, J.M.: *Differential effects of calcium channel blockers and stimulants on morphine withdrawal in vitro,* Eur. J. Pharmacol. **1988**, *152*, 175-178.

Basilico, L., Parolaro, D., Rubino, T., Gori, E., Giagnoni, G.: *Influence of ω-conotoxin on morphine analgesia and withdrawal syndrome in rats,* Eur. J. Pharmacol. **1992**, *218*, 75-81.

Beredek, G. and Szikszay, M.: *Potentiation of thermoregulatory and analgesic effects of morphine by calcium antagonists,* Pharmacol. Res. Commun. **1984**, *16*, 1009-1018.

Birnbaumer, L., Campbell, K.P., Catterall, W.A., Harpold, M.M., Hofmann, F., Horne, W.A., Mori, Y., Schwartz, A., Snutch, T.P., Tanabe, T., Tsien, R.W.: *The naming of voltage-gated calcium channels,* Neuron **1994**, *13*, 505-506.

Boldt, J., von Bormann, B., Kling, D., Russ, W., Ratthey, K., Hempelmann, G.: *Low-dose fentanyl analgesia modified by calcium channel blockers in cardiac surgery,* Eur. J. Anaesthesiology **1987**, *4*, 387-394.

Bongianni, F., Carla, V., Moroni, F., Pellegrini, D.: *Ca^{2+}-channel inhibitors prevent morphine withdrawal syndrome in rats,* Br. J. Pharmacol. **1985**, *86*, 529 P.

Bongianni, F., Carla, V., Moroni, F., Pellegrini-Giampietro, D.E.: *Calcium channel inhibitors suppress the morphine-withdrawal syndrome in rats,* Br. J. Pharmacol. **1986**, *88*, 561-567.

Bormann, von, B., Boldt, J., Sturm, G., Kling, D., Weidler, B., Lohmann, E., Hempelmann, G.: *Calcium-Antagonists in Anaesthesia,* Anaethesist **1985**, *34*, 429-434.

Bourinet, E., Soong, T.W., Stea, A., Snutch, T.P.: *Determinants of G-protein-dependent opioid modulation of neuronal calcium channels,* Proc. Natl. Acad. Sci. USA **1996**, *93*, 1486-1491.

Bowersox, S.S., Gadbois, Th., Singh, T., Pettus, M., Wang, Y.-X., Luther, R.R.: *Selective N-type neuronal voltage-sensitive calcium channel blocker, SNX – 111 , produces spinal antinociception in rat models of acute, persistent and neuropathic pain,* J. Pharmacol. Exper. Ther. **1996**, *279*, 1243-1249.

Bowersox, S., Tich, N., Mayo, M., Luther, R.: *SNX–111 [Ziconitide (USAN)],* Drugs Fut. **1998**, *23*, 152-160.

Brose, W.G., Gutlove, D.P., Luther, R.R., Bowersox, S.S., McGuire, D.: *Use of intrathecal SNX-111, a novel, N-type, voltage-sensitive, calcium channel blocker, in the management of intractable brachial plexus avulsion pain,* Clin. J. Pain, **1997**, *13*, 256-259.

Bustamante, D., Miranda, H.F., Pelissier, T., Paeile, C.: *Analgesic action of clonixin, nifedipine and morphine using the formalin test,* Gen. Pharmacol. **1989**, *20*, 319-322.

Carta, F., Bianchi, M., Argenton, S., Cervi, D., Marolla, G., Tamburini, M., Breda, M., Fantoni, A., Panerai, A.: *Effect of nifedipine on morphine-induced analgesia,* Anesth. Analg. **1990**, *70*, 493-498.

Catterall, W.A.: *Structure and function of voltage-gated ion channels,* Trends Neurosci. **1993**, *16*, 500-506.

Catterall, W.A. and Striessnig, J.: *Receptor sites for Ca^{2+} channel antagonist,* Trends Pharmacol. Sci. **1992**, *13*, 256-262.

Contreras, E., Tamayo, L., Amigo, M.: *Calcium channel antagonists increase morphine-induced analgesia and antagonize morphine tolerance,* Eur. J. Pharmacol. **1988**, *148*, 463-466.

Cox, B., Denyer, J.C.: *N-type calcium channel blockers in pain and stroke,* Exp. Opin. Ther. Patents **1998**, *8*, 1237-1250.

Del Pozo, E., Ruiz-Garcia, C., Baeyens, J.M.: *Analgesic effects of diltiazem and verapamil after central and peripheral administration in the hot-plate test,* Gen. Pharmac. **1990**, *21*, 681-685.

Diaz, A., Ruiz, F., Florez, J., Pazos, A., Hurlé, M.A.: *Regulation of dihydropyridine-sensitive Ca^{++} channels during opioid tolerance and supersensitivity in rats,* J. Pharmacol. Exper. Ther. **1995**, *274*, 1538-1544.

Diaz, A. and Dickenson, A.H.: *Blockade of spinal N- and P-type, but not L-type, calcium channels inhibits the excitability of rat dorsal horn neurones produced by subcutaneous formalin inflammation,* Pain **1997**, *69*, 93-100.

Dierssen, M., Florez, J., Hurlé, M.A.: *Calcium channel modulation by dihydropyridines modifies sufentanil-induced antinociception in acute and tolerant conditions,* Naunyn-Schmiedeberg's Arch. Pharmacol. **1990**, *342*, 559-565.

Dogrul, A., Yesilyurt, O., Isimer, A., Guzeldemir, M.E.: *L-type and T-type calcium channel blockade potentiate the analgesic effects of morphine and selective mu opioid agonist, but not to selective delta and kappa agonist at the level of the spinal cord in mice,* Pain **2001**, 93, 61-68.

Frink, M. Ch., Hennies, H.-H., Englberger, W., Haurand M., Wilffert, B.: *Influence of tramadol on neurotransmitter systems of the rat brain,* Arzneim.-Forsch./Drug Res. **1996**, 46, 1029-1036.

Garaulet, J.V., Laorden, M.L., Milanes, M.V.: *Effect of chronic administration of dihydropyridine Ca^{2+} channel ligands on sufentanil-induced tolerance to µ- and κ-opioid agonists in the guinea pig ileum myenteric plexus,* Regulatory Peptides **1996**, *63*, 1-8.

Glossmann, H. and Striessnig, J.: *Molecular properties of calcium channels,* Rev. Physiol. Biochem. Pharmacol. **1990**, *114*, 1-105.

Graudums, I., Winter, W., Frankus, E., Strassburger, W.W.A., Friderichs, E.J. (Grünenthal GmbH), *1-Phenyl-2-dimethylaminomethylcyclohexan-1-ol compounds as pharmaceutical active ingredients,* EP0780369 (**1997**), US5801201 (**1998**).

Gürdal, H., Sara, Y., Tulunay, F.C.: *Effects of Calcium Channel Blockers on formalin-induced nociception and inflammation in rats,* Pharmacology **1992**, *44*, 290-296.

Hasegawa, A.E. and Zacny, J.P.: *The influence of three L-type calcium channel blockers on morphine effects in healthy volunteers,* Anesth. Analg. **1997**, *85*, 633-638.

Heidelberger, R., Heinemann, C., Neher, E., Matthews, G.: *Calcium dependence of the rate of exocytosis in a synaptic terminal,* Nature **1994**, *371*, 513-515.

Herlitze, S., Garcia, D.E., Mackie, K., Hille, B., Scheuer, T., Catterall, W.A.: *Modulation of Ca^{2+} channels by G-protein βγ subunits,* Nature **1996**, *380*, 258-262.

Hisamoto M., Inaoka, Y., Sakaida, Y., Kagazaki, T., Enokida, R., Okazaki, T., Haruyama, H., Kinoshita, T., Matsuda, K.: *A-53930A and B, novel N-type Ca^{2+} channel blockers,* J. Antibiotics **1998**, *51*, 607-617.

Hoffmeister, F. and Tettenborn, D.: *Calcium agonists and antagonists of the dihydropyridine type: Antinociceptive effects, interference with opiate-µ-receptor agonists and neuropharmacological actions in rodents,* Psychopharmacology **1986**, *90*, 299-307.

Hunter, J.C.: *Voltage-gated ion channel modulators* in: Novel aspects of pain management. Opioids and beyond, edited by J. Sawynok and A. Cowan. Wiley-Liss. Inc., **1999**, 321-344.

Isom, L.L., De Jongh, K.S., Catterall, W.A.: *Auxillary subunits of Voltage-Gated Ion Channels,* Neuron **1994**, *12*, 1183-1194.

Kater, S.B., Mattson, M.P., Cohan, Ch., Connor J.: *Calcium regulation of the neuronal growth cone,* Trends Neurosci. **1988**, *11*, 315-321.

Kazuyuki, M., Kiyomi, K., Yoshitaka, A., Toshiyuki, K. (Shionogi & Co.), *P/Q type calcium channel antagonist,* WO9801121 (**1998**).

Lehmann, K.A., Kriegel, R., Ueki, M.: *Clinical relevance of drug interactions between opiates and calcium channel blockers,* Anaesthesist **1989**, 38, 110-115.

Linas, R.R., Steinberg, I.Z., Walton, K.: *Relationship between presynaptic calcium current and postsynaptic potential in squid giant synapse,* Biophys. J. **1981**, *33*, 323-351.

Linas, R.R., Sugimori, M., Silver, R.B.: *Microdomains of high calcium concentration in a presynaptic terminal,* Science, **1992**, *256*, 677-679.

Malmberg, A.B. and Yaksh, T.L.: *Voltage-sensitive calcium channels in spinal nociceptive processing: Blockade of N- and P-type channels inhibits formalin-induced nociception,* J. Neurosci. **1994**, *14*, 4882-4890.

Malmberg, A.B. and Yaksh, T.L.: *Effect of continuous intrathecal infusion of ω-conopeptides, N-type calcium-channel blockers, on behavior and antinociception in the formalin and hot-plate tests in rats,* Pain **1995**, *60*, 83-90.

Malone, T.C., Schelkun, R.M., Yuen, P.-W. (Warner-Lambert Co.), *Substituted phenols as novel calcium channel blockers*, WO9705125 (**1997**).

Marangos, P.J., Sullivan, B.W., Wiemann, T., Danks, A.M., Sragovicz, M., Makings, L.R. (Cypros Pharmaceutical Corp.), *Neuroprotective poly-guanidino compounds which block presynaptic N and P/Q calcium channels,* WO9836743 (**1998**).

McNaughton, N.C.L., White, C., Clark, B., Bath, C., Bleakman, D., Randall, A.D.: *Electrophysiological characterisation of the human N-type Ca^{2+} channel III: pH-dependent inhibition by a synthetic macrocyclic polyamine,* Neuropharmacology **1999**, *38*, 19-38.

Michaluk, J., Karolewicz, B., Antkiewicz-Michaluk, L., Ventulani, J.: *Effects of various Ca^{2+} channel antagonists on morphine analgesia, tolerance and dependence, and on blood pressure in the rat,* Eur. J. Pharmacol. **1998**, *352*, 189-197.

Miljanich, G.P. and Ramachandran, J.: *Antagonists of neuronal calcium channels: structure, function and therapeutic implications,* Ann. Rev. Pharmacol. Toxicol. **1995**, *35*, 707-734.

Miranda, H.F., Bustamante, D., Kramer, V., Pelissier, T., Saavedra, H., Paeile, C., Fernandez, E., Pinardi, G., *Antinociceptive effects of Ca^{2+} channel blockers,* Eur. J. Pharmacol. **1992**, *217*, 137-141.

Miranda, H.F., Pelissier, T., Scierralta, F.: *Analgesic effects of intracerebroventricular administration of calcium channel blockers in mice,* Gen. Pharmac. **1993**, *24*, 201-204.

Moises, H.C., Rusin, K., Macdonald, R.L.: *μ-opioid receptor-mediated reduction of neuronal calcium current occurs via a G$_o$-type GTP-binding protein,* J. Neurosci. **1994**, *14*, 3842-3851.

Murphy, K.M.M., Snyder, S.H.: *Calcium antagonist receptor binding sites labeled with [^{3}H] Nitrendipine,* Eur. J. Pharmacol. **1982**, *77*, 201-202.

Olivera, B.M., Rivier, J., Clark, C., Ramilo, C.A., Corpuz, G.P., Abogadie, F.C., Mena, E.E., Woodward, S.R., Hillyard, D.R., Cruz, L.J.: *Diversity of Conus neuropeptides,* Science **1990**, *249*, 257-263.

Olivera, B.M., Rivier, J., Scott, J.K., Hillyard, D.R., Cruz, L.J.: *Conotoxins,* J. Biol. Chem. **1991**, *266*, 22067-22070.

Omote, K., Sonoda, H., Kawamata, M., Iwasaki, H., Namiki, A.: *Potentiation of antinociceptive effects of morphine by calcium-channel blockers at the level of the spinal cord,* Anesthesiology **1993**, *79*, 746-752.

Pauwels, P.J., Leysen, J.E., Laduron, P.M.: *[^{3}H] Batrachotoxinin A20-α-benzoate binding to sodium channels in rat brain: characterization and pharmacological significance,* Eur. J. Pharmacol. **1986**, *124*, 291-298.

Pavone, F., Battaglia, M., Sansone, M.: *Nifedipine-morphine interaction: a further investigation on nociception and locomotor activity in mice,* J. Pharm. Pharmacol. **1992**, *44*, 773-776.

Penn, R.D. and Paice, J.A.: *Adverse effects associated with the intrathecal administration of Ziconotide,* Pain **2000**, *85*, 291-296.

Pereira, I.T., Prado, W.A., Dos Reis, M.P.: *Enhancement of the epidural morphine-induced analgesia by systemic nifedipine,* Pain, **1993**, *53*, 341-355.

Prado, W.A.: *Involvement of calcium in pain and antinociception,* Braz. J. Med. Biol. Res. **2001**, *34*, 449-461.

Ramkumar, V. and El-Fakahany, E.E.: *Increase in [^{3}H] Nitrendipine binding sites in the brain in morphine-tolerant mice,* Eur. J. Pharmacol. **1984**, *102*, 371-372.

Ramkumar, V. and El-Fakahany, E.E.: *Prolonged morphine treatment increases rat brain dihydropyridine binding sites: possible involvement in development of morphine dependence,* Eur. J. Pharmacol. **1988**, *146*, 73-83.

Reimann, W.S. (Grünenthal GmbH), *Compositions containing tramadol and a calcium channel antagonist – useful for the treatment of acute or chronic pain with reduced side-effects,* EP0835656 (**1998**), US5929122 (**1999**).

Reynolds, I.J., Gould, R.J., Snyder, S.H.: *[³H] Verapamil binding sites in brain and skeletal muscle: regulation by calcium,* Eur. J. Pharmacol. **1983**, *95*, 319-321.

Roca, G., Aquilar, J.G., Gornar, C., Mazo, V., Costa, J., Vidal, F.: *Nimodipine fails to enhance the analgesic effect of slow release morphine in the early phases of cancer treatment,* Pain **1996**, *68*, 239-243.

Ruiz, F.Dierssen, M., Florez, J., Hurlé, M.A.: *Potentiation of acute opioid-induced respiratory depression and reversal of tolerance by the calcium antagonist nimodipine in awake rats,* Naunyn Schmiedeberg's Arch. Pharmacol. **1993**, *348*, 633-637.

Santillán, R., Maestre, J.M., Hurlé, M.A., Flórez, J.: *Enhancement of opiate analgesia by nimodipine in cancer patients chronically treated with morphine: a preliminary report,* Pain **1994**, *58*, 129-132.

Santillán, R., Hurlé, M.A., Armijo, J.A., de los Mozos, R., Flórez, J.: *Nimodipine-enhanced opiate analgesia in cancer patients requiring morphine dose escalation: a double-blind, placebo-controlled study,* Pain **1998**, *76*, 17-26.

Schoemaker, H. and Langer, S.Z.: *[³H] Diltiazem binding to calcium channel antagonists recognition sites in rat cerebral cortex,* Eur. J. Pharmacol.**1985**, *111*, 273-277.

Shen, G.S., Layer, R.T., McCabe, R.T.: *Conopeptides: From deadly venoms to novel therapeutics,* Drug Discovery Today, **2000**, *5*, 98-106.

Smith, F.L. and Stevens, D.L.: *Calcium modulation of morphine analgesia: role of calcium channels and intracellular pool calcium,* J. Pharmacol. Exp. Ther. **1995**, *272*, 290-299.

Song, Y., Bowersox S.S., Connor, D.T., Dooley D.J., Lotarski S.M., Malone Th., Miljanich G., Millerman E., Rafferty M.F., Rock D., Roth B. D., Schmidt, J., Stoehr, S., Szoke, B. G., Taylor, Ch., Vartanian, M., Wang, Y.-X.: *(S)-4-Methyl-2-(methylamino)pentanoic acid [4,4-bis(4-fluorophenyl)-butyl]amide hydrochloride, a novel calcium channel antagonist, Is efficacious in several animal models of pain,* J. Med. Chem. **2000**, *43*, 3474-3477.

Spampinato, S., Speroni, E., Govoni, P., Pistacchio, E., Romagnoli, C., Murari, G., Ferri S.: *Effect of ω-conotoxin and verapamil on antinociceptive, behavioural and thermoregulatory responses to opioids in the rat,* Eur. J. Pharmacol. **1994**, *254*, 229-238.

Striessnig, J., Grabner, M., Mitterdorfer, J., Hering, S., Sinnegger, M.J., Glossmann, H.: *Structural basis of drug binding to L Ca^{2+} channels,* Trends Pharmacol. Sci. **1998**, *19*, 108-115.

Sundermann, B., Hennies, H.-H., Kögel, B.-Y., Buschmann, B. (Grünenthal GmbH): *3-Amino-3-arylpropan-1-ol compounds, their preparation and use,* EP1043306 (**2000**), US6288278 (**2001**).

Terlau, H., Shon,K.-J., Grilley, M., Stocker, M., Stühmer, W., Olivera, B.M.: *Strategy for rapid immobilization of prey by a fish-hunting marine snail,* Nature **1996**, *381*,148-151.

Tokuyama, S. and Ho, I.K.: *Effects of diltiazem, a Ca^{2+} channel blocker, on naloxone-precipitated changes in dopamine and its metabolites in the brains of opioid-dependent rats,* Psychopharmacol. **1996**, *125*, 135-140.

Tsien, R.W., Lipscombe, D., Madison, D.V., Bley, K.R., Fox, A.P.: *Multiple types of neuronal calcium channels and their selective modulation,* Trends Neurosci. **1988**, *11*, 431-438.

Tsien, R.W., Ellinor, P.T., Horne, W.A.: *Molecular diversity of voltage-dependent Ca^2 channels,* Trends Pharmacol. Sci. **1991**, *12*, 349-354.

Varadi, G., Mori, Y., Mikada, G., Schwartz, A.: *Molecular determinants of Ca^{2+} channel function and drug action,* Trends Pharmacol. Sci. **1995**, *16*, 43-49.

Wagner, J.A., Snowman, A.M., Biswas, A., Olivera, B.M., Snyder, S.H.: *ω-Conotoxin GVIA binding to a high-affinity receptor in brain : Characterization, calcium sensitivity, and solubilization*, J. Neurosci. **1988**, *8*, 3354- 3359.

Wang, Y-X., Gao, D., Pettus, M., Phillips, C., Bowersox, S.S.: *Interactions of intrathecally administered ziconotide, a selective blocker of neuronal N-type voltage-sensitive calcium channels, with morphine on nociception in rats,* Pain **2000**, *84*, 271-281.

Welch, S.P. and Olson, K.G.: *Opiate tolerance-induced modulation of free intracellular calcium in synaptosomes,* Life Sci., **1991**, *48*, 1853-1861.

Westenbroek, R.E., Hoskins, L., Catterall, W.A.: *Localization of Ca^{2+} channel subtypes on rat spinal motor neurons, interneurons, and nerve terminals,* J. Neurosci., **1998**, *18*, 6319-6330.

Williams, M., Kowaluk, E.A., Arneric, S.P.: *Emerging Molecular Approaches to Pain Therapy,* J. Med. Chem. **1999**, *42*, 1481-1500.

Wong, Ch. H., Dey, P., Yarmush, J., Wu, W.-H., Zbuzek, V.K.: *Nifedipine-induced analgesia after epidural injection in rats,* Anesth. Analg. **1994**, *79*, 303-306.

Yuen, P.-W. (Warner-Lambert Co.), *Substituted quinolines and isoquinolines as calcium channel blockers, their preparation and the use thereof,* US5767129 (**1998**).

Zamponi, G.W., Bourinet, E., Nelson, D., Nargeot, J., Snutch, T.P.: *Crosstalk between G proteins and protein kinase C mediated by the calcium channel α_1 subunit,* Nature **1997**, *385*, 442-446.

Zharkovsky, A., Töttermann, A.M., Moisio, J., Aktee, L.: *Concurrent nimodipine attenuates the withdrawal signs and the increase of cerebral dihydropyridine binding after chronic morphine treatment in rats,* Naunyn-Schmiedeberg's Arch. Pharmacol. **1993**, *347*, 483-486.

Zucker, R.S.: *Calcium and transmitter release,* J. Physiol. (Paris) **1993**, *87*, 25-36.

7 Glutamate Receptors

7.1 Metabotropic Glutamate Receptors

Klaus Schiene and Corinna Maul

Evidence from the last several decades indicates that the excitatory amino acid glutamate plays a significant role in nociceptive processing. Glutamate and glutamate receptors are located in areas of the brain, spinal cord and periphery which are involved in pain sensation and transmission (for a review see Fundytus 2001). Glutamate acts at several types of receptors, including ionotropic (directly coupled to ion channels) and metabotropic (directly coupled to intracellular second messengers via guanine nucleotide regulatory (G) proteins) receptors. In this chapter we are focussing on metabotropic glutamate receptors which modulate a variety of neuronal effects at both pre- and post-synaptic level in several brain regions.

Glutamate plays a significant role in nociceptive processing

Molecular cloning and pharmacological studies revealed the existence of at least eight mGlu receptor subtypes (mGlu1-mGlu8) which are classified into 3 groups based on sequence homology, signal transduction mechanisms and receptor pharmacology. Group I mGluRs which include mGluR1 and mGluR5 stimulate phosphatidylinositol (PI) hydrolysis, and activation of these receptors ultimately leads to activation of PKC, and increases in the level of intracellular Ca^{2+}. The increase in the level of intracellular Ca^{2+} may in turn trigger production of NO via Ca^{2+}/calmodulin activation of NOS. Group II (mGluR2 and mGluR3) and group III (mGluR 4,6,7,8) mGluRs are negatively coupled to adenylate cyclase, and activation of these receptors inhibits the production of cyclic adenosine-3',5'-monophosphate (cAMP).

group I	group II	group III
mGluR 1,5	mGluR 2,3	mGluR 4,6,7,8
PI-coupled	cAMP-coupled	cAMP-coupled

All mGluRs are characterized by a putative signal peptide, an unusually large (470 - 510 amino acids) extracellular amino terminal domain (ATD), seven membrane-spanning regions characteristic of the G protein-coupled receptor (GPCR) superfamily, and an intracellular carboxy terminal domain variable in size and amino acid composition among the various members of the family. Many of the mGlu receptors exist as various isoforms with different intracellular carboxy termini generated by alternative splicing of their pre-messenger RNA (Conn and Pin, 1997).

Sequence homology is in the range 65 - 70% between mGluRs belonging to the same group, but falls to 40 – 45 % among members of different groups. Conserved regions are found in the membrane-spanning regions and in a hydrophobic region located in the extracellular ATD. It is now generally accepted that mGluR receptors constitute, together with the Ca^{2+}-sensing receptor, a putative pheromone receptor, and $GABA_B$ receptors a distinct family (type C family) of GPCRs. Distinctive features of type C family are: an unusually large extracellular ATD, no homology with other GPCR families at the level of the transmembrane regions, and coupling with G-proteins localized at the level of the second and not the third intracellular loop. For group I mGluRs a molecular mechanism leading to domain closure has been postulated (Constantino et al., 1999).

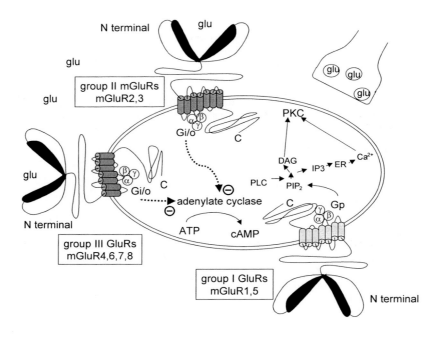

Figure 1: Second messenger coupling of mGluRs. Group II and group III mGluRs are negatively coupled to adenylate cyclase. Activity at group I mGluRs stimulates a phospholipase C (PLC)-catalyzed phosphoinositide (PIP_2) hydrolysis which leads to the production of inositol triphosphate (IP_3) and diacylglycerol (DAG). The production of IP_3 promotes the release of intracellular Ca^{2+} from its stores within the endoplasmatic reticulum (ER). The increased Ca^{2+} influx from either extracellular or intracellular sources, and production of DAG, are essential elements for the stimulation of the enzyme PKC.

Selective compounds for all groups as well as some subtype-selective compounds have been found which have been very useful in mGluR research during the last

decade. A selection of mGluR modulators is given in fig. 2
(for a review see Pin et al., 1999).

Group I mGluR modulators:

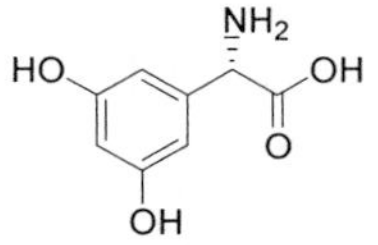

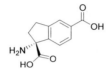

(S)-3,5-DHPG, selective
group I mGlu receptor agonist,
3,5-dihydroxy-phenylglycine

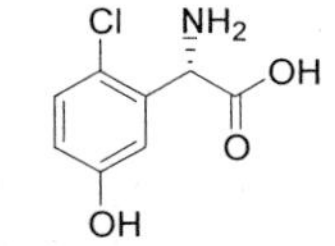

CHPG, selective mGlu5
receptor agonist,
2-chloro-5-hydroxy-phenylglycine

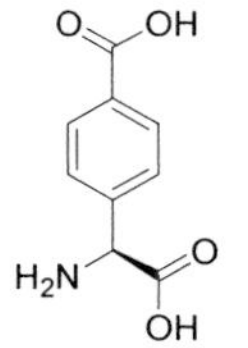

(S)-4-CPG, selective
group I antagonist, 4-Carboxy-
phenylglycine

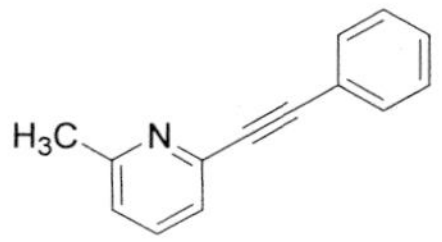

MPEP, selective
mGluR5 antagonist,
2-Methyl-6-phenyl-
ethynyl-pyridine

AIDA, selective
mGluR1 antagonist
1-Amino-indan-1,5-
dicarboxylic acid

CPCCOEt, selective mGluR1 antagonist,
2-Hydroxyimino-1a,2-dihydro-1*H*-7-
oxa-cyclopropa[*b*]naphthalene-7a-
carboxylic acid ethyl ester

Group II mGluR modulators:

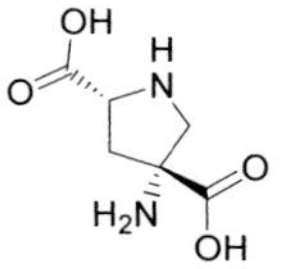

(2*R*,4*R*)-APDC
((2*R*,4*R*)-4-aminopyrrolidine-
2,4-carboxylic acid),
selective group II mGluR agonist

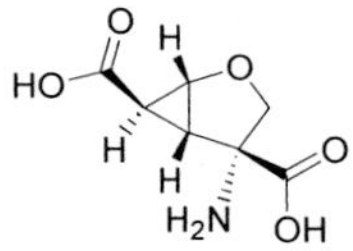

LY-379268
selective group II mGluR agonist
(Monn et al. 1999)

LY-354740
selective group II mGluR agonist
(Monn et al. 1997)

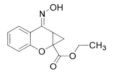

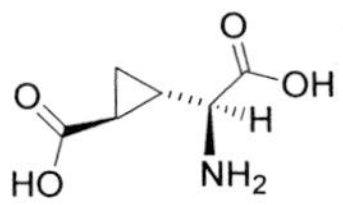

L-CCG 1, selective group II
mGluR agonist, 2-(Amino-
carboxy-methyl)-cyclopropane-
carboxylic acid

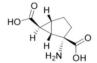

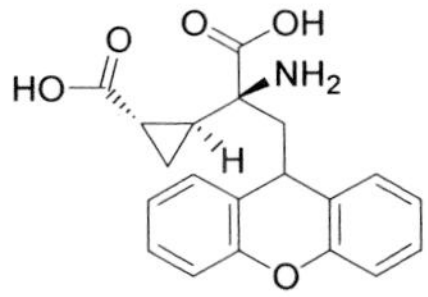

LY 341495, group II mGluR
antagonist (Ornstein et al. 1998)

Group II mGluR modulators:

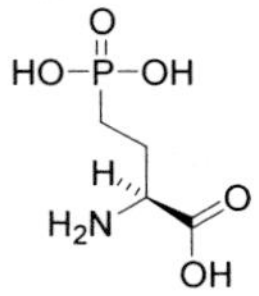

(S)-SOP, group III
mGluR agonist,
(S)-serine O-phosphate

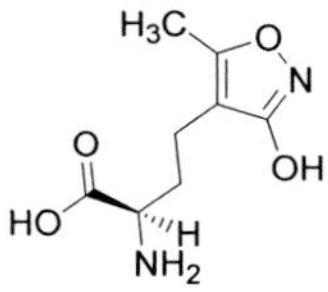

(S)-homo-AMPA,
mGluR6-selective agonist

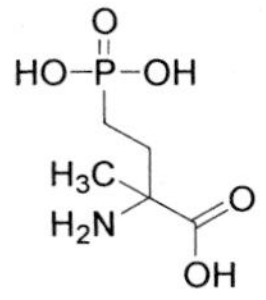

MSOP, group III mGluR
selective antagonist, (RS)-α-
Methylserine-O-phosphate

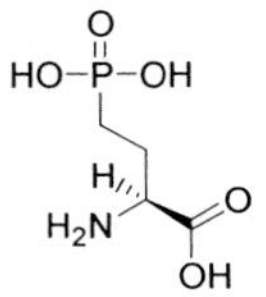

L-AP4, selective group III
mGluR agonist
(Monaghan et al. 1983)

Figure 2: Group I, II and II mGluR modulators.

Varying distributions of expression of the mRNA for the various subunits of mGluRs have been detected throughout the dorsal horn of the spinal cord, with the exception of mGluR2, mGluR6 and mGluR8, which are undetectable in rat spinal cord (Yashpal et al., 2001).

The coupling of group I mGluRs to PI hydrolysis suggests an influence on pain perception because of PKC activation

The coupling of group I mGluRs directly to PI hydrolysis suggests an influence on pain perception because this leads to the activation of PKC. PKC has been shown to contribute significantly to the development of persistent pain. Inhibition of PKC attenuates formalin-induced pain scores and mechanical hyperalgesia associated with a thermal injury (Coderre, 1992, Yashpal et al., 1995). Following nerve constriction injury, there is an increase in membrane-associated PKC in the spinal cord (Mao et al., 1992). PKCγ knockout mice were shown to have a significant reduction of mechanical and thermal allodynia following nerve constriction injury (Malmberg et al., 1997).

Electrophysiological data have shown that application of mGluR agonists to the brain, spinal cord and periphery induces neuronal depolarization (Zheng and Gallagher, 1992, Boxall et al., 1996) and resulted in long-lasting potentiation of synaptic transmission as well as acute neuronal cell death (Zheng et al., 1996). Iontophoretic application of the mGluR antagonist (R,S)-CHPG attenuates rat dorsal horn activity associated with repeated mustard oil application (Young et al., 1994, 1995). However, in vivo experiments do not show clear results in acute pain models. It has been shown that the effects of mGluR agonists may be different in normal animals compared with animals with carrageenan-induced inflammation. The non-selective mGluR agonist (1S,3R)-ACPD facilitates neuronal responses evoked by noxious stimuli in normal animals, but inhibits these responses in animals suffering from inflammation. The group I mGluR selective agonist 3,5-Dihydroxyphenylglycine (DHPG) produces mixed effects in normal animals and inhibition in animals with inflammation (Stanfa and Dickensen, 1998; Maione et al., 2000). However, antisense oligonucleotide knockdown of spinal mGluR1 significantly reduced cold hyperalgesia, heat hyperalgesia and mechanical allodynia in the ipsilateral (injured) hindpaw of neuropathic rats (Fundytus et al., 2001).

mGluR agonists do not show clear results in acute pain models

In a model of acute postoperative pain, several mGluR antagonists do not produce any reduction in hyperalgesia or allodynia indicating that mGluR antagonists play only a minor role in acute pain (Zahn and Brennan, 1998). In a recent study it was shown that intrathecal administration of the mGluR1/5 antagonist (S)-4CPG was unable to significantly reduce the nociceptive responses induced by formalin injection in the hindpaw. It was shown that (S)-

4CPG (i.t. administration) did not influence formalin-induced activation of spinal PKC. On the other hand it has been reported that group I mGluR antagonists show antinociceptive in the second phase of the formalin test (s.c. administration) (Bhave et al., 2001). However, Bhave et al. presented results indicating that peripheral group I mGluR activation is necessary for full expression of inflammatory hyperalgesia, and blockage of these receptors is sufficient to completely eliminate the effects of increased glutamate levels in the periphery. Peripherally applied glutamate, the endogenous agonist of mGluRs, increased thermal sensitivity. Injection of the group I mGluR antagonists MPEP or CPCOEt 15 min before glutamate injection completely blocked glutamate-induced thermal hypersensitivity. NMDA and group II and III mGluR antagonists had no effect. This suggests that glutamate released during inflammation may activate group I mGluRs leading to thermal hyperalgesia.

In contrast to its non-significant effects when administered i.t. in the formalin-test, i.t. treatment with (*S*)-4CPG was effective at significantly reducing neuropathic-like pain behavior in nerve-injured rats (Fisher et al., 1998; Yashpal et al., 2001; for a review see Fundytus, 2001). Consistent with the behavioural effects, there is evidence that chronic constriction injury induced increases in the translocation and activation of spinal PKC dependent on activity at mGlu1/5 receptors (Yashpal et al., 2001).

Antagonism of group I mGluRs appears to be particularly useful in the reduction of hyperalgesia and allodynia associated with chronic pain

In summary, it has been shown that group I mGluR antagonists can lead to antinociception, antihyperalgesia or anti-allodynia in models of chronic and inflammatory pain.

Inhibitory metabotropic GluRs (group II and III) also represent potential targets for new analgesics. Group II and group III mGluRs are present in the superficial dorsal horn, thalamus and cortical areas involved in pain processing. Furthermore, subtypes of mGluR II and III and their mRNA respectively have been shown to be upregulated in chronic pain states (Boxall et al., 1998; Azkue et al., 2001; Neto et al., 2001). There is growing evidence to suggest that selective agonists of group II and group III mGluRs have a potential for treatment of pain (Dolan and Nolan, 2000).

Group II and III mGluRs represent potential targets for new analgesics

Activation of the G-protein-coupled mGluR group II and group III has been shown to inhibit cAMP formation and reduce neuronal excitability and synaptic transmission (Gereau and Conn, 1995; Macek et al., 1996; Neugebauer et al., 1997; Miller, 1998; Bushell et al., 1999; Schoepp et al., 1999). Therefore agonists at these receptors may be useful in downregulating the enhanced responses of nociceptive neurons during the stages of the neuronal

Agonists at group II and group III mGlu receptors may be useful in downregulating the enhanced responses of nociceptive neurons during neuronal sensitization which involves the cAMP - PKA pathway

sensitization which involve the cAMP - PKA pathway. The group II agonists LCCG1 ((2S,1'S,2'S)-2-(carboxy-cyclopropyl)glycine), the highly potent, selective and systemically active ligand LY379268 ((-)-2-oxa-4-amino-bicyclo[3.1.0]hexane-4,6-dicarboxylate) and the group III agonist L-AP4 (L(+)-2-amino-4-phosphonobutyric acid) reversed the capsaicin-induced sensitization in primate spinothalamic tract cells. The group II GluRs may modulate the response of sensitized neurons, because, in contrast to L-AP4, the group II agonists have no effect on responses to cutaneous stimuli under control conditions but reversed the enhanced responses of sensitized spinothalamic tract cells (Neugebauer et al., 2000). Furthermore the inflammatory hyperalgesia after intra-plantar carrageenan injection as well as capsaicin-induced neurogenic thermal hyperalgesia was reduced after administration of LY379268 (Sharpe et al., 2002). Group II mGluRs may also play a role in the development of anti-nociceptive morphine tolerance. The systemically active group II mGluR LY354740 ((+)-2-aminobicyclo [3,1,0]hex-ane-2,6-dicarboxylic acid) inhibited the development of morphine tolerance in mice (Popik et al., 2000) and nalox-one-induced symptoms of morphine withdrawal (Klo-dzinska et al., 1999).

Furthermore, the group III agonist L-AP4 attenuated changes in mechanical thresholds after spinal cord injury (Mills et al., 2002) and produced dose dependent reduc-tions in spontaneous nociceptive behavior of rats induced by intrathecal (i.t.) administration of the selective group I mGluR agonist (RS)-3,5-dihydroxyphenylglycine ((RS)-DHPG) (Lefebvre et al., 2000).

Therefore mGluRs, particularly group I mGluRs may be useful targets for therapy of chronic inflammatory pain, neuropathic pain and as an adjunct to opioid analgesic treatment. During the last couple of years a number of patents claiming new analgesics affecting metabotropic glutamate receptors have been filed. A selection is given in fig. 3:

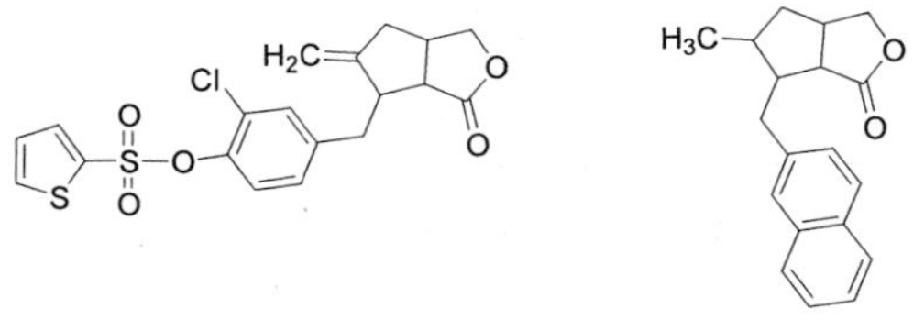

Stolle et al. (Bayer AG), WO 0104107, WO 9936418, WO 9936417, WO 9936419, mGluR1 antagonists

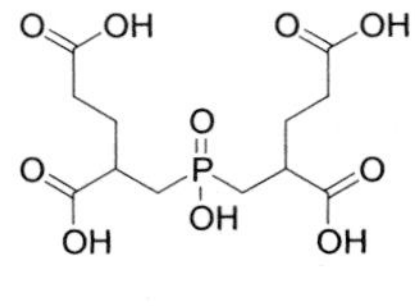

Kozikowski et al., WO 0064911 ligands for mGluRs

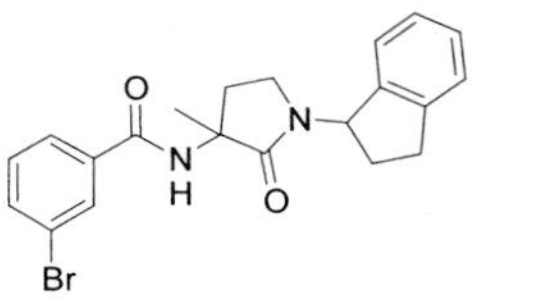

Clark et al. (Eli Lilly) WO 0069816
mGluR5 antagonists

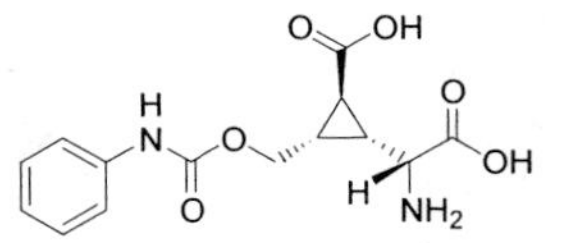

Colladocano et al. (Eli Lilly), WO 0192213,
mGluR agonists

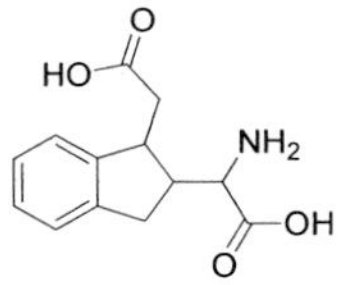

Curry (IGT Pharma),
WO 0102342, mGluR
modulators

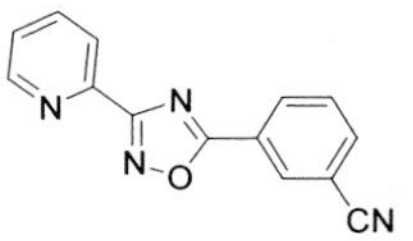

van Wagenen et al. (NPS Pharmaceuticals)
WO 0112627, mGluR5 antagonists

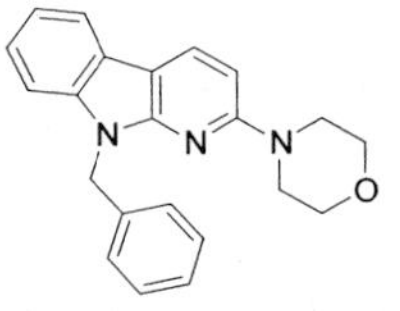

Jakobsen, P. (Novo Nordisk) US 5783575
mGluR1a antagonists

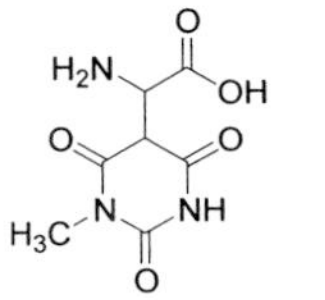

Curry, WO 0179185,
mGluR modulators

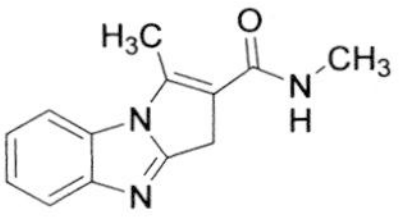

Hayashibe et al. (Yamanouchi)
WO 0059913

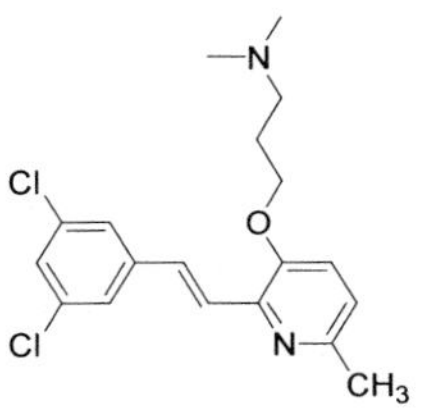

Allgeier et al. (Novartis) WO 9902497
mGluR5 antagonists

Figure 3: Further mGluR ligands.

References

Allgeier, H., Auberson, Y., Biollaz, M., Cosford, N. D., Gasparini, F., Endorn, R., Johnson, E. C., Kuhn, R., Varney, M. A., Velicelebi, G. (Novartis): *Pyridine derivatives*, WO 9902497.

Azkue, J..J., Murga, M., Fernandez-Capetillo, O., Mateos, J..M., Elezgarai, I., Benitez, R., Osorio, A., Diez, J., Puente, N., Bilbao, A., Bidaurrazaga, A., Kuhn, R., Grandes, P.: *Immunoreactivity for the group III metabotropic glutamate receptor subtype mGluR4a in the superficial laminae of the rat spinal dorsal horn*. J. Comp. Neurol. **2001**, *430*, 448-57.

Bhave, G., Karim, F., Carlton, S. M., Gereau, R. W.: *Peripheral group I metabotropic glutamate receptors modulate nociception in mice*, Nature Neurosci. **2001**, *4*, 417-423.

Boxall, S. J., Thompson, S. W., Dray, A., Dickenson, A. H., Urban, L.: *Metabotropic glutamate receptor activation contributes to nociceptive reflex activity in the rat spinal cord in vitro*, Neuroscience. **1996**, *4*, 13-20.

Boxall, S.J., Berthele, A., Laurie, D.J., Sommer, B., Zieglgansberger, W., Urban, L., Tolle, T. R.: *Enhanced expression of metabotropic glutamate receptor 3 messenger RNA in the rat spinal cord during ultraviolet irradiation induced peripheral inflammation*, Neuroscience. **1998**, *82*, 591-602.

Bushell, T. J., Lee C. C., Shigemoto R., Miller R. J.: *Modulation of synaptic transmission and differential localisation of mGlus in cultured hippocampal autapses*, Neuropharmacology. **1999**, *38*, 1553-1567.

Clark, B. P., Cwi, C. L., Harris, J. R., Kingston, A. E., Scott, W. L. (Eli Lilly): *Metabotropic glutamate receptor antagonists*, WO 0069816.

Coderre, T. J.: *Contribution of protein kinase C to central sensitization and persistant pain following tissue injury*, Neurosci. Letters **1992**, *140*, 181-184.

Colladocano, I., Gonzalez-Garcia, R., Lopez de Uralde-Garmendia, B. (Eli Lilly): *Excitatory amino acid receptor modulators*, WO 0192213.

Conn, P. and Pin, J.-P.: *Pharmacology and functions of metabotropic glutamate receptors*, Ann. Rev. Pharmacol. Toxicol. **1997**, *37*, 205-237.

Constantino, G. and Pelliciari, R.: *Homology modeling of metabotropic glutamate receptors. (mGluRs) Structural motifs affecting binding modes and pharmacological profile of mGluR1 agonists and competitive antagonists*, J. Med. Chem. **1996**, *39*, 3998-4006.

Constantino, G., Macchiarulo, A., Pellicciari, R.: *Modeling of amino-terminal domains of group I metabotropic glutamate receptors: structural motifs affecting ligand selectivity*, J. Med. Chem. **1999**, *42*, 5390-5401.

Curry, K., (IGT Pharma): *2-Aminoindane analogs*, WO 0102342.

Curry, K.: *Novel amino carboxy alkyl derivatives of barbituric acid,* WO 0179185.

Dolan, S. and Nolan, A.M.: *Behavioural evidence supporting a differential role for group I and II metabotropic glutamate receptors in spinal nociceptive transmission*, Neuropharmacology. **2000**, *39*, 1132-1138.

Mao, J., Price, D. D., Mayer, D. J.,Hayes, R. L.: *Pain-related increases in spinal cord membrane-bound proteinkinase C following peripheral nerve injury*, Brain Res. **1992**, *588*, 144-149.

Fundytus, M. E.: *Glutamate receptors and nociception*, CNS Drugs **2001**, *15*, 29-58.

Fundytus, M. E., Yashpal, K., Chabot, J.-G., Osborne, M. G., Lefebvre, C. D., Dray, A., Henry, J. L., Coderre, T. J.: *Knockdown of spinal metabotropic glutamate receptor 1 (mGluR1) alleviates pain and restores opioid efficacy after nerve injury in rats*, Br. J. Pharmacol. **2001**, *132*, 354-367.

Fisher, K., Fundytus, M. E., Cahill, C. M., Coderre, T. J.: *Intrathecal administration of the mGluR compound, (S)-4CPG, attenuates hyperalgesia and allodynia associated with sciatic nerve constriction injury in rats*, Pain **1998**, *77*, 59-66.

Gasparini, F. , Lingenhohl, K., Stoehr, N., Flor, P. J., Heinrich, M., Vranesic, I., Biollaz, M., Allgeier, H., Heckendorn, R., Urwyler, S., Varney, M. A., Johnson, E. C., Hess, S. D., Rao, S. P., Sacaan, A. I., Santori, E. M., Velicelebi, G., Kuhn, R.: *2-Methyl-6-(phenylethynyl)-pyridine (MPEP), a potent, selective and systemically active mGlu5 receptor antagonist*, Neropharmacology **1999**, *38*, 1493-1504.

Gereau, R.W. 4th and Conn, P.J.: *Roles of specific metabotropic glutamate receptor subtypes in regulation of hippocampal CA1 pyramidal cell excitability*, J Neurophysiol. **1995**, *74*, 122-129.

Hayashibe, S., Itahana, H., Okada, M., Kohara, A., Maeno, K., Yahiro, K., Shimada, I., Tanabe, K., Negoro, K., Kamikubo, T., Sakamoto, S. (Yamanouchi Pharmaceutical Co., ltd.): *Novel thiazolobenzimidazole derivatives*, WO 0059913.

Kozikowski, A. P., Wroblewski, J. T., Nan, F. (Georgetown University): *Ligands for metabotropic glutamate receptors*, WO 0064911.

Klodzinska, A., Chojnacka-Wojcik, E., Palucha, A., Branski, P., Popik, P., Pilc, A.: *Potential anti-anxiety, anti-addictive effects of LY 354740, a selective group II glutamate metabotropic receptors agonist in animal models,* Neuropharmacology. **1999**, *38*, 1831-1839.

Lefebvre, C., Fisher, K., Cahill, C. M., Coderre, T. J.: *Evidence that DHPG-induced nociception depends on glutamate release from primary afferent C-fibres,* Neuroreport. **2000**, *11*, 1631-1635.

Macek, T. A., Winder, D. G., Gereau, R. W. 4th, Ladd, C. O., Conn, P. J.: *Differential involvement of group II and group III mGluRs as autoreceptors at lateral and medial perforant path synapses*. J. Neurophysiol. **1996**, *76*, 3798-3806.

Maione, S., Marabese, I., Leyva, J.: *Characterization of mGluRs which modulate nociception in the PAG of the mouse*, Neuropharmacology **1998**, *37*, 1475-1483.

Maione, S., Oliva, P., Marabese, I., Palazzo, E., Rossi, F., Berrino, L., Rossi, F., Filipelli, A.: *Periaqueductal gray matter metabotropic glutamate receptors modulate formalin-induced nociception*, Pain **2000**, *85*, 183-189.

Malmberg, A. B., Chen, C. C., Tonegawa, S., Basbaum, A. I.: *Preserved acute pain and reduced neuropathic pain in mice lacking PKC gamma*, Science **1997**, *278*, 279-283.

Miller, R. J.: *Presynaptic receptors*, Annu. Rev. Pharmacol. Toxicol. **1998**, *38*, 201-27.

Mills, C. D., Johnson, K. M., Hulsebosch, C. E.: *Role of group II and group III metabotropic glutamate receptors in spinal cord injury*, Exp. Neurol. **2002**, *173*, 153-67.

Monaghan, D. T., McMills, M. C., Chamberlin, A. R., Cotman, C. W.: *Synthesis of [3H]2-amino-4-phosphonobutyric acid and characterization of its binding to rat brain membranes: a selective ligand for the chloride/calcium-dependent class of L-glutamate binding sites*, Brain Res. **1983**, *278*, 137-144.

Monn, J. A., Valli, M. J., Massey, S. M., Hansen, M. M., Kress, T. J., Wepsiec, J. P., Harkness, A. R., Grutsch, J. L., Wright, R. A., Johnson, B. G., Andis, S. L., Kingston, A., Tomlinson, R., Lewis, R., Griffey, K. R., Tizzano, J. P., Schoepp, D. D.: *Synthesis, pharmacological characterization, and molecular modeling of heterobicyclic amino acids related to (+)-2-aminobicyclo[3.1.0]hexane-2,6-dicarboxylic acid (LY354740): identification of two new potent, selective, and systemically active agonists for group II metabotropic glutamate receptors*, J. Med. Chem. **1999**, *42*, 1027-1040.

Monn, J. A., Valli, M. J., Massey, S. M., Wright, R. A., Salhoff, C. R., Johnson, B. G., Howe, T., Alt, C. A., Rhodes, G. A., Robey, R. L., Griffey, K. R., Tizzano, J. P., Kallman, M. J., Helton, D. R., Schoepp, D. D.: *Design, synthesis, and pharmacological characterization of (+)-2-aminobicyclo[3.1.0]hexane-2,6-dicarboxylic acid (LY354740): a potent, selective, and orally active group 2 metabotropic glutamate receptor agonist possessing anticonvulsant and anxiolytic properties*, J. Med. Chem. **1997**, *40*, 528-537.

Neto, F. L., Schadrack, J., Platzer, S., Zieglgansberger, W., Tolle, T. R., Castro-Lopes, J. M.: *Up-regulation of metabotropic glutamate receptor 3 mRNA expression in the cerebral cortex of monoarthritic rats*, J. Neurosci. Res. **2001**, *63*, 356-367.

Neugebauer, V., Keele, N. B., Shinnick-Gallagher, P.: *Epileptogenesis in vivo enhances the sensitivity of inhibitory presynaptic metabotropic glutamate receptors in basolateral amygdala neurons in vitro*, J. Neurosci. **1997**, *17*, 983-995.

Neugebauer, V., Chen, P. S., Willis, W. D.: *Groups II and III metabotropic glutamate receptors differentially modulate brief and prolonged nociception in primate STT cells*, J. Neurophysiol. **2000**, *84*, 2998-3009.

Ornstein, P. L., Bleisch, T. J., Arnold, M. B., Kennedy, J. H., Wright, R. A., Johnson, B. G., Tizzano, J. P., Helton, D. R., Kallman, M. J., Schoepp, D. D.: *2-Substituted (2SR)-2-amino-2((1SR,2SR)-2-carboxycycloprop-1-yl)glycines as potent and selective antagonists of group II metabotropic glutamate receptors. 2. Effects of aromatic substitution, pharmacological characterization, and bioavailability*, J. Med. Chem. **1998**, *41*, 358-378.

Pin J.P., De Colle C., Bessis A. S., Acher F.: *New perspectives for the development of selective metabotropic glutamate receptor ligands*, Eur. J. Pharmacol. **1999**, *375*, 277-294.

Popik, P., Kozela, E., Pilc, A.: *Selective agonist of group II glutamate metabotropic receptors, LY354740, inhibits tolerance to analgesic effects of morphine in mice*, Br. J. Pharmacol. **2000**, *130*, 1425-1431.

Schoepp, D. D., Jane, D. E., Monn, J. A.: *Pharmacological agents acting at subtypes of metabotropic glutamate receptors*, Neuropharmacology **1999**, *38*, 1431-1476.

Sharpe, E. F., Kingston, A. E., Lodge, D., Monn, J. A., Headley, P. M.: *Systemic pre-treatment with a group II mGlu agonist, LY379268, reduces hyperalgesia in vivo*, Br. J. Pharmacol. **2002**, *135*, 1255-1262.

Stanfa, L. C. and Dickensen, A. H.: *Inflammation alters the effects of mGlu receptor agonists in spinal nociceptive neurons*, Eur. J. Pharmacol. **1998**, *347*, 165-172.

Stolle, A., Antonicek, H.-P.,Lensky, S., Voerste, A., Müller, T., Baumgarten, J., von dem Bruch, K., Müller, G., Stropp, U., Horvath, E., de Vry, J.-M.-V., Schreiber, R. (Bayer AG): *Substituted α,β-anellated butyrolactones*, WO 0104107.

Stolle, A., Antonicek, H.-P.,Lensky, S., Voerste, A., Müller, T., Baumgarten, J., von dem Bruch, K., Müller, G., Stropp, U., Horvath, E., de Vry, J.-M.-V., Schreiber, R. (Bayer AG): *Substituted bicyclic lactones*, WO 9936418.

Stolle, A., Antonicek, H.-P.,Lensky, S., Voerste, A., Müller, T., Baumgarten, J., von dem Bruch, K., Müller, G., Stropp, U., Horvath, E., de Vry, J.-M.-V., Schreiber, R. (Bayer AG): *Substituted lactones as modulators of metabotropic glutamate receptors*, WO 9936419.

Stolle, A., Antonicek, H.-P.,Lensky, S., Voerste, A., Müller, T., Baumgarten, J., von dem Bruch, K., Müller, G., Stropp, U., Horvath, E., de Vry, J.-M.-V., Schreiber, R. (Bayer AG): *Substituted β,γ-anellated lactones*, WO 9936417.

van Wagenen, B. C., Stormann, T. M., Moe, S. T., Sheehan, S. M., McLeod, D. A., Smith, D. L., Isaac, M. B., Slassi, A. (NPS Pharmaceuticals): *Heteropolycyclic compounds and their use as metabotropic glutamate receptors*, WO 0112627.

Yashpal, K., Pitcher, G. M., Parent, A., Quirion, R., Coderre, T. J.: *Noxious thermal and chemical stimulation induce increases in ^{3}H-phorbol 12,13-dibutyrate binding in spinal cord dorsal horn as well as persistant pain and hyperalgesia, which is reduced by inhibition of protein kinase C*, J. Neurosci. **1995**, *15*, 3263-3272.

Yashpal, K., Fisher, K., Chabot, J.-G., Coderre, T. J.: *Differential effects of NMDA and group I mGluR antogonists on both nociception and spinal cord protein kinase C translocation in the formalin test and a model of neuropathic pain in rats*, Pain **2001**, *94*, 17-29.

Young, M. R., Fleetwood-Walker, S. M., Mitchell, R., Munro, F. E.: *Evidence for a role of metabotropic glutamate receptors in sustained nociceptive inputs to rat dorsal horn neurons*, Neuropharmacology **1994**, *33*, 141-144.

Young, M. R., Fleetwood-Walker, S. M., Mitchell, R., Dickinson, T.: *The involvement of metabotropic glutamate receptors and their intracellular signalling pathways in sustained nociceptive transmission in rat dorsal horn neurons*, Neuropharmacology **1995**, *34*, 1033-1041.

Zahn, P. K. and Brennan, T. J.: *Intrathecal metabotropic glutamate receptor antagonists do not decrease mechanical hyperalgesia in a rat model of postoperative pain*, Anesth. Analg. **1998**, *87*, 1354-1359.

Zheng, F., Gallagher, J.P. *Metabotropic glutamate receptor agonists potentiate a slow afterdepolarization in CNS neurons*, Neuroreport. **1992**, 3, 622-624.

Zheng, F., Gallagher, J.P., Connor, J.A. *Activation of a metabotropic excitatory amino acid receptor potentiates spike-driven calcium increases in neurons of the dorsolateral septum*, J. Neurosci. **1996**, 16, 6079-6088.

7.2 NMDA Receptor Antagonists

Werner Englberger, Michael Przewosny and Corinna Maul

The amino acid L-glutamate is the main excitatory neuro-transmitter of the central nervous system (Fonnum, 1984). Glutamate exerts its excitatory effects either by activation of several G-protein-coupled metabotropic glutamate receptors or by induction of ion fluxes by different classes of ionotropic receptors. The NMDA receptor is one of those glutamate-gated ion channels which got its name from its selective artificial agonist NMDA (N-methyl-D-aspartate) and which controls slow but persistent ion fluxes of Na^+, K^+, and Ca^{2+} across the cell membrane.

Kainate or AMPA receptors are further glutamate-gated, fast-conducting cation channels which owe their designations to their selective agonists kainate or AMPA (α-amino-3-hydroxy-5-methyl-4-isoxazole-propionic acid), respectively (for review see: Chapter 7.3, Collingridge and Lester, 1989; Seeburg 1993; Hollmann and Heinemann 1994; Ozawa et al. 1998; Parsons et al. 1998; Dingledine et al. 1999).

Glutamate (glutamic acid) (2S)-2-Amino-pentanedioic acid

NMDA (N-methyl-D-aspartate) (2R)-2-Methylamino-succinic acid

Molecular Diversity of NMDA Receptors

In addition to the multiplicity of receptor sites for glutamate, the NMDA receptors bear their own complexity as they are constructed as multimers from three distinguishable subunit classes (i.e. NR1, NR2 and NR3 subunit class). With regard to the stoichiometry of the NMDA receptor there is still some debate as to whether a native NMDA-gated ion channel within the cell membrane consists of either a tetramer or pentamer. More recently, it has been suggested that the tetramic stoichiometry is more probable (Laube et al., 1998; Hollmann, 1999).

From electrophysiological studies with *in vitro* expressed NMDA subunits in cellular systems, it has been concluded that a conventional NMDA receptor must consist of a mixed combination of NR1 splice variants and $NR2_{A-D}$ subunits in order to have full physiological activity (Monyer et al., 1992). This NR1/NR2 expression pattern has also been reported to be a prerequisite for adequate cell surface expression of NMDA receptors (McIlhinney et al., 1996). Given the tetrameric stoichiometry, any conventional NMDA receptor might consist of two NR1 and two NR2 subunits.

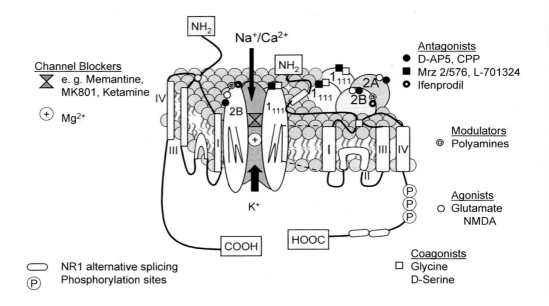

Figure 1: Model of NMDA receptor tetramer complex including the different pharma-cological effector sites (adapted from Danysz and Parsons (1998))

NR1 subunit class - one gene encoding for eight alternative splice variants

From rodent and human genomes one gene which encodes a single member of the NR1 subunit class (Moriyoshi et al., 1991; Zimmer et al., 1995) and four genes encoding $NR2_{A-D}$ of the NR2 subunit class have been cloned and have been assumed as essential NMDA receptor subunits (Ikeda et al., 1992; Kutsuwada et al., 1992; Meguro et al., 1992; Monyer et al., 1992). The mRNA of the NR1 subunit is further posttranslationally modified by alternative splicing of three exons yielding eight different splice variants (Nakanishi et al., 1992). In cDNA libraries different splice variants have been found. They show a varying expression pattern in rat brain and contribute to a different physiology of NMDA receptors (for review see Zukin and Bennett, 1995). Recently differential expression of splice variants after spinal cord injury has been reported (Prybylowski et al., 2001) and there is evidence for an interaction of the spliced N1 cassette of the NR1 subunit with zinc, protons and spermine as modulators of the NMDA receptor (for review see Dingle-dine, 1999). Yet the pharmacological relevance of the alternative NR1 splice variants is still relatively unclear.

NR2 subunit class four genes encoding for $NR2_{A-D}$

From molecular mutagenesis studies the glycine binding site has been found to be expressed on the NR1 subunit (Kuryatov et al., 1994; Wafford et al., 1995; Ivanovic et al.,

1998), whereas the NR2 subunits provide the binding sites for glutamate (Laube et al., 1997, Anson et al., 1998).

In addition, it can be assumed that there are further cooperative effects between NR1 and NR2 subunits as the affinity of ligands for the glycine$_B$ binding site of the NMDA receptor is dependent on the structure of the NR2 subunit (Honer et al., 1998).

More details regarding the physiological and pharmacological relevance of NR2$_{A-D}$ subunits have been obtained, at least in part from studies using NR2 subtype-selective antagonists. A high NR2$_B$ subtype-selectivity has been reported for ifenprodil-like antagonists (for review see: Chizh et al., 2001 and Zhuo, 2002). NR2$_B$-selective antagonists show a favorable efficacy to side-effect ratio which is thought to be partially due to a restricted distribution of the NR2$_B$-subtype. The NR2$_B$ subtype was found in the superficial layer of the spinal dorsal horn where it is thought to be putatively engaged in the transmission of nociceptive inputs. Additionally supraspinal sites seemed to be involved (Chizh et al., 2001). In contrast the NR2$_B$ subtype was not found in the cerebellum, which might in turn be responsible for the good tolerability in as much as no or rather little ataxia is caused by NR2$_B$-specific antagonists. Other NMDA antagonists have been shown to have at least a preference for inhibition of certain NR2 subunits (Sucher et al., 1996). The high affinity non-competitive antagonists MK-801 or phencyclidine with a preference for NR2$_A$ and therefore putatively with a high risk for psychotomimetic side-effects should be mentioned here. Whereas some low affinity non-competitive antagonists rather show a preference for NR2$_C$ with better tolerability in this respect (Monaghan et al., 1997). Further information about the pharmacology of the NMDA antagonists is given below in more detail.

Furthermore, in rodents a member of a third class of NMDA receptor subunits (NR3$_A$) has been cloned (Sucher et al., 1995). Expression of this NR3$_A$ subunit together with NR1 and NR2 subunits has been shown to cause *in vitro* an attenuation of the NMDA-induced ion fluxes and consequently NR3$_A$ knock-out mice show *in vivo* enhanced NMDA receptor activity (Das et al., 1998). Meanwhile a second member (NR3$_B$) of this third class of subunit with comparable features has been cloned from mouse genome (Nishi et al., 2001).

NR3 subunit class 2 genes encoding for NR3$_A$ or NR3$_B$

Very recently, Chatterton et al. (2002) reported that expression of NR1 with NR3$_A$ or NR3$_B$ without any NR2 subunit in xenopus oocytes results in the generation of functional active ion channels with unique physiological features. In particular, glycine alone seems to control the gating of the NR1/NR3 ion channel for small cations such as Na^+. Neither glutamate nor NMDA are needed as co-agonists for the activation of the channel.

Whereas the physiological role of the neurotransmitter glycine has so far been considered to be inhibitory (via strychnine-sensitive glycine receptors) the above interaction with NR1/NR3 ion channels indicates an excitatory role for glycine in addition to its co-agonistic function at the NMDA receptor. Further pecularities of the NR1/NR3 oligomers include the lack of voltage-dependent Mg^{2+} block (as shown subsequently for the conventional NMDA receptor combinations) and the antagonistic action of D-serine to these NR1/NR3 oligomers, whereas D-serine behaves as an alternative endogeneous co-agonist at the glycine binding site of conventional NR1/NR2 receptors (Chatterton et al., 2002). Since these findings are very recent, there is not sufficient data to discuss in more detail the physiology or even pharmacology of these novel NR1/NR3 oligomers.

Preliminary data support the existence of comparable sequences in the human genome, however, functional expression of human NR3 subunits has not been reported so far as far as we are aware.

In situ expression of NMDA receptors might be even more sophisticated in as much as NMDA receptor complexes might consist of a submixture of each different subunit class (for review see Béhé et al., 1999) possibly with new characteristic features. With the advent of the third NR3 subclass there might exist any mixture of all three subclasses of NR1, NR2, and NR3 subunits. In this respect NMDA receptor complexes might gain new functional characteristics as shown for the NR1/NR3 oligomers and there is obviously an urgent need for reconsideration of the NR3 contribution *in vivo*.

Functional Role of NMDA Receptors in Pain

Unfortunately a global knock-out of NR1 subunits (i.e. a total deficit of NMDA receptor functionality) produces non-viable offspring which die perinatally within hours (Forrest et al., 1994; Li et al., 1994). The non-viable offspring suffer from respiratory distress, cyanosis, and severe ataxia. In addition, due to neurophysiological abnormalities they do not develop any suckling reflex.

In this respect the development of conditional or regional knock-out mice proved to be a powerful tool for the elucidation of the functional role of NMDA receptors. By means of these techniques have provided significant evidence for the essential role of NMDA receptors in learning and memory processes within the hippocampus (Tsien et al., 1996) and thus those effects should therefore also be considered as typical adverse drug reaction of NMDA antagonists. Very recently a conditional knock-out of NR1 in the spinal cord has been reported to attenuate hyperalgesia in formalin-induced persistent pain models or in partial nerve injury models (South et al., 2001). These data are consistent with the previously shown attenuation of formalin-induced pain in regional NR1 knock-downs induced by intrathecal injection of NR1 antisense polynucleotides in rats (Garry et al., 2000).

Knock-out mice with depletion of $NR2_A$, $NR2_C$, or $NR2_D$ proved to be viable although global $NR2_B$ knock-outs also die perinatally due obviously to a missing suckling response (Kutsuwada et al., 1996). The $NR2_A$, $NR2_C$, or $NR2_D$ global knock-out mice show no severe symptomatology, are fertile, and have a normal life expectancy (Ikeda et al., 1995; Sakimura et al., 1995; Ebralidze et al., 1996). Most obvious in these knock-out mice is the deficit in spatial learning or memory (Morris water maze) obviously associated with an impaired synaptic plasticity (Sakimura et al., 1995). However, the combined knock-out of $NR2_A$ and $NR2_C$ worsens the symptomatology and causes severe motor impairment (Kadotani et al., 1996). So far only sparse data are available regarding the impact of the genetic NR2 knock-outs or genetic modifications on pain perception in animal models. A knock-out of $NR2_A$ abolishes a mechanical allodynia inducible by intrathecal injection of PGE_2 or NMDA totally, whereas $NR2_D$ knock-out mice behave like wild-type mice. However, the same authors reported that a comparable, mechanical allodynia induced by intrathecal injection of $PGF_{2\alpha}$ or AMPA showed the reverse phenomenon in as much as $NR2_A$ knock-out mice show allodynia like wild-type mice while the allodynic behavior is totally abolished in $NR2_D$ knock-outs (Minami et al., 2001). An overexpression of $NR2_B$ subunits in the forebrain results in an enhanced inflammatory pain perception (Wei et al., 2001) in addition to enhanced learning and memory capabilities (Tang et al., 2001). In addition, knocking out D-amino-acid oxidase, an enzyme involved in the catabolic degradation of D-amino acids and thus in the accumulation of the co-agonist D-serine of the NMDA receptor, results in potentiation of NMDA receptor function and in enhanced nocicepion (Wake et al., 2001).

Taken together there is some direct proof for a functional contribution of spinal NMDA receptors in the process of induction of hyperalgesia by conditional spinal NR1 knock-out animals or spinal NR1 knock-down experiments. While at least indirect evidence suggests a correlation between upregulation of the NMDA receptor activity and noci-ception, the interpretation of the impact of knocking out NR2 subunits needs further detailed research.

By far the most evidence for an essential role of NMDA receptor activation especially in chronic pain has been provided by pharmacological studies with NMDA receptor antagonists which is discussed below.

Physiology of NMDA Receptors Offers Several Therapeutic Target Approaches

Several functionally relevant binding sites at the NMDA receptor ion channel are suitable for therapeutical targeting (Wroblewski et al., 1989). These target sites comprise the primary recognition sites for the agonist glutamate or its artificial subsitute NMDA and the co-agonists glycine or D-serine as well as the modulatory polyamine sites or binding sites within the channel pore. They are discussed in more detail in the following sections.

(a) Competitive NMDA receptor antagonists

Obviously glutamate or its artificial substitute NMDA is a prerequisite for the activation of a conventional NMDA receptor. In the case of a postsynaptic NMDA receptor of a centrally-projecting neuron or interneuron within the substantia gelatinosa of the spinal dorsal horn, this might be provided by an innervating glutamatergic primary afferent fiber and a substantial release of glutamate into the synaptic cleft. This offers the glutamate binding site as a first target site for the so-called competitive glutamate antagonists which exert their antagonistic actions by competively displacing glutamate. The structures of those antagonists resemble closely the pharmacophores of glutamate. Usually they consist of an amino group which may be part of a heterocyclic system and an acidic moiety such as carboxylic acid or phosphoric acid.

AP5 and CPP are antagonists having a binding affinity for the NMDA receptor comparable to glutamate (Lehmann et al., 1987; Murphy et al., 1987). Spinally administered, both compounds exert antinociceptive effects (Coderre et al., 1994; Goettl et al., 1994; Kristensen et al., 1994; Leem et al., 1996). The limitation of such structures is of course their low lipophilicity which restricts their availability mainly to the periphery and usually requires spinal administration to obtain therapeutic efficacy.

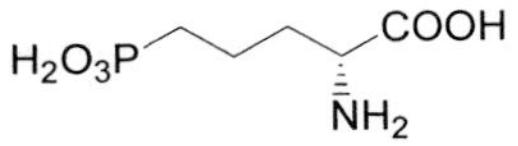

D-AP5 (D-norvaline)

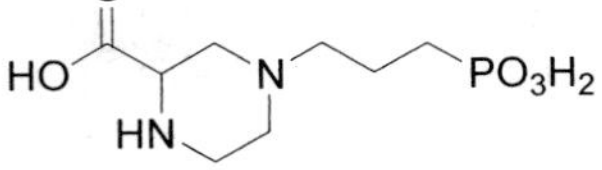

CPP, 4-(3-Phosphono-propyl)
-piperazine-2-carboxylic acid

Scheme 1: Structures of D-AP5 and CPP.

Incorporation of a nitrogen into heterocyclic structures (e.g. CPP, D-CPPene, or Selfotel) offers more lipophilic structures which in turn show a better blood - brain barrier (BBB) penetration (Kristensen et al., 1995; Herrling et al., 1997; Schmutz et al., 1997). Attempts to derivatize AP5/AP7 by introducing heterocyclic systems led to interesting structures with CNS availability and high potency. Examples are biphenylic derivatives such as SDZ-220,581 from the former Sandoz Pharma Ltd. (Urwyler et al., 1996), or others like PD-134,705 from the former Warner-Lambert Inc. (Ortwine et al., 1992), LY274614 from E. Lilly Inc. (Cheung et al.,1996), or WAY-126,090 from Wyeth-Ayerst (AHP) (Kinney et al., 1998) which is according to a company communication under preclinical development for neuropathic pain.

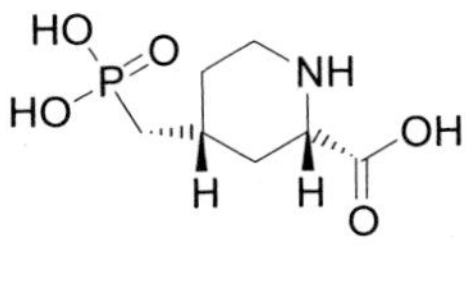

Selfotel (CGS-19,755)

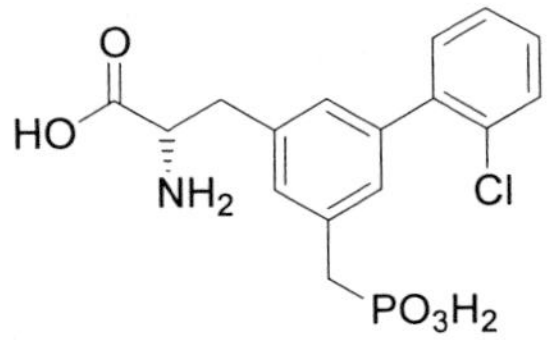

SDZ-220581

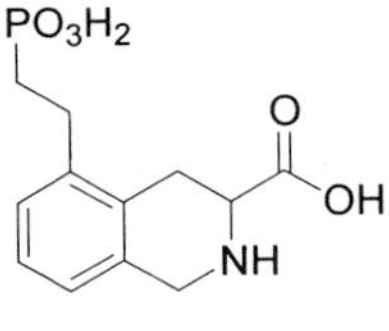

PD-134705

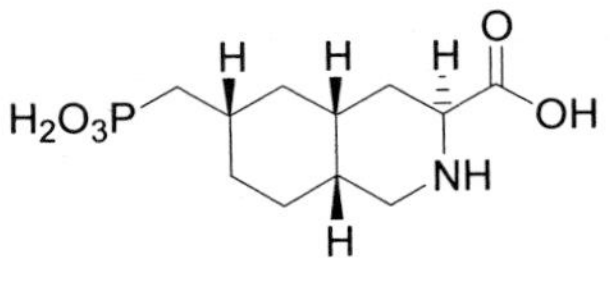

LY-274614

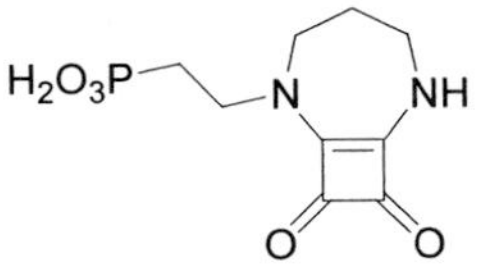

WAY-126090

Scheme 2: Examples for competitive NMDA receptor antagonists.

In a human case study concerning a severe intractable chronic pain state, racemic CPP (i.t.) has been shown to have analgesic efficacy (Kristensen et al., 1992). However, increasing the lipophilicity of competitive NMDA antagonists and hence their CNS availability in turn increases the risk of central adverse effects. Therefore administration of this class of antagonists should be restricted to local sites (Kristensen, 1997). This was also emphasized in clinical studies with the systemic administration of competitive NMDA antagonists (the main focus of drug development has been stroke therapy) which have been stopped because of intolerable CNS effects such as psychotomimesis among other reasons (Muir et al., 1995; Davis et al., 1997). Recently, inorganic iron complexes derived from degradation products of the nitric oxide donor nitroprusside have been shown to exert competitive NMDA antagonism with selective affinities in the nanomolar range. The inhibition does not seem to be due to generation of NO or to any interaction with a redox site but is probably the result of a steric hindrance mechanism. A new mechanism has been proposed involving an exchange of loosely bound H_2O/NH_3 species in the coordination sphere of the iron complex with an amino acid side chain in the vicinity of the competitive binding_site of glutamate. However, the significance of the latter findings for the pharmacology of NMDA receptors needs further evaluation (Neijt et al., 2001).

In addition, the presence of glycine as a further co-agonist is necessary for activation of conventional NR1/NR2 ion channels. Neither glutamate nor glycine on their own cause any essential activation so the simultaneous presence of both amino acids is an obligate requirement for activation (Johnson et al.1987, Kleckner et al.1988).

This co-agonistic excitatory glycine binding site is often designated as 'strychnine-insensitive glycine binding site of the NMDA receptor' to distinguish it from the inhibitory strychnine-sensitive glycine binding site. Following a pragmatic proposal by Danysz and Parsons (1998) in their comprehensive review of the physiology and prospective therapeutic significance of this glycine binding site of the NMDA receptor we prefer the terms glycine$_B$ site or glycine$_B$ antagonist or agonist for competitive effectors of this site. Besides glycine the non-proteinogenic amino acid D-serine has been found as a further endogenous agonist of the glycine$_B$ site (Danysz et al., 1990; Mothet et al., 2000). The distribution of endogeneous D-serine and its generating enzyme D-serine racemase in the CNS resembles the distribution of NMDA receptors (Wolosker et al., 1999; Mothet et al., 2000). Evidence for the

(b) Glycine$_B$ site antagonists

Glycine

D-Serine

physiological relevance of D-serine for nociception might be provided by the enhanced nociceptive behavior of mutant mice lacking the enzyme D-amino-acid oxidase, an enzyme involved in the catabolic degradation of D-amino acids (Wake et al., 2001). An interesting new approach for inhibition of NMDA receptor activation might therefore be any attenuation of D-serine concentrations for example by inhibition of D-serine racemase (Panizzutti et al., 2001).

Glycine_B site antagonists which have been shown to be effective in analgesic models can be divided into different chemical classes although so far any high affinity effector molecule of the glycine_B site bears more or less the structural motif of glycine within its molecular structure, as can be observed in the first example, kynurenic acid.

Because kynurenic acid is an endogeneous metabolite of tryptophan metabolism and has been found in mammalian brain (Moroni et al., 1988) it has been suggested that it might be a putative endogeneous antagonist (Stone, 1993). In the later course of the tryptophan metabolic pathway there are further putative harmful metabolites generated such as the oxygen radical generating 3-hydroxy-kynurenine and the NMDA receptor agonist quinolinic acid. Therefore inhibition of the generation of these harmful metabolites has been attempted by blocking kynurenine-3-hydroxylase activity thus allowing kynurenic acid to accumulate (for review see Stone, 2000). However, relatively high concentrations of kynurenic acid are necessary for inhibition of glycine_B site receptor binding or NMDA receptor ion fluxes (Bertolino et al.,1989; Danysz et al., 1989). But even metabolic inhibition of kynurenine-3-hydroxylase which provokes accumulation of kynurenic acid seems to have little physiological relevance (Urenjak et al., 2000). Kynurenic acid is further hampered by its relatively low selectivity.

Derivatization of kynurenic acid leads to far more potent and selective antagonists such as 7-chloro-kynurenic acid or 5,7-dichlorokynurenic acid (Kemp et al., 1988; Baron et al., 1990) which have been shown to inhibit glycine-induced tailflick facilitation (i.e attenuation of glycine-induced hyperalgesia) or the late phase of formalin-induced nociception when given intrathecally (Kolhekar et al., 1994, Chapman et al., 1995). Nevertheless kynurenic acid derivatives are still hampered by a poor blood - brain barrier penetration and hence a low CNS availability.

Kynurenic acid

3-Hydroxy-kynurenine

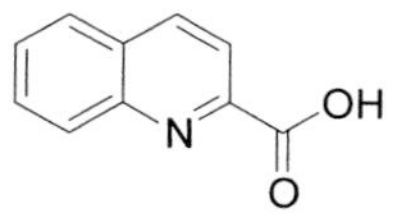

Quinolinic acid

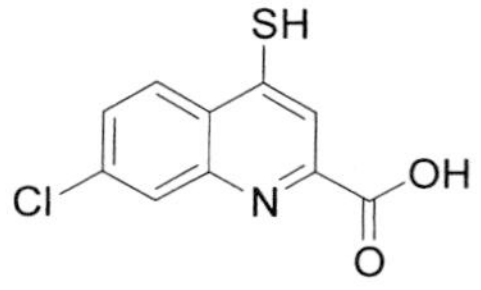

7-Chlorokynurenic acid 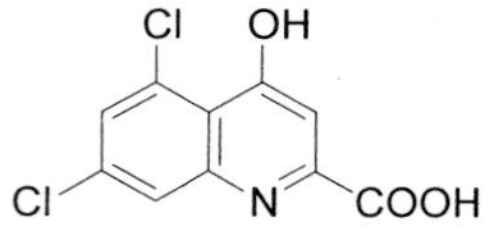   5,7-Dichlorokynurenic acid

Scheme 3: Structures of kynurenic acid derivatives.

7-Chlorothiokynurenic acid

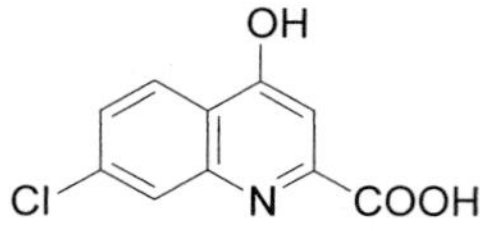

There have been further chemical attempts to improve CNS penetration such as the development of thio-kynurenic acids with improved CNS availability (Moroni et al., 1991; Chen et al., 1993).

Other attempts make use of the better CNS penetration of kynurenine which is converted enzymatically within the brain to kynurenic acid by kynurenine aminotransferase (Hokari et al., 1996) or the design of pro-drugs which enter the CNS more easily and are hydrolyzed within the brain e.g. glucosidic-linked 7-chlorokynurenic acid (Bonina et al., 2000).

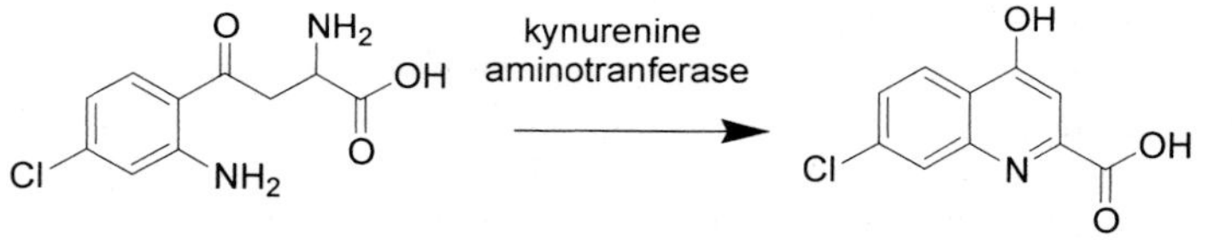

4-chlorokynurenine   7-chlorokynurenic acid

Scheme 4:   Enzyme-catalyzed formation of 7-chlorokynurenic acid.

Further systematic derivatization leads to selective and high affinity compounds such as the 4-aminotetrahydro-chinolin-carboxylate L-689,560 (Leeson et al., 1992) and to 4-hydroxyquinolin-2(1H)-ones (Rowley et al., 1993) of which L-701,324 has become the best known prototype which combines selective and high glycine$_B$ affinity and oral bioavailability (Kulagowski et al., 1994; Priestley et al., 1996).

L-701,324 has been shown to reverse the inflammation-induced mechanical hyperalgesia in rats without affecting the accompanying carrageenan-induced paw edema (Laird et al., 1996).

1,4-Dihydro-2,3-quinoxalinediones comprise another scaffold for glycine$_B$ antagonists with antinociceptive activity (Vaccarino et al., 1993; Woodward et al., 1995a; Lutfy and Weber, 1996; Lutfy and Weber, 1998; Lutfy et al., 1999) of which licostinel is a good example of a highly selective and highly potent member of this series (Woodward et al., 1995b).

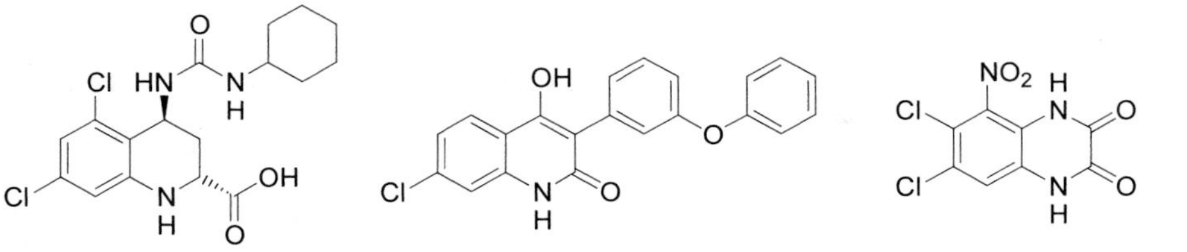

L-689560   L-701,324   Licostinel (ACEA-1021)

Scheme 5: Examples for glycine_B antagonists.

Whereas earlier quinoxalinediones derivatives comprise relatively similiar compounds which differ only in their side chain substitution pattern, the condensation of heteroarylic ring systems to the quinoxalinediones scaffold might offer the development of a broader range of highly potent and selective glycine_B antagonists such as CGP-68,730A (Pozza et al., 2000).

Indole-2-carboxylic acids represent another scaffold known for more than a decade as competitive glycine_B antagonists (Huettner, 1989). Structure - activity relationships favor the C4 and C6 position for substitutions with chlorine or other small electrophilic substituents to increase the binding affinity (Gray et al., 1991; Salituro et al., 1992) thus yielding for example the potent 4,6-dichloro-indole-2-carboxylate derivatives which closely resemble the 5,7-dichlorokynurenic acid pharmacophor.

A well-known, selective and high affinity example is MDL-105,519 which also represents the most frequently used radioligand for the glycine_B binding site (Siegel et al., 1996; Baron et al., 1997). Whereas the position of the halogenic substitutions and the carboxyl group seems to be restricted to fixed areas within the indole-2-carboxylate scaffold, a relatively bulky substitution at C3 is obviously possible or even favorable for high glycine_B affinity. This is also the case for the two advanced glycine_B antagonists synthesized by Glaxo Wellcome plc, Gavestinel (GV-150,526) and GV-196,771A from which the latter at least has been considered for clinical development in chronic pain therapy (Di Fabio et al., 2000).

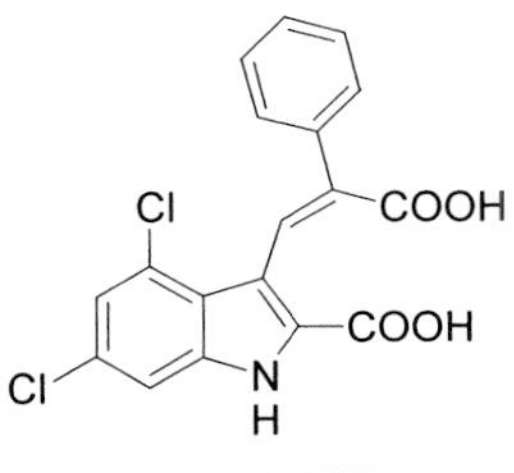

MDL-105519

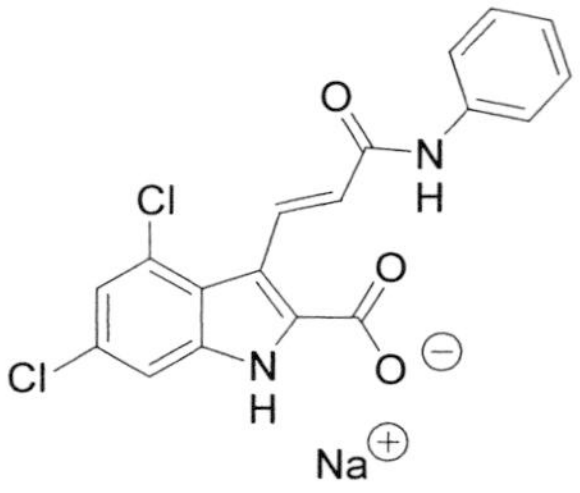

Gavestinel

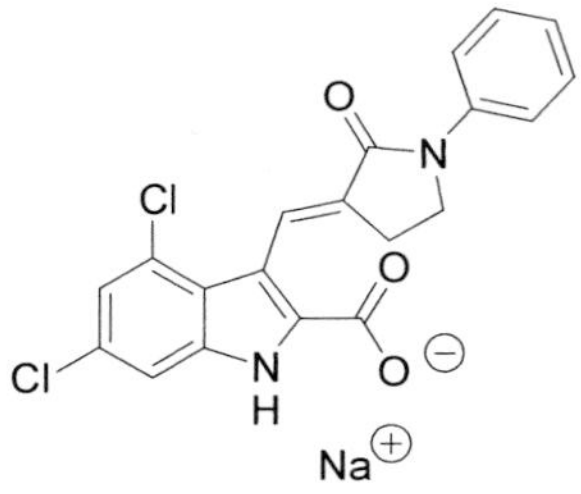

GV-196,771A

For GV-196,771 a basic schematic description of its synthesis is also given by Di Fabio et al. (2000). Both glycine$_B$ antagonists show a better fit with a two binding site model with Hill coefficients signifcantly lower than 1 (Chopra et al., 2000). The latter authors discuss possible steric hindrance of the binding of a second inhibitor molecule to the receptor oligomers thus resulting in negative cooperativity. GV-196,771A has been described to exert antihyperalgesic activity in either persistent formalin-induced pain models or in neuropathic sciatic nerve constriction models (Quartaroli et al., 1999, 2001). The modulation of nociceptive transmission in thalamic nuclei is obviously restricted to those neuropathic injury states which might result in an otherwise overall good tolerability of this compound (Bordi et al., 2000).

Quite diverse from the previously described chemical classes there are a series of more complex tricyclic glycine$_B$ antagonists of which the compound ZD-9,379 from Zeneca and MRZ-2/576 from Merz are good examples (Quiu et al., 1997; Parsons et al., 1997).

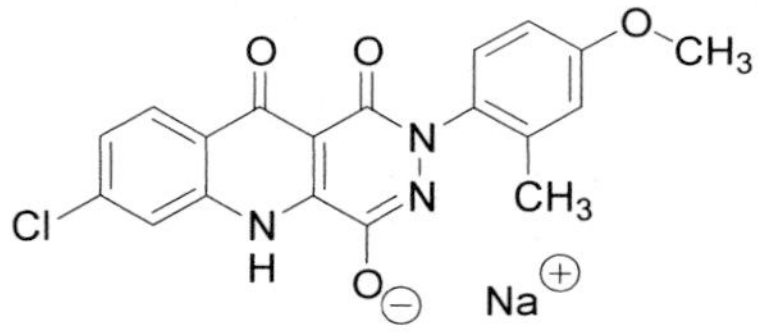

ZD-9379

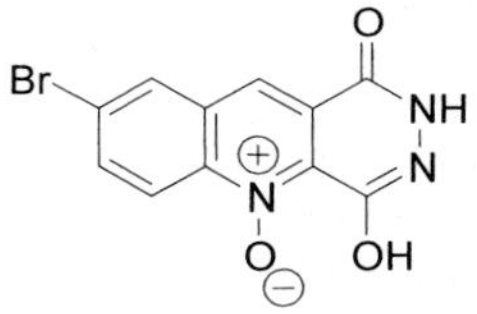

MRZ-2/576

Scheme 6: Examples for glycine$_B$ antagonists.

MRZ-2/576 has been demonstrated to cross the blood - brain barrier rapidly and to function centrally as a glycine$_B$ antagonist after systemic administration of doses within the relevant antinociceptive dose range. However, the compound is only short-acting within the CNS because of a relatively short half-life within this compartment (Parsons et al., 1997). The compound has antinociceptive properties and shows exceptionally good efficacy in a visceral pain model (McClean et al., 1998; Olivar et al., 1999).

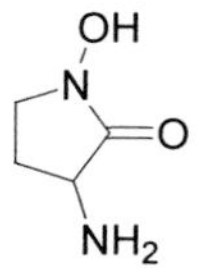

HA-966

Last but not least, an interesting class of functionally antagonistic glycine$_B$ effector molecules are the partial agonists of which (+)-HA-966 is the most important example. (+)-HA-966 has a low intrinsic agonistic activity (i.e. it yields on its own only a partial agonistic effect of about 10 - 40% of the possible maximal agonistic effect) but it has strong antagonistic activity which can 'neutralize' the effect of high efficacy agonists, such as glycine or D-serine (Hendersen et al., 1990; Singh et al., 1990; Danysz et al., 1998).

Thus partial agonists may allow some physiologically low level NMDA receptor activation while antagonizing high level excessive NMDA receptor activation and this may be the reason for the relatively good tolerability of such compounds.

The partial agonism of D-cycloserine has also been reported to be NR2-subunit dependent. Whereas D-cycloserine shows partial agonism in NR1-1a/NR2$_A$- or NR1-1a/NR2$_B$-expressing oocytes it has a higher intrinsic efficacy in NR1-1a/NR2$_C$-expressing oocytes in comparison to glycine (Sheinin et al., 2001).

(+)-HA-966 or D-cycloserine have been reported to exert antinociception in the late tonic pain phase of formalin-induced pain in rats and mice or to attenuate the thermal hyperalgesia in peripheral mononeuropathy in rats by sciatic nerve ligation (Mao et al., 1992; Millan and Seguin, 1993; Hunter and Singh, 1994; Millan and Seguin, 1994). Obviously partial agonists also reinforce the antinociceptive activity of either opioids or tachykinin NK1 antagonists (Seguin et al., 1994; Christensen et al., 1998) or might attenuate the development of morphine dependence during chronic treatment of neuropathic rats (Christensen et al., 2000).

Previously reported as a putative partial agonist at the glycine$_B$-site (Fossom et al., 1995) 1-aminocyclopropane-carboxylic acid has more recently been shown to act as a glycine$_B$-site agonist and concurrently as a glutamate-site antagonist (Nahum-Levy et al., 1999).

Of particular importance for the functionality of NMDA receptors is their voltage-dependent blockade by Mg^{2+}. At resting negative cell membrane potential in the presence of glutamate, glycine, and physiological Mg^{2+} concentrations the channel's ion flux is still blocked due to Mg^{2+} ions at a Mg^{2+} binding site within the ion channel pore. This block is not relieved until the cell membrane potential becomes sufficiently depolarized and in turn Mg^{2+} is released from its binding site within the pore (Novak et al., 1984; Li-Smerin et al., 1996). By mutagenesis studies one asparagine within the M2-segment of all NMDA subunits has been identified as being essential for this feature as an exchance of this asparagine strongly reduces the voltage-dependent block by Mg^{2+} ions (Burnashev et al.1992; Mori et al., 1992). In addition the channel conductivity for Ca^{2+} is also influenced by the same asparagine at this position (Burnashev et al., 1992; Sakurada et al., 1993). This Mg^{2+} block also varies with

D-Cycloserine

1-aminocyclo-propane-carboxylic acid

c) Blockade of the channel pore by Mg^{2+} and non-competitive NMDA channel blockers

the NR2 subunit composition of the NMDA receptor, indicating a stronger voltage dependency of NR1-NR2$_A$ or NR1-NR2$_B$ NMDA receptors compared to their NR2$_C$ or NR2$_D$ counterparts (Kuner et al., 1996; for review see Dingledine et al., 1999). A similiar pattern of NR2 subunit sensitivity has been found in the attenuation of the Mg^{2+} block by phosphorylation of NMDA receptors by protein kinase C (PKC) which has previously been proposed as a mechanism for the modulation of NMDA receptors (Chen et al., 1992; Wagner et al., 1996). However further detailed studies have raised doubts that this is the principal mechanism of the enhanced NMDA channel conductance (Zheng et al., 1999; for review see Dingledine et al., 1999). In addition a broad variety of other kinases besides PKC have been shown to phosphorylate multiple sites in the NMDA receptors (Lau et al., 1995; Suzuki et al., 1995; Omkumar et al., 1996; Leonard et al., 1997; Nakazawa et al., 2001).

Spatial or temporal summation of excitatory postsynaptic potentials from adjacent synapses activated by non-NMDA glutamate receptors or by other co-released neuropeptides of the sensory afferent fibers may be responsible for the depolarization which reverses the Mg^{2+} block. NMDA receptor-induced ion fluxes therefore need the simultaneous synaptical release of glutamate and its co-agonists glycine or D-serine in addition to the coincident activation of nearby excitatory synapses. Although the physiological Mg^{2+} concentrations are considered to cause an efficient NMDA receptor block at normal resting cell membrane potential there are several reports that high additional administration of Mg^{2+} might further attenuate the excitability of NMDA receptors and that Mg^{2+} can be used for treatment of hyperalgesic states. The significance of this Mg^{2+} block for chronic pain has been shown by the antihyperalgesic effects of spinally and also systemically administered Mg^{2+} in neuropathic pain or the second pain phase of the formalin-induced pain model in rats (Xiao and Bennett, 1994; et al., 2000; Takano et al., 2000). Spinally-administered, Mg^{2+} potentiates the antinociceptive effect of morphine (Kroin et al., 2000). Consequently, a Mg^{2+} deficiency in turn induces hyperalgesia which may be reversed by an NMDA antagonist (Dubray et al., 1997). Mg^{2+} has also been shown to mediate clinical analgesia in postoperative or neuropathic pain caused by cancer and other etiologies (Felsby et al., 1995; Traber et al., 1996; Koing et al., 1998; Crosby et al., 2000).

Within the channel pore there is also the binding site for the so-called open channel blockers which is also able to control ion currents through the receptor pore and is known as either MK-801 or phencyclidine (PCP) binding site, reflecting the nature of its well-known high-affinity ligands.

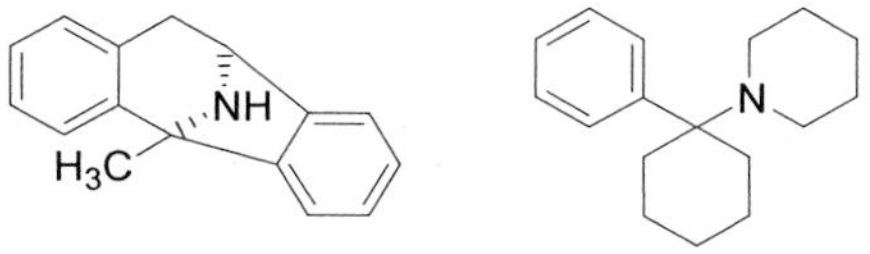

Dizocilpine (MK-801)   Phencyclidine

Scheme 7: Structures of MK-801 and phencyclidine.

Ligands of this binding site are called open channel blockers or non-competitive NMDA antagonists and due to their putative functionality i.e. steric hindrance of the ion fluxes only antagonism by such ligands has been described so far. An important feature of these antagonists is their so-called use-dependency (Huettner and Bean, 1988). In order to reach their binding site within the NMDA ion channel pore non-competitive NMDA antagonists (e.g. MK801, PCP, ketamine, memantine, see below) require an activated and open ion channel. In turn, once bound the channel blockers may become trapped within the channel pore when the NMDA receptor channel returns to its closed state (Sobolevsky et al., 2002).

High affinity open channel blockers like MK-801 or PCP (also known as 'angel dust' among drug abusers) cause intolerable psychotomimetic side-effects (Rogawski and Porter, 1990; Jentsch et al., 2000). In addition PCP and MK801 have been shown to cause neuronal vacuolization at least in rodents (Olney et al., 1989). There exists an inverse correlation between high binding affinity and the speed of the on and off kinetics among NMDA antagonists i.e. the higher the binding affinity the slower the on and off kinetics (Parsons et al., 1995; Black et al., 1996). Low affinity channel blockers with fast channel blocking kinetics and strong voltage dependency such as memantine, dextromethorphan, or remacemide offer a far more favorable efficacy to side-effect ratio than high affinity blockers with slow onset and offset kinetics such as MK-801 (Kemp et al., 1987; for review see Rogawski, 2000). The better tolerability of low to medium affinity, fast channel blockers is also emphasized by the fact that all clinically used non-competitive NMDA antagonists belong to this class (e.g. amantadine, memantine, dextromethorphan, ketamine). In addition there are some low affinity antagonists under clinical development for pain (Palmer and Widzowski, 2000).

The high affinity non-competitive antagonist MK-801 will be considered first (Wong et al., 1986; Huettner and Bean, 1988). Several analogs have been synthesized (Leeson et al., 1990) which have in common with other structural classes an amino nitrogen which can be protonated. MK-801 has been shown to inhibit thermal hyperalgesia, to reduce the hyperactivity and hyper-responsiveness of spinal dorsal horn neurons in neuropathic rats with unilateral sciatic nerve ligation, and to attenuate formalin-induced persistent pain in rats (Haley et al., 1990; Davar et al., 1991; Yamamoto et al., 1992; Chaplan et al., 1997; Sotgiu et al., 2000). However due to intolerable side-effects MK-801 has not been developed further (Koek et al., 1988; Tricklebank et al., 1989; Wozniak et al., 1990).

Ketamine

Synthesis (Kleemann et al., 1999):

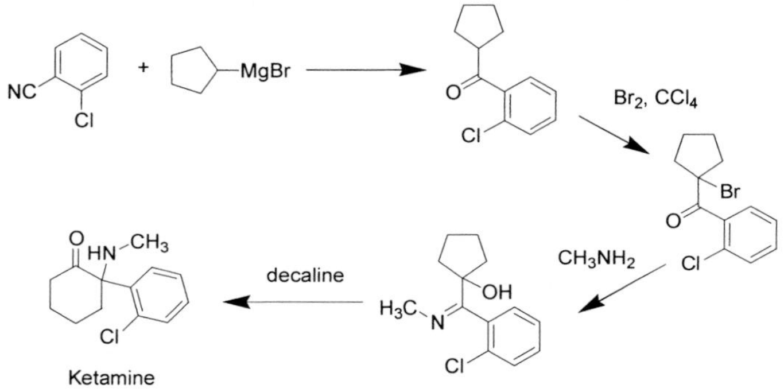

Ketamine

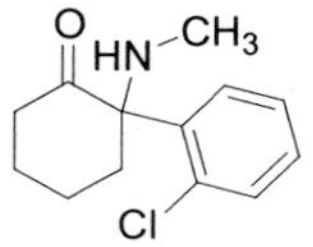

[6740-88-1]; 2-(2-Chloro-phenyl)-2-methylamino-cyclohexanone, $C_{13}H_{16}ClNO$, MW 237.73

Scheme 8: Synthesis of ketamine.

The structure of ketamine is similar to that of PCP. Keta-mine is an intermediate affinity fast channel blocker with a stereospecific preference for the S-(+)-enantiomer but with no selectivity for the NR1/NR2$_{A-D}$ heteromeric subunits (Yamakura et al., 2000). The majority of the clinical literature regarding NMDA antagonists is devoted to keta-mine. In addition to evidence of its preclinical antinoci-ceptive efficacy in animal pain models, there are many clinical studies and case reports substantiating the anal-gesic efficacy of ketamine. The therapeutic value of keta-mine, either used alone or as an adjuvant to other pain relief substances, seems to be in the treatment of chronic pain states, neuropathic pain, post-herpetic neuralgia, phantom limb pain, fibromyalgia, opioid-intractable cancer pain, burn-induced hyperalgesia, central post-stroke pain and other pain states (e.g. Eide et al., 1994; Max et al., 1995; Ilkjaer et al., 1996; Nicolajsen et al., 1996; Warncke et al., 1997; Davis, 1999; Fine, 1999; Finlay, 1999; Rabben et al., 1999; Graven-Nielsen et al., 2000; Mercadante et al., 2000; Vick et al., 2001). Despite the well-proven efficacy in several pain states the use of ketamine is hampered by psychotomimetic side-effects such as hallucinations, or sensory distortions and attenuation of memory (Davis, 1999; Newcomer et al., 1999; Shiigi et al., 1999). However one should also bear in mind that the pharmacology of ketamine is complex in as much as there are interactions with other binding sites (e.g. nicotinic and muscarinergic cholinergic and opioid sites, Na^+ and L-type Ca^{2+} ion channels) in addition to those involved in NMDA antagonism (for review see Kohrs et al., 1998).

Amantadine

Synthesis (Kleemann et al., 1999):

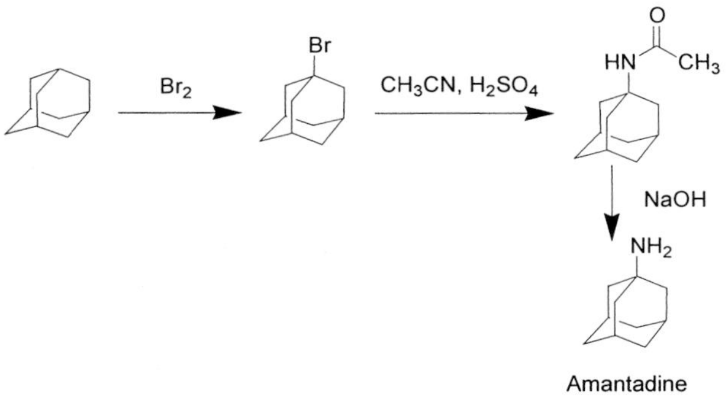

Scheme 9: Synthesis of amantadine.

Amantadine

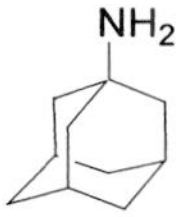

NH_2

(1-amino-adamantane), Tricyclo[3.3.1.1^{3,7}]decan-1-amine, $C_{10}H_{17}N$, MW151.25, [768-94-5],

A further class of compounds comprises the amino-adamantanes from which amantadine and memantine produced by Merz are well-known examples of drugs used for the long-term therapy of Parkinson's syndrome. Both compounds are examples of low to medium affinity, fast channel blockers with a strong voltage-dependency and a favorable efficacy to side-effect ratio (Parsons et al., 1995; Parsons et al., 1999a). Although amantadine has a low affinity for the NMDA receptor channel site and relatively high concentrations are necessary for specific interaction with the NMDA receptor (Parsons et al., 1995), amantadine reaches concentrations in the human brain which are considered to be high enough for NMDA antagonism

(Kornhuber et al., 1995) and has been described to relieve clinical neuropathic pain states (Pud et al., 1998).

Memantine

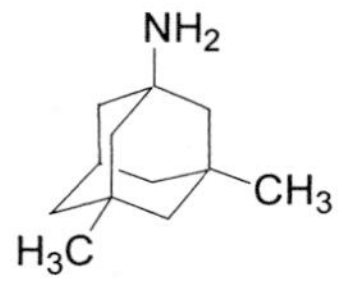

Synthesis (Kleemann et al., 1999):

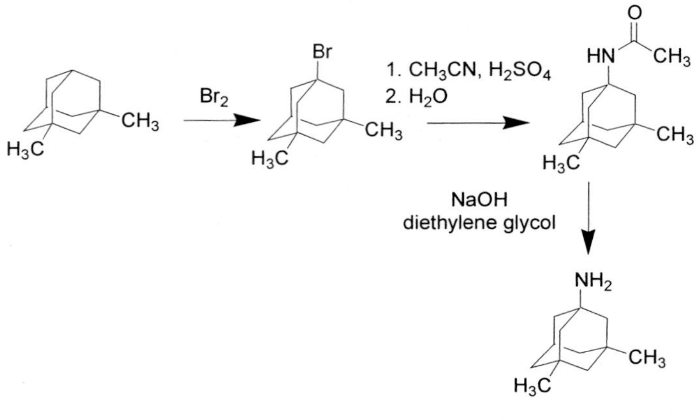

Memantine

(1-amino-3,5-dimethyladamantane), 3,5-dimethyl-tricyclo[3.3.1.1^{3,7}]decan-1-amine, $C_{12}H_{21}N$, MW 179,31, [19982-08-2];

Scheme 10: Synthesis of memantine.

In addition to antinociceptive activity in preclinical pain models such as carrageenan-induced thermal hyperalgesia or sciatic nerve constriction mononeuropathy in rats (Eisenberg et al., 1994; Suzuki et al., 2001) memantine has also shown analgesic efficacy in clinical studies and is under clinical development for neuropathic pain treatment (Eisenberg et al., 1998; Headley, 1999; Nikolajsen et al., 2000). There is evidence to show that memantine concentrations in the CNS reach levels which can effectively produce NMDA antagonism (Wesemann et al., 1980). In addition there is also evidence showing in situ NMDA antagonism of spinal neurons after ionto-phoretic administration of NMDA and systemic adminis-tration of memantine (Herrero et al., 1994).

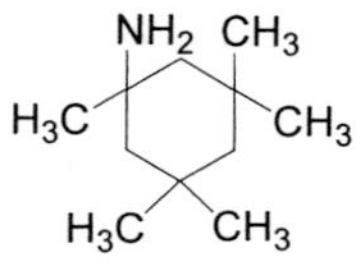

A series of amino-alkyl-cyclohexanes (e.g. MRZ-2/579) under recent development by Merz have been shown to attenuate the development of tolerance towards antinoci-ception by morphine in rats (Parsons et al., 1999b; Hough-ton et al., 2001).

MRZ-2/579

Remacemide from AstraZeneca is a pro-drug which is converted by hydrolysis and removal of glycine to its active desglycinyl derivative FPL-12,495 which is a low affinity fast kinetics channel blocker (Heyn et al., 1994; Subramaniam et al., 1996; Monaghan et al., 1997; Ahmed et al., 1999).

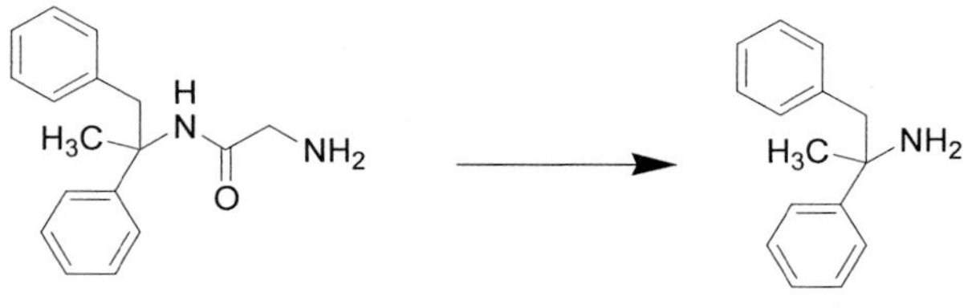

Remacemide   FPL-12,495

Scheme 11: Hydrolysis of remacemide.

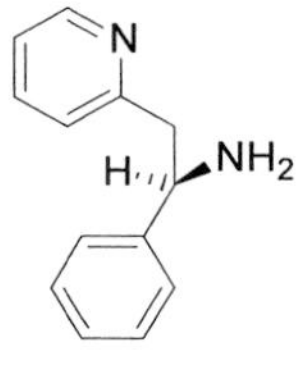

Both remacemide and its des-glycinyl-metabolite inhibit the inflammatory, mechanical hyperalgesia as well as the edema induced by injection of carrageenan or complete Freunds adjuvant into the rat hind paw (Asghar et al., 2000). As reported in a company communication, remacemide and its des-glycinyl-metabolite FPL-12,495 are not under further development although no obvious reason for this withdrawal is known (Schachter et al., 2000). A putative back-up of this structural class might be AR-R-15,896 which is at least in preclinical development by AstraZeneca (company communication). Compared to ketamine and memantine, AR-R-15,896 might have more favorable pharmacodynamic features (Mealing et al., 1999) which may be due to a stronger inhibition of NR1/NR2$_C$ and NR1/NR2$_B$ in comparison to NR1/NR2$_A$ NMDA receptor subtypes. This may also be the case for remacemide and its des-glycinyl-metabolite FPL-12,495 (Monaghan et al., 1997).

AR-R-15,896

Dextromethorphan

Synthesis (Kleemann et al., 1999):

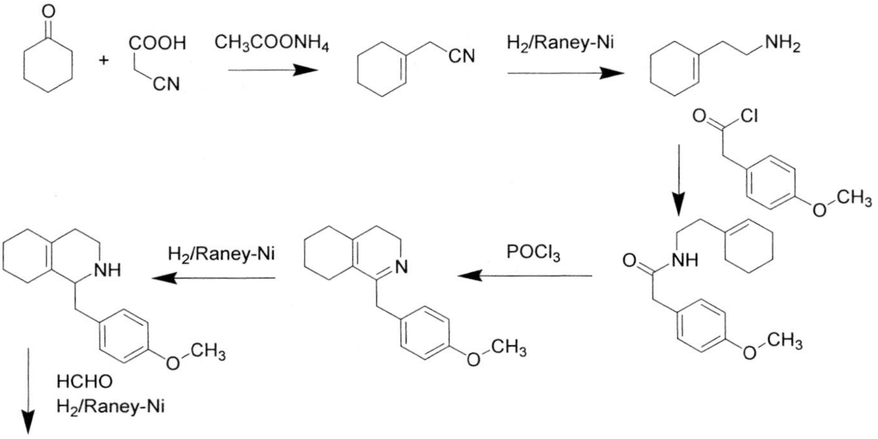

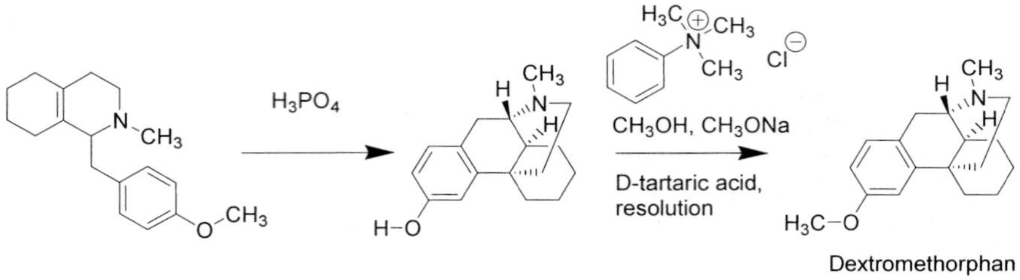

Scheme 12: Synthesis of dextromethorphan.

Dextromethorphan

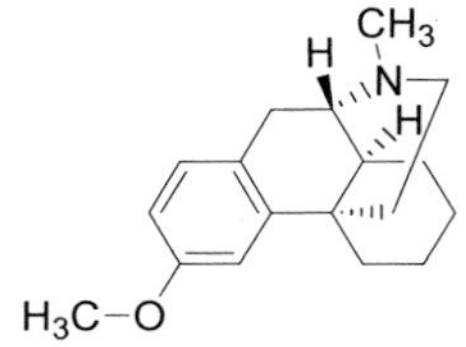

[125-71-3]; (9α,13α,14α)-3-methoxy-17-methyl-morphinan, MF $C_{18}H_{25}NO$, MW 271,40

Dextromethorphan and its O-demethylated metabolite dextrorphan (morphinans), are also low to medium affinity NMDA channel blockers. The former has been in clinical use as an antitussive for about 40 years and could therefore be considered as a very safe drug (Bem et al., 1992).

In addition to its NMDA antagonism in the micromolar range (Church et al., 1985; Wong et al., 1988; Netzer et al., 1993) dextromethorphan also inhibits 5HT and norepinephrine uptake in the submicromolar concentration range (Codd et al., 1995). It also has a high binding affinity for the sigma 1 binding site, a somewhat weaker affinity for the μ-opioid receptor and shows some inhibition of Na^+ and Ca^{2+} channels (Tortella et al., 1989; Zhou et al., 1991; Netzer et al., 1993; Codd et al., 1995). Dextromethorphan and its metabolite dextrorphan are antinociceptive in a variety of visceral, chronic neuropathic and inflammatory animal models (Mao et al., 1993; Tal et al., 1993; Elliott et al., 1995; Hao et al., 1996; Davidson et al., 1998). Dextromethorphan showed clinical analgesic efficacy in an experimental pain study and in the treatment of diabetic neuropathy, however it failed in postherpetic neuralgia and a further neuropathic pain study, a cancer pain treatment study, and in an experimental model for ischemic pain (McQuay et al., 1994; Price et al., 1994; Nelson et al., 1997; Mercadante et al., 1998; Plesan et al., 2000).

A further series which also originates from the opioid-descending structures comprises the benzomorphan scaffold as exemplified by BIII-277CL synthesized by Boehringer Ingelheim. This structural class includes both an affinity for the μ-opioid receptor site and the PCP-binding site of the NMDA receptor and has been optimized structurally to give selective NMDA interaction e.g. BIII-277CL (Carter et al., 1995; Grauert et al., 1997).

(d) Bifunctional molecules: μ-opioids with NMDA antagonistic activity

However, the above-mentioned benzomorphans and morphinans are not the only compounds reported to have affinity for both the NMDA receptor and the μ-opioid receptor. There have been several reports on the NMDA antagonistic features of known opioid compounds which have also been suggested to add favorable properties in addition to their analgesic effects to the respective opioids. In that respect dextropropoxyphen, ketobemidone, dextromethadone, and D-morphine have been reported to have affinity for the PCP-binding site within the NMDA receptor channel and to exert NMDA antagonistic effects (Ebert et al., 1995; Andersen et al., 1996; Gorman et al., 1997; Ebert et al., 1998; Davis et al., 1999; Stringer et al., 2000).

It has been proposed that both analgesic principles might act in a synergistic or at least additive manner thus reducing the necessary dose and in turn minimize adverse effects (Dickenson, 1997; Wiesenfeld-Hallin, 1998; Mao, 1999; Price et al., 2000). Following these assumptions there are combinations of dextromethorphan with opioids under clinical development (e.g. Morphidex™, a fixed combination of morphine with dextromethorphan) by the former Algos Pharmaceutical Corp. (Caruso, 2000; Katz, 2000). Many of the animal studies could be taken as a preclinical scientific basis for such clinical combination studies (Chapman et al., 1992; Advokat et al., 1995; Bernardi et al., 1996; Grass et al., 1996; Hoffmann et al., 1996; Honoré et al., 1996; Bhargava, 1997; Kauppila et al., 1998; Plesan et al., 1998; Allen et al., 2001).

Ketobemidone (see chapter 3.4)

Numerous reports have documented the favorable influence of NMDA antagonists (either non-competitive or competitive glycine$_B$ or glutamate antagonists) on the development of opioid tolerance and dependency during chronic use of opioids in a variety of different preclinical pain models or experimental paradigms (Marek et al., 1991; Tiseo et al., 1993; Mao et al., 1994; Elliott et al., 1994; Lutfy et al., 1995, 1996; Bilsky et al., 1996; Mao et al., 1996, 1999). The first clinical studies in humans for treatment or attenuation of physical dependency with NMDA antagonists are meanwhile under way (Bisaga et al., 2001). However, one should also bear in mind, that a combination of opioid agonism and NMDA antagonism might enhance the risk of developing a drug dependency. It is of particular importance to identify precisely the paradigms which are to be tested in the experimental models used to determine such relationships (Tzschentke et al., 1998). The reader is referred to some recently published reviews on this subject (Wolf, 1998; Vanderschuren et al., 2000; Trujillo, 2000).

As demonstrated for dextromethadone the pharmacological relevance of this additional NMDA component in addition to the remaining opioid component for antinociception after systemic administration needs further investigation. Dextromethadone has been shown to

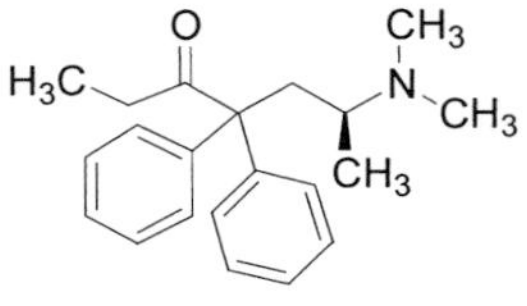

D-Methadone
(see chapter 3.4)

Sulfazocine

**(e) Ifenprodil-like, NR2B
specific antagonists**

reverse NMDA-induced hyperalgesia after intrathecal administration (Davis et al., 1999). However, following intravenous injection within the appropriate antinociceptive dose range, it could not be shown that dextromethadone specifically inhibited the electrically- or mechanically-induced spinal wind-up phenomenon or to inhibit the activity of spinal dorsal horn neurons evoked by iontophoretic administration of NMDA, whereas its antinociceptive and non-specific effects on the detectable inhibition of spinal neuronal activity could be fully antagonized by naloxone (Chizh et al., 2000).

However, methadone is considered by some authors to be a very useful drug because of its NMDA antagonistic effects for example for the treatment of cancer pain (Ayonrinde et al., 2000; Mancini et al., 2000).

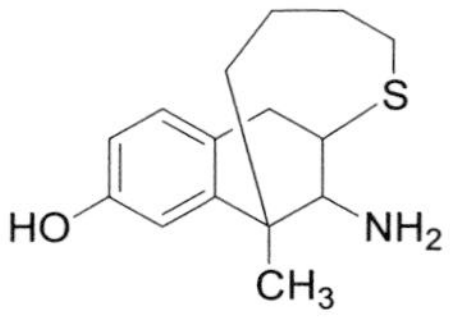

A very interesting approach might be the development of compounds whose structures give rise to a well-balanced NMDA antagonism and µ-opioid agonism. The former Biochem Pharma Corp. (today a subsidary of Shire) have developed such compounds of which sulfazocine is an example (Dimaio, WO 9703978; Dimaio et al., WO 9703979).

Recently there has been much interest in ifenprodil-like antagonists with regard to their potential role in pain relief, primarily because of the excellent tolerability of these NR2B subtype-specific drugs. Ifenprodil was the prototypical example of this NR2B-subclass-specific type of NMDA receptor antagonists (Williams, 1993; Avenet et al., 1996) and is the most often used high affinity ligand for this target site (Grimwood et al., 2000; Coughenour et al., 2001).

Ifenprodil

Ifenprodil

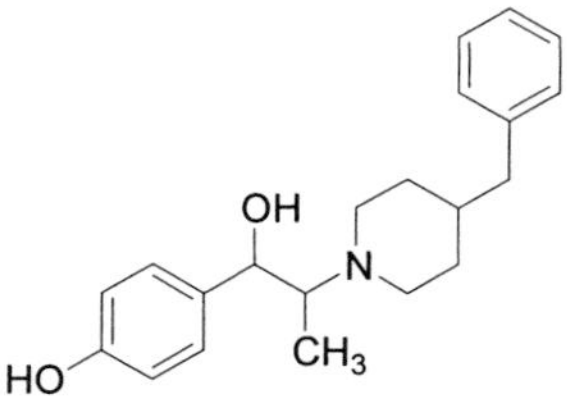

Synthesis (Kleemann et al., 1999):

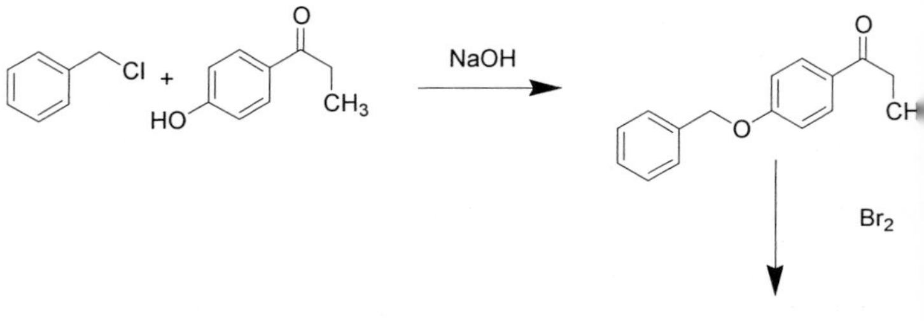

[23210-58-4]; 4-[2-(4-Benzyl-piperidin-1-yl)-1-hydroxy-propyl]-phenol, $C_{21}H_{27}NO_2$, MW 325.45

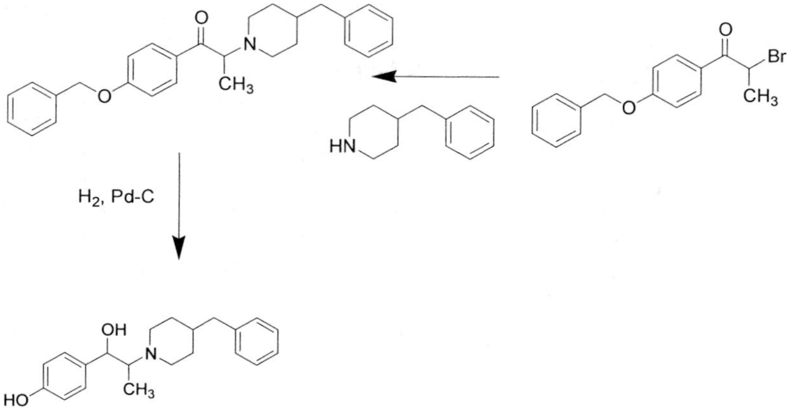

Scheme 13: Synthesis of ifenprodil.

In addition to its NMDA antagonistic activity, ifenprodil also interacts non-specifically with other receptor systems (e.g. sigma, 5HT3, α1; McCool et al., 1995; Moebius et al., 1997; Chenard et al., 1999). However, eliprodil, a back-up compound for ifenprodil and the newer NR2$_B$-specific antagonists proved to be far more specific (Chenard et al., 1991).

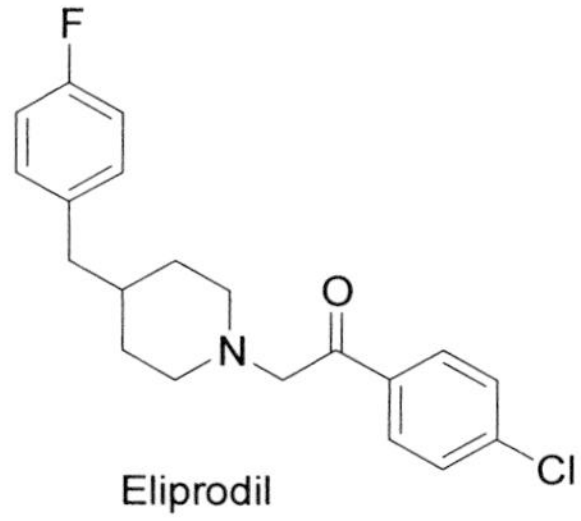

The inhibitory modulation of these drugs is restricted to NMDA receptor oligomers with at least one NR2$_B$ subunit. These subunit-specific antagonists might offer better efficacy and tolerability for pain treatment with particular emphasis on a lower risk of motor impairment in comparison to other NMDA receptor antagonist classes (Boyce et al., 1999; for a recent review see Chizh et al., 2001). In addition, genetic evidence has suggested that overexpression of NR2$_B$ in the forebrain enhances the nociception of formalin-induced pain (Wei et al., 2001; Zhuo, 2002). Since spinally mediated mechanisms appear to be unchanged in transgenic animals, this may provide evidence that central NMDA receptors are of significance in persistent inflammatory pain. Consistent with supraspinal pain modulation, ifenprodil could only be shown to inhibit single motor unit wind-up in non-spinalized rats, emphasizing the involvement of supraspinal mechanisms (Chizh et al., 2001). NR2$_B$ overexpression in the forebrain also enhances the processes of learning and memory (Tang et al., 1999, 2001). Therefore an attenuation might be expected as a putative side-effect of NR2$_B$-specific antagonists, although experimental studies have not shown any evidence for such side-effects so far (Fraser et al., 1996; Doyle et al., 1998). Yung (1998) provided evidence for the selective distribution of the $NR2_B$ subunit within laminae I - III in the dorsal spinal horn, but no $NR2_A$ or $NR2_C$ was detectable using immunohistological techniques. Obviously the $NR2_B$ subunit was expressed on the sensory presynaptic afferent fibers (Yung, 1998; Ma and Hargreaves, 2000). The lack of $NR2_B$ expression in the ventral spinal horn and in the cerebellum (Portera-Cailliau et al., 1996; Sasner et al., 1996) has been proposed as an explanation for the reduced motor side-effect profile of $NR2_B$ selective antagonists (Boyce et al., 1999). Obviously this class of NMDA antagonists bear no or only low potential for abuse in humans since eliprodil showed no evidence of reinforcing effects in non-human primates or PCP-discriminative stimulus effects in rats (Balster et al., 1994).

Ifenprodil as well as the $NR2_B$-specific antagonists CP-101,606 and Ro-25-6981 have been shown to be antinociceptive in a variety of pain models (Bernardi et al., 1996; Taniguchi et al., 1997; Boyce et al., 1999; Chizh et al., 2001; Minami et al., 2001). Of particular importance are their good putative therapeutic indices comparing analgesic and side-effect dose ranges. They inhibit mechanical allodynia in a neuropathic chronic constriction injury model in rats and reduce carrageenan-induced hyperalgesia. In comparison to other NMDA antagonists they produce little or no motor impairment within the respective antinociceptive dose ranges (Boyce et al., 1999).

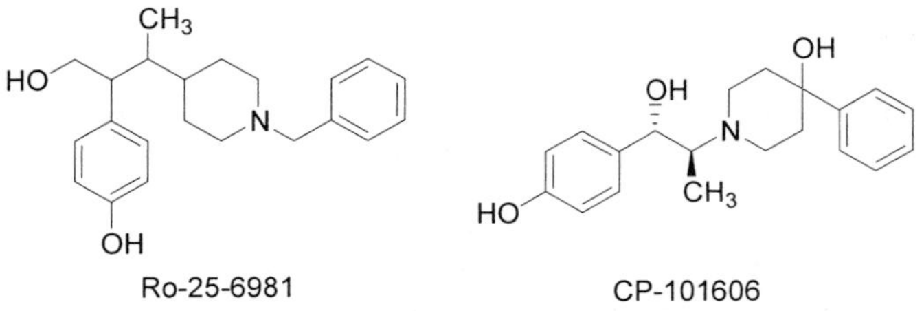

Ro-25-6981   CP-101606

Scheme 14: Examples for $NR2_B$-selective antagonists.

Obviously most of the known $NR2_B$-selective antagonists very closely resemble ifenprodil thus belonging to the same structural class. Well known examples of $NR2_B$-selective antagonists are eliprodil which was the follow-up compound to ifenprodil synthesized by Synthelabo (Avenet et al., 1997), CP-101,606 and analogs synthesized by Pfizer, and Roche's Ro 25-6981 (Fischer et al., 1997; Butler et al., 1998; Lynch et al., 2001).

Ifenprodil and its back-up compound eliprodil were under clinical development by Synthelabo but have been withdrawn because of cardiovascular side-effects. (i.e. HERG channel inhibition (Soldo et al., 2000)). According to communications by the respective companies the development of CP-101,606 and Ro 25-6981 has also been halted.

PD-196,860 is another NR2$_B$-specific antagonist which is under development by Purdue Pharma but still has the basic ifenprodil-like structure. It was only recently that new basic structures (e.g. iminopyrimidine) of NR2$_B$-specific antagonists were published (Claremon et al., 2002).

There is a broad literature concerning the involvement of NMDA receptor channels and the efficacy of NMDA antagonists in chronic pain treatment. Compounds like ketamine or dextromethorphan are well-characterized NMDA antagonists which have been in clinical use for decades. It has been shown in many case reports and in some clinical studies too, that these compounds might be clinically effective analgesics, however they are often associated with intolerable adverse effects. Thus the task is to develop safer NMDA antagonists with a better efficacy to side-effect ratio. The more recent advent of subtype-specific antagonists with strong analgesia but fewer side-effects looks to be a promising path towards new analgesics, especially for pain states which do not respond well to the conventional analgesics of today.

PD-196860

References

Advokat, C. and Rhein, F. Q.: *Potentiation of morphine-induced antinociception in acute spinal rats by the NMDA antagonist dextrorphan*, Brain Res. **1995**, *699*, 157-160.

Ahmed, M'. S., Mather, A., Enna, S. J.: *Binding of [³H]desglycinyl remacemide to rat brain membranes: association with the benzomorphan attachment site of the N-methyl-D-aspartic acid receptor channel*, Brain Res. **1999**, *8*, 46-50.

Allen, R. M. and Dykstra, L. A.: *N-Methyl-D-aspartate receptor antagonists potentiate the antinociceptive effects of morphine in squirrel monkeys*, J. Pharmacol. Exp. Ther. **2001**, *298*, 288-297.

Andersen, S., Dickenson, A. H., Kohn, M., Reeve, A., Rahman, W., Ebert, B.: *The opioid ketobemidone has a NMDA blocking effect*, Pain **1996**, *67*, 369-374.

Anson, L. C., Chen, P. E., Wyllie, D. J. A., Colquhoun, D., Schoepfer, R.: *Identification of amino acid residues of the NR2A subunit which control glutamate potency in recombinant NR1/NR2A NMDA receptors*, J. Neurosci. **1998**, *18*, 581-598.

Asghar, A. U. R., Hasan, S. S., King A. E.: *Actions of the anticonvulsant remacemide metabolite AR-R12,495AA on afferent-evoked spinal synaptic transmission in vitro and on models of acute and chronic inflammation in the rat*, J. Pharmacol. Exp. Ther. **2000**, *294*, 876-883.

Avenet, P., Léonardon, J., Besnard, F., Graham, D., Frost, J., Depoortere, H., Langer, S. Z., Scatton, B.: *Antagonist properties of the stereoisomers of ifenprodil at NR1A/NR2A and NR1A/NR2B subtypes of the NMDA receptor expressed in Xenopus oocytes*, Eur. J. Pharmacol. **1996**, *296*, 209-213.

414 Englberger, Przewosny and Maul

Avenet, P., Léonardon, J., Besnard, F., Graham, D., Depoortere, H., Scatton, B.: *Antagonist properties of eliprodil and other NMDA receptor antagonists at NR1A/NR2A and NR1A/NR2B receptors expressed in Xenopus oocytes*, Neurosci. Lett. **1997**, *223*, 133-136.

Ayonrinde, O. T. and Bridge, D. T.: *The rediscovery of methadone for cancer pain management*, Med. J. Aust. **2000**, *173*, 536-540.

Balster, R. L., Nicholson, K. L., Sanger, D. J.: *Evaluation of the reinforcing effects of eliprodil in rhesus monkeys and ist discriminative stimulus effects in rats*, Drug Alcohol Depend. **1994**, *35*, 211-216.

Baron, B. M., Harrison, B. L., Miller, F. P., McDonald, I. A., Salituro, F. G., Schmidt, C. J., Sorensen, S. M., White, H. S., Palfreyman, M. G.: *Activity of 5,7-dichlorokynurenic acid, a potent antagonist at the N-methyl-D-aspartate receptor-associated glycine binding site*, Mol. Pharmacol. **1990**, *38*, 554-561.

Baron, B. M., Harrison, B. L., Kehne, J. H., Schmidt, C. J., van Giersbergen, P. L. M., White, H. S., Siegel, B. W., Senyah, Y., McCloskey, T. C., Fadayel, G. M., Taylor, V. L., Murawsky, M. K., Nyce, P., Salituro, F. G.: *Pharmacological characterization of MDL 105,519, an NMDA receptor glycine site antagonist*, Eur. J. Pharmacol. **1997**, *323*, 181-192.

Begon, S., Pickering, G., Eschalier, A., Dubray, C.: *Magnesium and Mk-801 have a similiar effect in two experimental models of neuropathic pain*, Brain Res. **2000**, *887*, 436-439.

Béhé, P., Colquhoun, D., Wyllie, D. J. A.: *Activation of single AMPA- and NMDA-type glutamate-receptor channels*; in: Ionotropic glutamate receptors in the CNS, edited by P. Jonas and H. Monyer, Handbook of Experimental Pharmacology **1999**, *41*, 175-218.

Bem, J. L. and Peck, R.: *Dextromethorphan. An overview of safety issues*, Drug Safety **1992**, *7*, 190-199.

Bernardi, M., Bertolini, A., Szczawinska, K., Genedani, S.: *Blockade of the polyamine site of NMDA receptors produces antinociception and enhances the effect of morphine, in mice*, Eur. J. Pharmacol. **1996**, *298*, 51-55.

Bertolino, M., Vicini, S., Costa, E.: *Kynurenic acid inhibits the activation of kainic and N-methyl-D-aspartate acid-sensitive ionotropic receptors by a different mechanism*, Neuropharmacology **1989**, *28*, 453-457.

Bhargava H. N.: *Enhancement of morphine actions in morphine-naive and morphine-tolerant mice by LY 235959, a competitive antagonist of the NMDA receptor*, Gen. Pharmacol. **1997**, *28*, 61-64.

Bilsky E. J., Inturrisi, C. E., Sadée, W., Hruby, V. J., Porreca, F.: *Competitive and non-competitive NMDA antagonists block the development of antinociceptive tolerance to morphine, but not to selective μ or δ opioid agonists in mice*, Pain **1996**, *68*, 229-223.

Bisaga, A., Comer, S. D., Ward, A. S., Popik, P., Kleber, H., Fischman, M. W.: *The NMDA antagonist memantine attenuates the expression of opioid physical dependence in humans*, Psychopharmacology **2001**, *157*, 1-10.

Black, M., Lanthorn, T., Small, D., Mealing, G., Lam, V., Morley, P.: *Study of potency, kinetics of block and toxicity of NMDA receptor antagonists using fura-2*, Eur. J. Pharmacol. **1996**, *317*, 377-381.

Bonina, F. P., Arenare, L., Ippolito, R., Boatto, G., Battaglia, G., Bruno, V., de Caprariis, P.: *Synthesis, pharmacokinetics and anticonvulsant activity of 7-chlorokynurenic acid prodrugs*, Int. J. Pharm. **2000**, *202*, 79-88.

Bordi, F. and Quartaroli, M.: *Modulation of nociceptive transmission by NMDA/glycine site receptor in the ventroposterolateral nucleus of the thalamus*, Pain **2000**, *84*, 213-224.

Boyce, S., Wyatt, A., Webb, J. K., O´Donell, R., Mason, G., Rigby, M., Sirinathsinghji, D., Hill, R. G., Rupniak, N. M. J.: *Selective NMDA NR2B antagonists induce antinociception without motor dysfunction: correlation with restricted localisation of NR2B in dorsal horn*, Neuropharmacology **1999**, *38*, 611-623.

Burnashev, N., Schoepfer, R., Monyer, H., Ruppersberg, J. P., Günther, W., Seeburg, P. H., Sakmann, B.: *Control by asparagine reidues of calcium permeability and magnesium blockade in the NMDA receptor*, Science **1992**, *257*, 1415-1419.

Butler, T. W., Blake, J. F., Bordner, J., Butler, P., Chenard, B. L., Collins, M. A., DeCosta, D., Ducat, M. J., Eisenhard, M. E., Menniti, F. S., Pagnozzi, M. J., Sands, S. B., Segelstein, B. E., Volberg, W.,

White, W. F., Zhao, D.: *(3R,4S)-3-[4-(4-Fluorophenyl)-4-hydroxypiperidin-1-yl]chroman-4,7-diol: a conformationally restricted analoque of the NR2B subtype-selective NMDA antagonist (1S,2S)-1-(4-hydroxyphenol)-2-(4-hydroxy-4-phenylpiperidino)-1-propanol*, J. Med. Chem. **1998**, *41*, 1172-1184.

Carter, A. J., Bechtel, W. D., Grauert, M., Harrison, P., Merz, H., Stransky, W.: *BIII 277 CL is a potent and specific ion-channel blocker of the NMDA receptor-channel complex*, J. Pharmacol. Exp. Ther. **1995**, *275*, 1382-1389.

Caruso, F. S.: *Morphidex pharmacokinetic studies and single-dose analgesic efficacy studies in patients with postoperative pain*, J. Pain Symptom Manage. **2000**, *19*, S31-S36.

Chaplan, S. R., Malmberg, A. B., Yaksh, T. L.: *Efficacy of spinal NMDA-receptor antagonism in formalin hyperalgesia and nerve injury evoked allodynia in the rat*, J. Pharmacol. Exp. Ther. **1997**, *280*, 829-838.

Chapman, V. and Dickenson, A. H.; *The combination of NMDA antagonism and morphine produces profound antinociception in the rat dorsal horn*, Brain Res., **1992**, *573*, 321-323.

Chapman, V., Dickenson, A. H.: *Time-related roles of excitatory amino acid receptors during persistent noxiously evoked responses of rat dorsal horn neurones*, Brain Res., **1995**, *703*, 45-50.

Chatterton, J. E., Awobuluyi, M., Premkumar, L. S., Takahashi, H., Talantova, M., Shin, Y., Cui, J., Tu, S., Sevarino, K. A., Nakanishi, N., Tong, G., Lipton, S. A., Zhang, D.; *Excitatory glycine receptors containing the NR3 family of NMDA receptor subunits*, Nature **2002**, *415*, 793-798.

Chen, J., Graham, S., Moroni, F., Simon, R.: *A study of the dose dependency of a glycine receptor antagonist in focal ischemia*, J. Pharmacol. Exp. Ther. **1993**, *267*, 937-941.

Chen, L. and Huang, L.-Y. M.; *Protein kinase C reduces Mg^{2+} block of NMDA-receptor channels as a mechanism of modulation*, Nature **1992**, *356*, 521-523.

Chenard, B. L., Shalaby, I. A., Koe, I. A., Ronau, R. T., Butler, T. W., Prochniak, M. A., Schmidt, A. W., Fox, C. B.: *Separation of alpha 1 adrenergic and N-methyl-D-aspartate antagonist activity in a series of ifenprodil compounds*, J. Med. Chem. **1991**, *34*, 3085-3090.

Chenard, B. L. and Menniti, F. S.: *Antagonists selective for NMDA receptors containing the NR2B subunit*, Curr. Pharm. Des. **1999**, *5*, 381-404.

Cheung, N. S., O'Callaghan, D., Ryan, M. C., Dutton, R., Wong, M. G., Beart, P. M.: *Structure-activity relationships of competitive NMDA receptor antagonists*, Eur. J. Pharmacol. **1996**, *313*, 159-162.

Chizh, B. A., Schlütz, H., Scheed, M., Englberger, W.: *The N-methyl-D-aspartate antagonistic and opioid components of D-methadone antinociception in the rat spinal cord*, Neurosci. Lett. **2000**, *296*, 117-120.

Chizh, B. A., Headley, P. M., Tzschentke, T. M.: *NMDA receptor antagonists as analgesics: focus on the $NR2_B$ subtype*, Trends Pharmacol. Sci., **2001**, *22*, 637-643.

Chizh, B. A., Reißmüller, E., Schlütz, H., Scheede, M., Haase, G., Englberger, W.; *Supraspinal vs. Spinal sites of the antinociceptive action of the subtype-selective NMDA antagonist ifenprodil*, Neuropharmacology **2001**, *40*, 212-220.

Chopra, B., Chazot, P. L., Stephenson, F. A.: *Characterization of the binding of two novel glycine site antagonists to cloned NMDA receptors: evidence for two phamacological classes of antagonists*, Br. J. Pharmacol. **2000**, *130*, 65-72.

Christensen, D., Guilbaud, G., Kayser, V.: *The effect of the glycine/NMDA receptor antagonist, (+)-HA-966, on morphine dependence in neuropathic rats*, Neuropharmacology, **2000**, *39*, 1589-1595.

Christensen, D., Idänpään-Heikkilä, J. J., Guilbaud, G., Kayser V.; *The antinociceptive effect of combined systemic administration of morphine and the glycine/NMDA antagonist, (+)-HA-966 in a rat model of peripheral neuropathy*, Br. J. Pharmacol. **1998**, *125*, 1641-1650.

Claremon, D. A., McCauley, J. A., Liverton, N. J., Theberge, C. R., (Merck & Co Inc.*): New iminopyrimidine derivatives are NMDA NR2B inhibitors*, WO 0200629.

Codd, E. E., Shank, R. P., Schupsky, J. J., Raffa, R. B.: *Serotonin and norepinephrine uptake inhibiting activity of centrally acting analgesics: structural determinants and role in antinociception*, J. Pharmacol. Exp. Ther. **1995**, *274*, 1263-1270.

Coderre, T. J. and Van Empel, I.: *The utility of excitatory amino acid (EAA) antagonists as analgesic agents. Comparison of the antinociceptive activity of various classes of EAA antagonists in mechanical, thermal and chemical nociceptive tests*, Pain **1994**, *59*, 345-352.

Collingridge, G. L. and Lester, R. A. J.: *Excitatory amino acid receptors in the vertebrate central nervous system,* Pharmacol. Rev. **1989**, *40*, 145-210.

Coughenour L. L. and Barr, B. M.: *Use of trifluoroperazine isolates [³H]ifenprodil binding site in rat brain membranes with the pharmacology of the voltage-independent ifenprodil site on N-methyl-D-aspartate receptors containing NR2B subunits*, J. Pharmacol. Exp. Ther. **2001**, *296*, 150-159.

Crosby, V., Wilcock, A., Corcoran, R.: *The safety and efficacy of a single dose (500 mg or 1 g) of intraveneous magnesium sulfate in neuropathic pain poorly responsive to strong opioid analgesics in patients with cancer*, J. Pain Symptom Manage. **2000**, *19*, 35-39.

Danysz, W., Fadda, E., Wroblewski, J. T., Costa, E.: *Kynurenate and 2-amino-5-phosphonovalerate interact with multiple binding sites of the N-methyl-D-aspartate-sensitive glutamate receptor complex*, Neurosci. Lett. **1989**, *96*, 340-344.

Danysz, W., Fadda, E., Wroblewski, J. T., Costa, E.: *[3H]D-Serine labels strychnine-insensitive glycine recognition sites of rat central nervous system*, Life Sci. **1990**, *46*, 155-164.

Danysz, W. and Parsons, C. G.: *Glycine and N-methyl-D-aspartate receptors: Physiological significance and possible therapeutic applications*, Pharmacol. Rev. **1998**, *50*, 597-664.

Das, S., Sasaki, Y. F., Rothe, T., Premkumar, L. S., Takasu, M., Crandall, J. E., Dikkes, P., Conner, D. A., Rayudu, P. V., Cheung, W., Chen, H.-S., V., Lipton, S. A., Nakanishi, N.: *Increased NMDA current and spine density in mice lacking the NMDA receptor subunit NR3A*, Nature **1998**, *393*, 377-381.

Davar, G. Hama, A., Deykin, A., Vos, B., Maciewicz, R.: *MK-801 blocks the development of thermal hyperalgesia in a rat model of experimental painful mononeuropathy*, Brain Res. **1991**, 553, 327-330.

Davidson, E. M. and Carlton, S. M.: *Intraplantar injection of dextrorphan, ketamine, or memantine attenuates formalin-induced behaviors*, Brain Res. **1998**, *785*, 136-142.

Davis, S. M., Albers, G. W., Diener, H. C., Lees, K. R., Norris, J.: *Termination of acute stroke studies involving selfotel treatment. Assist steering committed.* Lancet **1997**, *349*, 32.

Davis, A. M. and Inturrisi, C. E.: *D-Methadone blocks morphine tolerance and N-methyl-D-aspartate-induced hyperalgesia*, J. Pharmacol. Exp. Ther. **1999**, *289*, 1048-1053.

Davis, S. R.: *Ketamine in chronic pain: a review*, Aust. J. Hosp. Pharm. **1999**, *28*, 94-98.

Dickenson, A. H.: *NMDA receptor antagonists: interactions with opioids*, Acta Anaesthesiol. Scand. **1997**, *41*, 112-115.

Di Fabio, R., Conti, N., Corsi, M., Donati, D., Gastaldi, P., Gaviraghi, G., Giacobbe, S., Pentassuglia, G., Quartaroli, M., Ratti, E., Trist, D. G., Ugolini, A. R.: *GV196771*, Drugs Fut. **2000**, *25*, 137-145.

Dimaio, J. (Biochem Pharma, Inc.): *Novel heterocyclic compounds for the treatment of pain and use thereof*, WO 9703978.

Dimaio, J. and Dixit, D. M. (Biochem Pharma, Inc*.)*: *Polycyclic alcaloid-derivatives as NMDA-receptor antagonists*, WO 9703979.

Dingledine, R., Borges, K., Bowie, D., Traynelis, S. F.: *The glutamate receptor ion channels*, Pharmacol. Rev. **1999**, *51*, 7-61.

Doyle, K. M., Feerick, S., Kirkby, D. L., Eddleston, A., Higgins, G. A.: *Comparison of various N-methyl-D-aspartate receptor antagonists in a model of short-term memory and a overt behaviour*, Behav. Pharmacol. **1998**, *9*, 671-681.

Dubray, C., Alloui, A., Bardin, L., Rock, E., Mazur, A., Rayssiguier, Y., Eschalier, A., Lavarenne, J.: *Magnesium deficiency induces an hyperalgesia reversed by the NMDA receptor antagonist MK801*, Neuroreport **1997**, *8*, 1383-1386.

Ebert, B., Andersen, S., Krogsgaard-Larsen, P.: *Ketobemidone, methadone, and pethidine are non-competitive N-methyl-D-aspartate (NMDA) antagonists in the rat cortex and spinal cord*, Neurosci. Lett. **1995**, *187*, 165-168.

Ebert, B., Andersen, S., Hjeds, H., Dickenson, A. H.: *Dextropropoxyphene acts as a noncompetitive N-methyl-D-aspartate antagonist*, J. Pain Symptom Manage. **1998**, *15*, 269-274.

Ebralidze, A. K., Rossi, D. J., Tonegawa, S., Slater, N. T.: *Modification of NMDA receptor channels and synaptic transmission by targeted disruption of the NR2C gene*, J. Neurosci. **1996**, *16*, 5014-5025.

Eide, P. K., Jorum, E., Stubhaug, A., Bremmes, J., Breivik, H.: *Relief of post-herpetic neuralgia with the N-methyl-D-aspartic acid receptor antagonist ketamine: a double-blind, cross-over comparison with morphine and placebo*, Pain **1994**, *58*, 347-354.

Eisenberg, E., LaCross, S., Strassman, A. M.:•*The effects of the clinically tested NMDA receptor antagonist memantine on carrageenan-induced thermal hyperalgesia in rats*, Eur. J. Pharmacol. **1994**, *255*, 123-129.

Eisenberg, E., Kleiser, A., Dortort, A., Haim, T., Yarnitsky, D.: *The NMDA (N-methyl-D-aspartate) receptor antagonist memantine in the treatment of postherpetic neuralgia: a double-blind, placebo-controlled study*, Eur. J. Pain **1998**, *2*, 321-327.

Elliott, K., Hynansky, A., Inturrisi, C. E.: *Dextromethorphan attenuates and reverses analgesic tolerance to morphine*, Pain **1994**, *59*, 361-368.

Elliott, K. J., Brodsky, M., Hynansky, A. D., Foley, K. M., Inturrisi, C. E.: *Dextromethorphan suppresses both formalin-induced nociceptive behavior and the formalin-induced increase in spinal cord c-fos mRNA*, Pain **1995**, *61*, 401-409.

Felsby, S., Nielson, J., Arendt-Nielson, L., Jensen, T. S.: *NMDA receptor blockade in chronic neuropathic pain: a comparism of ketamine and magnesium chloride*, Pain **1995**, *64*, 283-291.

Fine, P. G.: *Low-dose ketamine in the management of opioid nonresponsive terminal cancer pain*, J. Pain Symtom. Manage. **1999**, *17*, 296-300.

Finlay, I.: *Ketamine and its role in cancer pain*, Pain Rev. **1999**, *6*, 303-313.

Fischer, G., Mutel, V., Trube, G., Malherbe, P., Kew, J. N. C., Mohacsi, E., Heitz, M. P., Kemp, J. A.: *Ro 25-6981, a highly potent and selective blocker of N-methyl-D-aspartate, receptors containing the NR2B subunit. characterization in vitro*, J. Pharmacol. Exp. Ther. **1997**, *283*, 1285-1292.

Fonnum, F.: *Glutamate: A neurotransmitter in mammalian brain*, J. Neurochem. **1984**, *42*, 1-11.

Forrest, D, Yuzaki, M., Soares, H. D., Ng, L., Luk, D. C., Sheng, M., Stewart, C. L., Morgan, J. I., Connor, J. A., Curran, T.: *Targeted disruption of NMDA receptor I gene abolishes NMDA response and results in neonatal death*, Neuron, **1994**, *13*, 325-338.

Fossom, L. H., von Lubitz, D. K. J. E., Lin, R. C.-S., Skolnick, P.: *Neuroprotective actions of 1-aminocyclopropanecarboxylic acid, a partial agonist at strychnine-insensitive glycine sites*, Neurol. Res. **1995**, *17*, 265-269.

Fraser, C. M., Cooke, M. J., Fisher, A., Thompson, I. D., Stone, T. W.: *Interactions between ifenprodil and dizocilpine on mouse behaviour in models of anxiety and working memory*, Eur. J. Neuropsychopharmacol. **1996**, *6*, 311-316.

Garry, M. G., Malik, S., Yu, J., Davis, M. A., Yang, J.: *Knock down of spinal NMDA and formalin evoked behaviours in rat*, NeuroReport **2000**, *11*, 49-55.

Goettl, V. M. and Larson, A. A.: *Antinociception induced by 3-((+-)-2-carboxypiperazin-4-yl)-propyl-1-phosphonic acid (CPP), an N-methyl-D-aspartate (NMDA) competitive antagonist, plus 6,7-dinitroquinoxaline-2,3-dione (DNQX), a non-NMDA antagonist, differs from that induced by MK-801 plus DNQX*, Brain Res. **1994**, *642*, 334-33.

Gorman, A. L., Elliott, K. J., Inturrisi, C. E.: *The d- and l-isomers of methadone bind to the non-competitive site on the N-methyl-D-aspartate (NMDA) receptor in rat forebrain and spinal cord*, Neurosci. Lett. **1997**, *223*, 5-8.

Grass, S., Hoffmann, O., Xu, X.-J., Wiesenfeld-Hallin, Z.: *N-Methyl-D-aspartate receptor antagonists potentiate morphine´s antinociceptive effect in the rat*, Acta Physiol. Scand. **1996**, *158*, 269-273.

Grauert, M., Bechtel, W. D., Ensinger, H. A., Merz, H., Carter, A. J.: *Synthesis and structure-activity relationships of 6,7-benzomorphan derivatives as antagonists of the NMDA receptor-channel complex*, J. Med. Chem. **1997**, *40*, 2922-2930

Graven-Nielsen, T., Kendall, S. A., Henrikksson, K. G., Bengtsson, M., Sörensen, J., Johnson, A., Gerdle, B., Arendt-Niesen, L.: *Ketamine reduces muscle pain, temporal summation, and referred pain in fibromyalgia patients*, Pain **2000**, *85*, 483-491.

Gray N. M., Dappen, M. S., Cheng, B. K., Cordi, A.A., Biesterfeldt, J. P., Hood, W. F., Monahan, J. B.: *Novel indole-2-carboxylates as ligands for the strychnine-insensitive N-methyl-D-aspartate-linked glycine receptor*, J. Med. Chem. **1991**, *34*, 1283-1292.

Grimwood, S., Richards, P., Murray, F., Harrison, N., Wingrove, P. B., Hutson, P. H.: *Characterisation of N-methyl-D-aspartate receptor-specific [^{3}H]ifenprodil binding to recombinant human NR1a/NR2B receptors compared with native receptors in rodent brain membranes*, J. Neurosci. **2000**, *75*, 2455-2463.

Haley, J. E., Sullivan, A. F., Dickenson, A. H.: *Evidence for spinal NMDA receptor involvement in prolonged chemical nociception in rat*, Brain Res. **1990**, 518, 218-226.

Hao, J.-X. and Xu, X.-J.: *Treatments of a chronic allodynia-like response in spinally injured rats: effects of systemically administered excitatory amino acid receptor antagonists*, Pain **1996**, *66*, 279-285.

Headley, P. M.: *NMDA antagonists: unequal to each other or unequal to the task?*, Eur. J. Pain **1999**, 3, 185-187.

Henderson, G., Johnson, J. W., Ascher, P.: *Competitive antagonists and partial agonists at the glycine modulatory site of the mouse N-methyl-D-aspartate receptor*, J. Physiol. **1990**, *430*, 189-212.

Herrero, J. F., Headley, P. M., Parsons, C. G.: *Mementine selectively depresses NMDA receptor-mediated responses of rat spinal neurones in vivo*, Neurosci. Lett. **1994**, *165*, 37-40.

Herrling, P. L., Emre, M., Watkins, J. C.: *D-CPPene (SDZ EAA-494) – A competitive NMDA antagonist: Pharmacology and result in humans,* in: Excitatory amino acids – clinical results with antagonists, edited by P. Herrling, Academic Press, London, **1997**, 23-30.

Heyn, H., Gietl, Y., Bankmann, Anders, M.W.: *Tissue distribution and stereoselectivity of remacemide-glycine hydrolase*, Drug Metab. Dispos. **1994**, *22*, 973-974.

Hoffmann, O. and Wiesenfeld-Hallin, Z.: *Dextromethorphan potentiates morphine antinociception, but does not reverse tolerance in rats*, Neuroreport **1996**, 7, 838-840.

Hokari, M., Wu, H. Q., Schwarz, R., Smith, Q. R.: *Facilitated brain uptake of 4-chlorokynurenine and conversion to 7-chlorokynurenic acid*, Neuroreport **1996**, *8*, 15-18.

Hollmann, M: *Structure of ionotropic glutamate receptors;* in Ionotropic glutamate receptors in the CNS, edited by P. Jonas and H. Monyer, H., Handbook of Experimental Pharmacology **1999**, *41*, 1-98.

Hollmann, M. and Heinemann, S.; *Cloned glutamate receptors*, Annu. Rev. Neurosci. **1994**, *17*, 31-108.

Honer, M., Benke, D., Laube, B., Kuhse, J., Heckendorn, R., Allgeier, H., Angst, C., Monyer, H., Seeburg, P. H., Bet, H., Mohler, H.: *Differentiation of glycine antagonist sites of N-methyl-D-aspartate receptor subtypes*, J. Biol. Chem. **1998**, *273*, 11158-11163.

Honoré, P., Chapman, V., Buritova, J., Besson, J.-M.: *Concomitant administration of morphine and an N-methyl-D-aspartate receptor antagonist profoundly reduces inflammatory evoked spinal c-Fos expression*, Anaesthesiology **1996**, *85*, 150-160.

Houghton, A. K., Parsons, C. G., Headley, P. M.: *Mrz2/576, a fast kinetic NMDA channel blocker, reduces the development of morphine tolerance in awake rats*, Pain **2001**, *91*, 201-207.

Huettner, J. E. and Bean, B. P.: *Block of N-methyl-D-aspartate-activated current by the anticonvulsant MK-801: selective binding to open channels*, Proc. Natl. Acad. Sci. USA **1988**, *85*, 1307-1311.

Huettner, J. E.: *Indole-2-carboxylic acid: a competitive antagonist of potentiation by glycine at the NMDA receptor*, Science **1989**, *243*, 1611-1613.

Hunter, J. C. and Singh, L.: *Role of excitatory amino acid receptors in the mediation of the nociceptive response to formalin in the rat*, Neurosci. Lett. **1994**, *174*, 217-221.

Ikeda, K., Nakasawa, M., Mori, H., Araki, K., Sakimura, K., Watanabe, M., Inoue, Y., Mishina, M.: *Cloning and expression of the epsilon 4 subunit of the NMDA receptor channel*, FEBS Lett. **1992**, *313*, 34-38.

Ikeda, K., Araki, K., Takayama, C., Inoue, Y., Yagi, T., Aizawa, S., Mishina, M.: *Reduced spontaneous activity of mice defective in the ε4 subunit of the NMDA receptor channel*, Brain Res. Mol. Brain Res. **1995**, *33*, 61-71.

Ilkjaer, S., Petersen, K. L., Brennum, J., Wernberg, M., Dahl, J. B.: *Effect of systemic N-methyl-D-aspartate receptor antagonist (ketamine) on primary and secondary hyperalgesia in humans*, Br. J. Anaesth. **1996**, *76*, 829-834.

Ivanovic, A., Reiländer, H., Laube, B., Kuhse, J.: *Expression and initial characterization of a soluble glycine binding domain of the N-methyl-D-aspartate receptor NR1 subunit*, J. Biol. Chem. **1998**, *273*, 19933-19937.

Jentsch, J. D., Taylor, J. R., Roth, R. H.: *Phencyclidine model of frontal cortical dysfunction in nonhuman primates*, Neuroscientist **2000**, *6*, 263-270.

Johnson, J. W. and Ascher, P.: *Glycine potentiates the NMDA response in cultured mouse brain neurones*, Nature **1987**, *325*, 529-531.

Kadotani, H., Hirano, T., Masugi, M., Nakamura, K. Katsuki, M.,Nakanishi, S.: *Motor discoordination results from the combined disruption of the NMDA receptor NR2A and NR2C subunits, but not from single disruption of the NR2A or NR2C subunit*, J. Neurosci. **1996**, *16*, 7859-7867.

Katz, N. P.: *Morphidex (MS:DM) double-blind, multiple-dose studies in chronic pain patients*, J. Pain Symptom Manage. **2000**, *19*, S37-S41.

Kauppila, T., Xu, X.-J., Yu, W., Wiesenfeld-Hallin, Z.: *Dextromethorphan potentiates the effect of morphine in rats with peripheral neuropathy*, Neuroreport **1998**, *9*, 1071-1074.

Kemp, J. A., Foster, A. C., Wong, E. H. F.: *Noncompetitive antagonists of excitatory amino acid receptors*, Trends Neurosci., **1987**, *10*, 294-298.

Kemp, J. A., Foster, A. C., Leeson, P. D., Priestley, T., Tridgett, R., Iversen, L: L., Woodruff, G. N.: *7-Chlorokynurenic acid is a selective antagonist at the glycine modulatory site of the N-methyl-D-aspartate receptor complex*, Proc. Natl. Acad. Sci. USA **1988**, *85*, 6547-6550.

Kinney, W. A.; Abou-Gharbia, M.; Garrison, D. T.; Schmid, J.; Kowal, D. M.; Bramlett, D. R.; Miller, T. L.; Tasse, R. P.; Zaleska, M. M.; Moyer, J. A.: *Design and synthesis of [2-(8,9-dioxo-2,6-diazabicyclo[5.2.0]non-1(7)-en-2-yl)- ethyl]phosphonic acid (EAA-090), a potent N-methyl-D-aspartate antagonist, via the use of 3-cyclobutene-1,2-dione as an achiral amino acid bioisostere*, J. Med. Chem. **1998**; *41*, 236-246.

Kleckner, N. W. and Dingledine, R.: *Requirement for glycine in activation of N-methyl-D-aspartic acid receptors expressed in Xenopus oocytes*, Science **1988**, *241*, 835-837.

Kleemann, A., Engel, J., Kuscher, B., Reichert, D.: *Pharmaceutical substances*, **1999**, Georg Thieme Verlag, Stuttgart.

Koek, W., Woods, J. H., Winger, G. D.: *MK-801, a proposed noncompetitive antagonist of excitatory amino acid neurotransmission, produces phencyclidine-like behavioral effects in pigeons, rats and rhesus monkeys*, J. Pharmacol. Exp. Ther., **1988**, *245*, 969-974.

Kohrs, R. and Durieux, M. E.: *Ketamine: teaching an old drug new tricks*, Anesth. Analg., **1998**, *87*, 1186-1193.

Koinig, H., Wallner, T., Marhofer, P., Andel, H., Hörauf, K., Mayer, N.; *Magnesium sulfate reduces intra- and postoperative analgesic requirements*, Anesth. Analg. **1998**, *87*, 206-210.

Kolhekar, R., Meller, S. T., Gebhart, G. F.: *N-Methyl-D-aspartate receptor-mediated changes in thermal nociception: allosteric modulation at glycine and polyamine sites*, Neuroscience **1994**, *63*, 925-936.

Kornhuber, J., Quack, G., Danysz, W., Jellinger, K., Danielcczyk, W., Gsell, W., Riederer, P.: *Therapeutic brain concentration of the NMDA receptor antagonist amantadine*, Neuropharmacology **1995**, *34*, 713-721.

Kristensen, J. D., Svensson, B., Gordh, T. J.: *The NMDA receptor antagonist CPP abolishes neurologic ´wind-up pain´ after intrathecal administration in humans*, Pain **1992**, *51*, 249-253.

Kristensen, J. D., Karsten, R., Gordh, T., Berge, O.-G.: *The NMDA antagonist 3-(2-carboxypiperazin-4-yl)propyl-1-phosphonic acid (CPP) has antinociceptive effect after intrathecal injection in the rat*, Pain **1994**, *56*, 59-67.

Kristensen, J. D., Hartvig, P., Karlsten, R., Gordh, T., Halldin, M.: *CSF and plasma pharmacokinetics of the NMDA antagonist CPP after intrathecal, extradural and i.v. administration in anaesthetiized pigs*, Br. J. Anaesth. **1995**, *74*, 193-200.

Kristensen, J. D.: *Intrathecal administration of a competitive NMDA receptor antagonist for pain treatment, in: Excitatory amino acids – clinical results with antagonists*, Ed. Herrling, P., Academic Press, London, **1997**, 23-30.

Kroin, J. S., McCarthy, R. J., von Roenn, N., Schwab, B., Tuman, K. J., Ivankovich, A. D.: *Magnesium sulfate potentiates morphine antinociception at the spinal level*, Anesth. Analg., **2000**, *90*, 913-917.

Kulagowski, J. J., Baker, R., Curtis, N. R., Leeson, P. D., Mawer, I. M., Moseley, A. M., Ridgill, M. P., Rowley, M., Stansfield, I., Foster, A. C., Grimwood, S., Hill, R. G., Kemp, J. A., Marshall, H. R., Saywell, K. L., Tricklebank, M. D.: *3´-(Arylmethyl)- and 3´-(Aryloxy)-3-phenyl-4-hydroxyquinolin-2(1H)-ones: orally active antagonists of the glycine site on the NMDA receptor*, J. Med. Chem. **1994**, *37*, 1402-1405.

Kuner, T. and Schoepfer, R.: *Multiple structural elements determine subunit specificity of Mg^{2+} block in NMDA receptor channels*, J. Neurosci. **1996**, *16*, 3549-3558.

Kuryatov, A., Laube, B., Betz, H., Kuhse, J.: *Mutational analysis of the glycine binding site of the NMDA receptor: Structural similiarity with bacterial amino acid binding proteins*, Neuron **1994**, *12*, 1291-1300.

Kutsuwada, T., Kashiwabuchi, N., Mori, H., Sakimura, K., Kushiya, K., Araki, K., Meguro, H., Masaki, H., Kumanishi, T., Arakawa M., Mishina, M.: *Molecular diversity of the NMDA receptor channel*, Nature **1992**, *358*, 36-41.

Kutsuwada, T., Sakimura, K., Manabe, T., Takayama, C., Katakura, N., Kushiya, E., Natsume, R., Watanabe, M., Inoue, Y., Yagi, T., Aizawa, S., Arakawa, M., Takahashi, T., Nakamura, Y., Mori, H., Mishina, M.: *Impairment of suckling response, trigeminal neuronal pattern formation, and hippocampal LTD in NMDA receptor ε2 subunit mutant mice*, Neuron **1996**, *16*, 333-344.

Laird, J. M. A., Mason, G. S., Webb, J., Hill, R. G., Hargreaves, R. J.: *Effects of a partial agonist and a full antagonist acting at the glycine site of the NMDA receptor on inflammation-induced mechanical hyperalgesia in rats*, Br. J. Pharmacol. **1996**, *117*, 1487-1492.

Lau, L.-F. and Huganir, R. L.: *Differential tyrosine phosphorylation of N-methyl-D-aspartate receptor subunits*, J. Biol. Chem., **1995**, *270*, 20036-20041.

Laube, B., Hirai, H., Sturgess, M., Betz, H., Kuhse, J.: *Molecular determinants of agonist discrimination by NMDA receptor subunits: Analysis of the glutamate binding site on the NR2B subunit*, Neuron **1997**, *18*, 493-503.

Laube, B., Kuhse, J., Betz, H.: *Evidence for a tetrameric structure of recombinant NMDA receptors*, J. Neurosci. **1998**, *18*, 2954-2961.

Leem, J. W., Choi, E. J., Park, E. S., Paik, K. S.: *N-methyl-D-aspartate (NMDA) and non-NMDA glutamate receptor antagonists differentially suppress dorsal horn neuron responses to mechanical stimuli in rats with peripheral nerve injury*, Neurosci. Lett. **1996**, *211*, 37-40.

Leeson, P. D., Carling, R. W., James, K., Smith, J. D., Moore, K. W., Wong, E. H. F., Baker, R.: *Role of hydrogen binding in ligand interaction with the N-methyl-D-aspartate receptor ion channel*, J. Med. Chem. **1990**, *33*, 1296-1305.

Leeson, P. D., Carling, R. W., Moore, K. W., Moseley, A. M., Smith, J. D., Stevenson, G., Chan, T., Baker, R., Foster, A. C., Grimwood, S., Kemp, J. A., Marshall, G. R., Hoogsteen, K.: *4-Amino-2-carboxytetrahydrochinolines. Structure-activity relationships for antagonism at the glycine site of the NMDA receptor*, J. Med. Chem. **1992**, *35*, 1954-1968.

Lehmann, J., Schneider, J., McPherson, S., Murphy, D. E., Bernard, P., Tsai, C., Bennett, D. A., Pastor, G., Steel, D. J., Boehm, C., Cheney, D. L., Liebman, J. M., Williams, M., Wood, P. L.: *CPP, a selective N-methyl-D-aspartate (NMDA)-type receptor antagonist: characterization in vitro and in vivo*, J. Pharmacol. Exp. Ther. **1987**, *240*, 737-746.

Leonard, A. S. and Hell, J. W.: *Cyclic AMP-dependent protein kinase and protein kinase C phosphorylate N-methyl-D-aspartate receptors at different sites*, J. Biol. Chem. **1997**, *272*, 12107-12115.

Li, Y., Erzurumlu, R. S., Chen, C., Jhaveri, S., Tonegawa, S.: *Whisker-related neuronal patterns fail to develop in the trigeminal brainstem nuclei of NMDAR1 knockout mice*, Cell **1994**, *76*, 427-437.

Li-Smerin, Y. and Johnson, J. W.: *Kinetics of the block by intracellular Mg^{2+} of the NMDA-activated channel in cultered rat neurons*, J. Physiol. **1996**, *491*, 121-135.

Lutfy, K., Shen, K.-Z., Kwon, I.-S., Cai, S. X., Woodward, R. M., Keana, J. F. W., Weber, E.: *Blockade of morphine tolerance by ACEA-1328, a novel NMDA receptor/glycine site antagonist*, Eur. J. Pharmacol. **1995**, *273*, 187-189.

Lutfy, K., Shen, K.-Z., Woodward, R. M., Weber, E.: *Inhibition of morphine tolerance by NMDA receptor antagonists in the formalin test,* Brain Res. **1996**, *731*, 171-181.

Lutfy, K. and Weber, E.: *Attenuation of nociceptive responses by ACEA-1021, a competitive NMDA receptor/glycine site antagonist, in the mice,* Brain Res. **1996**, *743*, 17-23.

Lutfy, K. and Weber, E.: *Tolerance develops to the antinociceptive and motor impairing effects of ACEA-1416, a NMDA receptor antagonist, in the formalin and rotarod tests in mice,* Pharmacol. Res. **1998**, *37*, 295-302.

Lutfy, K., Doan, P., Nguyen, M., Weber, E.: *Effects of ACEA-1328, a NMDA receptor/glycine site antagonist, on U-50,488H-induced antinociception and tolerance*, Eur. J. Pharmacol. **1999**, *384*, 1-5.

Lynch, D. R., Shim, S. S., Seifert, K. M., Kurapathi, S., Mutel, V., Gallagher, M. J., Guttmann, R. P.: *Pharmacological characterization of interactions of Ro 25-6981 with the NR2B(ε2) subunit*, Eur. J. Pharmacol. **2001**, *416*, 185-195.

Ma, Q. P. and Hargreaves, R. J.: *Localization of N-methyl-D-aspartate NR2B subunits on primary sensory neurones that give rise to small-caliper sciatic nerve fibers in rats*, Neuroscience **2000**, 101, 699-707.

Mancini, I., Lossignol, D. A., Body, J. J.: *Opioid switch to oral methadone in cancer pain*, Curr. Opin. Oncol., **2000**, *12*, 308-312.

Mao, J., Price, D. D., Hayes, R. L., Lu, J., Mayer, D. J.; *Differential roles of NMDA and non-NMDA receptor activation in induction and maintenance of thermal hyperalgesia in rats with painful peripheral mononeuropathy*, Brain Res. **1992**, *598*, 271-278.

Mao, J., Price, D. D., Hayes, R. L., Lu, J., Mayer, D. J., Frenk, H.. *Intrathecal treatment with dextrophan or ketamine potently reduces pain-related behaviors in a rat model of peripheral mononeuropathy*, Brain Res. **1993**, *605*, 164-168.

Mao, J., Price, D. D., Mayer, D. J.: *Thermal hyperalgesia in association with the development of morphine tolerance in rats: roles of excitatory amino acid receptors and protein kinase C*, J. Neurosci. **1994**, *14*, 2301-2312.

Mao, J., Price, D. D., Caruso, F. S., Mayer, D. J.: *Oral administration of dextromethorphan prevents the development of morphine tolerance and dependence in rats*, Pain **1996**, *67*, 361-368.

Mao, J.: *NMDA and opioid receptors: their interactions in antinociception, tolerance and neuroplasticity*, Brain Res. Rev. **1999**, *30*, 289-304.

Marek, P., Ben-Eliyahu, S., Vaccarino, A. L., Liebeskind, J. C.: *Delayed application of MK-801 attenuates development of morphine tolerance in rats*, Brain Res. **1991**, *558*, 163-165.

Max, M. B., Byas-Smith, M. G., Gracely, R. H., Bennett, G. J.: *Intravenous infusion of the NMDA antagonist, ketamine, in chronic posttraumatic pain with allodynia: a double-blind comparison to alfentanil and placebo*, Clin. Neuropharmacol. **1995**, *18*, 360-368.

McQuay, H. J., Carroll, D., Jadad, A. R., Glynn, C. J., Jack, T., Moore, R. A., Wiffen, P. J.: *Dextromethorphan for the treatment of neuropathic pain: a double-blind randomised controlled crossover trial with integral n-of-1 design*, Pain **1994**, *59*, 127-133.

McClean, M., Chizh, B. A., Headley, P. M.: *Effects of NMDA receptor antagonists on nociceptive responses in vivo: comparism of antagonists acting at the glycine site with uncompetitive antagonists*, Amino Acids **1998**, *14*, 217-221.

McCool, B. A. and Lovinger, D. M.: *Ifenprodil inhibition of the 5-hydroxytryptamine3 receptor*, Neuropharmacology **1995**, *34*, 621-629.

McIlhinney, R. A. J., Molnar, E., Atack, J. R., Whiting, P. J.: *Cell surface expression of the human N-methyl-D-aspartate receptor subunit 1a requires the co-expression of the NR2A subunit in transfected cells*, Neuroscience **1996**, *70*, 989-997.

Mealing, G. A. R., Lanthorn, T. H., Murray, C. L., Small, D. L., Morley, P.: *Differences in degree of trapping of low-affinity uncompetitive N-methyl-D-aspartic acid receptor antagonists with similiar kinetics of block*, J. Pharmacol. Exp. Ther. **1999**, *288*, 204-210.

Meguro, H., Mori, H., Araki, K., Kushiya, E., Kutsuwada, T., Yamazaki, M., Kumanishi, T., Arakawa, M., Sakimura, K., Mishina, M.: *Functional characterization of a heteromeric NMDA receptor channel expressed from cloned cDNAs*, Nature **1992**, *357*, 70-74.

Mercadante, S., Casuccio, A., Genovese, G.: *Ineffectiveness of dextromethorphan in cancer pain*, J. Pain Symptom Manage. **1998**, *16*, 317-322.

Mercadante, S., Arcuri, E., Tirelli, W.-, Casuccio, A.: *Analgesic effect of intravenous ketamine in cancer patients on morphine therapy: a randomized, controlled, double-blind, crossover, double-dose study*, J. Pain Symptom. Manage. **2000**, *20*, 246-252.

Millan, M. J. and Seguin, L.: *(+)-HA 966, a partial agonist at the glycine site coupled to NMDA receptors, blocks formalin-induced pain in mice*, Eur. J. Pharmacol. **1993**, *238*, 445-447.

Millan, M. J. and Seguin, L.: *Chemically-diverse ligands at the glycineB site coupled to N-methyl-D-aspartate (NMDA) receptors selectively block the late phase of formalin-induced pain in mice*, Neurosci. Lett. **1994**, *178*, 139-143.

Minami, T., Matsumura, S., Okuda-Ashitaka, E., Shimamoto, K., Sakimura, K., Mishina, M., Mori, H., Ito, S.: *Characterization of the glutamatergic system for induction and maintenance of allodynia*, Brain Res. **2001**, *895*, 178-185.

Moebius, F. F., Reiter, R. J., Hanner, M., Glossmann, H.: *High affinity of sigma$_1$-binding sites for sterol isomerization inhibitors: evidence for a pharmacological relationship with the yeast sterol C_8-C_7 isomerase*, Brit. J. Pharmacol. **1997**, *121*, 1-6.

Monaghan, D. T. and Larsen, H.: *NR1 and NR2 subunit contributions to N-methyl-D-aspartate receptor channel blocker pharmacology*, J. Pharmacol. Exp. Ther. **1997**, *280*, 614-620.

Monyer, H., Sprengel, R., Schoepfer, R., Herb, A., Higuchi, M., Lomeli, H., Burnashev, N., Sakman, B., Seeburg, P. H.: *Heteromeric NMDA receptors: molecular and functional distinction of subtypes*, Science **1992**, *256*, 1217-1221.

Mori, H., Masaki, H., Yamakura, T., Mishina, M.: *Identification by mutagenesis of a Mg^{++}-block site of the NMDA receptor channel*, Nature, **1992**, *358*, 673-675.

Moriyoshi, K., Masu, M., Ishii, T., Shigemoto, R., Mizuno, N., Nakanishi, S.; *Molecular cloning and characterization of the rat NMDA receptor*, Nature **1991**, *354*, 31-37.

Moroni, F., Alesiani, M., Galli, A., Mori, F., Pecorari, R., Carla, V., Cherici, G., Pellicciari, R.: *Thiokynurenates: a new group of antagonists of the glycine modulatory site of the NMDA receptor*, Eur. J. Pharmacol. **1991**, *199*, 227-232.

Moroni, F., Russi, P., Lombardi, G., Beni, M., Carla, V.: *Presence of kynurenic acid in the mammalian brain*, J. Neurochem. **1988**, *51*, 177-180.

Mothet, J.-P., Parent, A. T., Wolosker, H., Brady, R. O., Linden, D. J., Ferris, C. D., Rogawski, M. A., Snyder, S. H.: *D-Serine is an endogenous ligand for the glycine site of the N-methyl-D-aspartate receptor*, Proc. Natl. Acad. Sci. U.S.A. **2000**, *97*, 4926-4931.

Muir, K. W. and Lees, K. R.: *Clinical experience with excitatory amino acid antagonist drugs*, Stroke **1995**, *26*, 503-513.

Murphy, D. E., Schneider, J., Boehm, C., Lehmann, J., Williams, M.: *Binding of [3H]3-(2-carboxypiperazin-4-yl)propyl-1-phosphonic acid to rat brain membranes: a selective, high-affinity ligand for N-methyl-D-aspartate receptors*, J. Pharmacol. Exp. Ther. **1987**, *240*, 778-784.

Nahum-Levy, R., Fossom, L. H., Skolnick, P., Benveniste, M.: *Putative partial agonist 1-aminocyclo-propanecarboxylic acid acts as a glycine-site agonist and a glutamate-site antagonist at N-methyl-D-aspartate receptors*, Mol. Pharmacol. **1999**, *56*, 1207-1218.

Nakanishi, N., Axel, R., Schneider, N. A.: *Alternative splicing generates functionally distinct N-methyl-D-aspartate receptors*, Proc. Natl. Acad. Sci. USA **1992**, *89*, 8552-8556.

Nakazawa, T., Komai, S., Tezuka, T., Hisatsune, C., Umemori, H., Semba, K., Mishina, M., Manabe, T., Yamamoto, T.: *Characterization of Fyn-mediated tyrosine phosphorylation sites on GluRε2 (NR2B) subunit of the N-methyl-D-aspartate receptor*, J. Biol. Chem. **2001**, *276*, 693-699.

Neijt, H., Koller, M., Urwyler, S.: *Inorganic iron complexes derived from the nitric oxide donor nitroprusside: competitive N-methyl.D-aspartate receptor antagonists with nanomolar affinity*, Biochem. Pharmacol. **2001**, *61*, 343-349.

Nelson, K. A., Park, K. M., Robinovitz, E., Tsigos, C., Max, M. B.: *High-dose oral dextromethorphan versus placebo in painful diabetic neuropathy and postherpetic neuralgia*, Neurology **1997**, *48*, 1212-1218.

Netzer, R., Pflimlin, P., Trube, G.: *Dextromethorphan blocks N-methyl-D-aspartate-induced currents and voltage-operated inward currents in cultured cortical neurones*, Eur. J. Pharmacol. **1993**, *238*, 209-216.

Newcomer, J. W., Farber, N. B., Jevtovic-Todorovic, V., Selke, G., Melson, A. K., Hershey, T., Craft, S., Olney, J. W.: *Ketamine-induced NMDA receptor hypofunction as a model of memory impairment and psychosis*, Neuropsychopharmacol. **1999**, *20*, 106-118.

Nikolajsen, L., Hansen, C. L., Nielsen, J., Keller, J., Arendt-Nielsen, L., Jensen, T. S.: *The effect of ketamine on phantom pain: a central neuropathic disorder maintained by peripheral input*, Pain **1996**, *67*, 69-77.

Nikolajsen, L., Gottrup, H., Kristensen, A. G. D., Jensen, T. S.: *Memantine (a N-methyl-D-aspartate receptor antagonist) in the treatment of neuropathic pain after amputation or surgery: a randomized, double-blinded, cross-over study*, Anesth. Analg. **2000**, *91*, 960-966.

Nishi, M, Heather, H., Lu, H.-P., Kawata, M., Hayashi, Y.: *Motoneuron-specific expression of NR2B, a novel NMDA-type glutamate receptor subunit that works in a dominant-negative manner*, J. Neurosci. **2001**, *21*, RC185 (1-6).

Novak, L., Bregestovski, P., Ascher, P., Herbet, A., Prochiantz, A.: *Magnesium gates glutamate-activated channels in mouse central neurones*, Nature (London), **1984**, *307*, 462-465.

Olivar, T., Laird, J. M.; *Differential effects of N-methyl-D-aspartate receptor blockade on nociceptive somatic and visceral reflexes*, Pain **1999**, *79*, 67-73.

Olney, J. W., Labruyere, J., Price, M. T.: *Pathological changes induce in cerebrocortical neurons by phencyclidine and related drugs*, Science **1989**, *244*, 1360-1362.

Omkumar, R. V., Kiely, M. J., Rosenstein, A. J., Min, K.-T., Kennedy, M. B.: *Identification of a phosphorylation site for calcium/calmodulin-dependent protein kinase II in the NR2B subunit of the N-methyl-D-aspartate receptor*, J. Biol. Chem. **1996**, *271*, 31670-31678.

Ortwine D. F., Malone, T. C., Bigge, C. F., Drummond, J. T., Humblet, C., Johnson, G., Pinter, G. W.: *Generation of N-methyl-D-aspartate agonist and competitive antagonist pharmacophor models.*

Design and synthesis of phosphonoalkyl-substituteed tetrahydroisochinolines as novel antagonoists, J. Med. Chem. **1992**, *35*, 1345-1370.

Ozawa, S., Kamiya, H., Tsuzuki, K.: Glutamate receptors in the mammalian central nervous system, Progr. Neurobiol. **1998**, *54*, 581-618.

Palmer, G. C. and Widzowski, D.: *Low affinity use-dependent NMDA receptor antagonists show promise for clinical development*, Amino Acids **2000**, *19*, 151-155.

Panizzutti, R., Miranda, J. de, Ribeiro, C. S., Engelender, S., Wolosker, H.: *A new strategy to decrease N-methyl-D-aspartate (NMDA) receptor coactivation: inhibition of D-serine synthesis by converting serine racemase into an eliminase*, Proc. Natl. Acad. Sci. USA **2001**, *98*, 5294-5299.

Parsons, C. G., Quack, G., Bresink, I., Baran, L., Przegalinski, E., Kostowski, W., Krzascik, P., Hartmann, S., Danysz, W.: *Comparison of the potency, kinetics, and voltage-dependency of a series of uncompetitive NMDA receptor antagonists in vitro with anticonvulsive and motor impairment activity in vivo*, Neuropharmacology **1995**, *34*, 1239-1258.

Parsons, C. G, Danysz, W., Quack, G.: *Glutamate in CNS disorders as a target for drug development: an update*, Drugs News Perspect. **1998**, *11*, 523-569.

Parsons, C. G, Danysz, W., Quack, G.: *Memantine is a clinically well tolerated N-methyl-D-aspartate (NMDA) receptor antagonist – a review of preclinical data*, Neuropharmacology **1999a**, *38*, 735-767.

Parsons, C. G., Danysz, W, Bartmann, A., Spielmanns, P., Frankiewicz, T., Hesselink, M., Eilbacher, B., Quack, G.: *Amino-alkyl-cyclohexanes are novel uncompetitive NMDA receptor antagonists with strong voltage-dependency and fast blocking kinetics: in vitro and in vivo characterization*, Neuropharmacol. **1999b**, *38*, 85-108.

Plesan, A., Hedman, U., Xu, X.-J., Wiesenfeld-Hallin, Z.: *Comparison of ketamine and dextromethorphan in potentiating the antinociceptive effect of morphine in rats*, Anesth. Analg. **1998**, *86*, 825-829.

Plesan, A., Sollevi, A., Segerdahl, M.: *The N-methyl-D-aspartate-receptor antagonist dextromethorphan lacks analgesic effect in a human experimental ischemic pain model*, Acta Anaesthesiol. Scand. **2000**, *44*, 924-928.

Portera-Cailliau, C., Price, D. L., Martin, L. J.: *N-Methyl-D-aspartate receptor proteins NR2A and NR2B are differentially distributed in the developing rat central nervous sytem as reveiled by subunit-specific antibodies*, J. Neurochem. **1996**, *66*, 692-700.

Pozza, M. F., Zimmermann, K., Bischoff, S., Lingenhöhl, K.: *Electrophysiological characterization of CGP68730A a N-methyl-D-aspartate antagonist acting at the strychnine-insensitive glycine site*, Prog. Neuropsychopharmacol. Biol. Psychiatry **2000**, *24*, 547-670.

Price, D. D., Mao, J., Frenk, H., Mayer, D. J.: *The N-methyl-D-aspartate receptor antagonist dextromethorphan selectively reduces temporal summation of second pain in man*, Pain **1994**, *59*, 165-174.

Price, D. D., Mayer, D. J., Mao, J., Caruso, F. S.: *NMDA receptor antagonists and opioid receptor interactions as related to analgesia and tolerance*, J. Pain Symptom Manage. **2000**, *19*, S7-S11.

Priestley, T., Laughton, P., Macaulay, A. J., Hill, R. G., Kemp, J. A.: *Electrophysiological characterisation of the antagonist properties of two novel NMDA receptor glycine site antagonists, L-695,902 and L-701,324*, Neuropharmacology **1996**, *35*, 1573-1581.

Prybylowski, K. L., Grossman, S. D., Wrathall, J. R., Wolfe, B. B.: *Expression of splice variants of the NR1 subunit of the N-methyl-D-aspartate receptor in the normal and injured rat spinal cord*, J. Neurochem. **2001**, *76*, 797-805.

Pud, D., Eisenberg, E., Spitzer, A., Adler, R., Fried, G., Yarnitsky, D.: *The NMDA receptor antagonist amantadine reduces surgical neuropathic pain in cancer patients: a double blind, randomized, placebo controlled trial*, Pain **1998**, *75*, 349-354.

Quartaroli, M., Carignani, C., Dal Forno, G., Mugnaini, M., Ugolini, A., Arban, R.; Bettelini, L., Maraia, G., Belardetti, F., Reggiani,A., Trist, D. G., Di Fabio, R., Corsi, M.: *Potent antihyperalgesic activity without tolerance produced by glycine site antagonist of N-methyl-D-aspartate receptor GV196771A*, J. Pharmacol. Exp. Ther. **1999**, *290*, 158-169.

Quartaroli, M., Fasdelli, N., Bettelini, L., Maraia, G., Corsi, M.: *GV196771A, an NMDA receptor/glycine site antagonist, attenuates mechanical allodynia in neuropathic rats and reduces tolerance induced by morphine in mice*, Eur. J. Pharmacol. **2001**, *430*, 219-227.

Rabben, T., Skjelbred, P., Oye, I.: *Prolonged analgesic effect of ketamine, an N-methyl-D-aspartate receptor inhibitor, in patients with chronic pain*, J. Pharmacol. Exp. Ther. **1999**, *289*, 1060-1066.

Rigby M., Le Bourdellès, B., Heavens, R. P., Kelly, S., Smith, D., Butler, A., Hammans, R., Hills, R., Xuereb, J. H., Hill, R. G., Whiting, P. J., Sirinathsinghji, D. J. S.: *The messenger RNAs for the N-methyl-D-aspartate receptor subunits show region-specific expression of different subunit composition in the human brain*, Neuroscience **1996**, *73*, 429-447.

Rogawski, M. A.: *Low affinity channel blocking (uncompetitive) NMDA receptor antagonists as therapeutic agents – towards an understanding of their favorable tolerability*, Amino Acids **2000**, *19*, 133-149.

Rogawski, M. A. and Porter, R. J.: *Antiepileptic drugs: pharmacological mechanisms and clinical efficacy with consideration of promising developmental stage compounds*, Pharmacol. Rev. **1990**, *42*, 223-285.

Rowley, M., Leeson, P. D., Stevenson, G. I., Moseley, A. M., Stansfield, I., Sanderson, I., Robinson, L., Baker, R., Kemp, J. A., Marshall, G. R., Foster, A. C., Grimwood, S., Tricklebank, M. D., Saywell, K. L.: *3-Acyl-4-hydroxyquinolin-2(1H)-ones. Systemically active anticonvulsants acting by antagonism at the glycine site of the N-methyl-D-aspartate receptor complex*, J. Med. Chem. **1993**, *36*, 3386-3396.

Sakimura, K., Kutsuwada, T., Ito, I., Manabe, T., Takayama, C., Kushiya, E., Yagi, T., Aizawa, S., Inoue, Y., Sugiyama, H., Mishina, M.: *Reduced hippocampal LTP and spatial learning in mice lacking NMDA receptor $\varepsilon 2$ subunit*, Nature **1995**, *373*, 151-155.

Sakurada, K., Masu, M., Nakanishi, S.: *Alteration of Ca^{++} permeability and sensitivity to Mg^{++}- and channel blockers by a single amino acid substitution in the N-methyl-D-aspartate receptor*, J. Biol. Chem. **1993**, *268*, 410-415.

Salituro, F. G., Harrison, B. L., Baron, B. M., Nyce, P. L., Stewart, K. T., Kehne, J. H., White, H. S., McDonald, I. A.: *3-(2-Carboxyindol-3-yl)propionic acid-based antagonists of the N-methyl-D-aspartic acid receptor associated glycine binding site*, J. Med. Chem. **1992**, *35*, 1791-1799.

Sasner, M. and Buonnanno, A.: *Distinct N-methyl-D-aspartate receptor 2B subunit gene sequences confer neural and developmental specific expression*, J. Biol. Chem. **1996**, *271*, 21316-21322.

Schacter, S. C. and Tarsy, D.: *Remacemide: current status and clinical applications*, Expert Opin. Investig. Drugs **2000**, *9*, 871-883.

Schmutz, M., Arthur, A., Falek, H., Karsson, G., Kotake, A., Lantwicki, L., Larure, L., Markabi, S., Murphy, D., Powell, M., Sauer, D.: *Selfotel (CGS19755), in: Excitatory amino acids – clinical results with antagonists*, edited by P. Herrling, Academic Press, London, **1997**, 1-6.

Seeburg, P. H.: *The molecular biology of mammalian glutamate receptor channels*, Trends Neurosci. **1993**, *16*, 359-365.

Seguin, L. and Millan, M. J.: *The glycine B receptor partial agonist, (+)-HA 966, enhances induction of antinociception by RP 67580 and CP-99,994*, Eur. J. Pharmacol. **1994**, *253*, R1-R3.

Sheinin, A, Shavit, S., Benveniste, M.: *Subunit specificity and mechanism of action of NMDA partial agonist D-Cycloserine*, Neuropharmacology **2001**, *41*, 151-158.

Shiigi, Y. and Casey, D. E.: *Behavioral effects of ketamine, an NMDA antagonist, in non-human primates*, Psychopharmacology **1999**, 146, 67-72.

Siegel, B. W., Sreekrishna, K., Baron, B. M.: *Binding of the radiolabelled glycine site antagonist [^{3}H]MDL 105,519 to homomeric NMDA.NR1a receptors*, Eur. J. Pharmacol. **1996**, *312*, 357-365.

Singh, L., Donald, A. E., Foster, A. C., Hutson, P. H., Iversen, L. L., Iversen, S. D., Kemp, J. A., Leeson, P. D., Marshall, G. R., Oles, R. J., Priestley, T., Thorn, L., Tricklebank, M. D., Vass, C. A., Williams, B. J.: *Enantiomers of HA-966 (3-amino-1-hydroxypyrrolid-2-one) exhibit distinct central nervous system effects: (+)-HA-966 is a selective glycine/N-methyl-D-aspartate receptor antagonist, but (-)-HA-966 is a potent g-butyrolactone-like sedative*, Proc. Natl. Acad. Sci. USA **1990**, *87*, 347-351.

Sobolevsky, A. I., Beck, C., Wollmuth, L. P.: *Molecular rearrangements of the extracellular vestibule in NMDAR channels during gating*, Neuron **2002**, *33*, 75-85.

Soldo, B. L. and Rock, D. M.: Ifenprodil and eliprodil, subtype selective NMDA antagonists, suppress HERG channel function, FASEB J. **2000**, *14*, A1359.

Sotgiu, M. L. and Biella, G.: *Differential effects of MK-801, a N-methyl-D-aspartate non-competitive antagonist, on the dorsal horn neuron hyperactivity and hyperexcitability in mononeuropathic rats*, Neurosci. Lett. **2000**, *283*, 153-156.

South, S., Bogulavsky, J., Franklin, S., Martin, D., Vissel, B., Sailer, A., Malkmus, S., Masuyama, T., Horner, P., Gage, F., Tonegawa, S., Yaksh, T., Heinemann, S., Inturrisi, C. E.: *A conditional knockout (KO) of the NMDAR1 subunit in spinal cord dorsal horn attenuates hyperalgesia*, Abstr. Society of Neurosciences Meeting, **2001**.

Stone, T. W.: *Neuropharmacology of quinolinic and kynurenic acids*, Pharmacol. Rev. **1993**, *45*, 310-378.

Stone, T. W.: *Development and therapeutic potential of kynurenic acid and kynurenine derivatives for neuroprotection*, Trends Pharmacol. Sci. **2000**, *21*, 149-154.

Stringer, M., Makin, M. K., Miles, J., Morley, J. S.: *D-Morphine, but not L-morphine, has low micromolar affinity for the non-competitive N-methyl-D-aspartate site in rat forebrain. Possible clinical implications for the management of neuropathic pain*, Neurosci. Lett. **2000**, *295*, 21-24.

Subramaniam, S., Donevan, S. D., Rogawski, M. A.: *Block of the N-methyl-D-aspartate receptor by remacemide and its des-glycine metabolite*, J. Pharmacol. Exp. Ther. **1996**, *276*, 161-168.

Sucher, N. J., Akbarian, S., Chi, C. L., Leclerc, C. L., Awobuluyi, M., Deitcher, D. L., Wu, M. K., Yuan, J. P., Jones, E. G., Lipton, S. A.: *Developmental and regional expression pattern of a novel NMDA receptor-like subunit (NMDAR-L) in the rodent brain*, J. Neurosci. **1995**, *15*, 6509-6520.

Sucher, N. J., Awobuluyi, M., Choi, Y.-B., Lipton, S. A.: *NMDA receptors: from genes to channels*, Trends Pharmcol. Sci. **1996**, *17*, 348-355.

Suzuki, R., Matthews, E. A., Dickensen, A. H.: *Comparison of the effects of MK-801, ketamine and memantine on responses of spinal dorsal horn neurones in a rat model of mononeuropathy*, Pain **2001**, *91*, 101-109.

Suzuki, T. and Okumura-Noji, K.: *NMDA receptor subunits e1 (NR2A) and e2 (NR2B) are substrates for Fyn in the postsynaptic density fraction isolated from the rat brain*, Biochem. Biophys. Res. Comm. **1995**, *216*, 582-588.

Takano, Y., Sato, E., Kaneko, T., Sato, I.: *Antihyperalgesic effects of intrathecally administered magnesium sulfate in rats*, Pain **2000**, *84*, 175-179.

Tal, M. and Bennett, G. J.: *Dextrorphan relieves neuropathic heat-evoked hyperalgesia in the rat*, Neurosci. Lett. **1993**, *151*, 107-110.

Tang, Y.-P., Shimizu, E., Dube, G. R., Rampon, C., Kerchner, G. A., Zhuo, M., Liu, G., Tsien, J. Z.: *Genetic enhancement of learning and memory in mice*, Nature **1999**, *401*, 63-69.

Tang, Y.-P., Wang, H., Feng, R., Kyin, M., Tsien, J. Z.: *Differential effects of enrichment on learning and memory function in NR2B transgenic mice*, Neuropharmacology **2001**, *41*, 779-790.

Taniguchi, K., Shinjo, K., Mizutani, M., Shimada, K., Ishikawa, T., Menniti, F. S., Nagahisa, A.: *Antinociceptive activity of CP-101,606, an NMDA receptor NR2B subunit antagonist*, Brit. J. Pharmacol. **1997**, *122*, 809-812.

Tiseo, P. L. and Inturrisi, C. E.: *Attenuation and reversal of morphine tolerance by the competitive N-methyl-D-aspartate receptor antagonist, LY274614*, J. Pharmacol. Exp. Ther. **1993**, *264*, 1090-1096.

Tortella, F. C., Pellicano, M., Bowery, N. G.: *Dextromethorphan and neuromodulation: old drug coughs new activities*, Trends Pharmacol. Sci. **1989**, *10*, 501-507.

Tramer, M. R., Schneider, J., Marti, R.-A., Rifat, K.: *Role of magnesium sulfate in postoperative analgesia*, Anaesthesiology **1996**, *84*, 340-347.

Tricklebank, M. D., Singh, L., Oles, R. J., Preston, C., Iversen, S. D.: *The behavioural effects of MK-801: a comparison with antagonists acting non-competitively at the NMDA receptor*, Eur. J. Pharmacol. **1989**, *167*, 127-135.

Trujillo, K. A.: *Are NMDA receptors involved in opiate-induced neural and behavioral plasticity? A review of preclinical studies*, Psychopharmacology **2000**, *151*, 121-141.

Tsien, J. Z., Huerta, P. T., Tonegawa, S.: *The essential role of hippocampal CA1 NMDA receptor-dependent synaptic plasticity in spatial memory*, Cell, **1996**, *87*, 1327-1338.

Tzschentke T. M. and Schmidt, W. J.: Does the noncompetitive NMDA receptor antagonist dizocilpine (MK801) really block behavioural sensitization associated with repeated drug administration?, Trends Pharmacol. Sci. **1998**, *19*, 447-451.

Urenjak, J. and Obrenovitch, T. P.: *Kynurenine 3-hydroxylase inhibition in rats: Effects on extracellular kynurenic acid concentration and N-methyl-D-aspartate-induced depolarisation in the striatum*, J. Neurochem. **2000**, *75*, 2427-2433.

Urwyler, S., Campell, E., Fricker, G., Jenner, P., Lemaire, M., McAllister, K. H., Neijt, H. C., Park, C. K., Perkins, M., Rudin, M., Sauter, A., Wiederhold, K.-H., Müller, W.: *Biphenyl-derivatives of 2-amino-7-phosphono-heptanoic acid: A novel class of potent competitive N-methyl-D-aspartate receptor antagonists: II. Pharmacological characterization in vivo*, Neuropharmacology **1996**, *35*, 655-669.

Vaccarino, A. L., Marek, P., Kest, B., Weber, E., Keana, J. F. W., Liebeskind, J. C.; *NMDA receptor antagonists, MK-801 and ACEA-1011, prevent the development of tonic pain following subcutaneous formalin*, Brain Res. **1993**, *615*, 331-334.

Vanderschuren, L. J. M. J., Kalivas, P. W.: *Alterations in dopaminergic and glutaminergic transmission in the induction and expression of behavioral sensitization: a critical review of preclinical studies*, Psychopharmacology **2000**, *151*, 99-120.

Vick, P. G. and Lamer, T. J.: *Treatment of central post-stroke pain with oral ketamine*, Pain **2001**, *92*, 311-313.

Wafford, K. A., Kathoria, M., Bain, C. J., Marshall, G., Lebourdelles, B., Kemp, J. A., Whiting, P. J.: *Identification of amino acids in the N-methyl-D-aspartate receptor NR1 subunit that contribute to the glycine binding site*, Mol. Pharmacol. **1995**, *47*, 374-380.

Wagner, D. A. and Leonard, J. P.: *Effect of protein kinase-C activation on the Mg^{2+}-sensitivity of cloned NMDA receptors*, Neuropharmacology **1996**, *35*, 29-36.

Wake, K., Yamazaki, H., Hanzawa, S., Konno, R., Sakio, H., Niwa, A., Hori, Y.: *Exaggerated responses to chronic nociceptive stimuli and enhancement of N-methyl-D-aspartate receptor-mediated synaptic transmission in mutant mice lacking D-amino-acid oxidase*, Neurosci. Lett. **2001**, *297*, 25-28.

Warncke, T., Stubhaug, A., Jorum, E.: *Ketamine, an NMDA receptor antagonist, suppresses spatial and temporal properties of burn-induced secondary hyperalgesia in man: a double-blind, cross-over comparison with morphine and placebo*, Pain **1997**, *72*, 99-106.

Wei, F., Wang, G.-D., Kerchner, G. A., Kim, S. J., Xu, H.-M., Chen, Z.-F., Zhuo, M.: *Genetic enhancement of inflammatory pain by forebrain NR2B overexpression*, Nature Neurosci. **2001**, *4*, 164-169.

Wesemann, W., Sturm, G., Fünfgeld, E. W.: *Distribution of metabolism of the potential anti-Parkinson drug memantine in the human*, J. Neural Transm. **1980**, *16*, Suppl., 143-148.

Wiesenfeld-Hallin, Zsuzsanna; *Combined opioid-NMDA antagonist therapies. What advantages do they offer for the control of pain syndromes*, Drugs, **1998**, *55*, 1-4.

Williams, K.: *Ifenprodil discriminates subtypes of the N-methyl-D-aspartate receptor: selectivity and mechanisms at recombinant heteromeric receptors*, Mol. Pharmacol. **1993**, *44*, 851-859.

Wolf, M. E.: *The role of excitatory amino acids in behavioral sensitization to psychomotor stimulants*, Progr. Neurobiol. **1998**, *54*, 679-720.

Wolosker, H., Blackshaw, S., Snyder, S. H.: *Serine racemase: a glial enzyme synthesizing D-serine to regulate glutamate-N-methyl-D-aspartate neurotransmission*, Proc. Natl. Acad. Sci. USA **1999**, *96*, 13409-13414.

Wong, B. Y., Coulter, D. A., Choi, D. W., Prince, D. A.: *Dextrorphan and dextromethorphan, common antitussives, are antiepileptic and antagonise N-methyl-D-aspartate in brain slices*, Neurosci. Lett. **1988**, *85*, 261-266.

Wong, E. H. F., Kemp, J. A., Priestley, T., Knight, A. R., Woodruff, G. N., Iversen, L. L.: *The anticonvulsant MK-801 is a potent N-methyl-D-aspartate antagonist*, Proc. Natl. Acad. Sci. USA **1986**, *83*, 7104-7108.

Woodward, R. M., Huettner, J. E., Tran, M., Guastella, J., Keana, J. F. W., Weber, E.: *Pharmacology of 5-chloro-7-trifluoromethyl-1,4-dihydro-2,3-quinoxalinedione: a novel sytemically active ionotropic glutamate receptor antagonist*, J. Pharmacol. Exp. Ther. **1995a**, *275*, 1209-1218.

Woodward, R. M., Huettner, J. E., Guastella, J., Keana, J. F. W., Weber, E.: *In vitro pharmacology of ACEA-1021 and ACEA-1031: systemically active quinoxalinedioneswith high affinity and selectivity for N-methyl-D-aspartate receptor glycine sites*, Mol. Pharmacol. **1995b**, *47*, 568-581.

Wozniak, D. F., Olney, J. W., Kettinger III, L., Miller, J. P.: *Behavioral effects of MK-801 in the rat*, Psychopharmacology **1990**, *101*, 47-56.

Wroblewski, J. T. and Danysz, W.: *Modulation of glutamate receptors: molecular mechanisms and functional implications*, Annu. Rev. Pharmacol. Toxicol. **1989**, *29*, 441-474.

Xiao, W. H. and Bennett, G. J.: *Magnesium suppresses neuropathic pain responses in rats via a spinal site of action*, Brain Res. **1994**, *666*, 168-172.

Yamakura, T. and Shimoji, K.: *Subunit- and site-specific pharmacology of the NMDA receptor*, Progr. Neurobiol. **1999**, *59*, 279-298.

Yamakura, T., Sakimura, K., Shimoji, K.: *The stereoselective effects of ketamine isomers on heteromeric N-methyl-D-aspartate receptor channels*, Anesth. Analg. **2000**, 225-229.

Yamamoto, T. and Yaksh, T. L.: *Studies on the spinal interaction of morphine and the NMDA antagonist MK-801 on the hyperesthesia observed in a rat model of sciatic mononeuropathy*, Neurosci. Lett. **1992**, *135*, 67-70.

Yung, K. K. L.: *Localization of glutamate receptors in dorsal horn of rat spinal cord*, Neuroreport **1998**, *9*, 1639-1644.

Zheng, X., Zhang, L., Wang, A. p., Bennett, M. V. L., Zukin, S.: *Protein kinase C potentiation of N-methyl-D-aspartate receptor activity is not mediated by phosphorylation of N-methyl-D-aspartate receptor subunits*, Proc. Natl. Acad. Sci. USA **1999**, *96*, 15262-15267.

Zimmer, M., Fink, T. M., Franke, Y., Lichter, P., Spiess, J.: *Cloning and structure of the gene encoding the human NMDA receptor (NMDAR-1)*, Gene **1995**, *159*, 219-223.

Zhou, G.-Z. and Musacchio, J. M.: *Computer-assisted modeling of multiple dextromethorphan and sigma binding sites in guinea pig brain*, Eur. J. Pharmacol. **1991**, *206*, 261-269.

Zhuo, M.: *Glutamate receptors and persistent pain: targeting forebrain NR2B subunits*, Drug Discov. Today **2002**, *7*, 259-267.

Zukin, R. S. and Bennett, M. V. L.: *Alternatively spliced isoforms of the NMDAR1 receptor subunit*, Trends Neurosci. **1995**, *18*, 306-313.

7.3 AMPA and Kainate Receptors

Corinna Maul and Bernd Sundermann

Introduction

Glutamate is the major exitatory neurotransmitter in the mammalian central nervous system and its interactions with membrane receptors play a critical role in nearly every aspect of brain function, including cognition, memory and sensation.

Glutamate receptors are classified in two main categories:

- ionotropic receptors (iGluRs) directly coupled to ion channels

- metabotropic receptors (mGluRs) coupled to intracellular second messengers via guanine nucleotide regulatory proteins (G-proteins; see Chapter 7.1)

iGluRs include those selectively sensitive to N-methyl-D-aspartate (NMDA; see Chapter 7.2), AMPA and kainate. AMPA and kainate selective receptors are often referred to as non-NMDA receptors. Their potential use in pain therapy is the topic of this chapter (for a comprehensive overview see Fundytus, 2001).

Expression studies have verified that there are further subtypes of all non-NMDA receptors. The subunits GluR1 to GluR4 bind AMPA with higher affinity than kainate, while GluR5 to GluR7 are kainate-selective (Gasic and Holleman, 1992). There is also a family of kainate-binding proteins (KA1, KA2) which bind kainate with high affinity, but are not functional receptor channels and have little sequence similarity with the GluR genes. AMPA and kainate receptors have four transmembrane-spanning domains, similar to other ligand-gated ion channels. In neurons expressing GluR2 with other subunits there are no Ca^{2+} currents, but in the absence of the GluR2 subunit glutamate can trigger Ca^{2+} influx.

Glutamate (Glutamic acid)
(2S)-2-Amino-pentanedioic acid

NMDA
(2R)-2-Methylamino-succinic acid

Kainate (Kainic acid)
(2S,3S,4R)-3-Carboxy-methylpyrrolidine-2,4-dicarboxylic acid

AMPA
(2S)-2-Amino-3-(5-methyl-3-oxo-2,3-dihydro-isoxazol-4-yl)-propionic acid

AMPA/Kainate and Pain

The role of non-NMDA receptor modulators in pain is not as clear as the role of NMDA receptors, but there is evidence to indicate that AMPA and kainate receptors may be involved in nociceptive processing.

Recently, it has been shown that spinal neurons express functional kainate receptors which contribute to synaptic transmission between primary afferent fibers and dorsal horn neurons (Li et al., 1999). Administration of the AMPA/kainate antagonist CNQX to the spinal cord

CNQX (7-Nitro-2,3-dioxo-1,2,3,4-tetrahydro-quinoxaline-6-carbonitrile)

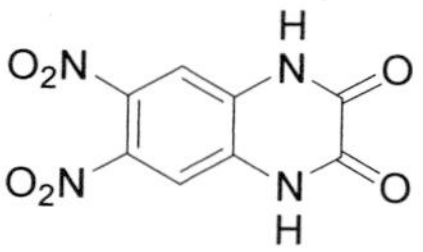

DNQX (6,7-Dinitro-1,4-
dihydroquinoxaline-2,3-
dione)

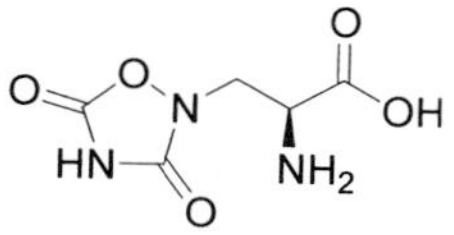

Quisqualic acid
glutamate receptor agonist
acting at AMPA receptors
and group I mGluRs

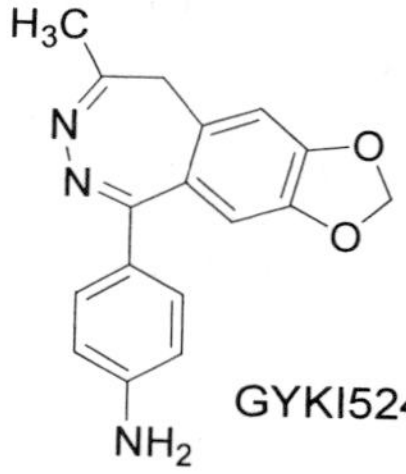

GYKI52466

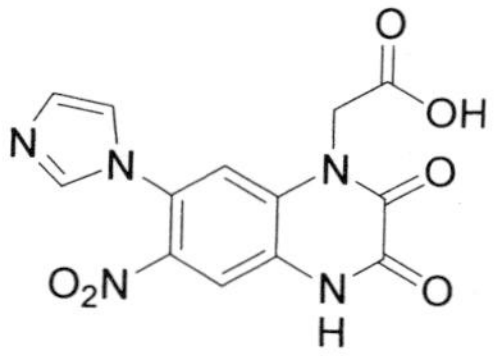

YM-872

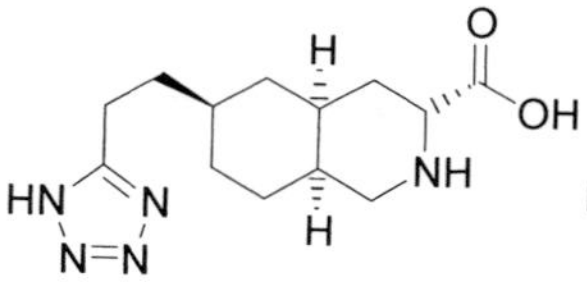

diminishes dorsal horn neuronal responses induced by non-noxious and noxious mechanical stimulation (Neugebauer et al., 1993).

Following inflammation there is a 10-fold increase in axons expressing AMPA or kainate receptors (Coggeshall and Carlton, 1999). In anaesthetized rats, antagonism of AMPA/kainate receptors inhibits dorsal horn neuronal responses induced by innocuous and noxious mechanical stimulation of a chronically inflamed ankle (Neugebauer et al., 1994). Application of kainate to the rat hindpaw induces activation of primary afferent neurons, an effect that is reduced by the AMPA/kainate antagonist DNQX (Ault and Hildebrand, 1993).

Several animal studies suggest that modulation of AMPA and kainate receptors can significantly affect pain transmission at diverse targets in the nervous system (Coderre and Melzack, 1992, Procter et al., 1998). Intrathecal administration of AMPA or kainate receptor agonists (e.g. AMPA, kainate, quisqualic acid) produce spontanous nociceptive behaviors, thermal and mechanical hyperalgesia, and allodynia (Sun et al., 1991; Okano et al., 1993; Yezierski et al., 1998). The AMPA/kainate receptor antagonist GYKI52466 was found to be fairly potent in rat tail flick and mouse phenylquinone writhing assays (Szekely et al., 1997). YM872, another AMPA receptor antagonist, also showed effects on acute pain (Nishiyama et al., 1999).

The AMPA/kainate antagonist LY-293558 (GluR5/GluR2) caused antinociceptive and ataxic effects in the formalin test, whereas the selective GluR5 antagonist LY-382884 exhibited antinociceptive effects without ataxia, while the GluR2-preferring antagonist LY-302679 caused ataxia but did not produce antinociceptive effects. These findings suggest an involvement of GluR5 in the processing of nociceptive information (Simmons et al., 1998). Moreover, there is evidence that kainate receptors can act as the induction trigger for long-term changes in synaptic transmission (Bortolotto et al., 1999).

LY-293558 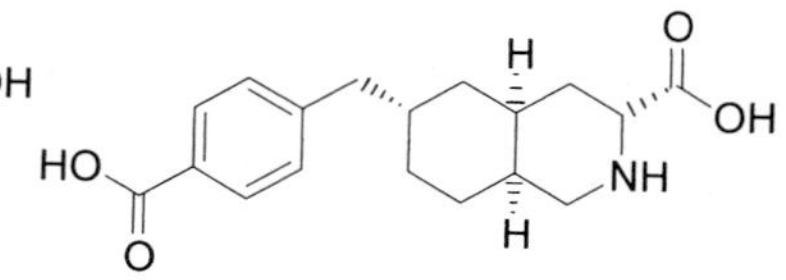   LY-382884

Scheme 1: AMPA/Kainate antagonists.

There is also evidence that AMPA/kainate receptors may be involved in chronic pain: following peripheral nerve injury AMPA receptor expression is upregulated and peaks 2 weeks after nerve ligation (Harris et al., 1996). Furthermore, GYKI52466 potently inhibits hyperalgesia in Freund adjuvant-induced chronic arthritis (Szekely et al., 1997).

(2*S*,4*R*)-Methylglutamate (SYM2081), a selective GluR5 and GluR6 desensitizing agonist showing 500 - 2000-fold selectivity for homomeric kainate receptors (composed of GluR5 and GluR6 subunits) over AMPA receptors (composed of GluR1, GluR2 or GluR3 subunits) (Zhou et al., 1997), reduces allodynia and hyperalgesia in CCI rats (Sutton et al., 1999) and freeze injury model of neuropathic pain (Ta et al., 2000). The location of the methyl group at the 4 position of glutamate is critical for kainate receptor agonist activity as glutamate analogs with the methyl group at the 2 or 3 position had negligible activity (Donevan et al., 1998).

Analgesia after intrathecal administration of the glutamate antagonist NBQX supports a site of action at AMPA/kainate receptors in the superficial laminae of the spinal dorsal horn (Furuyama et al., 1993). In addition to this spinal action, injection of the glutamate antagonist CNQX into the rat hindpaw reverses hyperalgesia and allodynia caused by pharmacologic activation of AMPA and kainate receptors, thus suggesting a peripheral action (Zhou et al., 1996). Finally, the ubiquity of AMPA/kainate receptors in the brain leaves open the possibility that their antagonists may mediate analgesia by blocking excitatory neurotransmission at supraspinal sites.

There is evidence that AMPA/kainate antagonists also reduce clinical pain. Intravenous LY293558 (0.4 or 1.2 mg/kg) proved to reduce postoperative pain in human volunteers (Gilron et al., 2000). It strongly antagonizes both AMPA receptors (particularly GluR2) and kainate receptors (particularly GluR5). By January 2000, LY-293558 was undergoing phase II trials for pain and other CNS indications. Data from the first studies provide early evidence for its analgesic efficacy at doses that are well tolerated. The most striking side-effect was hazy vision, described as white clouds in the periphery with sparing central vision (Gilron, 2001).

SYM-2081

NBQX (6-Nitro-2,3-dioxo-1,2,3,4-tetrahydro-benzo[f]quinoxaline-7-sulfonic acid amide)

LY-293558

6-[2-(1H-Tetrazol-5-yl)-ethyl]-decahydro-isoquinoline-3-carboxylic acid, $C_{13}H_{21}N_5O_2$, MW 279.34, 154652-83-2

Further Compounds

Some AMPA/kainate antagonists are in clinical trials for several indications based on their neuroprotective and anticonvulsive properties. A selection is given below.

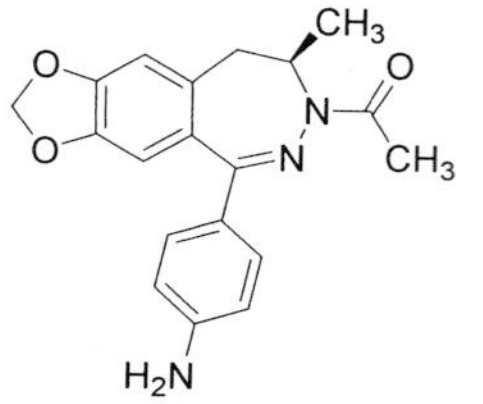

Talampanel, phase II
clinical trials for epilepsy
and Parkinson's disease
(Eli Lilly)

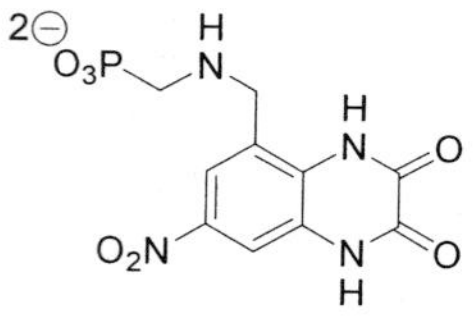

AMP-397A, phase I clinical
trials for epilepsy (Novartis)

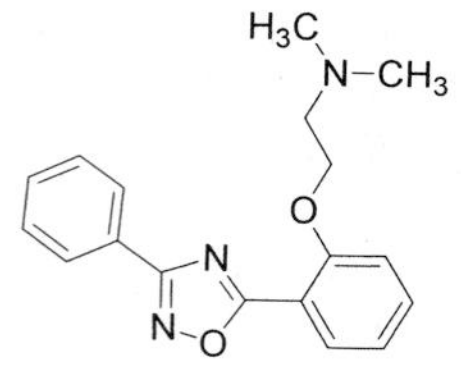

Irampanel, phase II clinical trials for
cerebral ischemia, combined AMPA
receptor/sodium channel antagonist
(Weiser et al. (Boehringer Ingelheim),
1999)

Scheme 2: Compounds in clinical trials.

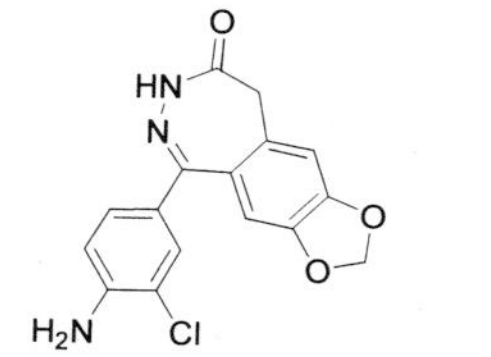

AMPA receptor antagonist
Xia et al., 1999 (CoCensys)

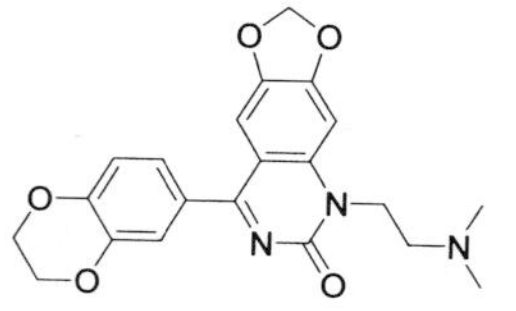

AMPA receptor modulator
Upasani et al., 1999 (CoCensys)

Although AMPA and kainate antagonists have been less extensively studied in pain models than NMDA receptor antagonists, recent evidence suggests that they may also be useful in the treatment of clinical pain. Studies suggest that antagonism of multiple types of glutamate receptors might be necessary to achieve effective pain relief since NMDA, AMPA and kainate are all involved in peripheral pain transmission (Lutfy et al., 1997).

With respect to recent patent applications the neuroprotective properties of non-NMDA antagonists are still in the focus of pharmacetical research, but the majority of patents does not propose that they should be used for pain relief. However, the continuing interest in AMPA/kainate receptor modulators might also lead to further investigations of their analgesic properties. Two examples of AMPA receptor modulators recently claimed for pain are shown.

References:

Ault, B. and Hildebrand, L.M.: *Activation of nociceptive reflexes by peripheral kainate receptors*, J. Pharmacol. Exp. Ther. **1993**, *265*, 927-932.

Bortolotto, Z.A., Clarke, V.R., Delany, C.M., Parry, M.C., Smolders, I., Vignes, M., Ho, K.H., Miu, P., Brinton, B.T., Fantaske, R., Ogden, A., Gates, M., Ornstein, P.L., Lodge, D., Bleakman, D., Collongridge, G.L.: *Kainate receptors are involved in synaptic plasticity*, Nature **1999**, *402*, 297-301.

Coderre, T.J. and Melzack, R.: *The contribution of excitatory amino acids to central sensitization and persistent nociception after formalin-induced tissue injury*, J. Neurosci. **1992**, *12*, 3665-3670.

Coggeshall, R.E. and Carlton, S.M.: *Evidence for an inflammation-induced change in the local glutamaterig regulation of postganglionic sympathetic efferents*, Pain **1999**, *83*, 163-168.

Donevan, S.D., Beg, A., Gunther, J.M., Twyman, R.E.: *The methylglutamate, SYM 2081, is a potent and highly selective agonist at kainate receptors*, J. Pharmacol. Exp. Ther. **1998**, *285*, 539-545.

Fundytus, M.E.: *Glutamate receptors and nociception*, CNS Drugs **2001**, *15*, 29-58.

Furuyama, T., Kiyama, H., Sato, K., Park, H.T., Maeno, H., Takagi, H., Tohyama, M.: *Region-specific expression of subunits of ionotropic glutamate receptors (AMPA-type, KA-type, and NMDA receptors) in the rat spinal cord with special reference to nociception*, Brain Res. Mol. Brain Res. **1993**, *18*, 141-151.

Gasic, G.P. and Holleman, M.: *Molecular neurobiology of glutamate receptors*, Ann. Rev. Physiol. **1992**, *54*, 507-536.

Gilron, I., Max, M.B., Lee, G., Booher, S.L., Sang, C.N., Chappell, A.S., Dionne, R.A.: *Effects of the 2-amino-3-hydroxy-5-methyl-4-isoxazole-propionic acid/kainate antagonist LY293558 on spontaneous and evoked postoperative pain*, Clin. Pharmacol. Ther. **2000**, *68*, 320-327.

Gilron, I.: *LY-293558*, Curr. Opin. Invest. Drugs **2001**, *2*, 1273-1278.

Harris, J.A., Corsi, M., Quartaroli, M., Arban, R., Bentivoglio, M.: *Upregulation of spinal glutamate receptors in chronic pain*, Neuroscience **1996**, *74*, 7-12.

Li, P., Wilding, T.J., Kim, S.J., Calejesan, A.A., Huettner, J.E., Zhuo, M.: *Kainate-receptor-mediated sensory synaptic transmission in mammalian spinal cord*, Nature **1999**, *397*,161-164.

Lutfy, K., Cai, S.X., Woodward, R.M., Weber, E.: *Antinociceptive effects on NMDA and non.NMDA receptor antagonists in the tail flick test in mice*, Pain **1997**, *76*, 31-40.

Neugebauer, V., Lucke, T., Schaible, H.G.: *Differential effects of N-methyl-D-aspartate (NMDA) and non-NMDA receptor antagonists on the responses of rat spinal neurons with joint input*, Neurosci. Lett. **1993**, *155*, 29-32.

Neugebauer, V., Lucke, T., Grubb, B., Schaible, H.G.: *The involvment of N-methyl-D-aspartate (NMDA) and non-NMDA receptors in the responsiveness of rat spinal neurons with input from the chronically inflamed ankle*, Neurosci. Lett. **1994**, *170*, 237-240.

Nishiyama, T., Gyermek, L., Lee, C., Kawasaki-Yatsugi, S., Yamaguchi, T.: *The spinal antinociceptive effects of a novel competitive AMPA receptor antagonist, YM872, on thermal or formalin-induced pain in rats*, Anesth. Analg. **1999**, *89*, 143-147.

Okano, K., Kuraishi, Y., Satoh, M.: *Pharmacological evidence for involvement of excitatory amino acids in aversive responses induced by intrathecal substance P in rats*, Biol. Pharm. Bull. **1993**, *16*, 861-865.

Procter, M. J., Houghton, A.K., Faber, E.S., Chizh, B.A., Omstein, P.L., Lodge, D., Headley, P.M.: *Actions of kainate and AMPA selective glutamate receptor ligands on nociceptive processing in the spinal cord*, Neuropharmacology **1998**, *37*, 1287-1297.

Simmons, R.M., Li, D.L., Hoo, K.H., Deverill, M., Ornstein, P.L., Iyengar, S.: *Kainate GluR5 receptor subtype mediates the nociceptive response to formalin in the ra*t, Neuropharmacology **1998**, *37*, 25-36.

Sun, X.F. and Larson, A.A.: *Behavioral sensitization to kainic acid and quisqualic acid in mice: comparison to NMDA and substance P responses*, J. Neurosci. **1991**, *11*, 3111-3123.

Sutton, J.L., Maccecchini, M.L., Kajander, K.C.: *The kainate receptor antagonist 2S,4R-4-methylglutamate attenuates mechanical allodynia and thermal hyperalgesia in a rat model of nerve injury*, Neuroscience **1999**, *91*, 283-292.

Szekely, J.I., Kedves, R., Mate, I., Torok, K., Tarnawa, I.: *Apparent antinociceptive and anti-inflammatory effects of GYKI 52466*, Eur. J. Pharmacol. **1997**, *336*, 143-154.

Ta, L.E., Dionne, R.A., Fricton, J.R., Hodges, J., Kajander, K C.: *SYM-2081 a kainate receptor antagonist reduces allodynia and hyperalgesia in a freeze injury model of neuropathic pain*, Brain Res. **2000**, *858*, 106-120.

Upsani, R., Lan, N., Wang, Y., Field, G., Fick, D.B. (CoCensys), *Substituted quinazolines and analogs and the use thereof*, WO9944612 (**1999**).

Weiser, T., Brenner, M., Palluk, R., Bechtel, W.D., Ceci, A., Brambilla, A., Ensinger, H.A., Sagrada, A., Wienrich, M.: *BIIR 561 CL: A novel combined antagonist of α-amino-3-hydroxy-5-methyl-4-isoxazolepropionic acid receptors and voltage-dependent sodium channels with anticonvulsive and neuroprotective properties*, J. Pharmacol. Exp. Ther. **1999**, *289*, 1343-1349.

Yezierski, R.P., Liu, S., Ruenes, G.L., Kajander, K.J., Brewer, K.L.: *Excitotoxic spinal cord injury: behavioral and morphological characteristics of a central pain model*, Pain **1998**, 75, 141-155.

Xia, H., Cai, S.X., Field, G., Lan, N.C., Wang, Y. (CoCensys): *Substituted 2,3-benzodiazepin-4-ones and the use thereof*, US5891871 (**1999**).

Zhou, S., Bonasera, L., Carlton, S.M.: *Peripheral administration of NMDA, AMPA or KA results in pain behaviors in rats*, Neuroreport **1996**, 7, 895-900.

Zhou, L.M., Gu, Z.Q., Costa, A.M., Yamada, K.A., Mansson, P.E., Giordano, T., Skolnick, P., Jones, K.A.: *(2S,4R)-4-methylglutamic acid (SYM 2081): a selective, high-affinity ligand for kainate receptors*, J. Pharmacol. Exp. Ther. **1997**, 280, 422-427.

8 Acetylcholine Receptors

8.1 Nicotinic Acetylcholine Receptors

Bernd Sundermann and Corinna Maul

Introduction

Nicotinic acetylcholine receptors (nAChRs) form a family of pentameric ligand-gated ion channels (Hucho and Weise, 2001). A range of subtypes is known due to the occurrence of different subunits forming the ion channel (Jones et al., 1999; Clementi et al., 2000; Cordero-Erausquin et al., 2000; Picciotto et al., 2000). α- and β-subunits are most common, especially for neuronal nACh receptors, but γ-, δ- and ε-subunits have also been described. Tissue distribution of specific receptor subtypes varies distinctively, especially between the CNS and peripheral tissues. Neuronal nAChRs interact with various neurotransmitter systems besides the cholinergic system, including noradrenergic, GABAergic and dopaminergic systems (Williams and Arneric, 1996; Soreq, 1998). How neuronal nAChRs influence pain perception and signaling is not completely understood (Bai et al., 1997; Khan et al., 1997; Flores, 2000).

Although the antinociceptive potential of the natural product nicotine, an unselective nAChR agonist, was noticed as early as 1932 (Davis et al., 1932; Sahley and Berntson, 1979; Aceto et al., 1997; Rao et al., 1996; review: Badio et al., 1995) interest in antinociceptive nicotinic agents was virtually non-existent for several decades. This changed dramatically in 1992 when another natural nACh receptor agonist was discovered and reported to be at least 200 times more potent than morphine (Spande et al., 1992; Holladay et al., 1997; Flores et al., 1999; Decker et al., 2001):

Starting in 1964 Daly and his co-workers at the National Institute of Health collected poison-dart frogs in the Pacific highlands of Ecuador in collaboration with Myers' group. They were looking for pharmacologically active alkaloids (Spande et al., 1992; Daly et al., 2000) and in 1974 collected and extracted alkaloid-containing samples from the skins of *Epipedobates tricolor* specimens among others. The pooled samples were fractioned by HPLC (Daly et al., 1980) and when mice were injected with specific fractions they swiftly raised and arched their tails. This was interpreted as a typical Straub-tail effect characteristic of μ-opioids (Spande et al., 1992; Daly, 1993). Two years later Daly collected more frogs, but subsequent extractions of the frog skins yielded less than1 mg of the active compound, so it was not possible to

(*S*)-Nicotine, a tobacco alkaloid:

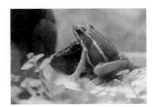

Figure 1: *Epipedobates tricolor.*

Sundermann and Maul

elucidate its chemical structure at that time. Coincidentally a newly signed international treaty to protect endangered species prohibited further collection of *Epipedobates tricolor* specimens. On the other hand skin extracts from frogs collected from other venues or raised in captivity did not contain the desired compound, so it was assumed that this compound - or its precursor - was derived from an unknown specific dietary source (Daly et al., 1997; 2000).

Identification of a natural compound as the first potent nicotinic analgesic – discovery of EPIBATIDINE

The extraordinary antinociceptive potency of the unknown compound was determined in a mouse model of acute nociception, the hot plate test. Despite the Straub-tail effect observed earlier, the antinociceptive effect of the compound could not be not antagonized with the μ-opioid receptor antagonist naloxone but with the nAChR antagonist mecamylamine, so the unknown compound was deduced to be a potent nicotinic analgesic (Spande et al., 1992; Qian et al., 1993; Badio and Daly, 1994; Sullivan and Bannon, 1996).

Elucidation of the structure of epibatidine – more than a decade after its initial discovery

Epibatidine

The race for nicotinic analgesics

Only in 1990 were the remains of the original extract stored by Daly subjected to modern analytical methods and the structure of the compound - which was named *epibatidine* - finally elucidated by spectroscopic methods, especially IR and NMR techniques (Spande et al., 1992; Daly, 1993; Daly et al., 2000). This was published in 1992 - 12 years after the initial publication on *Epipedobates tricolor* extracts (Daly et al., 1980) and very shortly after Daly and co-workers had filed patents on epibatidine and close structural analogs (see *Epibatidine*).

With the discovery of this first potent (Ki ≤ 100 pm) but non-selective neuronal nAChR agonist, being extremely efficacious in animal models of pain, a race not only for the synthesis of the scarce compound (Dehmlow, 1995) but for nicotinic agonists as potential analgesics ensued. Although several dozen publications on the total synthesis of epibatidine were published in the 1990s, original total syntheses of epibatidine are still a stimulating topic of academic research (Roy et al. 2001).

Boyce et al. 2000: Analgesic and toxic effects of ABT-594 resemble epibatidine and nicotine in rats

While the findings of Daly et al. where initially met with euphoria, today only limited work is carried out with respect to nicotinic analgesics. The promise of finding a non-opioid treatment for severe acute pain with a potency that is at least comparable to μ-opioid full agonists has not been fulfilled. This is in general due to either dose limiting toxic effects or insufficient potency (Boyce et al., 2000; also see: Bai et al., 1997; Francis 1999; Kesingland et al., 2000). It has been speculated, but not proven, that these problems might be overcome with nAChR subtype-selective compounds (Marks et al., 1998; Bannon et al.,

1998; Marubio et al., 1999; Williams et al., 1999). This speculation is corroborated by data suggesting that only neuronal nAChRs are important for the antinociceptive effects of epibatidine, while toxic effects might be mediated by peripheral nAChRs (Sullivan et al., 1994).

On the other hand ABT-594, a nicotinic agonist presumed to be selective for the $\alpha_2\beta_4$-subtype of the neuronal nACh receptor (Khan et al., 1997, 1998; Kowaluk and Arneric, 1998; Thatte, 2000), is reported to be in clinical development against neuropathic pain, a pain state that often cannot be effectively treated with opioids or other medications (Lawand et al., 1999; Gilbert et al., 2001).

Can neuropathic pain be effectively treated with nicotinic agonists?

Epibatidine

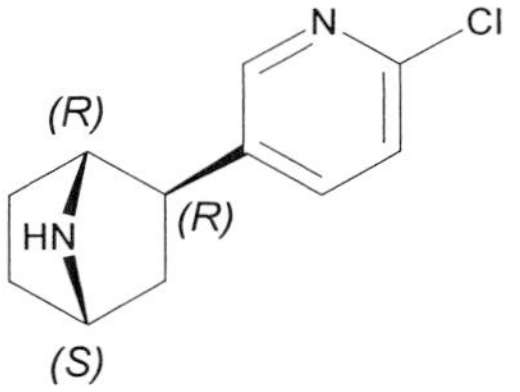

The natural product epibatidine was the starting point for worldwide activities towards the discovery of nicotinic analgesics. Besides its unusual antinociceptive potency (review: Bai et al., 1997) its exceptional structure combines a scarce chloropyridine moiety with a 7-aza-norbornane (7-azabicyclo[2.2.1]heptane) bicycle which has never before been found in a natural product before. In 1994 the absolute configuration of natural (+)-epibatidine was determined to be 1R,2R,4S (Fletcher et al., 1994). Initial patents on epibatidine and close structural analogs were filed by the U.S. Department of Health (Daly et al., 1993, 1995).

Epibatidine's antinociceptive effect can be antagonized by pretreatment with the centrally active nAChR antagonist mecamylamine, but not with the peripheral antagonist hexamethonium, so the activation of central nAChRs is presumed to be essential for nicotinic analgesics (Sullivan et al., 1994). The high toxicity of epibatidine has been attributed to its lack of selectivity for specific neuronal nAChR subtypes and has precluded its development as a therapeutic agent.

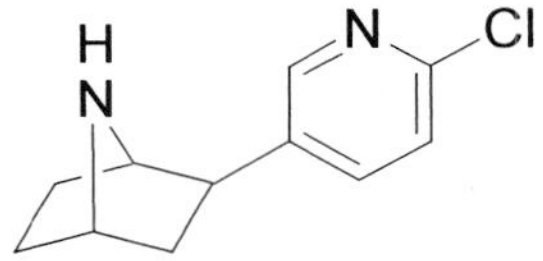

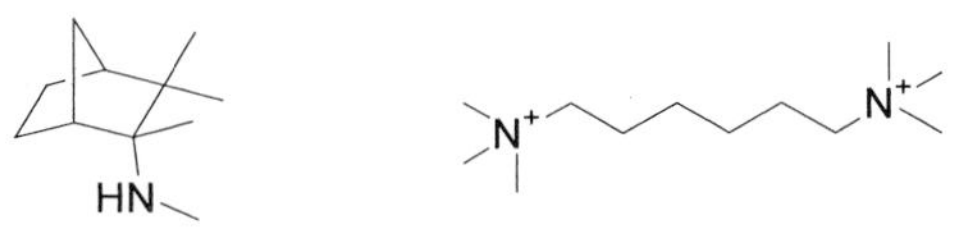

[140111-52-0];
(+)-(1R,2R,4S)-2-(6-Chloropyridin-3-yl)-7-azabicyclo[2.2.1]heptane, $C_{11}H_{13}ClN_2$, M_r 208.69

Figure 2: nAChR antagonists.

Mecamylamine

Hexamethonium

While Dehmlow's review details a variety of efforts towards the total synthesis of epibatidine (Dehmlow, 1995) the synthesis of this natural product is still an intriguing challenge for academic research. More than three dozen

Total syntheses of epibatidine

(formal) total syntheses have been published in the past decade (Roy et al., 2001). A production route has not been developed so the following scheme is intended only to give an exemplary overview of successful early synthetic strategies:

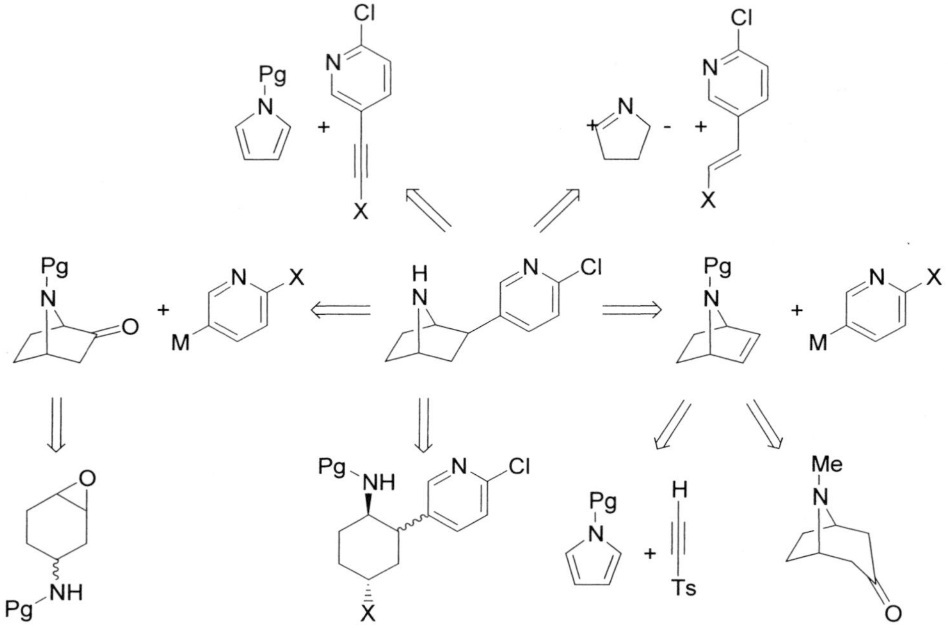

Pg, protecting group; M, metal (complex); X, activating/leaving group.

Figure 3: Retrosynthetic strategies for the total synthesis of epibatidine.

Epibatidine – a very potent but highly toxic nicotinic analgesic

Epibatidine was shown to be a very potent and selective agonistic ligand of nicotinic acetylcholine receptors. This natural product is effective in various animal models of pain through a pronounced nAChR agonistic mechanism (Ki < 100 pm) which is accompanied by severe and nACh-related side-effects (Corey et al. 1993; Rupniak et al., 1994; Boyce et al., 2000). A clear differentiation between antinociceptive activity in animal models of pain and toxic side-effects cannot be determined. Nevertheless there is some activity directed towards the development of epibatidine as an analgesic (Bai et al., 1997).

Structure-activity relationship of epibatidine and structural analogs

Remarkably, there is very little difference between the natural and unnatural enantiomer of epibatidine with respect to their antinociceptive potency in various animal models (Sullivan et al., 1994; Bai et al., 1997).

The *exo* position of the chloropyridine is essential for the antinociceptive potency of epibatidine – its racemic *endo* diastereoisomer is inactive. Also inactive are amides derived from epibatidine through acylation of the secondary amine function (R = C(O)R'). On the other hand the potency of 7-methylepibatidine (R = Me) is comparable to epibatidine itself, so a basic nitrogen but not necessarily a secondary amine is needed for activity (Li et al., 1993).

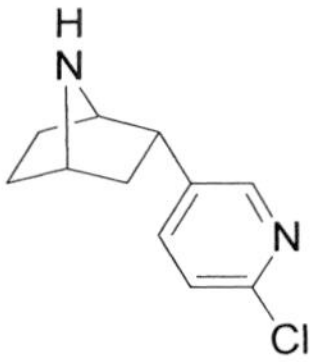

Several attempts have been made to synthesize less toxic and/or more potent epibatidine analogs through the variation of its aromatic moiety. Selected examples are displayed in the following scheme (Badio et al., 1997; Carroll et al., 2001; Che et al., 2001):

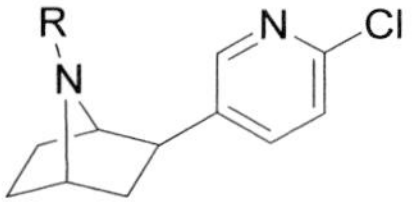

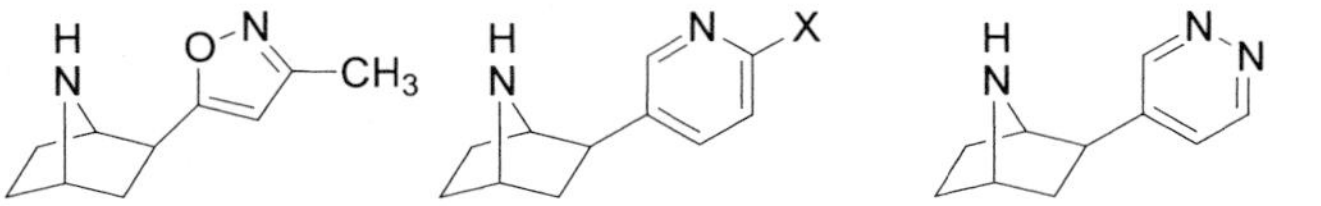

endo-epibatidine

epibatidine derivatives

(±)-eboxidine,   epibatidine derivatives,   epibatidine derivatives,
Badio et al., 1997   Carroll et al., 2001   Che et al., 2001

Figure 4: Variations in the aromatic moiety of epibatidine.

The analogs synthesized by Che et al. (Bayer AG) are reported to be in the preclinical stage directed towards the development of new analgesics (Pharmaprojects No. 31767).

The biochemical properties of epibatidine have been compared to the ring-enlarged 8-azabicyclo[3.2.1]octane derivative homoepibatidine and several 2-azabicyclo-[2.2.1]heptanes (Cox et al., 2001).

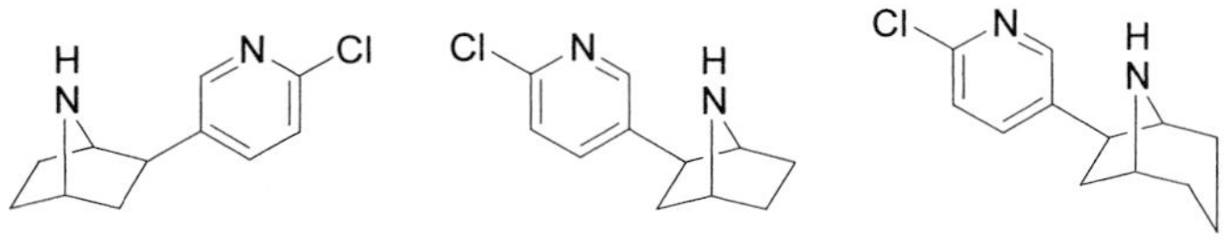

Modifications to the azabicycloalkane skeleton

(+)-epibatidine,   (-)-epibatidine,   (±)-homoepibatidine,
Ki 19 pM   Ki 20 pM   Ki 230 pM

Figure 5: nACh receptor affinities of the epibatidine enantiomers and (±)-homoepibatidine (α2β4 subtype).

exo-Homoepibatidine was found to be only slightly less active than epibatidine itself, but the 2-azabicyclo[2.2.1]-heptane derivatives behave differently: both 5-*exo*- and 6-*exo*-(6-Chloropyridin-3-yl)-2-azabicyclo[2.2.1]heptane are inactive while both *endo*-diastereoisomers are active. This was hypothesized to result from the spatial relationship between the nitrogen atoms.

Biochemical properties of 2-azabicyclo[2.2.1]heptane analogs of epibatidine

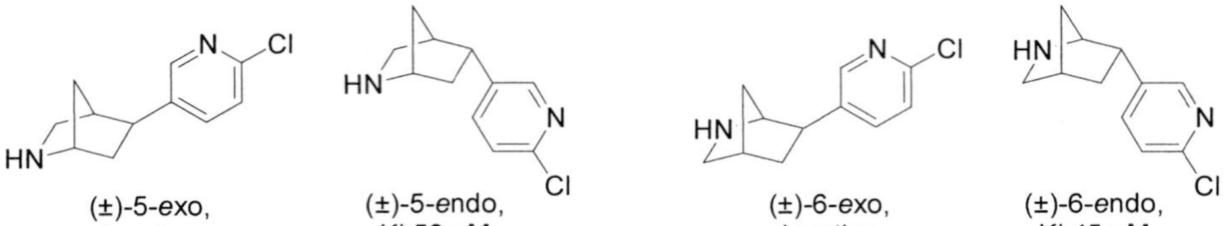

| (±)-5-*exo*, inactive | (±)-5-*endo*, Ki 56 pM | (±)-6-*exo*, inactive | (±)-6-*endo*, Ki 45 pM |

Figure 6: nACh receptor affinities of 5- and 6-(6-Chloropyridin-3-yl)-2-azabicyclo[2.2.1]-heptanes ($\alpha_2\beta_4$ subtype).

ABT-594

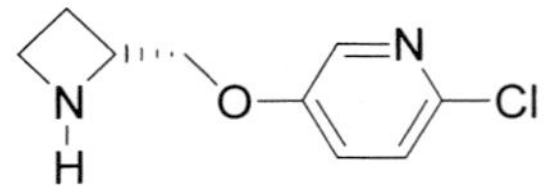

[198283-73-7]; (R)-5-(Azetidin-2-yl-methoxy)-2-chloropyridine, $C_9H_{11}ClN_2O$, M_r 198,65

ABT-594 is reported to be in clinical trials for the treatment of neuropathic pain (Thatte, 2000; Sorbero et al. 2001). Its precursor (R)-N-Boc-azetidin-2-yl-methanol is accessible in a short sequence starting from commercially available D-aspartic acid dibenzyl ester. The synthesis is concluded by Mitsunobu coupling with 6-chloropyridin-3-ol and subsequent acidic deprotection. On a larger scale the primary alcohol is activated as a mesylate prior to coupling with 6-chloropyridin-3-ol in the presence of potassium hydroxide, so that Mitsunobu conditions can be avoided (Meyer et al., 2000).

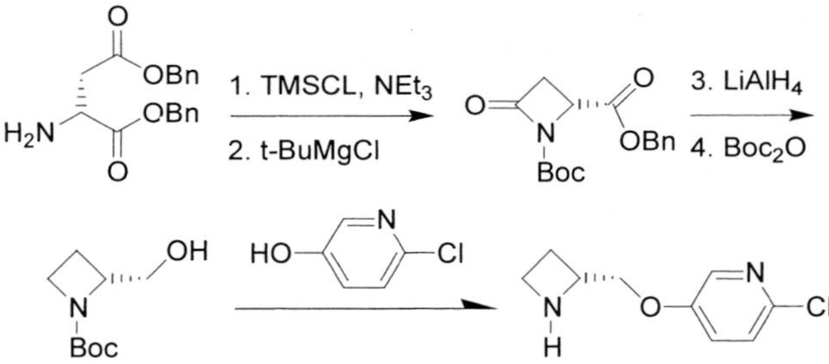

Figure 7: Synthesis of ABT-594.

The properties of ABT-594, the most advanced compound derived from the discovery of epibatidine, are well documented in the literature (Decker et al., 1998; Thatte, 2000). Its antinociceptive potential has been proven in various animal models, but according to Boyce et al. (2001) the side-effect profile of ABT-594 does not represent a significant improvement compared to other potential nicotinic analgesics.

Other Compounds

The race to find nicotinic analgesics has - in a very few years - resulted in a cornucopia of potential clinical candidates. The following scheme is intended to give an overview of the most striking examples:

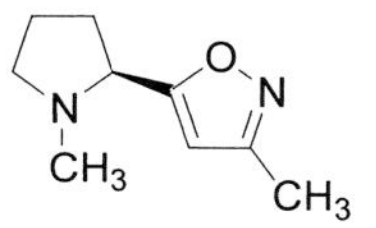
ABT-418

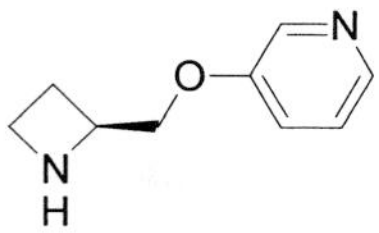
A-85380

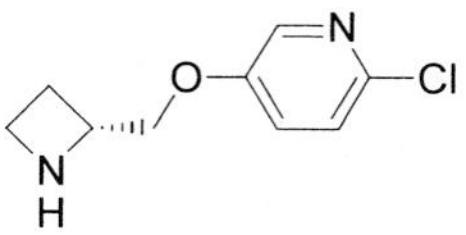
ABT-594,
phase II (pain)

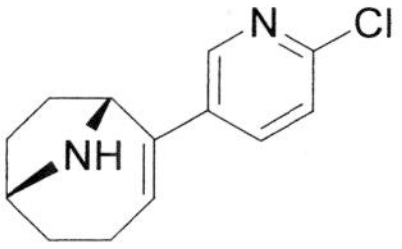
UB-165

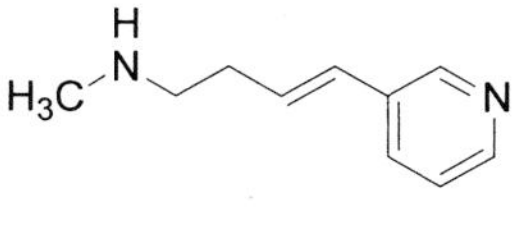
RJR-2403
"metanicotine"

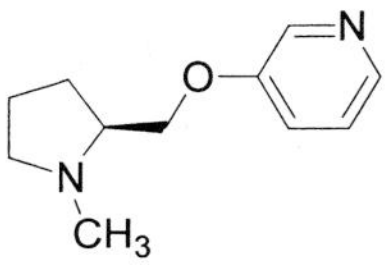
A-84543

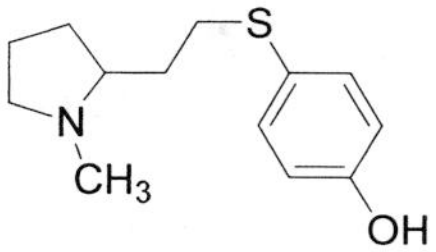
SIB-1553A

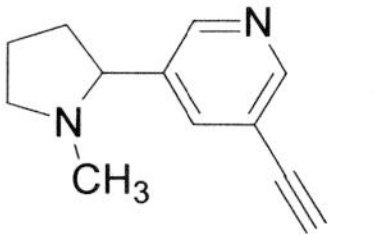
SIB-1785

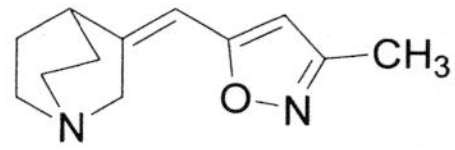
NNC 90-0270

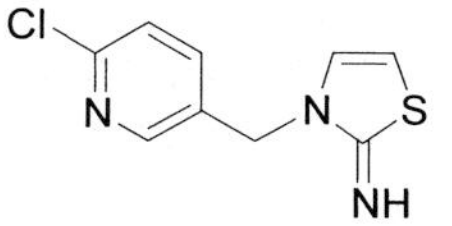
Latli and Casida,
University of California,
WO0170733

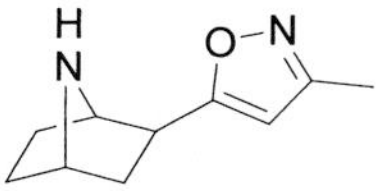
eboxidine,
Badio et al., 1997

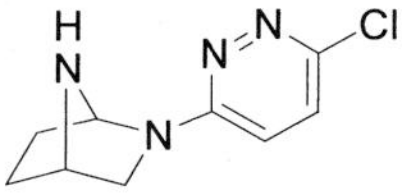
DBO-83

Figure 8: Potential nicotinic analgesics.

Recently disclosed patent applications comprise related structures designated to be nAChR modulators/antagonist. Also recently a patent was granted to Advanced Medicine Inc. covering so-called multibinding compounds for the treatment of pain, consisting of two to 10 covalently bound known nAChR agonists (Natarajan et al. (Advanced Medicine), US6288055 (2001)).

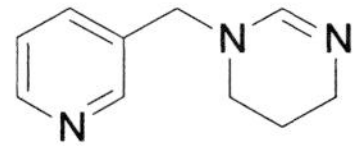
Imoto et al.,
Suntory, WO0181334

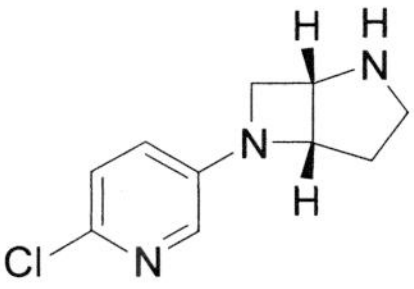
Schrimpf et al.,
Abbott, WO0181347

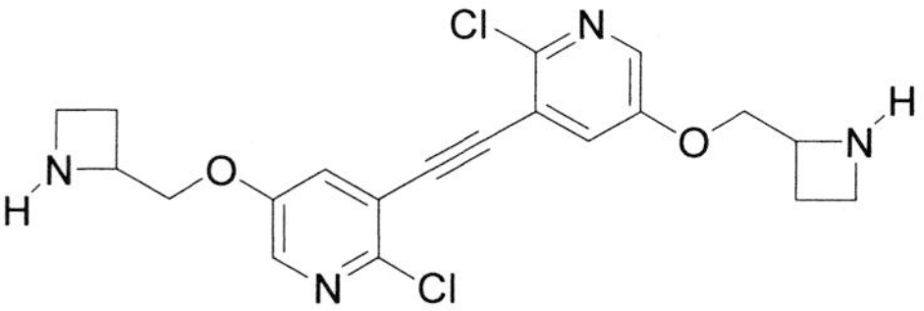
Natarajan, Advanced Medicine Inc., US6288055, 2001

An overview of available biochemical data on more than 20 nACh receptor ligands has recently been published (Sharples and Wonnacott, 2001).

References

Aceto, M. D., Awaya, H., Martin, B. R., May, E. L.: *Antinociceptive action of nicotine and its methoiodide derivatives in mice and rats*, Br. J. Pharmacol. **1983**, *79*, 869-876.

Bai, D., Xu, R., Zhu, X.: *Epibatidine*, Drugs Fut. **1997**, *22*, 1210-1220.

Badio, B., Daly, J. W.: *Epibatidine, a potent analgesic and nicotinic agonist*, Mol. Pharmacol. **1994**, *45*, 563-569.

Badio, B., Shi, D., Garraffo, H. M., Daly, J. W.: *Antinociceptive effects of the alkaloid epibatidine: Further studies on involvement of nicotinic receptors*, Drug Dev. Res. **1995**, *36*, 46-59.

Badio, B., Garraffo, H. M., Plummer, C. V., Padgett, W. L., Daly, J. W.: *Synthesis and nicotinic activity of eboxidine: an isoxazole analogue of epibatidine*, Eur. J. Pharmacol. **1997**, *321*, 189-194.

Bannon, A. W., Decker, M. W., Holladay, M. W., Curzon, P., Donnelly-Roberts, D. L., Puttfarcken, P. S., Bitner, R. S., Diaz, A., Dickenson, A. H., Porsolt, R. D., Williams, M., Arneric, S. P.: *Broad-spectrum, non-opioid analgesic activity by selective modulation of neuronal nicotinic acetylcholine receptors*, Science **1998**, *279*, 77-81.

Boyce, S., Webb, J. K., Shepheard, S. L., Russell, M. G. N., Hill, R. G., Rupniak, N. M. J.: *Analgesic and toxic effects of ABT-594 resemble epibatidine and nicotine in rats*, Pain **2000**, *85*, 443-450.

Carroll, F. I., Liang, F., Navarro, H. A., Brieaddy, L. E., Abraham, P., Damaj, M. I., Martin, B. R.: *Syntheses, nicotinic acetylcholine receptor binding, and antinociceptive properties of 2-exo-2-(2'-Substituted 5-pyridinyl)-7-azabicyclo[2.2.1]heptanes. Epibatidine-analogues*, J. Med. Chem. **2001**, *44*, 2229-2237.

Che, D., Wegge, T., Stubbs, M. T., Seitz, G., Meier, H., Methfessel, C.: *exo-2-(Pyridazin-4-yl)-7-azabicyclo[2.2.1]heptanes: Syntheses and nicotinic acetylcholine receptor agonist activity of potent pyridazine analogues of (±)-epibatidine*, J. Med. Chem. **2001**, *44*, 47-57.

Clementi, F., Fornasari, D., Gotti, C.: *Neuronal nicotinic receptor, important new players in brain function*, Eur. J. Pharmcol. **2000**, *393*, 3-10.

Cordero-Erausquin, M., Marubio, L. M., Changeux, J.-P.: *Nicotinic receptor function: new perspectives from knockout mice*, Trends Pharmacol. Sci. **2000**, *21*, 211-217.

Corey, E. J., Loh, T.-P., Rao, S. A., Daley, D. C., Sarshar, S.: *Stereocontrolled total synthesis of (+)- and (-)-epibatidine.*, J. Org. Chem. **1993**, *58*, 5600-5602.

Cox, C. D., Malpass, J. R., Gordon, J., Rosen, A.: *Synthesis of epibatidine isomers: endo-5- and 6-(6'-chloro-3'-pyridyl-2-azabicyclo[2.2.1]heptanes*, J: Chem. Soc., Perkin Trans. 1 **2001**, 2372-2379.

Daly, J. W.: *Epibatidine*, Alkaloids **1993**, *43*, 255-256.

Daly, J. W., Garraffo, H. M., Meyers, C. W.: *The origin of frog skin alkaloids: an enigma*, Pharmaceut. News **1997**, *4*, 9-14.

Daly, J. W., Garraffo, H. M., Spande, T. F., Decker, M. W., Sullivan, J. P., Williams, M.: *Alkaloids from frog skin: the discovery of epibatidine and the potential for developing novel non-opioid analgesics*, Nat. Prod. Rep. **2000**, *17*, 131-135.

Daly, J. W., Spande, T. F., Garraffo, H. M. (Dept. Health Human Services [USA]): *Epibatidine and derivatives, compositions and methods of treating pain*, US5314899 (**1993**): also see WO9318037, EP629200, JP95505149.

Daly, J. W., Spande, T. F., Garraffo, H. M. (Dept. Health Human Services [USA]): *Epibatidine and derivatives, compositions and methods of treating pain*, US5462956 (**1995**).

Daly, J. W., Tokuyama, T., Fujiwara, T., Highet, R. J., Karle, I. L.: *A new class of indolizidine alkaloids from the poison frog, Dendrobates tricolor. X-ray analysis of 8-hydroxy-8-methyl-6-(2'-methylhexylidene)-1-azabicyclo[4.3.0]nonane*, J. Am. Chem. Soc. **1980**, *102*, 830-836.

Davis, L., Pollock, L. J., Stone, T. T.: *Visceral pain*, Surg. Gynecol. Obstet. **1932**, *55*, 418-426.

Decker, M. W., Meyer, M. D., Sullivan, J. P.: *The therapeutic potential of nicotinic acetylcholine receptor agonists for pain control*, Exp. Opin. Invest. Drugs **2001**, *10*, 1819-1830.

Decker, M. W., Curzon, P., Holladay, M. W., Nikkel, A. L., Bitner, R. S., Bannon, A. W., Donnelly-Roberts, D. L., Puttfarcken, P. S., Kuntzweiler, T. A., Briggs, C. A., Williams, M., Arneric, S. P.: *The role of neuronal nicotinic acetylcholine receptors in antinociception: Effects of ABT-594*, J. Physiol. (Paris) **1998**, *92*, 221-224.

Dehmlow, E. V.: *Epibatidine competition: synthetic work on a novel natural analgetic.*, J. Prakt. Chem. **1995**, *337*, 164-174.

Fletcher, S. R., Baker, R., Chambers, M. S., Herbert, R. H., Hobbs, S. C., Thomas, S. R., Verrier, H. M., Watt, A. P., Ball, R. G.:*Total Synthesis and determination of the absolute configuration of epibatidine*, J. Org. Chem. **1994**, *59*, 1771-1778.

Flores, C. M.: *The promise and pitfalls of nicotinic cholinergic approach to pain management*, Pain **2000**, *88*, 1-6.

Flores, C. M., Hargreaves, K. M.: *Neuronal nicotinic receptors: New targets in the treatment of pain*, in Neuronal nicotinic receptors: Pharmacology and therapeutic opportunities, edited by S. P. Arneric, J. D. Brioni. Wiley-Liss, New York, **1999**, 359-373.

Francis, P.: *RJR-2403*, Curr. Opin. CPNS Drugs **1999**, *1*, 378-382.

Gilbert, S. D., Clark, T. M., Flores, C. M.: *Antihyperalgesic activity of epibatidine in the formalin model of facial pain*, Pain **2001**, *89*, 159-165.

Holladay, M. W., Dart, M. J., Lynch, J. K.: *Neuronal nicotinic acetylcholine receptors as targets for drug discovery*, J. Med. Chem. **1997**, *40*, 4169-4194.

Hucho, F., Weise, C.: *Ligand-gated ion channels*, Angew. Chem. Int. Ed. Engl. **2001**, *40*, 3100-3116.

Imoto, M., Iwanami, T., Akabane, M. (Suntory Ltd.): *Use of cyclic amidine compounds as nicotinic acetylcholine receptor modulators*, WO0181334 (**2001**).

Jones, S., Sudweeks, S., Yakel, J. L.: *Nicotinic receptors in the brain: correlating physiology with function*, Trends Neurosci. **1999**, *22*, 555-561.

Kesingland, A. C., Gentry, C. T., Panesar, M. A., Vernier, J.-M., Cube, R., Walker, K., Urban, L.: *Analgesic profile of the nicotinic acetylcholine receptors agonists, (+)-epibatidine and ABT-594 in models of persistent inflammatory and neuropathic pain*, Pain **2000**, *86*, 113-118.

Khan, I. M., Buerkle, H., Taylor, P., Yaksh, T. L.: *Nociceptive and antinociceptive responses to intrathecally administered nicotinic agonists*, Neuropharmacology **1998**, *37*, 1515-1525.

Khan, I. M., Yaksh, T. L. , Taylor, P.: *Epibatidine binding sites and activity in the spinal cord*, Brain Res. **1997**, *753*, 269-282.

Kowaluk, E. A., Arneric, S. P.: *Novel molecular approaches to analgesia*, Ann. Rep. Med. Chem. **1998**, *33*, 11-20.

Latli, B, Casida, J. E. (University of California): *Di-substituted iminoheterocyclic compounds*, WO0170733 (**2001**).

Lawand, N. B., Lu, Y., Westlund, K. N.: *Nicotinic cholinergic receptors: potential targets for inflammatory pain relief*, Pain **1999**, *80*, 291-299.

Li, T., Qian, C., Eckman, J., Huang, D. F., Shen, T. Y.: *The analgesic effect of epibatidine and isomers*, Bioorg. Med. Chem. Lett. **1993**, *3*, 2759-2764.

Marks, M. J., Smith, K., W., Collins, A., C.: *Differential agonist inhibition identifies multiple epibatidine binding sites in mouse brain*, J. Parmacol. Exp. Ther. **1998**, *285*, 377-386.

Marubio, L. M., del Mar Arroyo-Jimenez, M., Cordero-Erausquin, M., Lena, C., Le Novere, N., de Kerchove d'Exaerde, A., Huchet, M., Damaj, M. I.: *Reduced antinociception in mice lacking neuronal nicotinic receptor subunits*, Nature **1999**, *398*, 805-810.

Meyer, M. D., Anderson, D. J., Campbell, J. E., Carroll, S., Marsh, K. C., Rodrigues, A. D., Decker, M. W.: *Preclinical pharmacology of ABT-594: A nicotinic acetylcholine receptor agonist for the treatment of pain*, CNS Drug Rev. **2000**, *6*, 183-194.

Natarajan, M., Jenkins, T.E., Grifiin, J.H. (Advanced Medicine, Inc.): *Analgesics Agents*, US6288055 (**2001**).

Picciotto, M. R., Caldarone, B. J., King, S. L., Zachariou, V.: *Nicotinic receptors in the brain: Links between molecular biology and behaviour*, Neuropsychopharmacology **2000**, *22*, 451-465.

Qian, C., Li, T., Shen, T. Y., Libertine-Graham, L., Eckman, J., Biftu, T., Ip, S.: *Epibatidine is a nicotinic analgesic*, Eur. J. Pharmacol. **1993**, *250*, R13-R14.

Rao, T. S., Correa, L. D., Reid, R. T., Lloyd, G. K.: *Evaluation of anti-nociceptive effects of neuronal nicotinic acetylcholine receptor (nAChR) ligands in the rat tail-flick assay*, Neuropharmacology **1996**, *35*, 393-405.

Roy, B., Watanabe, H., Kitahara, T.: *Simple synthesis of (±)-epibatidine*, Heterocycles **2001**, *55*, 861-871; see reference 6.

Rupniak, N. M. J., Patel, S. Marwood, R., Webb, J., Traynor, J. R., Elliott, J., Freedman, S. B., Fletcher, S. R., Hill, R. G.: *Antinociceptive and toxic effects of (+)-epibatidine oxalate attributable to nicotinic agonist activity*, Br. J. Pharmacol. **1994**, *113*, 1487-1493.

Sahley, T. L., Berntson, G. G.: *Antinociceptive effects of central and systemic administration of nicotine in the rat*, Psychopharmacology **1979**, *65*, 279-283.

Schrimpf, M.R., Tietje, K.R., Toupence, R.B., Ji, J., Basha, A. (Abbott Laboratories): *New N-substituted diazabicyclic compounds are nicotinic acetylcholine receptor antagonists*, WO0181347 (**2001**).

Sharples, C. G. V., Wonnacott, S.: *Neuronal nicotinic receptors*, Tocris Reviews No. 19 **2001.**

Sorbera, L.A., Revel, L., Leeson, P.A., Castaner, J: *ABT-594*, Drugs Fut. **2001**, *26*, 927-934.

Soreq, H.: *Cholinergic Mechanisms – Tenth International Symposium*, IDrugs **1998**, *1*, 787-793.

Spande, T. F., Garraffo, H. M., Edwards, M. W., Yeh, H. J. C., Pannell, L., Daly, J. W.: *Epibatidine: a novel (chloropyridyl)azabicycloheptane with potent analgesic activity from an Ecuadorian poison frog*, J. Am. Chem. Soc. **1992**, *114*, 3475-3478.

Sullivan, J. P., Bannon, A. W.: *Epibatidine: Pharmacological properties of a novel nicotinic acetylcholine receptor agonist and analgesic agent*, CNS Drug Rev. **1996**, *2*, 21-39.

Sullivan, J. P., Briggs, C. A., Donnelly-Roberts, D., Brioni, J. D., Radek, R. J., McKenna, D. G., Campbell, J. E., Arneric, S. P., Decker, M. W.: *(+)-Epibatidine can differentially evoke responses mediated by putative subtypes of nicotinic acetylcholine receptors (nAChR) ligands in the rat tail-flick assay*, Med. Chem. Res. **1994**, *4*, 502-516.

Thatte, U.: *ABT-594*, Curr. Opin. CPNS Drugs **2000**, *2*, 227-234.

Williams, M., Arneric, S. P.: *Beyond the tobacco debate: dissecting the therapeutic potential of nicotine*, Exp. Opin. Invest. Drugs **1996**, *5*, 1035-1045.

Williams, M., Kowaluk, E. A., Arneric, S. P.: *Emerging molecular approaches to pain therapy*, J. Med. Chem. **1999**, *42*, 1481-1500.

8.2 Muscarinic acetylcholine receptors

Corinna Maul and Bernd Sundermann

Introduction

The neurotransmitter acetylcholine (ACh) binds to two types of cholinergic receptors: the ionotropic family of nicotinic receptors and the metabotropic family of muscarinic receptors. Nicotinic receptors are ligand-gated ion-channels which modulate cell membrane potentials. Muscarinic acetylcholine receptors (mAChRs) belong to the large superfamily of membrane-bound G-protein coupled receptors (GPCRs). Five subtypes of muscarinic receptors (M_1-M_5) have been cloned and sequenced from a variety of mammalian and nonmammalian species. They show a remarkably high degree of sequence similarities across species as well as across receptor subtypes. Like all GPCRs, muscarinic acetylcholine receptors are characterized by seven transmembrane regions connected by intra- and extracellular loops. Between the fifth and sixth transmembrane region muscarinic receptors possess a large intracytoplasmatic loop which is considered to be responsible for G-protein coupling selectivity and which exhibits high divergence between the different subtypes.

Acetylcholine

Muscarine

Nicotine

Receptor Localization

The M_1-M_5 muscarinic receptors are expressed predominantly within the parasympathetic nervous system, which exerts excitatory and inhibitory control over central and peripheral tissues, and participate in a number of physiological functions such as the function of heart and smooth muscles, glandular secretion, release of neurotransmitters, gene expression and cognitive functions such as learning and memory. Availability of molecular probes and receptor subtype-selective antibodies has provided detailed knowledge of receptor distribution. A significant presence in a wide variety of brain regions and peripheral tissues has been described.

Pilocarpine

Muscarinic Agonists and Antagonists

Muscarinic agonists such as muscarine and pilocarpine and antagonists such as atropine, the racemic form of natural hyoscyamine, have been known for more than a century. Only recently more selective ligands have been found that will hopefully generate a better understanding of the role mAChR subtypes in physiological processes and especially brain function.

Atropine

mAChR Subtypes

First pharmacological evidence for the presence of multiple subtypes of muscarinic receptors appeared in the early 1950s and became more evident as differences in tissue responses to various muscarinic ligands were observed. On pharmacological criteria, only four distinct subtypes of muscarinic acetylcholine receptors have been identified by use of selective antagonists.

Genes encoding M_1-M_5 receptors were identified in the mid 1980s (Kubo et al., 1986; Bonner et al., 1987); numbers were assigned in the order of discovery. The M_5 muscarinic receptor gene was the last to be found. It is present in the brain and viscera, but only in very low concentrations. No selective high-affinity ligands or toxins for the M_5 receptor have been found, and no tissues with predominant concentrations of M_5 receptors have been identified (Yeomans et al., 2001).

mACh Receptor Function

mAChR subtypes activate different second messenger transduction systems, with M_1, M_3 and M_5 acting through the phosphoinositol cascade via the α subunits of the G_q family, whereas M_2 and M_4 mainly lower cAMP levels via G_i and $G_{0\alpha}$ (Caulfield and Birdsall, 1998).

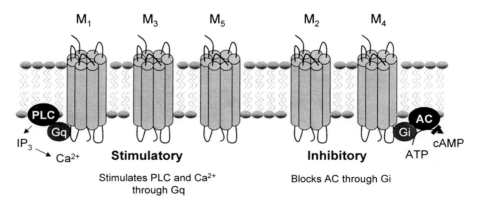

Figure 1: The muscarinic acetylcholine receptor family. IP_3, inositol triphosphate; PLC, phospholipase C; AC, adenylate cyclase (adapted from Felder et al. 2000).

Muscarinic receptors play a key role in many functions in the periphery and the central nervous system. In the periphery, muscarinic receptors are involved in cardiac function, glandular secretion, and smooth muscle contractility. Central muscarinic receptors modulate pain perception, motor control and memory processes (Bymaster et al., 2001).

The psychological effects of muscarinic drugs have been exploited for religious or recreational purposes for a long time (Shulgin, 1982). The recreational use probably requires some deeper interests in psychedelics - there seems to be a general consensus that the effects are not purely pleasurable.

Abuse of muscarinics

Natural Muscarinics

Many of the earliest known ligands for muscarinic acetylcholine receptors were of natural origin, typically from plants such as deadly nightshade, thorn apple and tobacco, which is particularly rich in muscarinic toxins such as the closely related antagonists atropine (see above), scopolamine (see below) and hyoscyamine. Other natural muscarinic acetylcholine receptor ligands are toxins from snakes, particularly mambas, which are selective for M_1, M_2 and M_4 receptors. They consist of 63 to 66 amino acids and four disulfide bridges which form loops. They are members of a large group of snake toxins which are called three-finger toxins: three loops are extended like the middle fingers of a hand, and the disulfides and the shortest loop are in the palm of the hand. For example M_1-toxin1, isolated from the venom of the East African green mamba, is highly specific for M_1 receptors and binds irreversibly to it. It appears to be completely specific for M_1 receptors and is one of the most specific ligands ever found for any target protein (Potter, 2001). A possible explanation for the good selectivity is that the toxins bind to an allosteric site, but because of their size they probably also bind to extracellular parts of the receptors which are rather different in the various subtypes (Karlsson, 2000).

Hyoscyamine

Snake toxins are potent (irreversible) muscarinic ligands

Muscarinics in Clinical Use

A number of muscarinic agonists and antagonists are launched or in clinical trials, especially as antiemetics (e.g. scopolamine), as treatment for urinary incontinence (e.g. tolterodine), glaucoma (pilocarpine), and airway diseases (e.g. ipratropium bromide), but, to the best of our knowledge, only few are used as adiuvants in analgesic compositions, e.g. tiemonium iodide which is used in various combinations with analgesics like paracetamol or metamizole (Coffalon®, Viscéralgine®).

Tiemonium iodide used as an adiuvant in analgesic compositions (Labrid et al., 1976)

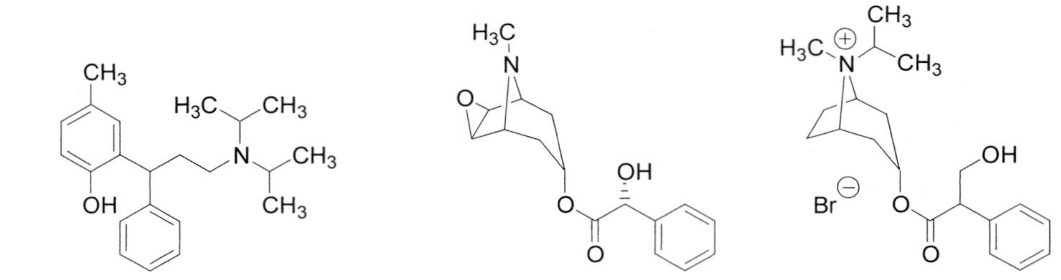

Tolterodine, muscarinic
antagonist, launched for
the treatment of urinary incontinence
(Crandall, 2001; Nilvebrant, 2001)

Scopolamine, muscarinic
antagonist, used clinically
as an antispasmodic,
antiemetic drug (Kovac, 2000)

Ipratropium bromide,
bronchodilator
(Disse, 2001)

Figure 2: Muscarinics drugs.

Potential Use of Subtype Selective mAChR Agonists and Antagonists

In the last couple of years, subtype-selective ligands of mAChRs were investigated for further therapeutic areas: M_1 (M_3) agonists as well as M_2 antagonists attracted interest in the treatment of Alzheimer's disease (Davis et al., 1995), which is accompanied by a shortage of acetylcholine and therefore an understimulation of muscarinic receptors (Zlotos et al., 1999; Lachowicz et al., 2001; Wienrich et al., 2001). For subtype-selective antagonists, the treatment of peripheral smooth muscle disorders such as bladder, airway and bowel disorders with M_3 antagonists has been of particular interest, while antagonists of M_2 and M_4 receptors have been suggested as treatments for movement disorders (Salamone et al., 2001), dementia, cardiac disorders, and pain (Felder et al., 2000).

Analgesic potential of mAChR modulators

Acetylcholine is generally considered to be an algogenic agent because it has been shown to produce burning pain when applied to human skin. Nonetheless, it is still unknown whether ACh appears in inflammatory exudates or under other painful conditions, but possible extraneuronal sources of ACh in the close vicinity of primary afferent terminals have been identified. In the cornal epithelial cells for example, high concentrations of ACh have been found that may be released after injury, and ACh has been shown to excite corneal nerve endings. Furthermore it has been shown that human keratinocytes are able to synthesize and secrete ACh. Here ACh plays a role in regulating cell-cell attachment, but in addition it may be released in larger amounts after cutaneous injury. Moreover, the ability of dorsal root ganglia (DRG) to synthesize ACh has been reported (Tata et al., 1994).

An electrophysiological study has shown that muscarine treatment of C-units left them with a marked and sustained desensitization to mechanical and heat stimuli (Bernadini et al., 2001). The mechanical desensitization is in agreement with preceeding results where the ACh analog carbachol was shown to excite C-nociceptors and at the same time produced desensitization to mechanical stimulation lasting up to 45 minutes (Steen and Reeh, 1993).

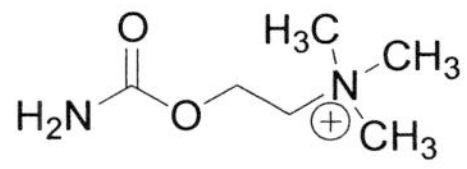

Carbachol

Furthermore, it is well documented that mAChRs are involved in the modulation of central nociception (see Yaksh et al., 1985, Hartvig et al., 1989, Bartolini et al., 1992):

Modulation of central nociception through mAChRs

Centrally administered acetylcholine has been found to cause antinociception, which was proposed to depend on the activation of descending pathways (Hartvig et al., 1989). M_1 as well as M_3 muscarinic receptors have been shown to play an essential role in the modulation of pain perception (Naguib and Yaksh, 1997). Cholinergic antinociception induced both directly, through muscarinic agonists, and indirectly, by enhancing extracellular ACh levels through cholinesterase inhibitors, is prevented, in a dose-related manner, by i.c.v. administration of antisense DNA to the M_1 gene coding for the mouse M_1 receptor (Ghelardini et al., 2000). On the other hand, studies using muscarinic agonists lacking M_1 agonistic activity in tissues and M_1 cell lines showed that M_1 agonistic activity is not required for antinociception (Sheardown et al., 1997).

Muscarinic agonists and pain - M_1 and M_3 receptors

Experiments with muscarinic M_2 and M_4 knock-out mice indicate a crucial role of especially M_2 receptors in mediating antinociception. Analgesic activity of oxotremorine, an unselective muscarinic agonist, was reduced significantly when administered to M_2 knock-out mice (tail-flick, hot plate). However, oxotremorine-induced analgesia was not completely abolished in M_2 -/- mice indicating that the M_2 receptor is not the only muscarinic receptor subtype involved in 'muscarinic analgesia' (Gomeza et al., 2001). In another study it was shown by antagonization with a specific toxin that antinociception induced by muscarinic agonists, e.g. CMI-936 derived from epibatidine (see nAChRs), is mediated via muscarinic M_4 receptors (Ellis et al., 1999). The following figure shows muscarinic agonists with antinociceptive properties. Among others, the compounds arecoline, aceclidine, xanomyeline, and oxotremorine are active in the tail-flick, hot plate, writhing, and grid-shock assay (Sheardown et al., 1997):

Muscarinic agonists and pain - M_2 and M_4

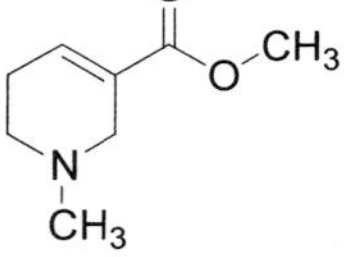

Arecoline 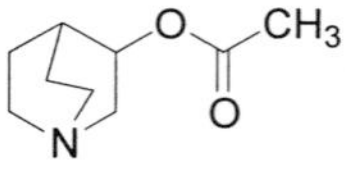   Aceclidine 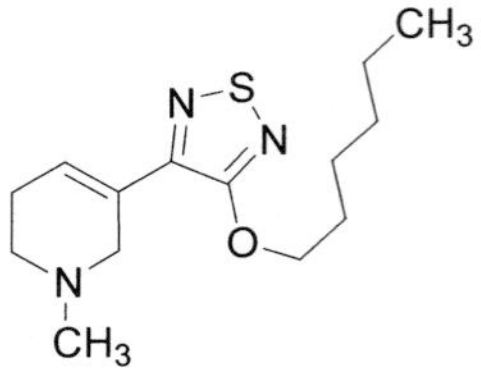   Xanomeline 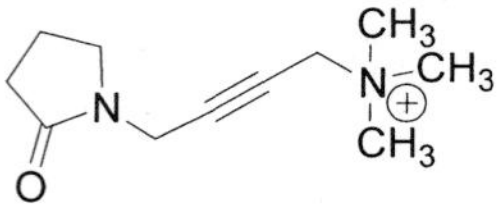   Oxotremorine

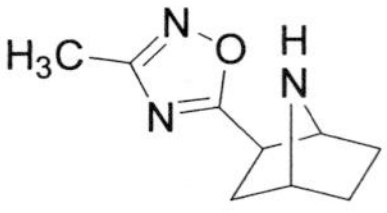

CMI-936
(Ellis et al., 1999)

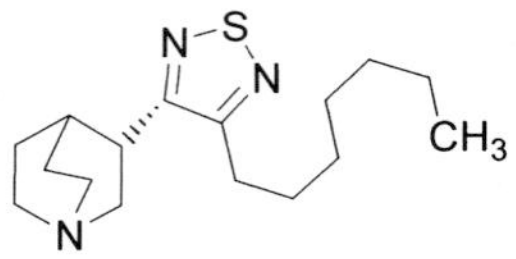

LY297802, agonist at M_1, partial agonist/antagonist
at M_2/M_3, equiefficacious to morphine in producing
antinociception in animals (Shannon et al., 1997)

Figure 3: Muscarinic agonists with antinociceptive properties.

Muscarinic antagonists and pain

On the other hand, investigations on the antinociceptive effects of muscarinic antagonists, namely pirenzepine (M_1), AF-DX116 (M_2) and 4-DAMP (M_3), showed that the M_3 antagonist can inhibit the second phase of formalin-induced nociception (Honda et al., 2000).

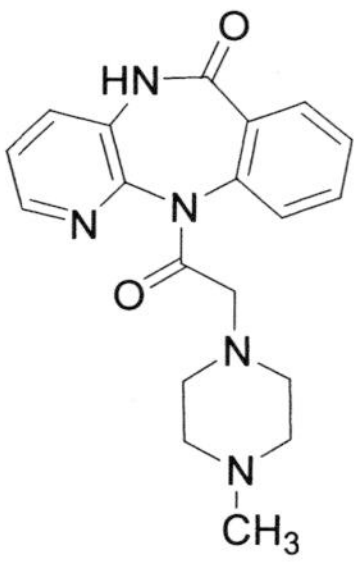

Pirenzepine
M_1 muscarinic receptor
antagonist

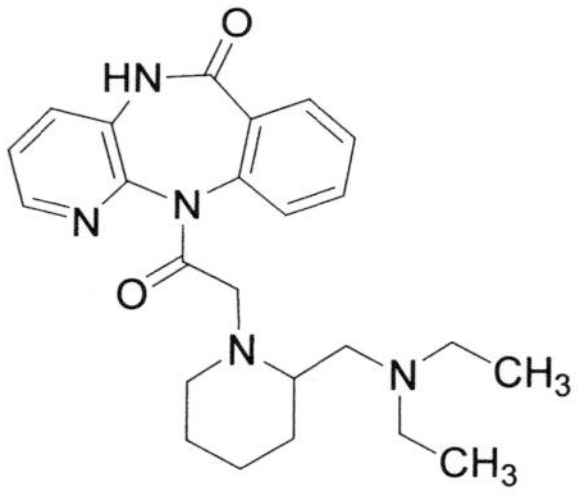

AF-DX 116
M_2 muscarinic receptor
antagonist

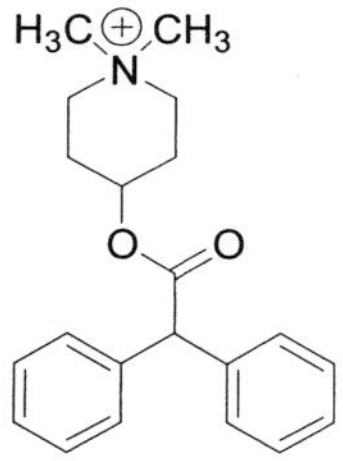

4-DAMP
M_3 muscarinic receptor
antagonist

Potential use of allosteric modulators

A further possibility for affecting muscarinic receptors are allosteric modulators. They act at a site apart from the common binding site of the receptor protein. Depending on the allosteric modulator, the type of ligand and the receptor subtype, ligand binding can be elevated, reduced or remain unchanged. Used as enhancers of acetylcholine action, allosteric modulators might be benificial for the treatment of pain (Holzgrabe and Mohr, 1998).

Outlook

Although serious efforts have been directed towards the discovery of muscarinic acetylcholine receptor modulators, to the best of our knowledge the promising results concerning antinociceptive properties, especially of muscarinic agonists, in animal models have not led to a marketed drug by now. During the last years only few patent applications on muscarinic modulators have been filed for the treatment of pain. A selection is given in the following figure:

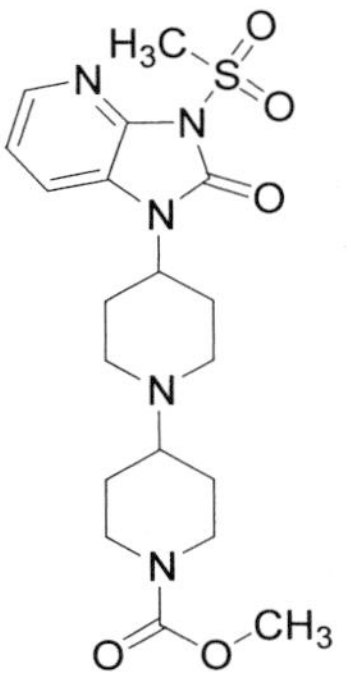

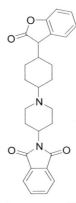

Yamawaka et al., Banyu,
M_4 agonist, WO0127104

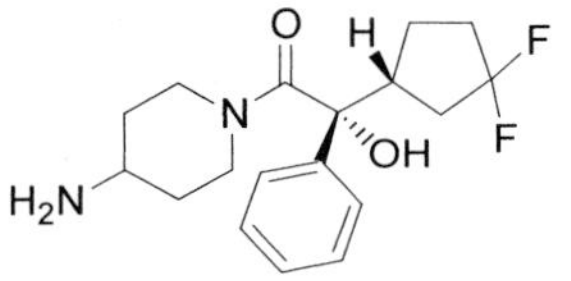

Tsuchiya et al., Banyu, M_3 antagonist,
useful in pain accompanied by smooth
muscle twitch of digestive organs,
WO9940070

Dantanarayana, Alcon,
muscarinic modulator, WO9932479

References

Bartolini, A., Ghelardini, C., Fantetti, L., Malcangio, M., Malmberg-Aiello, P., Giotti, A..: *Role of muscarinic receptor subtypes in central antinociception*, Br. J. Pharmacol. **1992**, *105*, 77-82.

Bonner, T.I., Buckley, N. J., Young, A. C., Brann, M. R.: *Identification of a family of muscarinic acetylcholine receptor genes*, Science **1987**, *237*, 527-532.

Bernardini, N., Sauer, S. K., Haberberger, R., Fischer, M. J. M., Reeh, P. W.: *Excitatory nicotinic and desensitizing muscarinic (M_2) effects on C-nociceptors in isolated rat skin*, J. Neurosci. **2001**, *21*, 3295-3302.

Caulfield, M. P. and Birdsall, N. G. M.: *International union pharmacology XVII. Classification of muscarinic acetylcholine receptors*, Pharmacol. Rev. **1998**, *50*, 279-290.

Crandall, C.: *Tolterodine: a clinical review*, J. Womens Health Gend. Based Med. **2001**, *10*, 735-743.

Dantanarayana, A. (Alcon Laboratories, Inc.): *Phtalimide-piperidine, -pyrrolidine and -azepine derivatives, their preparation and their use as muscarinic receptor (ant)agonists*, WO9932479 (**1999**).

Davis, R. E., Doyle, P. D., Carroll, R. T., Emmerling, M. R., Jaen, J.: *Cholinergic therapies for Alzheimer's disease*, Arzneim.-Forsch./Drug Res. **1995**, *45*, 425-431.

Disse, B.: *Antimuscarinic treatment for lung diseases. From research to clinical practice*, Life Sci. **2001**, *68*, 2557-2564.

Ellis, J. L., Harman, D., Gonzalez, J., Spera, M. L., Liu, R., Shen, T. Y., Wipij, D. M., Zuo, F.: *Development of muscarinic analgesics derived from epibatidine: role of the M_4 receptor subtype*, J. Pharmacol. Exp. Ther. **1999**, *288*, 1143-1150.

Felder, C. C., Bymaster, F. P., Ward, J., DeLapp, N.: *Therapeutic opportunities for muscarinic receptors in the central nervous system*, J. Med. Chem. **2000**, *43*, 4333-4353.

Ghelardini, C., Galeotti, N., Bartolini, A.: *Loss of muscarinic antinociception by antisense inhibition of M_1 receptors*, Br. J. Pharmacol. **2000**, *129*, 1633-1640.

Gomeza, J., Zhang, L., Kostenis, E., Felder, C.C., Bymaster, F.P., Brodkin, J., Shannon, H., Xia, B., Duttaroy, A., Heng, C.-X., Wess, J.; *Generation and pharmacological analysis of M_2 and M_4 muscarinic receptor knockout mice*, Life Sci. **2001**, *68*, 2457-2466.

Hartvig, P., Gillberg, P. G., Gordh, T., Post, C.: *Cholinergic mechanisms in pain and analgesia*, Trends Pharmacol. Sci. **1989**, *10*, suppl., 75-79.

Honda, K., Harada, A., Takano, Y., Kamiya, H.: *Involvement of M_3 muscarinic receptors of the spinal cord in formalin-induced nociception in mice*, Brain Res. **2000**, *859*, 38-44.

Karlsson, E., Jolkkonen, M., Mulugeta, E., Onali, P., Adem, A.: *Snake toxins with high selectivity for subtypes of muscarinin acetylcholine receptors*, Biochimie **2000**, *82*, 793-806.

Kovac, A.L.: *Prevention and treatment of postoperative nausea and vomiting*, Drugs **2000**, *59*, 213-243.

Kubo, T., Fukuda, K., Mikami, A., Maeda, A., Takahashi, H., Mishina, M., Haga, T., Haga, K., Ichiyama, A., Kangawa, K.: *Cloning, sequencing, and expression of complementary DNA encoding the muscarinic acetylcholine receptor*, Nature **1986**, *323*, 411-416.

Labrid, C., Dureng, G., Bert, H., Duchene-Malluraz, P.: *Different membrane mechanisms of action for tiemonium; a comparison with atropine and papaverine*, Arch. Int. Pharmacodyn. Ther. **1976**, *223*, 231-245.

Lachowicz, J. E., Duffy, R. A., Ruperto, V., Kozlowski, J., Zhou, G., Clader, J., Billard, W., Binch, H., Crosby, G., Cohen-Williams, M., Strader, C. D., Coffin, V.: *Facilitation of acetylcholine release and improvement in cognition by a selective M_2 muscarinic antagonist, SCH 72788*, Life Sci. **2001**, *68*, 2585-2592.

Nilvebrant, L.: *Clinical experiences with tolterodine*, Life Sci. **2001**, *68*, 2549-2556.

Naguib, M. and Yaksh, T.L.: *Characterization of muscarinic receptor subtypes that mediate antinociception in the rat spinal cord*, Anesth. Analg. **1997**, *85*, 847-853.

Potter, L.T.: *Snake toxins that bind specifically to individual subtypes of muscarinic receptors*, Life Sci. **2001**, *68*, 2541-2547.

Shannon, H. E., Sheardown, M. J., Bymaster, F. P., Calligaro, D. O., Delapp, N. W., Gidda, J., Mitch, C. H., Sawyer, B. D., Stengel, P. W., Ward, J. S., Wong, D. T., Olesen, P. H., Suzdak, P. D., Sauerberg, P., Swedberg, M. D. B.: *Pharmacology of Butylthio[2.2.2] (LY297802/NNC11-1053): A novel analgesic with mixed muscarinic receptor agonist and antagonist activity*, J. Pharmacol. Exp. Ther. **1997**, *281*, 884-894.

Shulgin, A. T.: *Chemistry of psychomimetics*, in Handbook of Experimental Pharmacology, vol. 55/III, **1982**, edited by F. Hoffmeister and G. Stille, Springer-Verlag, Berlin.

Salamone, J. D., Correa, M., Carlson, B. B., Wisniecki, A., Mayorga, A. J., Nisenbaum, E., Nisenbaum, L., Felder, C.: *Neostriatal muscarinic receptor subtypes involved in the generation of tremulous jaw movements in rodents. Implications for cholinergic involvement in Parkinsonism*, Life Sci. **2001**, *68*, 2579-2584.

Sheardown, M. J., Shannon, H. E., Swedberg, M. D. B., Suzdak, P. D., Bymaster, F. P., Olesen, P. H., Mitch, C. H., Ward, J. S., Sauerberg, P.: *M_1 receptor agonist activity is not a requirement for muscarinic antinociception*, J. Pharmacol. Exp. Ther. **1997**, *281*, 868-875.

Steen, K. H. and Reeh, P. W.: *Actions of cholinergic agonists on sensory nerve endings in rat skin, in vitro*, J. Neurophysiol. **1993**, *70*, 397-405.

Tata, A. M., Plateroti, M., Cibati, M., Biagioni, S., Augusti-Tocco, G.: *Cholinergic markers are expressed in developing and mature neurons of chick dorsal root ganglia*, J. Neurosci. Res. **1994**, *37*, 247-255.

Tsuchiya, Y., Nomoto, T., Ohsawa, H., Kawakami, K., Ohwaki, K., Nishikibe, M. (Banyu Pharmaceutical Co.): *Preparation of N-acyl cyclic amine derivatives as selective antagonists of muscarine M_3 receptor*, WO9940070 (**1999**).

Wienrich, M., Meier, D., Ensinger, H.A., Gaida, W., Raschig, A., Walland, A., Hammer, R.: *Pharmacodynamic profile of the M_1 agonist talsaclidine in animals and man*, Life Sci. **2001**, *68*, 2593-2600.

Yaksh, T. L., Dirksen, R., Harty, G. J.: *Antinociceptive effects of intrathecally injected cholinomimetic drugs in the rat and cat*, Eur. J. Pharmacol. **1985**, *117*, 81-88.

Yamakawa, T., Ando, M.; Koito, S., Ohwaki, K., Kimura, T., Saeki, T., Miyaji, M., Iwahori, Y., Fujikawa, T., Otake, N., Noguchi, K. (Banyu Pharmaceutical Co.): *Preparation of substituted imidazolidinone derivatives as agonists of muscarinic acetylcholine receptor M4*, WO0127104 (**2001**).

Yeomans, J., Forster, G., Blaha, C.: *M_5 muscarinic receptors are needed for slow activation of dopamine neurons and for rewarding brain stimulation*, Life Sci. **2001**, *68*, 2449-2456.

Zlotos, D. P., Bender, U., Holzgrabe, U.: *Muscarinic receptor agonists and antagonists*, Exp. Opin. Ther. Patents **1999**, *9*, 1029-1053.

9 Further Opioid Receptors[1]

9.1 The δ Opioid Receptor

Claudia Pütz

Introduction

Among the variety of pharmacological effects related to the activation of the opioid system the ability of opioids to relieve pain for centuries was considered to be the most relevant clinical aspect. Drugs selectively activating μ receptors are well known to be potent analgesics and still represent the gold standard for the treatment of a variety of pain conditions. The clinical utility of these drugs is, however, limited by undesirable side effects including respiratory depression, constipation and physical dependence (Zenz and Willweber-Strumpf, 1993; Dondio et al., 1997). In the search for potent and safe analgesics to replace the existing μ agonists a great deal of research effort has been dedicated to the discovery of drugs selective for the δ opioid receptor (Dondio et al., 1997, 1999).

The existence of the δ opioid receptor was first demonstrated by Lord, Waterfield, Hughes and Kosterlitz in 1977 (Lord et al., 1977). Their experiments, which showed a differential rank order of potency between morphine alkaloids and the opioid peptides Leu-enkephalin, Met-enkephalin (Hughes, 1975) and β-endorphin in bioassays on guinea pig ileum (GPI) and mouse vas deferens (MVD), led them to postulate that the peptides acted at the δ opioid receptors in the mouse vas deferens and μ opioid receptors in the guinea pig ileum. This receptor differentiation was supported by studies showing that approximately 10 times as much of the opioid antagonist naloxone was needed to antagonize actions at the δ opioid receptor compared with the μ opioid receptor. However, naloxone is a rather nonselective antagonist, so the synthesis of the δ opioid receptor selective antagonist naltrindole (NTI, see below) spawned the hope that pharmacologists would uncover the secrets of the δ opioid receptor and perhaps allow an assignment of different opiate effects to the activation of different opioid receptor types.

Discovery of the δ opioid receptor

H-Tyr-Gly-Gly-Phe-X
Leu-enkephalin: X = Leu
Met-enkephalin: X = Met

---

[1] The so far unsuccessful attempts towards the development of selective κ-opioid agonists are summarised in Chapter 3.1. Clinically relevant opioids with affinity to the κ-opioid receptor are discussed in Chapter 3.4.

Cloning of the δ receptor

Attempts to clone opioid receptors failed for a long time due to the paucity of their mRNAs in brain tissues and the lack of an appropriate cloning strategy. Two groups (Evans et al., 1992; Kieffer et al., 1992) simultaneously used very similar expression cloning strategies to identify the δ receptor gene. The advent of a powerful expression cloning method in mammalian cells allowed both groups to succeed in cloning the mouse δ opioid receptor from the mouse neuroblastoma/rat glioma hybrid cell NG108-15.

The δ receptor belongs to the GPCR superfamily

The δ opioid receptor sequence comprises 372 amino acids with seven putative transmembrane domains. The δ receptor belongs to the GPCR superfamily. The alignment of mouse, rat and human δ opioid receptor sequences shows highly homologous sequences among these species (Knapp et al., 1994; Jin et al., 1999).

Receptor distribution

The distribution of δ receptors appears to be best conserved across mammalian species. δ Receptors are most densely distributed in forebrain structures and sparse to non-existent in most midbrain and brainstem areas. This relationship is particularly evident in the nigrostriatal system where moderate to dense δ receptor binding is observed in the caudate-putamen of the rat, guinea pig, hamster, and monkey (Yaksh et al., 1997).

Evidence for two δ receptor subtypes

The availability of a number of potent and selective δ ligands, agonists and antagonists, gave great impact to the investigation of δ opioid receptor pharmacology. A wide array of pharmacological evidence supports the existence of two subtypes within the δ receptor class.

DPDPE
H-Tyr-D-Pen-Gly-Phe-D-Pen-OH
[D-Pen^2,D-Pen^5]enkephalin

Studies on the antinociceptive effects of various highly selective peptidic δ agonists, particularly [D-Pen^2,D-Pen^5]enkephalin (DPDPE) (Mosberg et al., 1983) and [D-Ala^2,Glu^4]deltorphin, sometimes referred to as deltorphin II (Erspamer et al., 1989; Kreil et al., 1989; Jiang et al., 1990; Lazarus et al., 1999) and the distinct reversal of their action by the two nonequilibrium δ-opioid antagonists [D-Ala^2,Leu^5,Cys^6]enkephalin (DALCE) (Bowen et al., 1987) and naltrindole-5′-isothiocyanate (5′NTII) or by the reversible antagonists 7-benzylidenenaltrexone (BNTX) and naltriben (NTB), have provided the basis for the δ receptor subtypes δ$_1$ and δ$_2$. Further studies on cross-tolerance, electrophysiological recordings and measurements of adenylate cyclase activity in brain tissues strengthened the hypothesis of a δ$_1$ receptor that would be preferentially activated by DPDPE and blocked by BNTX, and a δ$_2$ receptor that responds to deltorphin II and is inhibited by NTB (Jiang et al., 1991; Sofuoglu et al., 1991).

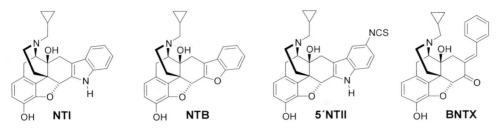

Figure 1: Non-peptidic tool compounds for the δ opioid receptor (antagonists).

While *in vivo* data supports the existence of δ receptor subtypes, the results from radioligand binding studies have generally been less conclusive. The possibility of a single receptor with two affinity states cannot be excluded (Negri et al., 1991; Xu et al., 1991; Fang et al., 1994). Furthermore, only a single molecular form of the δ receptor has been isolated so far. Based upon binding and adenylate cyclase inhibition experiments with the cloned receptor, the latter seems to represent the δ_2 subtype. Another line of evidence based on antisense oligonucleotide experiments again supports the hypothesis that the cloned δ opioid receptor corresponds to that classified pharmacologically as δ_2 (Hul et al., 1994; Zaki et al., 1996).

> Antisense oligonucleotide experiments supports the hypothesis that the cloned δ opioid receptor corresponds to the subtypes classified pharmacologically as δ_2

An additional aspect of the pharmacology of δ opioid receptor ligands has been referred to as a modulatory action on the effects of μ opioid receptor agonists such as morphine (Heyman et al., 1986, 1989; Porreca et al., 1992) in a variety of endpoints, including antinociception in mice and rats. Porreca and coworkers, using the mouse tail-immersion test, have confirmed that δ receptor agonists at sub-antinociceptive doses increase antinociceptive responses to μ opioid receptor agonists. Thus administration of the selective δ agonist DPDPE, at a dose that produces no antinociception, potentiates the analgesic activity of i.c.v. morphine (Porreca et al., 1992).

> δ opioid receptor ligands modulatate the effects of μ opioid receptor agonists

Biphalin

> Biphalin - one of the most potent opioids

The peptide biphalin, a dimeric enkephalin analog, shows equal affinity for both μ and δ receptors. Biphalin is bioactive and crosses the blood brain barrier but is not very stable. Biphalin has been shown to be one of the most potent opioids ever identified in eliciting antinociception after central administration in the mouse: its potency in the tail flick test was almost seven times greater than that of i.c.v. etorphine, at least two orders of magnitude greater than that of i.c.v. carfentanyl, sufentanyl or fentanyl, and three orders of magnitude greater than the antinociceptive potency of i.c.v. morphine or alfentanyl. Nevertheless, after i.t. administration it only produces a 60% maximal antinociceptive effect in the tail flick test, even at doses three orders of magnitude higher than those effective i.c.v., suggesting that it may in part act on the putative opioid receptor complex of physically or functionally interacting μ and δ opioid receptors (Horan et al., 1993).

Potential Clinical Applications of δ Opioid Agonists

Furthermore, studies with agonists at the δ opioid receptor uncovered that the δ opioid system is involved in many biological processes, and thus δ opioid based medications may have great therapeutic potential for the treatment of a variety of disorders (Coop and Rice, 2000).

- respiratory disorders

Those related to the respiratory apparatus are of special interest: DPDPE causes a dose dependent increase in foetal respiratory activity which was blocked by administration of naloxone (Cheng et al., 1992). These stimulatory effects of selective δ agonists may be of clinical value in treating respiratory disorders such as apnoea.

- gastrointestinal disorders

I.c.v. and i.t. administration of the δ opioid agonist deltorphin II in rodents inhibits diarrhea and colonic bead expulsion in a dose-dependent manner but does not delay small intestine transit time. δ agonists have been found to mediate mainly antisecretory effects and influence gut motility only marginally. These effects can be antagonized by pretreatment with NTI (Shook et al.1989).

- immunological disorders

DPDPE has been found to have marked *in vitro* immunostimulant activity in patients suffering from leprosy and tuberculosis, enhancing antigen-stimulated proliferation of peripheral blood mononuclear cells and T-cell rosetting. DPDPE has been found to enhance cytokine production by T-helper cells, IL-6 production by macrophages and NK cell activity in murine splenocytes, suggesting immunostimulatory activity at low *in vitro* concentrations (Mazumder et al., 1993; House et al., 1996; Rogers et al., 2000).

I.c.v. administration of DPDPE results in inhibition of spontaneous bladder contraction in the rat (Tsushima et al., 1993).

- urinary incontinence

In mice DPDPE enhances the hypoxic conditioning-induced increase in survival time. Furthermore, DPDPE also increases survival time in naive mice, independent of hypoxic conditioning. This effect can be blocked by BNTX but not by NTI, indicating that the mechanism of acute hypoxic adaptation involves an endogenous δ_1 opioid pathway. δ agonists therefore can be considered as promising therapeutic agents to reduce the morbidity and mortality associated with clinical hypoxia in settings such as drowning, head injury, apnoea and complicated childbirths. The mechanism of neuroprotection induced by activation of the δ opioid receptors seems to involve decreasing body temperature, thereby mimicking the natural acute adaptation to hypoxia (Kalivas and Stewart, 1991; Suzuki et al., 1994).

- hypoxia

Selective δ agonists have been shown to exert potent cardioprotective effects in intact animals and cardiac myocytes via activation of $G_{i/o}$ proteins, protein kinase C, and ultimately the mitochondrial K_{ATP} channel (Warltier et al., 2000; Schultz et al., 2001).

- cardioprotective effects

In addition to their use as pharmacological tools, selective δ opioid antagonists may have clinical potential in the treatment of a variety of disorders where endogenous opioids play a modulatory role, e.g. disorders of food intake, shock, constipation, mental disorders, CNS injury, alcoholism, drug addiction and immune function (Spetea et al., 2001). It is also worth mentioning that δ antagonists have been shown to possess an antitussive effects in rodents, thus indicating another possible clinical application for these compounds (Kamei et al., 1994).

Potential clinical applications of δ opioid antagonists

The development of acute tolerance and dependence evoked in mice by morphine can be suppressed by pretreatment with NTI. Multiple administration of either NTI or 5′NTII before and during chronic implantation with morphine pellets also substantially inhibits the development of morphine tolerance and dependence. These results suggest the use of δ antagonists to be useful for the prevention of opioid tolerance and physical dependence without compromising the antinociceptive potency of μ opioid receptor agonists (Abdelhamid et al., 1991).

Prevention of μ-opioid tolerance and physical dependence by δ antagonists

Non-peptide δ ligands

Following a flurry of medicinal chemistry activity in the late 1980s, a number of non-peptide pharmacological tools selective for the δ opioid receptors, became available to challenge the pre-eminent position occupied by the existing peptide δ ligands. The first non-peptide δ antagonist NTI represented a breakthrough in this field that was followed by the discovery of several selective δ agonists - TAN-67, BW373U86 and SNC80 (Scheideler, 2000).

Rational design of non-peptide δ opioid ligands - the message address concept

Essential progress for the discovery of non-peptide δ ligands came from rational design: the message address concept proposed by Schwyzer in 1977 that subsequently was re-elaborated by Portoghese (Portoghese et al., 1988). This concept attributes the role of the opiate message to the N-terminal Tyr[1] present in the endogenous peptide δ ligands Leu-enkephalin and Met-enkephalin (Tyr-Gly-Gly-Phe-X), whereas the δ address resides in the amino acid sequence starting from Phe-Leu or Phe-Met respectively. The Gly-Gly sequence is interpreted as a spacer maintaining an adequate distance between Tyr and Phe. Based on this rationale, the first non-peptide selective δ opioid ligand naltrindole (NTI) was discovered (Portoghese et al., 1988).

NTI shows subnanomolar affinity for the δ opioid receptor along with a very potent antagonistic activity in the mouse vas deferens

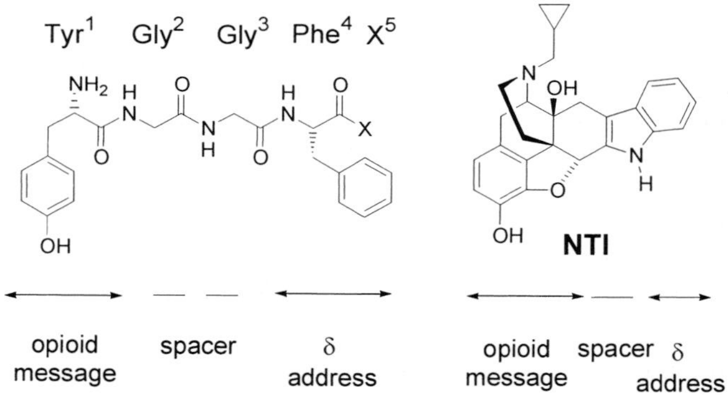

Figure 2: The message address concept.

NTI – starting point for the design of novel potent and selective δ opioid ligands

Portoghese and coworkers also considered other naltrindole derivatives substituted in position 6 or 7 with aryl, benzyl or aniline moieties to evaluate the effect of flexible aryl groups on selectivity, but obtained non-selective compounds only. This result demonstrates that the conformational flexibility of these aryl groups causes them to reside preferentially in regions of space that are not accepted by the δ opioid receptor (Portoghese et al., 1994). A more rigid compound however, 7-benzylidene-naltrindole (BNTX) proved to be a potent and highly selective δ_1 antagonist ($K_i(\delta_1)$ = 0.1 nM; $K_i(\delta_2)$ = 10.8 nM; Portoghese et al., 1992). The isothiocyanate derivative 5'-NTII was designed as a non-equilibrium δ-selective antagonist (Portoghese et al., 1990).

Another approach to producing δ-selective antagonists is the fragmentation of the indolomorphinan framework. Resulting indolooctahydroisoquinoline derivatives were first disclosed by Toray. Eight months later, SmithKline Beecham disclosed the same compounds, but also derivatives featuring diverse five-membered ring spacers and different substitution patterns at the phenolic moiety (Dondio et al. (SmithKline Beecham), 1994).

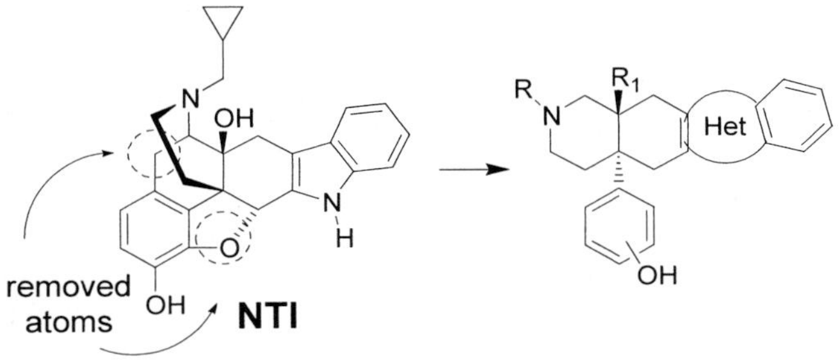

removed atoms / **NTI**

Figure 3: Fragmentation of the indolomorphinan framework.

Substitution of N-cyclopropylmethyl (CPM) for N-methyl in general results in a shift from opioid antagonist to agonist. Applied to spiromorphinans the spiroindanyloxymorphone SIOM was discoverd, a potent δ ligand characterized as a full agonist in the MVD (IC_{50} 19 nM; antagonized by NTI). *In vivo* data however showed that SIOM possesses the unusual feature of acting as a δ antagonist at low dose and as a δ agonist at higher dose (Portoghese et al., 1993).

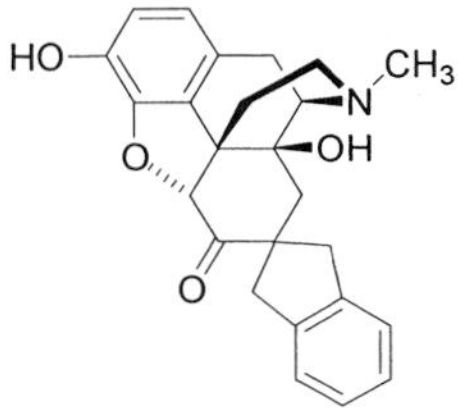

Introduction of a six-membered ring into the octahydroisoquinoline series resulted in the discovery of a new class of potent and selective δ agonists (Dondio et al., 1995). Toray and SmithKline Beecham disclosed similar octahydroisoquinolines bearing an aromatic six-membered ring spacer. TAN-67 is the most interesting derivative to emerge from this (Nagase et al., 1994, 2001; Knapp et al., 1995). The pharmacological properties of the two enantiomers of TAN-67 were investigated by Dondio (Dondio et al., 1995). SB213698 (also named (-)-TAN-67 by Toray) is the active enantiomer displaying subnanomolar affinity for the δ receptor, being far less potent at μ and κ opioid receptors. SB213698 is a full δ agonist in the MVD (IC_{50} 62 nM). The corresponding (+)-

SIOM

Octahydroisoquinolines:

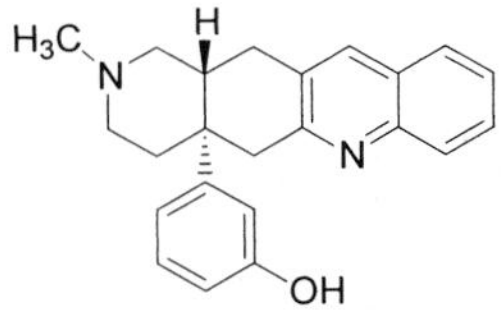

TAN-67 – the prototype of a new class of potent and selective δ agonists

enantiomer is inactive in this test up to a concentration of 1 µM.

BW373U86: Extension of the message address concept to non-aromatic moieties

In 1992 Glaxo Wellcome disclosed BW373U86 (Lee et al., 1992), a new selective δ agonist structurally unrelated to the previously known δ ligands. BW373U86, although not very selective in binding assays, is the most potent δ agonist in isolated tissue bioassays displaying a remarkable µ/δ selectivity ratio of 715 and is reported to be a potent analgesic that does not produce physical dependence (Lee et al., 1992).

SNC80 dose dependently produces antinociception in the mouse warm water tail flick test (i.c.v., i.t. and i.p.)

SNC80, the optically pure enantiomer of the methyl ether of BW373U86, exhibits a remarkable µ/δ selectivity in both receptor binding and *in vitro* bioassays (Calderon et al., 1994, 1997). In mice, SNC80 administered i.c.v., i.t. and i.p. dose dependently produces antinociception in the mouse warm water tail flick test with ED_{50} values of 105 and 69 nmol/mouse and 57 mg/kg, respectively. After i.c.v. administration SNC80 is active in the mouse hot plate test (ED_{50} 92 nmol/mouse). Studies with selective µ and δ opioid antagonists revealed that the antinociceptive activity elicited by SNC80 is mediated by the selective activation of the δ receptor. However, high doses caused brief, non-lethal seizures. Glaxo Wellcome has discontinued development of SNC80 for the treatment of pain. The project was terminated in 1995.

BW373U86 (R = H)
SNC80   (R = Me)

DPI-3290

DPI-3290 (Chang et al. (Ardent Pharmaceuticals), 1994), another compound from the piperazine series, is a mixed δ/µ opioid receptor agonist under development by Ardent Pharmaceuticals as an analgesic for the relief of severe intra- and post-operative pain. The i.v. formulation is licensed to Organon Teknika. In preclinical models DPI-3290 significantly reduces levels of respiratory depression, nausea and emesis of narcotic drugs. Phase II i.v. trials in severe pain in AIDS patients are underway. In Phase I trials DPI-3290 induced potent analgesia equal to morphine. A sublingual formulation is also in Phase I trials.

cpd. 1

AstraZeneca is developing a series of selective non-peptidic δ opioid receptor agonists for the treatment of neuropathic pain. The compounds (e.g. cpd., 1) are in preclinical studies. *In vivo*, they are effective analgesics with negligible tolerance and dependence. They have parenteral and oral activity with suitable pharmacokinetics and pharmacodynamics.

The δ opioid receptor agonist AR-M390 is under development by AstraZeneca for the treatment of neuropathic pain. It is designed to overcome unwanted side-effects of opioid analgesics. In rats, it shows naltrindole-reversible antiallodynic activity but no efficacy against physiological pain. There is no seizure activity. AR-M390 has an oral bioavailability of 90 – 100% (221 ACS (San Diego), 2001, MEDI 185).

AR-M390

Other δ ligands that have been disclosed include aryltetrahydroacridinemethanamines (Pütz et al. (Grünenthal), 1998) like cpd. 2, aminomethylphenylcycohexanes (Pütz et al. (Grünenthal), 2000) like cpd. 3, but also compounds from a heterocyclic benzocycloalkene series (Zimmer et al. (Grünenthal), 1997) like cpd. 4. These compounds are claimed to be δ agonists and especially useful for the treatment of pain.

cpd. 2   cpd. 3   cpd. 4

In conclusion, the investigation of peptidic and non-peptidic tool compounds for the δ receptor have demonstrated the potential use of δ agonists and antagonists for a variety of clinical applications, especially for the treatment of pain. Full exploitation of this potential will however only be possible with ideal non-peptidic compounds having high potency, selectivity and, above all, optimal drug metabolism and pharmacodynamic characteristics.

Non-peptide δ compounds hold substantial potential for the mediation of a variety of pharmacological effects

References

Abdelhamid, E.E., Sultana, M., Portoghese, P.S., Takemori, A.E.: *Selective blockage of delta opioid receptors prevents the development of morphine tolerance and dependence in mice*, J. Pharmacol. Exp. Ther. **1991**, *258*, 299-303.

Bowen, W.K., Hellewell, S.B., Keleman, M., Huey, R., Stewart, D.: *Affinity labelling of δ-opiate receptors using [D-Ala², Leu⁵, Cys⁶]enkephalin: covalent attachment via thiol-disulfide exchange*, J. Biol. Chem. **1987**, *262*, 13434-13439.

Calderon, S.N., Rothman, R.B., Porreca, F., et al.: *Probes for narcotic receptor-mediated phenomena. Synthesis of SNC80: a highly selective non-peptide δ opioid receptor agonist*, J. Med. Chem. **1994**, *37*, 2125-2128 (Disclosure of SNC80).

Calderon, S.N., Rice, K .C., Rothman, R.B. et al.: *Probes for narcotic receptor mediated phenomena. 23. Synthesis, opioid receptor binding and bioassay of the highly selective δ agonist SNC80 and related novel nonpeptide δ opioid receptor ligands*, J. Med. Chem. **1997**, *40*, 695-704.

Chang, K.-J., Bubacz, D.G., Davis, A.O., McNutt, R.W., Collins, M.A., Bishop, M.J. (Delta Pharmaceuticals): *Opioid Compounds*, US5681830 (**1994**).

Cheng, P.Y., Wu, D.L., Decena, J., et al.: *Central opioid modulation of breathing dynamics in the fetal lamb: effects of DPDPE and partial antagonism by naltrindole*, J. Pharmacol. Ther. **1992**, *262*, 1004-1010.

Coop, A. and Rice, K.C.: *Role of delta opioid receptors in biological processes*, Drugs News Perspect. **2000**, *13*, 481-487.

Dondio, G., Clarke, G.D., Giardina, G., et al.: *Potent and selective non-peptidic delta opioid ligands based on the novel heterocycle-condensed octahydroisoquinoline structure*, Reg. Pept. **1994**, *1*, 43-44.

Dondio, G. and Ronzoni, S. (SmithKline Beecham Farmaceutici S.p.A.): *Hydroisoquinoline Derivatives*, W09504734 (**1995**).

Dondio, G., Clarke, G.D., Giardina, G., et al.: *The role of the spacer in the octahydroisoquinoline series: discovery of SB 213698, a non-peptidic, potent and selective delta opioid agoni*st, Analgesia **1995**, *1*, 394-399.

Dondio, G., Ronzoni, S., Petrillo, P.: Non-peptide δ opioid agonists and antagonists, Exp. Opin. Ther. Patents **1997**, *7*, 1075-1098.

Dondio, G., Ronzoni, S., Petrillo, P.: *Non-peptide delta opioid agonists and antagonists (Part II)*, Exp. Opin. Ther. Patents **1999**, *9*, 353-374.

Erspamer, V., Melchiorri, P., Falconieri-Erspamer, G., Negri, L., Corsi, R., et al.: *Deltorphins: a family of naturally occurring peptides with high affinity and selectivity for δ opioid binding sites,* Proc. Natl. Acad. Sci. USA **1989,** *86*, 5188-5192.

Evans, C.J., Keith, D.E., Morrison, H., Magendzo, K., Edwards, R.H.: *Cloning of the δ opioid receptor by functional expression*, Science **1992**, *258*, 1952-1955.

Fang, L., Knapp, R.J., Horvath, R., Matsunaga, T. O., Haaseth, R. C., Hruby, V. J., Porreca, F., Yamamura, H. I.: *Characterization of [^{3}H]naltrindole binding to delta opioid receptors in mouse brain and mouse vas deferens: Evidence for delta opioid receptor heterogeneity*, J. Pharmacol. Exp. Ther. **1994**, *268*, 836-846.

Heyman, J.S., Vaught, J.L., Mosberg, H.I., Haaseth, R.C., Porreca, F.: *Modulation of μ-mediated antinociception by δ agonists in the mouse: selective potentiation of morphine and normorphine by DPDPE*, Eur. J. Pharmacol. **1986**, *165*, 1-10.

Heyman, J.S., Jiang, Q., Rothman, R.B., Mosberg, H.I., Porreca F.: *Modulation of μ-mediated antinociception by δ agonists: charaterization with antagonists,* Eur. J. Pharmacol. **1989**, *169*, 43-52.

Horan, P.J., Edward, A.M., Lipkowski, A.W., Hruby, V. J., Porreca, F., et al. : *Antinociceptive profile of biphalin, a dimeric enkephalin analog*, J. Pharmacol. Exp. Ther. **1993**, *265*, 1446-1454.

House, R.V., Thomas, P.T., Bhargava, H.N.: *A comparative study of immunmodulation produced. by in vitro exposure to delta opioid receptor agonist peptides*, Peptides **1996**, *17*, 75-81.

Hughes, J.: *Isolation of an endogenous compound from the brain with pharmacological properties similar to morphine*, Brain Res. **1975**, *88*, 205-308.

Hul, G.R., Childers, S., Pasternak, G., *An opiate-receptor gene family reunion*, Trends Neurosci. **1994**, *17*, 89-93.

Jiang, Q., Mosberg, H.I., Porreca, F.: *Antinociceptive effects of deltorphin II, a highly selective δ agonist in vivo*, Life Sci. Pharmacol. Lett. **1990**, *47*, 43-47.

Jiang, Q., Takemori, A.E., Sultana, M., et al.: *Differential antagonism of opioid delta antinociception by [D-Ala^2,Leu^5,Cys^6]enkephalin and naltrindole 5´-isothiocyanate: evidence for delta receptor subtypes*, J. Pharmacol. Exp.Ther. **1991**, *257*, 1069-1095.

Jin, X.-L. Zhou, D.-H., Chi, Z.-Q.: *Recent progress on the study of delta opioid receptor*, Chin. Pharmacol. Bull. **1999**, *15*, 1-4.

Kalivas, P.W. and Stewart, J.: *Dopamine transmission in drug- and stress-induced behavioral sensitization*, Brain Res. Rev. **1991**, *16*, 223-244.

Kamei, J., Iwamoto, Y., Suzuki, T., et al.: *Involvement of δ₁-opioid receptor antagonism in the antitussive effect of δ-opioid receptor antagonists*, Eur. J. Pharmacol. **1994**, *251*, 291-294.

Kieffer, B.L., Befort, K., Gaveriaux-Ruff, C., Hirth, C.G.: *The δ opioid receptor, isolation of cDNA clone by expression cloning and pharmacological characterization*, Proc. Natl. Acad. Sci. USA **1992**, *89*, 12048-12052.

Knapp, R.J., Malatynska, E., Fang, L., Li, X., Babin, E., Nguyen, M., Santoro, G., Varga, E. V., Hruby, V. J., Roeske, W. R., et al.: *Identification of a human delta opioid receptor: cloning and expression*, Life Sci. **1994**, *54*, 463-469.

Knapp, R.J., Landsman, R., Waite, Malatynska, E., Varga, E., Haq, W., Hruby, V. J., Roeske, W. R., Nagase, H., Yamamura, H. I.: *Properties of TAN 67, a nonpeptidic δ-opioid receptor agonist at cloned human δ- and μ-opioid receptors*, Eur. J. Pharmacol. **1995**, *291*, 129-134.

Kreil, G., Barra, D., Simmaco, M., Erspamer, V., Erspamer, G. F., Negri, L., Severini, C., Corsi, R., Melchiorri, P.: *Deltorphin, a novel amphibian skin peptide with high selectivity and affinity for δ opioid receptors*, Eur. J. Pharmacol. **1989**, *162*, 123-128.

Lazarus, L.H., Bryant, S.D., Cooper, P.S., Salvadori, S.: *What peptides these deltorphines be*, Prog. Neurobiol. **1999**, *57*, 377-420.

Lee, P.H.K., McNutt, R.W, Chang, K.J.: *A non peptidic deltaopioid receptor agonist, BW373U86, suppresses naloxone-precipitated morphine abstinence*, Abstracts of the **1992** College on Problems of Drug-Dependence-International Narcotics Research Conference, Abstract 34. (First disclosure of BW373U86).

Lord, J.A., Waterfield, A.A., Hughes, J., Kosterlitz, H.W.: Nature **1977**, *267*, 495-499.

Mazumder S., Nath I., Dhar M.M., *Immunomodulation of human T cell responses with receptor selective enkephalines,* Immunol. Lett. **1993**, *35*, 33-38.

Mosberg, H. I., Hurst, R., Hruby, V. J., Gee, K., Akiyama, K., Yamamura, H. I., Galligan, J. J., Burks, T. F.: *Cyclic penicillamine containing enkephalin analog display profound δ receptor selectivities*, Life Sci. **1983**, *33*, 447-450.

Nagase, H., Wakita, H., Kawai, K.: *Synthesis of non-peptidic delta opioid agonists and their structure activity relationships*, Jpn. J. Pharmacol. **1994**, *64*, 35.

Nagase, H., Yajima, Y., Fujii, H., Kawamura, K., Narita, M., Kamei, J., Suzuki, T.: *The pharmacological profile of delta opioid receptor ligands, (+) and (-) TAN 67 on pain modulation*, Life Sci. **2001**, *68*, 2227-2231.

Negri, L., Potenza, R.L., Corsi, R. Melchiorri, P.: *Evidence for two subtypes of delta opioid receptors in rat brain*, Eur. J. Pharmacol. **1991**, *196*, 335-336.

Porreca, F., Takemori, A.E., Portoghese, P.S., Sultana, M., Bowen, W.D.: *Modulation of μ-mediated antinociception by a subtype of opioid δ receptor in the mouse*, J. Pharmacol. Exp. Ther. **1992**, *263*, 147-152.

Portoghese, P.S., Sultana, M., Nagase, H., Takemori, A.E.: *Application of the message-address concept in the design of highly potent and selective non-peptide δ opioid receptor antagonists*, J. Med. Chem. **1988**, *31*, 281-282.

Portoghese, P.S., Sultana, M., Takemori, A.E.: *Naltrindole 5′isothiocyanate: a nonequilibrium, highly selective δ opioid receptor antagonist*, J. Med. Chem. **1990**, *33*, 1547-1548.

Portoghese, P.S., Sultana, M., Nagase, H., Takemori, A.E.: *A highly selective δ₁-opioid antagonist: 7-benzylidenenaltrexone*, Eur. J. Pharmacol. **1992**, *218*, 195-196.

Portoghese, P.S., Moe, S.T., Takemori, A.E.: *A selective δ1 opioid receptor agonist derived from oxymorphone. Evidence for separate recognition sites for δ1 opioid receptor agonists and antagonists*, J. Med. Chem. **1993**, *36*, 2572-2574.

Portoghese, P.S., Sultana, M., Moe, S.T., Takemori, A.E.: *Synthesis of naltrexone-derived δ-opioid antagonists. Role of conformation of the δ address moiety*, J. Med. Chem. **1994**, *37*, 579-585.

Pütz, C.K., Straßburger, W., Kögel B.-Y. (Grünenthal GmbH): *Preparation of aminomethylphenylhexenes and analogs as analgesics* , WO01049651(**2001**).

Pütz, C.K., Straßburger, W., Zimmer, O., Englberger, W. (Grünenthal GmbH): *Preparation of aryltetrahydroacridinemethanamines as δ-opioid receptor ligands*, EP970949 (**1998**).

Rogers, T.J., Steele, A.D., Howard, O.M., Oppenheim, J.J.: *Bidirectional heterologous desensitization of opioid and chemokine receptors*, Ann. NY Acad. Sci. **2000**, *917*, 19-28.

Scheideler, M.A.: *Evidence for the role of delta opioid agonists in pain signaling*, Curr. Opin. CPNS Invest. Drugs **2000**, *2*, 171-177.

Schultz, J.E.J. and Gross, G. J.: *Opioids and cardioprotection*, Pharmacol. Ther. **2001**, *89*, 123-127.

Schwyzer, R.: *ACTH: a short introductory review*, Ann. NY Acad. Sci. **1977**, *297*, 3-26.

Shook, J.E., Lemcke, P.K., Gehrig, C.A., Hruby, V.J., Burks, T.F.: *Antidiarrheal properties of supraspinal mu and delta and peripheral mu, delta and kappa opioid receptors: inhibition of diarrhea without constipation*, J. Pharmacol. Exp. Ther. **1989**, *249*, 83-90.

Sofuoglu, M., Portoghese, P.S., Takemori, A.E.: *Differential antagonism of δ opioid agonists by naltrindole and its benzofuran analog (NTB) in mice: evidence for δ opioid receptor subtypes*, J. Pharmacol. Exp. Ther. **1991**, *257*, 676-680.

Spetea, M., Harris, H. E., Berzetei-Gurske, I. P., Klareskog, L., Schmidhammer, H.: *Binding, pharmacological and immunological profiles of the delta-selective opioid receptor antagonist HS 378*, Life Sci. **2001**, *69*, 1775-1782.

Suzuki, T., Mori, T., Funda, M., Misawa, M., Nagase, H.: *Attenuation of the discriminative stimulus properties of cocaine by delta opioid receptor antagonists*, Eur. J. Pharmacol. **1994**, *263*, 207-211.

Tsushima, H., Mori, M., Matsuda, T.: *Effects of DPDPE, microinjected into the supraoptic and paraventricular nuclei, on outflow rate*, Jpn. J. Pharmacol. **1993**, *63*, 181-186.

Warltier, D.C., Pagel, P.S., Kersten, J.R.: *Approaches to the prevention of perioperative myocardial ischemia*, Anesthesiology **2000**, *92*, 253-259.

Xu, H., Ni, Q., Jakobson, A.E., Rice, K.C., Rothman, R.B.: *Preliminary ligand binding data for subtypesof the delta opioid receptor in rat brain membranes*, Life Sci. **1991**, *49*, 141-146.

Yaksh, T.L.: *Pharmacology and mechanism of opioid analgesic activity*, Acta Anaesthesiol. Scand. **1997**, *41*, 97-111.

Zaki, P. A., Bilsky, E. J., Vanderath, T. W., Lai, J., Evans, C. J., Porreca, F. : *Opioid receptor types and subtypes: the δ receptor as a model*, Ann. Rev. Pharmacol. Toxicol. **1996**, *36*, 379-401.

Zenz, M. and Willweber-Strumpf, A.: *Opiophobia and cancer pain in Europe*, Lancet **1993**, *341*, 1075-1076.

Zimmer, O., Straßburger, W., Pütz, C.K., Kögel B.-Y. (Grünenthal GmbH): *Substituted heterocyclic benzocycloalkenes and their use as analgesics*, EP922703 (**1997**).

9.2 Opioid-Receptor-Like 1 (ORL1)

*Bernd Sundermann and
Corinna Maul*

Introduction

Following the discovery of the orphan G-protein-coupled human receptor ORL1 (Mollereau et al., 1994), later classified as the fourth opioid receptor subtype in addition to μ, κ, and δ, its endogenous agonist, the heptadeka-peptide nociceptin (orphanin FQ) was identified simultaneously by Meunier et al. and Reinscheid et al. in 1995. Early studies indicated an important role for ORL1 in a range of physiological processes, implicating selective agonists or antagonists of this receptor to have potential for the treatment of pain and anxiety, the control of appetite, influencing memory and learning and other uses (Mogil et al., 1996a; Pomonis et al., 1996; Ueda et al., 1997; Jenck et al., 1997; Yu et al., 1997; Manabe et al., 1998; for reviews see: Meunier 1997, 2000; Darland et al. 1998, Barlocco et al. 2000; Mogil and Pasternak 2001). The pharmacology of nociceptin in particular has put ORL1 in the spotlight of pain research (see *Nociceptin*).

IUPHAR recommended nomenclature:

- **OP$_1$** (δ)
- **OP$_2$** (κ)
- **OP$_3$** (μ)
- **OP$_4$** (ORL1)

The nomenclature in this field is nonuniform. ORL1 designates the human receptor specifically; its equivalents in other species have different names. Use of the term OP$_4$ for all species has been recommended by IUPHAR; in a comprehensive review on ORL1 by Mogil and Pasternak (2001) the term NOP$_1$ is used. Herein the terms ORL1 and nociceptin will be used exclusively.

Some receptors similar to (or identical with) ORL1:

- rat: ROR-C, XOR, LC132
- mouse: MOR-C, KOR-3

Receptor Localization and Signaling

ORL1 is widely distributed in the CNS (Mollereau et al., 1994) and is also present in some peripheral tissues. The gene encoding the rat variant of ORL1 has been shown to give rise to several receptor forms by alternative splicing (Curró et al., 2001). Similar to other opioid receptors activation of ORL1 results in inhibition of cAMP synthesis, N-type voltage-gated calcium channels and neurotransmitter release as well as activation of inwardly rectifying potassium channels (review: Ronzoni et al., 2001).

In general the classical opioid ligands, e.g. morphine and fentanyl, do not bind to ORL1. Known exceptions include the μ-selective nonpeptidic ORL1 agonists buprenorphine (Wnendt et al., 1999), lofentanil and etorphine (Butour et al., 1997). Naloxone benzoylhydrazone (NalBzOH) has been found to be a non-selective ORL1 antagonist with moderate affinity (Ozaki et al., 2000b). In addition to nociceptin as a peptide agonist compound and certain

Table 1: Ligands for ORL1.

receptor affinity	ORL1 Ki/nM	μ Ki/nM
bupren-orphine	8.4	0.51
lofentanil	24	0.023
etorphine	530	0.18

(Thomsen and Hohlweg, 2000)

other peptides (Topham et al., 1998, Bigoni et al., 2000, Ronzoni et al., 2001), drug discovery projects aimed at the identification of potent and selective nonpeptidic ligands for ORL1 have identified antagonists from two different structural classes (J-113397, JTC-801) and some closely structurally related agonists – spiropiperidines such as Ro 64-6198 and NNC 63-0532 – which can be used today to elaborate on the physiological role of ORL1 in preclinical studies (Ronzoni et al., 2001; Thomsen 2001; see *ORL1 Antagonists* and *ORL1 Agonists*).

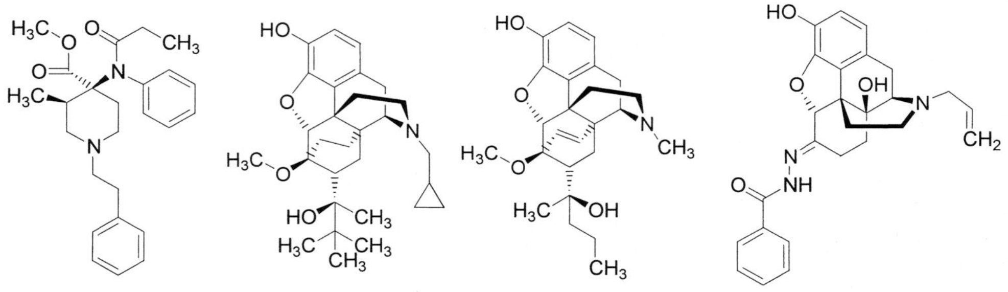

| Lofentanil | Buprenorphine | Etorphine | NalBzOH |

Figure 1: Non-selective ORL1 ligands.

Nociceptin (Orphanin FQ)

Nociceptin:

FGGFTGARKSARKLANQ

[170713-75-4]

The heptadecapeptide nociceptin has some structural similarity to dynorphin A (YGGFLRRIRPKLKWDNQ; Darland et al., 1998), but bears an N-terminal phenylalanine (F) instead of tyrosine (Y) which is essential for the activation of classical opioid receptors (μ, κ, δ). It was named nociceptin (NC) by Meunier et al. (1995) to indicate its initially observed hyperalgesic effect and is the endogenous agonist of ORL1.

Nociceptin's pain modulating properties

The role of nociceptin in pain modulation has been extensively studied, but opposite effects have been observed depending upon dose and route of administration (Barlocco et al., 2000):

Supraspinal anti-opioid effects of NC?

In mice NC has been reported to cause hyperalgesia in the hot-plate (Meunier et al., 1995) and tail-flick test (Reinscheid et al., 1995) after i.c.v. administration, but these observations may rather be due to a reduction of opioid-mediated stress-induced analgesia (attributable to the i.c.v. route of administration) than to a genuine hyperalgesic effect of NC (Mogil et al., 1996a). This anti-opioid function of supraspinal NC has been shown to antagonize antinociception produced by opioid agonists (Mogil et al., 1996b). On the other hand Rossi et al.,

(1996) have reported naloxone-sensitive analgesia after i.c.v. administration of NC in mice.

After intrathecal (i.t.) administration of NC in rats hyperalgesia (Okuda-Ashitaka et al., 1996) was observed as well as naloxone- or naltrexone-reversible antinociception potentially caused by NC-induced release of endogenous opioids (King et al., 1997; Jhamandas et al., 1998). These bidirectional effects may be dose dependent with antinociception being predominant at higher doses (Tian et al., 1997). In mice both Reinscheid et al. (1995) and Grisel et al. (1996) did not observe antinociception but paralysis after i.t. administration of NC. Jhamandas et al., (1998) report an opioid-like antinociceptive effect of intrathecal NC as well as antagonism of morphine-induced antinociception. These and further contradicting early reports on the pharmacology of NC have been reviewed by Zaki and Evans (1998). Contradictory finding have also been reported with knockout mice (review: Mogil and Pasternak 2001).

Spinal pro- and antinociception by NC?

Keeping in mind the peptidic nature of NC, two basic conclusions can be drawn: ORL1 and NC do play an important role in pain transmission and thorough investigations of potent and selective small molecule ORL1 agonists and antagonists are needed to elucidate whether a potential new analgesic should block or activate the ORL1 receptor.

Potent and selective ORL1 ligands as potential analgesics

ORL1 Antagonists

The first potent and selective nonpeptidic ORL1 antagonist was described by Kawamoto et al. (1999, 2001; (Banyu Pharmaceutical Co.), 2000). J-113397 is the result of a lead optimization effort based on a screening hit (cpd. 1) with submicromolar affinity for ORL1.

J-113397

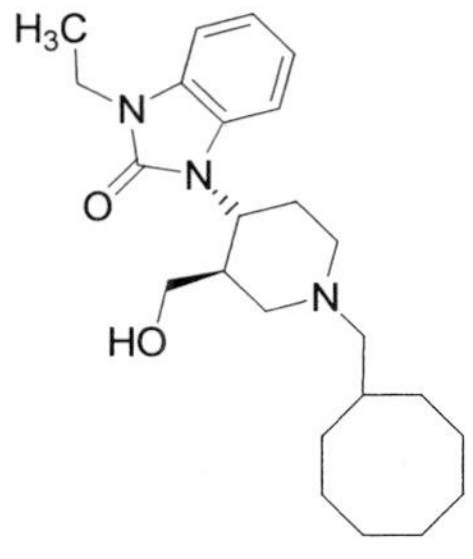

Table 2: Opioid receptor affinities of J-113397 and related compounds.

receptor affinity (Ki/nM)	ORL1	μ	κ	δ
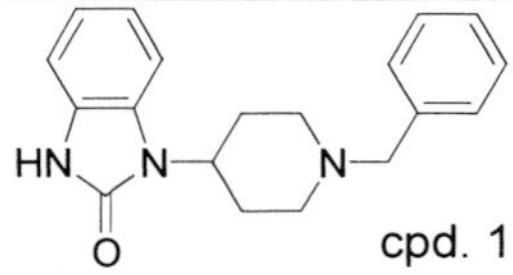 cpd. 1	200	1700	110	>10000
J-113397	2.3	2200	1400	>10000
ent-J-113397	820	3300	2600	>10000

[256640-45-6] 1-[(3R,4R)1-Cyclooctylmethyl-3-hydroxy-methyl-piperidin-4-yl]-3-ethyl-1,3-dihydro-benzoi-midazol-2-one, $C_{24}H_{37}N_3O_2$, M_r 399.57

An alternative to the initial 11-step synthesis of J-113397 with improved yield was developed by De Risi et al. (2001)

JTC-801

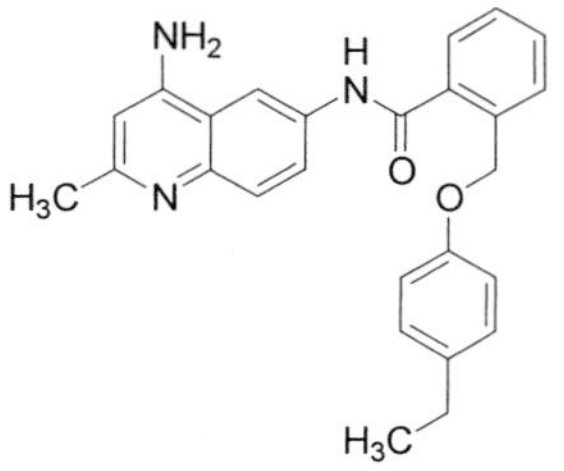

[244218-51-7] N-(8-Amino-6-methyl-naphthalen-2-yl)-2-(4-ethyl-phenoxymethyl)-benzamide, $C_{27}H_{26}N_2O_2$, M_r 410.20

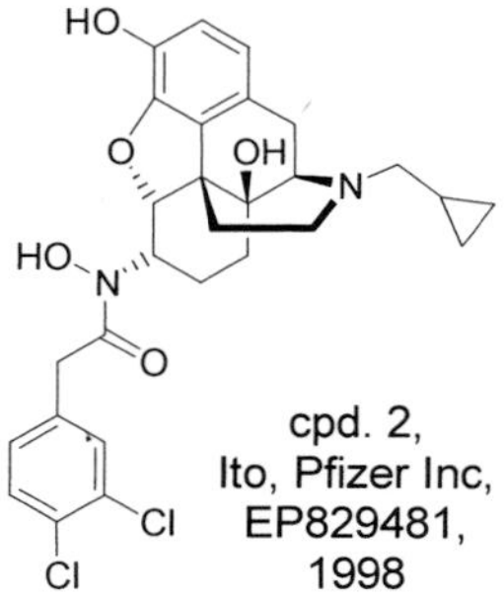

cpd. 2,
Ito, Pfizer Inc,
EP829481,
1998

Pharmacological investigations have proven J-113397 to be the most potent ORL1 antagonist known today (Ozaki et al., 2000a, b; Bigoni et al., 2000; Ichikawa et al., 2001). J-113397 is reported to be active in the formalin test, but inactive against pain responses to thermal and mechanical stimuli (Okuda et al., 2000).

The achiral ORL1 antagonist JTC-801 again is a result of lead optimisation efforts, in this case starting from a 4-aminoquinoline derivative that has not been disclosed. In pharmacological evaluations JTC-801 has been reported to antagonize nociceptin-induced allodynia and to show antinociceptive properties *in vivo* (mouse hot plate and rat formalin test; Shinkai et al. (Japan Tabacco), 1999; Shinkai et al., 2000; Yamada et al., 2002). The potential of JTC-801 as a novel type of analgesic is reported to be under clinical evaluation (Japan Tabacco web page).

Table 3: Opioid receptor affinities of JTC-801.

receptor affinity (Ki/nM)	ORL1	μ	κ	δ
JTC-801	8.1	103	1060	8650

Further ORL1 antagonists include a series of NalBzOH analogs where the benzoylhydrazone moiety is replaced by hydroxylamides (cpd. 2). These compounds are also claimed to have agonistic activity at μ, κ and δ receptors.

Similar compounds have been disclosed by Toray Industries (Nagase et al., JP2000053572). Cpd. 3 and 4 are specifically claimed to be ORL1 antagonists:

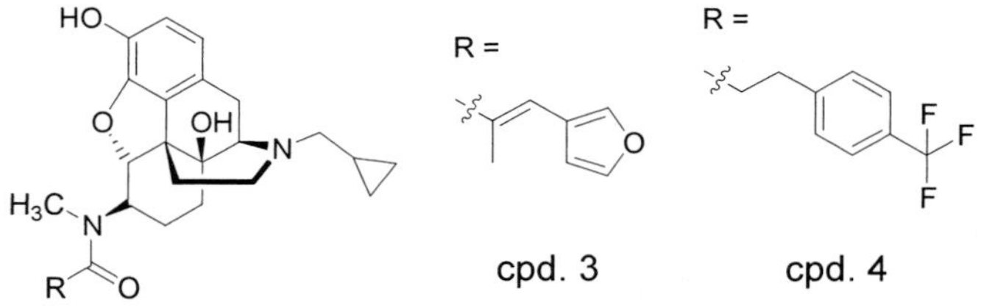

Figure 2: ORL-1 antagonists.

ORL1 Agonists

High throughput screening at Roche revealed cpd. 5, bearing some resemblance to lofentanil (see Introduction) and having pronounced affinity for ORL1. Optimization efforts led to the spiropiperidine cpd. 6 with 10-fold selectivity for ORL1 over μ and ultimately gave rise to the discovery of Ro 64-6198 (Wichmann et al., 1999; Röver et al., 2000; Adam et al. (Roche), 1998, 1999, 2000; Cesura et al. (Roche), 2000).

Table 4: Opioid receptor affinities of selected ORL-1 ligands.

receptor affinity (Ki/nM)	ORL1	μ	κ	δ
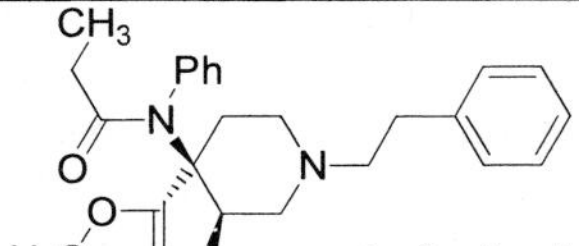 Lofentanil	25	0.13	5.0	0.79
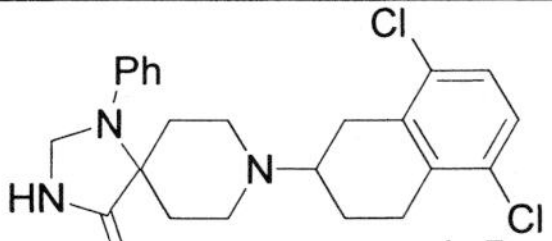 cpd. 5	5.0	7.9	40	630
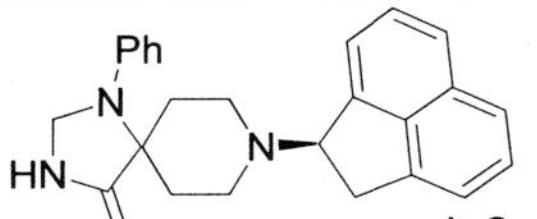 cpd. 6	0.25	4.0	20	100
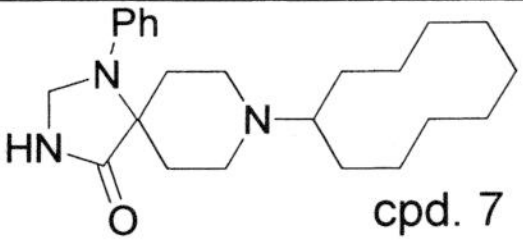 cpd. 7	0.082	0.63	2.0	50
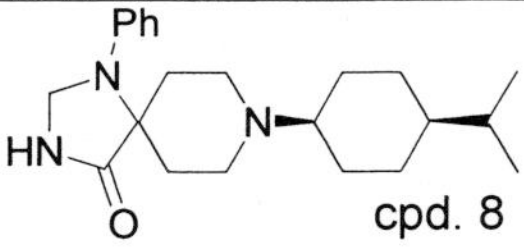 cpd. 8	0.079	3.2	25	250
Ro 64-6198	0.40	50	79	>1000

Ro 64-6198

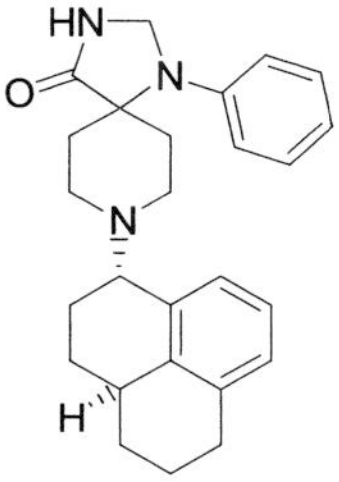

[280783-56-4] 8-[(1S,3aS)-2,3,3a,4,5,6-Hexahydro-1H-phenalen-1-yl]-1-phenyl-1,3,8-triaza-spiro[4.5]decan-4-one, $C_{26}H_{31}N_3O$, M_r 401.54

In this series of spiro-piperidines selectivity was achieved by replacement of the initial substituted tetra-hydronaphthalene moiety (cpd. 5) by acenaphthenyl (10-fold; cpd. 6) and finally by hexahydro-1H-phenalene (100-fold; Ro 64-6198)

The cyclodecyl- and *cis*-4-isopropylcyclohexyl derivatives (cpds. 7 and 8) are the most potent, but only moderately selective small molecule ORL1 agonists known today

Ro 64-6198 has 100-fold selectivity for ORL1 and thus is the most selective small molecule ORL1 agonist known today. Oral bioavailability is poor (4 %), but the compound crosses the blood-brain barrier. Ro 64-6198 is reported to be in clinical trials for the treatment of anxiety. At anxiolytic doses (~1 mg/kg) Ro 64-6198 has no effect on the perception of acute (tail-flick) or inflammatory pain in rats, at higher doses severe neurological side-effects dominate (Jenck et al., 2000; Wichmann et al., 2000; Higgins et al., 2001). Since no neurological impairment was observed in ORL1 knockout mice treated with Ro64-6198, these effects may well pose a general limitation to the clinical use of ORL1 agonists.

In vitro characterization of Ro 64-6198: (Dautzenberg et al., 2001; Rizzi et al., 2001)

NNC 63-0532

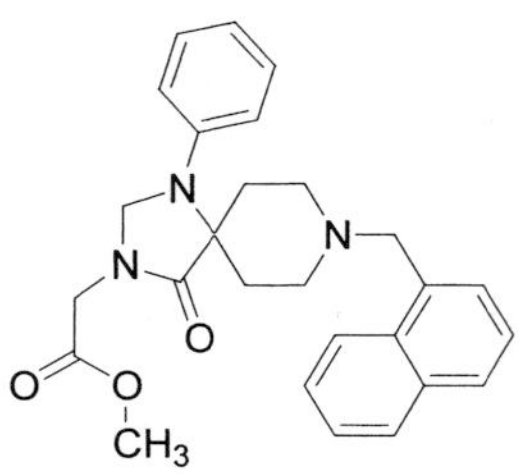

Watson et al.,
Novo Nordisk, WO9959997

[250685-44-0] (8-
Naphthalen-1-ylmethyl-4-
oxo-1-phenyl-1,3,8-triaza-
spiro[4.5]dec-3-yl)-acetic
acid methyl ester,
$C_{27}H_{29}N_3O_3$, M_r 443.54

At Novo Nordisk, a 3D search performed on lofentanil predicted that the 5-HT_{1A} agonist spiroxatrine was also an ORL1 ligand. Actually spiroxatrine was found to have moderate affinity for ORL1 (Ki 118 nM). A lead optimization effort led to the potent ORL1 agonist NNC 63-0532 (Thomsen and Hohlweg, 2000). While its oral bioavailability (20%) is reported to be considerably improved with respect to Ro 64-6198 (4%), *in vivo* studies suggest NNC 63-0532 to be not sufficiently selective for ORL1 (Ki 7.3 nM) over µ (Ki 140 nM). Further synthetic studies have led to more selective compounds (cpd. 9), but in contrast to NNC 63-0532 these do not cross the blood-brain barrier (Thomsen, 2001).

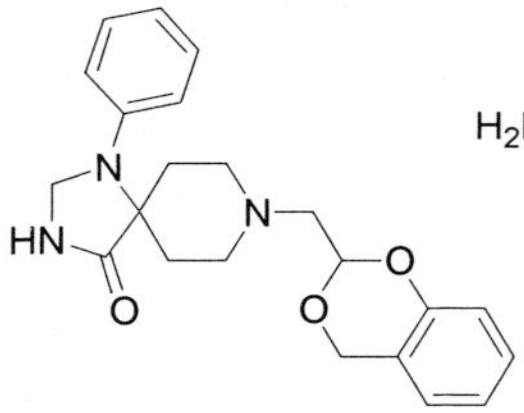

Spiroxatrine 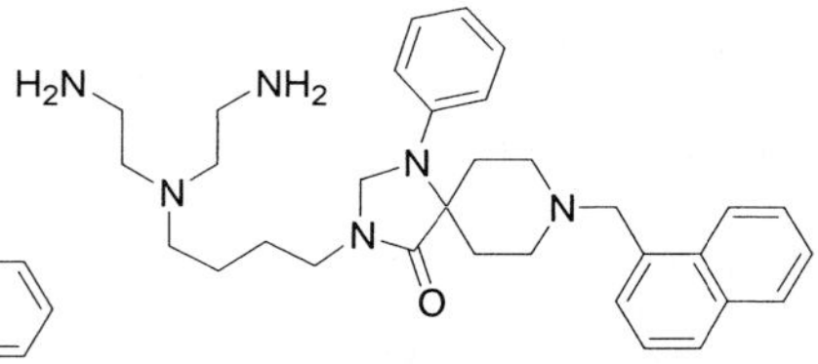   cpd. 9, Hohlweg et al.,
                           Novo Nordisk, WO0136418

Scheme 3: ORL1 ligands discovered by Novo Nordisk.

Other Compounds

Other ORL1 ligands that have been disclosed with little details include several benzimidazoles (cpds. 10-12), but also compounds from other structural classes (cpds. 13-16). Some of these compounds are claimed to be ORL1 agonists and especially useful for the treatment of pain.

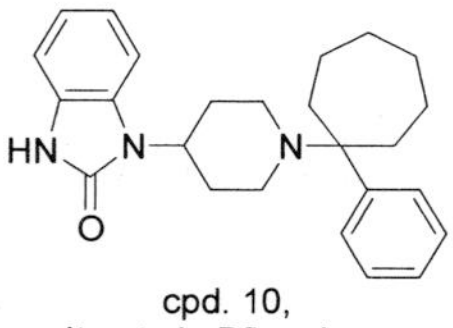

cpd. 10,
Ito et al., Pfizer Inc.,
WO9936421

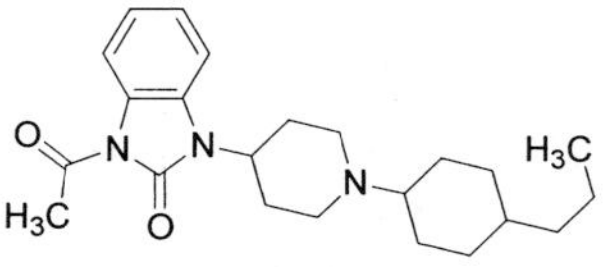

cpd. 12, Kyle et al.,
Euroceltique, WO0139775

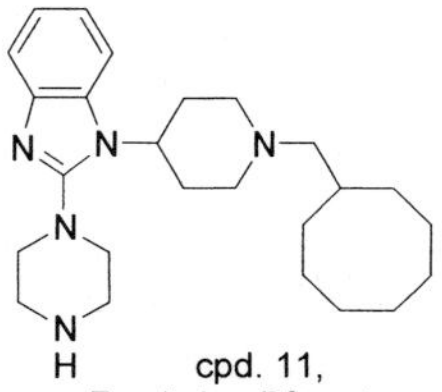

cpd. 11,
Fumitaka, Pfizer Inc.,
US6340681, 2001

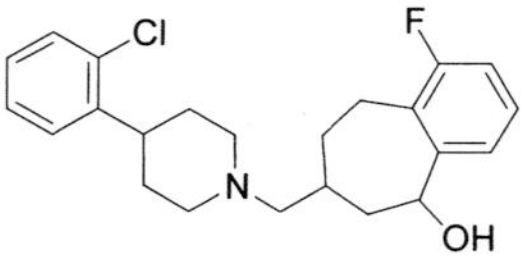

cpd. 13, Barlocco et al.,
SmithKline Beecham, WO0183454

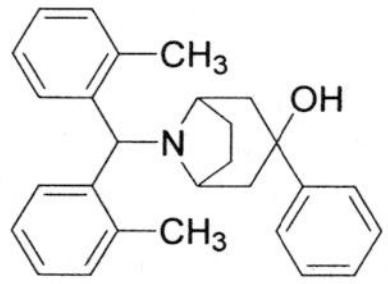

cpd. 15, Tulshian et al.,
Schering Corp., WO0006545

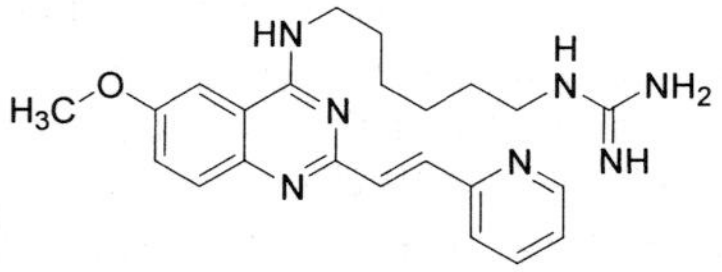

cpd. 16, Okana and Mori,
Nippon Shinyaku, WO0172710

Scheme 4: Further ORL-1 ligands.

References

Adam, G., Cesura, A., Galley, G., Jenck, F., Monsma, F., Röver, S., Wichmann, J. (F. Hoffmann-La Roche AG): *8-Substituted-1,3,8-triazaspiro[4.5]decan-4-on derivatives*, EP856514 (**1998**).

Adam, G., Cesura, A., Galley, G., Jenck, F., Röver, S., Wichmann, J. (F. Hoffmann-La Roche AG): *Piperidine derivatives*, WO9929696 (**1999**a).

Adam, G., Cesura, A., Galley, G., Jenck, F., Röver, S., Wichmann, J. (F. Hoffmann-La Roche AG): *1,3,8-Triazaspiro[4.5]decan-4-on derivatives*, EP921125 (**1999**b).

Adam, G., Cesura, A., Kolczewski, S., Roever, S., Wichmann, J. (F. Hoffmann-La Roche AG): *Di- or triaza-spiro(4,5)decane derivatives*, EP963985 (**1999**c).

Adam, G., Dautzenberg, F., Kolczewski, S., Roever, S., Wichmann, J. (F. Hoffmann-La Roche AG): *Spiro(piperidine-4,1'-pyrrolo(3,4-c)pyrrole)*, EP963987 (**1999**d).

Adam, G., Cesura, A., Jenck, F., Kolczewski, S., Roever, S., Wichmann, J. (F. Hoffmann-La Roche AG): *Diaza-spiro[3.5]nonane derivatives*, EP970957 (**2000**).

Barlocco, D., Cignarella, G., Giardina, G.A.M., Toma, L.: *The opioid-receptor-like 1 (ORL-1) as a potential target for new analgesics*, Eur. J. Med. Chem. **2000**, *35*, 275-282.

Barlocco, D., Cignarella, G., Giardina, G., Grugni, M. (SmithKline Beecham): *Benzosuberonylpiperidine compounds as analgesics*, WO0183454 (**2001**).

Bigoni, R., Calo, G., Rizzi, A., Guerrini, R., De Risi, C., Hashimoto, Y., Hashiba, E., Lambert, D.G., Regoli, D.: In vitro *characterization of J-113397, a non-peptide nociceptin/orphanin FQ receptor antagonist*, Naunyn-Schmiedeberg's Arch. Pharmacol. **2000**, *361*, 565-568.

Butour, J.-L., Moisand, C., Mazaruil, H., Mollereau, C., Meunier, J.-C.: *Recognition and activation of the opioid receptor-like ORL1 receptor by nociceptin, nociceptin analogs and opioids*, Eur. J. Pharmacol. **1997**, *321*, 97-103.

Cesura, A., Hoffmann, T., Roever, S., Wichmann, J. (F. Hoffmann-La Roche AG): *Piperidine derivatives*, WO0014067 (**2000**).

Curró, D., Hyeon, J., Anderson, M., Song, I., Del Valle, J., Owyang, C.: *Molecular cloning of the orphanin FQ receptor gene and differential tissue expression of splice variants in rats*, Gene **2001**, *266*, 139-145.

Darland, T., Heinricher, M.M.; Grandy, D.K.: *Orphanin FQ/nociceptin: a role in pain and analgesia, but so much more*, Trends Neurosci. **1998**, *21*, 215-221.

Dautzenberg, F.M., Wichmann, J., Higelin, J., Py-Lang, G., Kratzeisen, C., Malherbe, P., Kilpatrick, G.J., Jenck, F.: *Pharmacological characterization of the novel nonpetide orphanin FQ / nociceptin receptor agonist Ro 64-6198: Rapid and reversible desensitization of the ORL1 receptor in vitro and lack of tolerance in vivo*, J. Pharmacol. Exp. Ther. **2001**, *298*, 812-819.

De Risi, C., Pollini, G.P., Trapella, C., Peretto, I., Ronzoni, S., Giardina, G.A.M.: *A new synthetic approach to 1-[(3R,4R)-1-Cyclooctylmethyl-3-hydroxymethyl-4-piperidyl]-3-ethyl-1,3-dihydro-benzimidazol-2-one (J-113397), the first non-peptide ORL-1 receptor antagonist*, Bioorg. Med. Chem. **2001**, *9*, 1871-1877.

Fumitaka, I. (Pfizer Inc.): *New 2-benzimidazoylamine compounds are ORL-1 receptor agonists*, US6340681 (**2001**).

Grisel, J.E., Mogil, J.S., Belknap, J.K., Grandy, D.K.: *Orphanin FQ acts as a supraspinal, but not a spinal, anti-opioid peptide*, Neuroreport **1996**, *7*, 2125-2129.

Higgins, G.A., Grottick, A.J., Ballard, T.M., Richards, J.G., Messer, J., Takeshima, H., Pauly-Evers, M., Jenck, F., Adam, G., Wichmann, J.: *Influence of the selective ORL1 receptor agonist, Ro64-6198, on rodent neurological function*, Neruopharmacology **2001**, *41*, 97-107.

Hohlweg, R., Watson, B.T., Petterson, I. (Novo Nordisk): *Novel triazaspirodecanones with high affinity for opioid receptor subtypes*, WO0136418 (**2001**).

Ichikawa, D., Ozaki, S., Azuma, T., Nambu, H., Kawamoto, H., Iwasawa, Y., Takeshima, H., Ohta, H.: In vitro *inhibitory effects J-113397 on nociceptin/orphanin FQ-stimulated [^{35}S]GTPγS binding to mouse brain*, Neuroreport **2001**, *12*, 1757-1761.

Ito, F. (Pfizer Inc.): *Preparation of morphinan hydroxamic acid derivatives*, EP829481 (**1998**).

Ito, F., Kondo, H., Noguchi, H., Ohashi, Y. (Pfizer Inc.): *4-(2-Keto-1-benzimidazolinyl)piperidine compounds as ORL1-receptor agonists*, WO9936421 (**1999**).

Jhamandas, K.H., Sutak, M., Henderson, G.: *Antinociceptive and morphine modulatory actions of spinal orphanin FQ*, Can. J. Physiol. Pharmacol. **1998**, *76*, 314-324.

Jenck, F., Moreau, J.-L., Martin, J.R., Kilpatric, G.J., Reinscheid, R.K., Monsma Jr., F.J., Nothacker, H.-P., Civelli, O.: *Orphanin FQ acts as an anxiolytic to attenuate behavioral response to stress*, Proc. Natl. Acad. Sci. USA **1997**, *94*, 14854-14858.

Jenck, F., Wichmann, J., Dautzenberg, F.M., Moreau, J.-L., Ouagazzal, A.M., Martin, J.R., Lundstrom, K., Cesura, A.M., Poli, S.M., Roever, S., Kolczewski, S., Adam, G., Kilpatrick, G.: *A synthetic agonist at the orphanin FQ/nociceptin receptor ORL1: anxiolytic profile in the rat*, Proc. Natl. Acad. Sci. USA **2000**, *97*, 4938-4943.

Kawamoto, H., Ozaki, S., Itoh, Y., Miyaji, M., Arai, S., Nakashima, H., Kato, T., Ohta, H., Iwasawa, Y.: *Discovery of the first potent and selective small molecule opioid receptor-like (ORL1) antagonist: 1-[(3R,4R)-1-Cyclooctylmethyl-3-hydroxymethyl-4-piperidyl]-3-ethyl-1,3-dihydro-2H-benzimidazol-2-one (J-113397)*, J. Med. Chem. **1999**, *42*, 5061-5063.

Kawamoto, H., Ozaki, S., Ito, Y., Iwasawa, Y., (Banyu Pharmaceutical Co.): *Preparation of 2-oxoimidazole derivatives as antagonists of nociceptin ORL1 receptors*, WO0031061(**2000**).

Kawamoto, H., Nakashima, H., Kato, T., Arai, S., Kamata, K., Iwasawa, Y.: *Synthesis of J-113397, the first potent and selective ORL1 antagonist*, Tetrahedron **2001**, *57*, 981-986.

King, M.A., Rossi, G.C., Chang, A.H., Williams, L., Pasternak, G.W.: *Spinal analgesic activity of orphanin FQ/nociceptin and its fragments*, Neurosci. Lett. **1997**, *223*, 113-116.

Kyle, D., Goehring, R.R., Shao, B. (Euroceltique): *Benzimidazole compounds having nociceptin receptor affinity*, WO0139775 (**2001**).

Manabe, T., Noda, Y., Mamiya, T., Katagiri, H., Houtani, T., Nishi, M., Noda, T., Takahashi, T., Sugimoto, T., Nabeshima, T., Takeshima, H.: *Facilitation of long-term potentiation and memory in mice lacking nociceptin receptors*, Nature **1998**, *394*, 577-581.

Meunier, J.-C., Mollereau, C., Toll, L., Suaudeau, C., Moisand, C., Alvinerie, P., Butour, J.-L., Guillemot, J.-C., Ferrara, P., Monsarrat, B., Mazargil, H., Vassart, G., Parmentier, M., Costentin, J.: *Isolation and structure of the endogenous agonist of the opioid receptor-like ORL1 receptor*, Nature **1995**, *377*, 532-535.

Meunier, J.-C.: *Nociceptin / orphanin FQ and the opioid receptor-like ORL1 receptor*, Eur. J. Pharmacol. **1997**, *340*, 1-15.

Meunier, J.-C.: *The potential therapeutic value of nociceptin receptor agonists and antagonists*, Exp. Opin. Ther. Patents **2000**, *10*, 371-388.

Mollereau, C., Parmentier, M., Mailleux, P., Butour, J.-L., Moisand, C., Chalon, P., Caput, D., Vassart, G., Meunier, J.-C.: *ORL1, a novel member of the opioid receptor family. Cloning, functional expression and localization*, FEBS Lett. **1994**, *341*, 33-38.

Mogil, J.S., Grisel, J.E., Reinscheid, R.K., Civelli, O., Belknap, J.K., Grandy, D.K.: *Orphanin FQ is a functional anti-opioid peptide*, Neuroscience (Oxford) **1996**a, *75*, 333-337.

Mogil, J.S., Grisel, J.E., Zhangs, G., Belknap, J.K., Grandy, D.K.: *Functional antagonism of $\mu-$, $\delta-$, $\kappa-$opioid antinociception by Orphanin FQ*, Neurosci. Lett. **1996**b, *214*, 131-134.

Mogil, J.S. and Pasternak, G.W.; *The molecular and behavioral pharmacology of the orphanin FQ/nociceptin peptide and receptor family*, Phamacol. Rev. **2001**, *53*, 381-415.

Nagase, H., Endo, T., Kawamura, K., Yamane, S., Suzuki, T., Sato, K. (Toray Industries): *Morphinan analogs as ORL1 (opioid orphan) receptor antagonists*, JP2000053572 (**2000**).

Okana, M., Mori, K. (Nippon Shinyaku): *Heterocycle derivatives and drugs*, WO0172710 (**2001**).

Okuda, S, Tanaka, T., Miyaji, M., Nishino, M., Iguchi, T., Ozaki, S. Kawamoto, H., Ito, Y., Iwasawa, Y., Ohta, H.: *Pharmacological profiles of J-113397, a novel nociceptin (orphanin FQ) antagonist in pain regulation*, 30th Meet. Soc. Neurosci. **2000**, Abs. 435.13.

Okuda-Ashitaka, E., Tachibana, S., Houtani, T., Minami, T., Masu, Y., Nishi, M., Takeshima, H., Sugimoto, T., Ito, S.: *Identification and characterization of an endogenous ligand for opioid receptor homologue ROR-C: its involvement in allodynic response to innocuous stimulus*, Brain Res. Mol. Brain Res. **1996**, *43*, 96-104.

Ozaki, S., Kawamoto, H., Itoh, Y., Miyaji, M., Iwasawa, Y., Ohta, H.: *A potent and highly selective nonpeptidyl nociceptin/orphanin FQ receptor (ORL1) antagonist: J-113397*, Eur. J. Pharmacol. **2000**a, *387*, R17-R18.

Ozaki, S., Kawamoto, H., Itoh, Y., Miyaji, M., Azuma, T., Ichikawa, D., Nambu, H., Iguchi, T., Iwasawa, Y., Ohta, H.: *In vitro and in vivo pharmacological characterization of J-113397, a potent and selective non-peptidyl ORL1 receptor antagonist*, Eur. J. Pharmacol. **2000**b, *402*, 45-53.

Pomonis, J.D., Billington, C.J., Levine, A.S.: *Orphanin FQ, agonist of orphan opioid receptor ORL1, stimulates feeding in rats*, NeuroReport **1996**, *8*, 369-371.

Reinscheid, R.K., Nothacker, H.-P., Bourson, A., Ardati, A., Hennigsen, R.A., Bunzow, J.R., Grandy, D.K., Langen, H., Monsma Jr., F.J., Civelli, O.: *Orphanin FQ: A neuropeptide that activates an opioid like G protein-coupled receptor*, Science **1995**, *270*, 792-794.

Rizzi, D., Bigoni, R., Rizzi, A., Jenck, F., Wichmann, J., Guerrini, R., Regoli, D., Calo, C.: *Effects of Ro 64-6198 in nociceptin/orphanin FQ-sensitive isolated tissues*, Naunyn-Schmiedeberg's Arch. Pharmacol. **2001**, *363*, 551-555.

Röver, S., Adam, G., Cesura, A.M., Galley, G., Jenck, F., Monsma Jr., F.J., Wichmann, J., Dautzenberg, F.M.: *High affinity, non-peptide agonists for the ORL1 (Orphanin FQ/Nociceptin) receptor*, J. Med. Chem. **2000**a, *43*, 1329-1228.

Röver, S., Wichmann, J., Jenck, F., Adam, G., Cesura, A.M.: *ORL1 receptor ligands: Structure-activity relationships of 8-cycloalkyl-1-phenyl-1,3,8-triaza-dpiro[4.5]decan-4-ones*, Bioorg. Med. Chem. Lett. **2000**b, *10*, 831-834.

Ronzoni, S., Peretto, I., Giardina, G.A.M.: *Lead generation and lead optimisation approaches in the discovery of selective, non-peptide ORL-1 receptor agonists and antagonists*, Exp. Opin. Ther. Patents **2001**, *11*, 525-546.

Rossi, G., Leventhal, L., Pasternak, G.W.: *Naloxone sensitive orphanin FQ-induced analgesia in mice*, Eur. J. Pharmacol. **1996**, *311*, R7-R8.

Shinkai, H., Ito, T., Yamada, H. (Japan Tobacco): *New amide compounds are nociceptin antagonists – useful as analgesics e.g. for post-operative pain*, WO9948293 (**1999**).

Shinkai, H., Ito, T., Iida, T., Kitao, Y., Yamada, H., Uchida, I.: *4-Aminoquinolines: Novel nociceptin antagonists with analgesic activity*, J. Med. Chem. **2000**, *43*, 4667-4677.

Thomsen, C.: *Nociceptin receptor agonists*, Drugs Fut. **2001**, *26*, 1059-1064.

Thomsen, C. and Hohlweg, R.: *(8-Naphthalen-1-ylmethyl-4-oxo-1-phenyl-1,3,8-triaza-spiro[4.5]dec-3-yl)-acetic acid methyl ester (NNC 63-0532) is a novel potent nociceptin receptor agonist*, Br. J. Pharmacol. **2000**, *131*, 903-908.

Tian, J.H., Xu, W., Fangy, Y., Mogil, J.S., Grisel, J.E., Grandy, D.K., Han, J.-S.: *Bidirectional modulatory effect of orphanin FQ on morphine-induced analgesia: antagonism in brain and potentiation in spinal cord of the rat,* Br. J. Pharmacol. **1997**, *120*, 676-680.

Topham, C.M., Moulédous, L., Poda, G., Maigret, B., Meunier, J.-C.: *Molecular modelling of the ORL1 receptor and its complex with nociceptin*, Protein Engineering **1998**, *11*, 1163-1179.

Tulshian, D, Silverman, L.S., Matasi, J.J., McLeod, R.L., Hey, J.A., Capman, R.W., Bercovici, A. (Schering Corp.): *High affinity ligands for nociceptin receptor ORL-1*, WO0006545 (**2000**).

Ueda, H., Yamaguchi, T., Tokuyama, S., Inoue, M., Nishi, M., Takeshima, H.: *Partial loss of tolerance liability to morphine analgesia in mice lacking the nociceptin receptor gene*, Neuroscience Lett. **1997**, *237*, 136-138.

Watson, B.T., Hohlweg, R., Thomsen, C. (Novo Nordisk): *Novel 1,3,8-triazaspiro[4.5]decanones with high affinity for opioid recetor subtypes*, WO9959997 (**1999**).

Wichmann, J., Adam, G., Röver, S., Cesura, A.M., Dautzenberg, F.M., Jenck, F.: *8-Acenaphthen-1-yl-1-phenyl-1,3,8-triazasdpiro[4.5]decan-4-one derivatives as orphanin FQ receptor agonists*, Bioorg. Med. Chem. Lett. **1999**, *9*, 2343-2348.

Wichmann, J., Adam, G., Röver, S., Hennig, M., Scalone, M., Cesura, A.M., Dautzenberg, F.M., Jenck, F.: *Synthesis of (1S,3aS)-8-(2,3,3a,4,5,6-hexahydro-1H-phenalen-1-yl) -1-phenyl-1,3,8-triaza-spiro[4.5]decan-4-one, a potent and selective orphanin FQ (OFQ) receptor agonists with anxiolytic-like properties*, Eur. J. Med. Chem. **2000**, *35*, 839-851.

Wnendt, S., Krüger, T., Janocha, E., Hildebrandt, D, Englberger, W.: *Agonistic effect of buprenorphine in a nociceptin/OFQ receptor triggered reporter gene assay*, Mol. Pharmacol. **1999**, *56*, 334-338.

Yamada, H., Nakamoto, H., Suzuki, Y, Ito, T., Aisaka, K.: *Pharmacological profile of a novel opioid receptor-like 1 (ORL₁) receptor antagonist, JTC-801*, Br. J. Pharmacol **2002**, *135*, 323-332.

Yu, T.-P., Fein, J., Phan, T., Evans, C.J., Xie, C.-W.: *Orphanin FQ inhibits synaptic transmission and long-term potentiation in rat hippocampus*, Hippocampus **1997**, *7*, 88-94.

Zaki, P.A. and Evans, C.J.: *ORL-1: an awkward child of the opioid receptor family*, The Neuroscientist **1998**, *4*, 172-184.

10 Adenosine

Corinna Maul, Helmut Buschmann and Bernd Sundermann

In the 20 years since Daly reported the potential of adenosine receptors as drug targets (Daly, 1982), considerable advances have been made in the field of purinergic receptor-related research. Although a range of neurotransmitters is known, today there is no doubt that adenosine and adenosine 5'-triphosphate (ATP) also play an important role in the process of cell to cell communication. This function leads to multiple potential indications for research on adenosine and ATP, e.g. neurodegeneration or cardiovascular diseases, but here the focus lies on adenosine's role in pain (see also review by Salter and Sollevi, 2001).

Transmission of somatosensory information is normally initiated in the periphery through stimulation of endings of primary afferent neurons encoding information by an action potential discharge which is propargated into the central nervous system (CNS). The first level of central processing for most somatosensory information is the dorsal horn of the spinal cord or the homologous region of the trigeminal nucleus. The perception of this information as pain depends, among other things, on the actions and interactions of numerous neurotransmitter/neuromodulator systems at peripheral and central sites. Multiple lines of evidence support roles for adenosine and adenosine-5'-triphosphate (ATP) in the transmission of sensory information in the periphery and the dorsal horn (Salter and Sollevi, 2001).

Adenosine nucleosides and nucleotides exert a variety of effects through the activation of specific membrane receptors which are generally referred to as purinoreceptors. Burnstock defined two major classes of purinoreceptors named P1 and P2 (Burnstock, 1978). It was found that P1 purinoreceptors (adenosine receptors) are more responsive to adenosine. Adenosine receptors are the only extracellular nucleoside membrane receptors that have been described so far. P2 purinoreceptors (ATP-receptors) are more responsive to ATP and ADP as physiological agonists (Müller, 1996; Baraldi et al., 1999).

Today four subtypes of adenosine receptors - A_1, A_{2a}, A_{2b} and A_3 - are known, all of which are members of the G-protein coupled receptor (GPCR) family. While A_{2a} and A_{2b} receptors stimulate adenylyl cyclase and consequently lead to an increase of cAMP levels, A_1 and A_3 receptors produce the opposite effect upon activation.

Adenosine

ATP

P1 receptors = adenosine receptors

P2-receptors = ATP-receptors

Four adenosine receptor subtypes: A_1, A_{2a}, A_{2b} and A_3

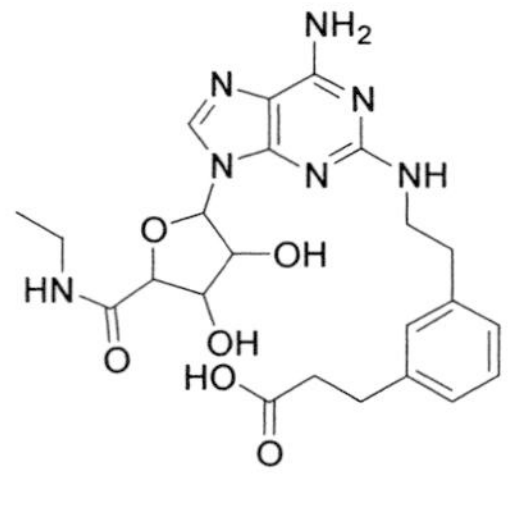

CGS-21680

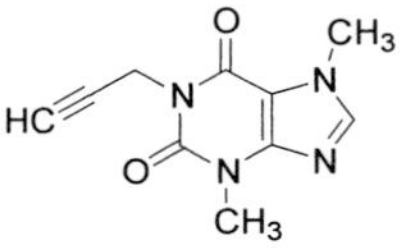

DMPX

The peripheral actions of adenosine itself have been found to be pro- or antinociceptive in behavioral tests. In human subjects pain is evoked when adenosine is administered locally, e.g. into the coronary artery (Lagerquist et al., 1990). Algogenic or pronociceptive effects have also been seen in animal models (Karlsten et al., 1992). Pharmacological studies indicate that the pro-nociceptive effects of peripherally administered adenosine are mediated by interaction with A_2-like adenosine receptors. The A_{2A}-selective agonist CGS 21680 enhances formalin-induced nociceptive behavior only during the latter phase of the test, while the low affinity A2-selective antagonist DMPX has the opposite effect (Doak and Sawynok, 1995). A_{2A}-selective antagonists (Fig. 1) are well studied in neuroprotective indications (Phillis, 2002) and there are (or have been) compounds in clinical trials which makes them the most important class of potential future drugs influencing P1 receptors, and some of them are claimed to be useful against pain (Gillespie et al. (Vernalis Research)), while A_{2A} agonists are reported to be useful against inflammatory diseases (Chan et al. (Glaxo Group), 1999, Linden et al. (University of Virginia), 2000). A_{2B} receptors have not been investigated as thoroughly as A_{2A} receptors and their role in pain management has not yet been elucidated.

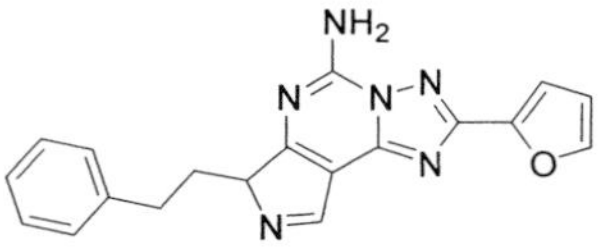

SCH-58261, neuroprotective, A_1 287 nM,
A_{2A} 0,6 nM (human) (Schering-Plough),
for analogs see Baraldi et al., 2002

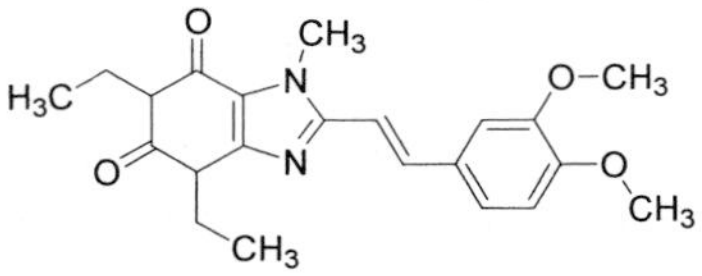

KW-6002, Phase II Parkinson,
A_1 580 nM, A_{2A} 13 nM (rat) (Kyowa Hakko)

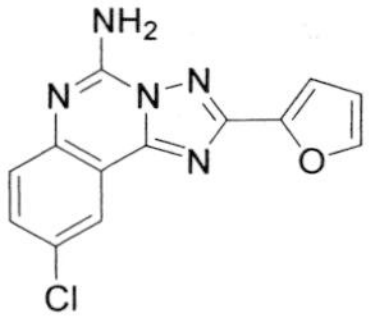

CGS 15943, discontinued,
vasoprotectant , A_1 3,5 nM, A_{2A} 0,4
nM (human) (Novartis)

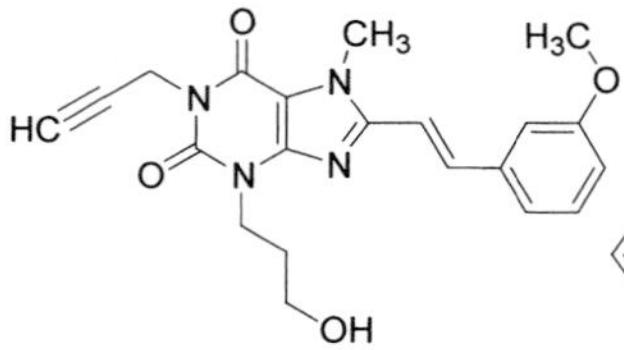

MSX-2, A_1 2500 nM,
A_{2A} 8 nM (human)
(Sauer et al., 2000)

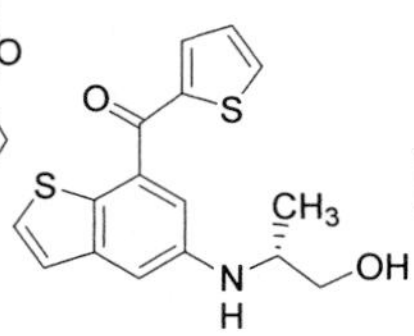

A_{2A} 2 nM (Gillespie et al.,
Vernalis Res.,
WO 0102409)

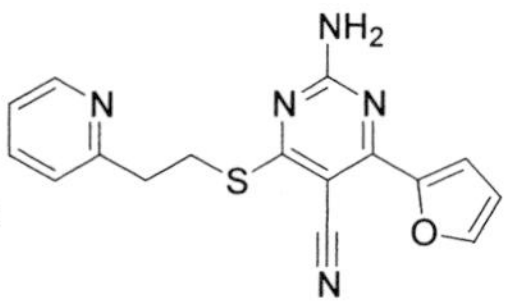

A_{2A} 0,8 nM (Borroni et
al.,Hoffmann La Roche,
WO 0162233)

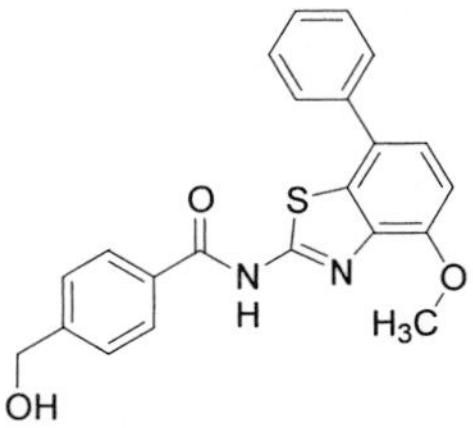

A_{2A} (Alanine et al.,
Hoffmann La Roche,
WO 0197786)

Figure 1: A_{2A} receptor antagonists

Additional antinociceptive potential of adenosine may arise from its antiinflammatory effects. These effects have been attributed to peripheral activation of A_2-like receptors which, among other actions, inhibits neutrophil adhesion and prevents the secretion of proinflammatory cytokines. Thus, while the activation of A_2 receptors might be involved in pronociception, antiinflammatory effects which may lead to diminished post-inflammatory pain have also been observed.

The A_1 receptor is distributed preferentially in most regions of the CNS, where adenosine acts as a neuromodulator inhibiting the release of neurotransmitters via prejunctional A_1 receptors. In electrophysiological recordings from DRG cell bodies adenosine has been shown to inhibit high voltage-gated Ca^{2+} currents, an effect mediated mainly through the activation of A_1 receptors. Presynaptic inhibitory effects of adenosine in the CNS are well known and may suppress Ca^{2+} currents as well as transmitter release processes not dependent upon Ca^{2+} influx (Dolphin et al., 1986; Macdonald et al., 1986).

In contrast to the local algogenic effects of adenosine, systemic administration of adenosine at low dosage has been shown to induce analgesia in humans. The activation of peripheral A_1 adenosine receptors induces antinociception in animal models of inflammatory or neuropathic pain. Tissue adenosine levels are elevated in conditions of ischemia and inflammation. The peripheral administration of A_1 antagonists increases pain behavior in nociceptive tests while A_1 agonists can produce antinociception, so it has been suggested that adenosine may activate peripheral A_1 receptors which then participate in reducing post-inflammatory pain. Some A_1 receptor agonists, all of them adenosine analogs with an intact sugar moiety, have proven to be analgesics. The adenine binding site at the A1 receptor has been investigated intensively (IJzerman et al., 1995; Rivkees et al., 1999).

Evidence for A_1 receptor agonists to be analgesics

UP202-32, analgesic, no development
reported since 1997 (BMS)

GR 79236, analgesic, discontinued
after phase 1 (Glaxo Wellcome)

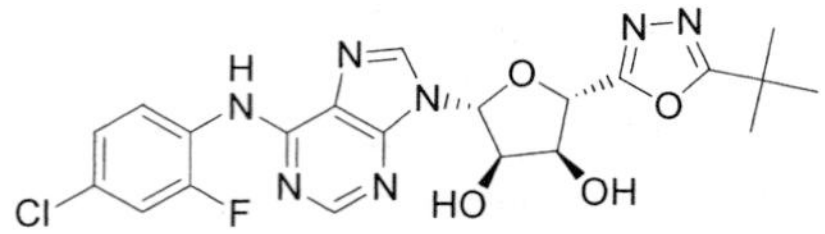

Glaxo Group WO99/67262, analgesic, several patent
applications for combinations with other analgesics recently
published (Bountra et al 2001)

Figure 2: A_1 receptor agonists.

Combination of A_1 agonistic and antagonistic action in one molecule

Some developments have been made towards the combination of A_1 agonist and antagonist structures in one molecule and these molecules were reported to have analgesic properties (Reddy et al., 1998), but further progress has not yet been published.

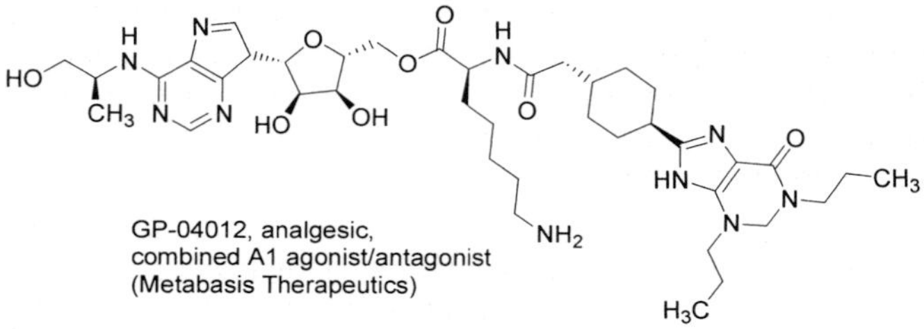

GP-04012, analgesic,
combined A1 agonist/antagonist
(Metabasis Therapeutics)

Figure 3: Combination of A_1 receptor agonist and antagonist.

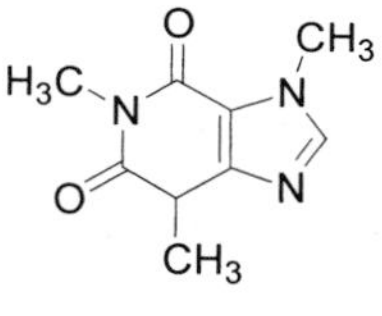

caffeine

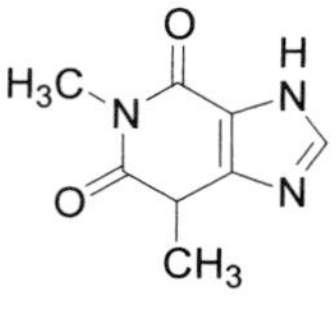

The most prominent mixed A_1/A_2 receptor antagonist is caffeine which is currently used clinically as an adjunctive analgesic in combination with acetaminophen and other NSAIDs. Its adjuvant activity has been demonstrated in both clinical and preclinical studies and it is extremely successful on the OTC market. Other mixed A_1/A_2 receptor antagonist are currently being investigated in preclinical studies (Akahane et al. (Fujisawa Pharm Co), 2001).

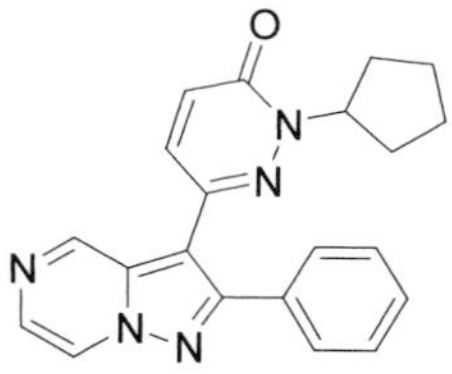

theophylline

A_1 0,1nM, A_{2a} 0,84 nM
(Akahane et al., Fujisawa, WO 0140230)

Figure 4: A_1/A_{2A} antagonist.

The fourth receptor of the adenosine receptor family - A_3 - has not yet been thoroughly investigated. The activation of A_3 receptors is not antagonized by xanthines like theophylline. The A_3 receptor shows low sequence homology between species: while the amino acid sequence homology of other adenosine receptors is usually in the range of 85% up to >90%, homology of the rat and human A_3 receptor is only about 74%. This may cause problems in drug development because data transfer from animal models to humans might be difficult.

There is some evidence that adenosine also participates in modulating peripheral somatosensory function through A_3 receptors on immune cells. A predominant response to the activation of A_3 receptors is degranulation of mast cells causing the release of multiple proinflammatory mediators (IL-6/IL-10/IL-12). Further involvement of A_3 receptors in pain and inflammation may be a result of adenosine-mediated inhibition of the release of tumor necrosis factor α (TNF-α), a proinflammatory cytokine produced by monocytes and macrophages.

The A_1 and A_3 receptor agonists known today are adenosine analogs and the sugar moiety has usually only minor modifications at 3'- and 5'-position. Moreover, there are various examples of N^6-substituted A_1-selective adenosine analogs reported in the literature. Exceptions which do not possess a sugar moiety are methanocarbocyclic analogs of adenosine where the A_1 and A_3 receptor agonists are claimed to be useful against pain (Jacobsen et al., 2001).

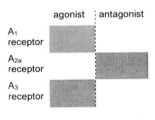

Functionality at P1 receptors of compounds useful for pain management (grey)

K_i values [nM]:
A_1 141, A_{2A} 732, A_3 2,2

K_i values [nM]:
A_1 8,7, A_{2A} 3390, A_3 466

Figure 5: A_3/A_1 receptor agonists.

Adenosine levels can also be influenced through indirect mechanisms mediated by adenosine kinase, adenosine deaminase and the nucleoside transport protein.

Indirect mechanisms influencing adenosine levels

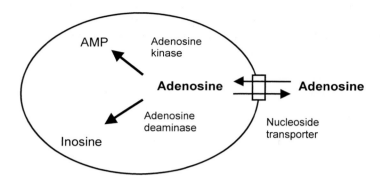

Figure 6: Indirect mechanisms for influencing adenosine levels.

Adenosine kinase

Among these potential pain targets only adenosine kinase has been intensively investigated preclinically as well as clinically. Adenosine kinase is a cytosolic enzyme catalyzing the phosphorylation of adenosine to adenosine-5'-monophosphate (AMP) and thus plays an important role in adenosine metabolism. Inhibition of intracellular adenosine kinase decreases the cellular reuptake of adenosine, thereby increasing the concentration of adenosine in the extracellular compartement. Antinociceptive effects of adenosine kinase inhibitors have been demonstrated pharmacologically with 5-iodotubercidin and 5'-deoxy-5-iodotubercidin which are efficacious in animal models of acute pain. Some adenosine kinase inhibitors with adenosine-related structure have been reported to be in clinical trials as potential pain killers. Non-nucleoside adenosine kinase inhibitors are also known: ABT-702 is reported not only to produce antinociception in both acute and chronic animal models of pain but furthermore can be administered by the oral route.

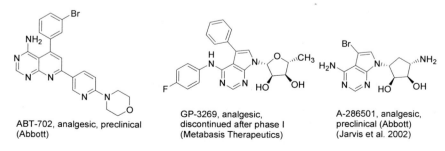

ABT-702, analgesic, preclinical
(Abbott)

GP-3269, analgesic,
discontinued after phase I
(Metabasis Therapeutics)

A-286501, analgesic,
preclinical (Abbott)
(Jarvis et al. 2002)

Figure 7: Adenosine kinase inhibitors

Severe side-effects (hemorrhages in rats and dogs brain) have been reported after systemic application of several selected adenosine kinase inhibitors (Erion, 2000). Nevertheless, ABT-702 in particular is still reported to be in preclinical development.

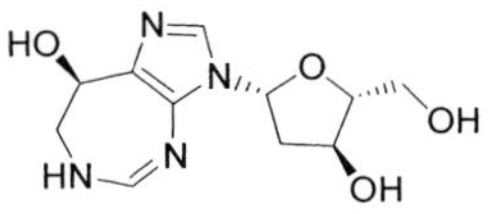

2'-deoxycoformycin

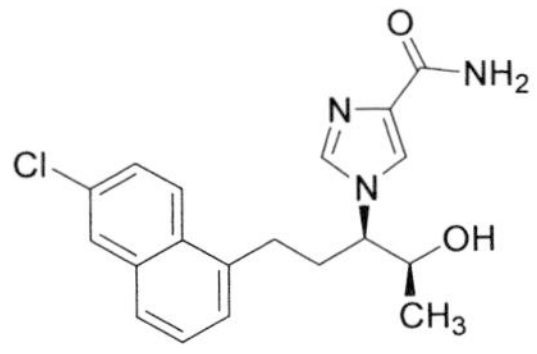

Tsuji et al.,
Fujisawa Pharmaceuticals,
WO 0153271

Figure 8: Adenosine deaminase inhibitors

Adenosine deaminase catalyzes the hydrolytic deamination of adenosine and 2'-deoxyadenosine to inosine and 2'-deoxyinosine respectively. Inhibition of adenosine deaminase leads to an accumulation of its substrates which results in adenosine receptor-mediated effects. Most inhibitors are not reported to have antinociceptive properties, but 2'-deoxycoformycin was proven to have an inhibitory effect on pain transmission (Poon and Sawynok, 1999), and Fujisawa Pharmaceuticals claim adenosine deaminase inhibitors to be active against chronic pain.

Adenosine deaminase: potential target for chronic pain

An increase of intracellular adenosine levels can also be achieved by inhibition of nucleoside transport proteins. Mammalian nucleoside transport processes can be classified into two types on the basis of their thermodynamic properties. These classes are the concentrative, Na^+-dependent transport processes and the equilibrative, Na^+-independent processes. The corresponding transporters are called CNTs (concentrative nucleoside transporters) and ENTs (equilibrative nucleoside transporters) (Pastor-Anglada and Baldwin, 2001).

Nucleoside transport inhibitors, active in neuropathic pain?

Some adenosine nucleoside transport inhibitors have been reported to be useful against pain, especially neuropathic pain (animal models) (Meert and van Belle (Janssen Pharm), 1998; Deleo and Schubert, 2000).

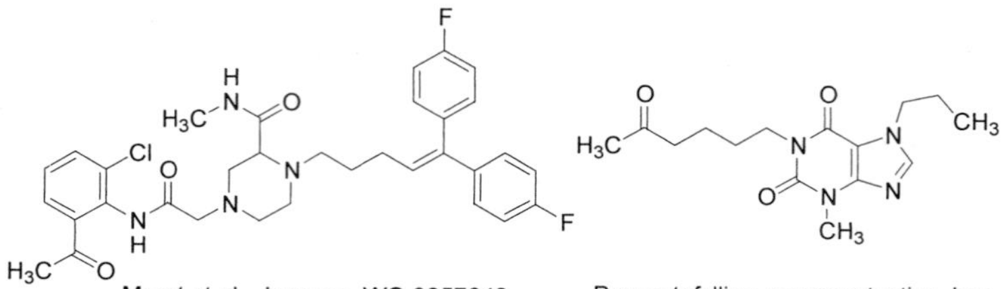

Meert et al., Janssen, WO 9857643
active in chronic pain

Propentofylline, neuroprotective, has
proven to be active in neuropathic pain

Figure 9: Nucleoside transport inhibitors.

Enhancement of the binding
of agonists to the receptor
by allosteric enhancers

A further possibility to modulate physiological adenosine
or agonistic effects could be allosteric enhancement.
Allosteric enhancers described so far enhance the binding
of several agonists by up to two-fold so they bind more
efficiently, and lower concentrations of the agonist are
needed (Bruns et al., 1990). Some of the compounds are
claimed to have analgesic properties (Baraldi, 1999) or
reported to be active in neuropathic pain (Li et al., 2002).

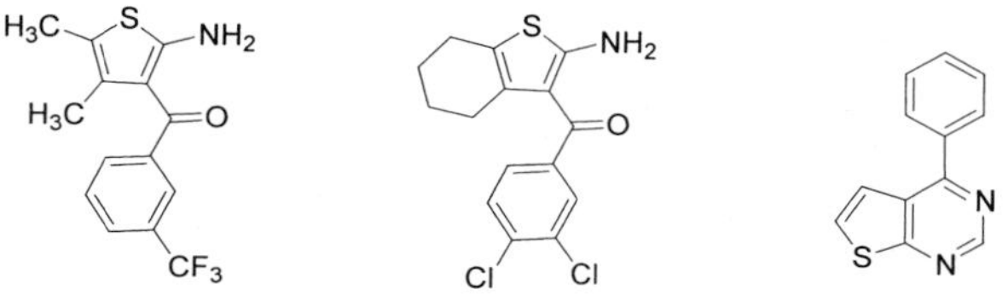

PD 81,723
(Parke-Davis)

van der Klein et al. 1999

Baraldi, US5939432
(1999)

Figure 10: Allosteric enhancers for the A1 receptor.

Clinical investigations to date have focussed on effects of
adenosine in experimentally-induced pain as well as
clinical pain states. These studies have shown that
adenosine administration reduces pain primarily in
situations that involve enhanced excitability and
nociceptive transmission in the CNS. Since centrally-
mediated enhanced excitability is considered to be an
important factor in chronic pain conditions, adenosine-
induced pain relief in patients with neuropathic pain
suggests that adenosine and adenosine analogs are of
special importance for future research.

References:

For reviews see

Baraldi, P. G., Cacciari, B., Romagnoli, R., Spalluto, G.: *A1 and A3 adenosine receptor agonists: an
overview*, Exp. Opin. Ther. Patents **1999**, *9*, 515-527.

Broadley, K. J.: *Drugs modulating adenosine receptors as potential therapeutic agents for cardiovascular
deseases*, Exp. Opin. Ther. Patents **2000**, *10*, 1669-1692.

Jacobson, K. A., van Galen, P. J. M., Williams, M.: *Adenosine receptors: pharmacology, structure-activity relationships, and therapeutic potential*, J. Med. Chem. **1992**, *35*, 407-422.

Kaiser, S. M., Quinn, R.J.: *Adenosine receptors as potential therapeutic targets*, DDT **1999**, *4*, 542-551.

Müller, C. E., Stein, B.: *Adenosine Receptor Antagonists: Structures and Potential Therapeutic Applications*, Curr. Pharmaceut. Design **1996**, *2*, 501-530.

Müller, C. E.: *Adenosine receptor ligands – recent developments part I. agonists*; Curr. Med. Chem. **2000**, *7*, 1269-1288.

Salter, M. W. and Sollevi, A.: *Roles of purines in nociception and pain*, Handbook of Experimental Pharmacology **2001**, 371-401.

Alanine, A., Flohr, A., Miller, A. K., Norcross, R. D., Riemer, C. (Hoffmann-La Roche), *Benzothiazole derivatives*, WO 0197786.

Akahane, A. et al.(Fujisawa Pharmaceutical Corporation, Ltd): Pyrazolopyrazines and their use as adenosine antagonists, WO 0140230, *Pyrazolopyrazines as adenosine antagonists*, WO 0024742.

Burnstock, G.: *A basis for distinguishing two types of purinergic receptor*. In: Cell membrane receptors for drugs and hormones: A multidisciplinary approach. New York, Raven Press **1978**, 107-118.

Baraldi, P. G. (Medco Research Inc.): Thiophenes useful for modulating the adenosine receptor, US 5939432 (1999).

Baraldi, P. G., Cacciari, B., Romagnoli, R., Spalluto, G., Monopoli, A., Ongini, E., Varani, K., Borea, P. A.: *7-Substituted 5-amino-2-(2-furyl)pyrazolo[4,3-e]-1,2,4-triazolo[1,5-c]pyrimidines as A2A adenosine receptor antagonists: a study on the importance of modifications at the side chain on the activity and solubility*, J. Med. Chem. **2002**, *45*, 115-126.

Borroni, E. M., Huber-Trottmann, G., Kil-Patrick, G.J., Norcross, R.D. (Hoffmann La Roche), *Adenosine receptor modulators*, WO 0162233.

Bountra, C., Clayton, N. M., Naylor, A. (Glaxo Group Ltd): *Formulations of Adenosine A1 Receptors*, WO 0145684, WO 0145683, WO 0145715.

Chan, C. et al. (Glaxo Group Ltd): *2-(Purin-9-yl)-tetrahydrofuran-3-4-diol derivatives*, WO 9941267, WO 9938877.

Daly, J. W.: *Adenosine receptors: Targets for future drugs*, J. Med. Chem. **1982**, *25*, 197-207.

Deleo, J. A., Schubert, P. (Trustees of Dartmouth College): *Compositions and method for decreasing neuropathic pain*, WO 0071128.

Doak, G. J. and Sawynok, J.: *Complex role of peripheral adenosine in the genesis of response to subcutaneous formalin in the rat*, Eur. J. Pharmacol. **1995**, *281*, 311-318.

Dolphin, A.C., Forda, S. R., Scott, R. H.: *Calcium-dependent currents in cultured rat dorsal root ganglion neurones are inhibited by an adenosine analog*, J. Physiol.**1986**, *373*, 47-61.

Erion, M., Purines 2000 (Conference), Madrid, July 12.

Gillespie, R. J., Giles, P. R., Lerpiniere, J., Dawson, C. E., Bebbington, D. (Vernalis Research, Ltd), *Thieno- and furopyrimidine derivatives as A2a-receptor antagonists*, WO0102409.

IJzerman, A.P., van Galen, P. J. M., van der Wenden, E. M.: *Molecular modelling of the adenosine A1 receptor*, New Perspectives in Drug Design **1995**, 121-136.

IJzerman, A.P., Kourounakis, A., van der Klein, P., *Allosteric modulation of G-protein-coupled receptors*, II Farmaco **2001**, *56*, 67-70.

Jacobsen, K. and Marquez, V., (The government of the United States of America, Department of Health and Human Services), *Methanocarba cycloalkyl nucleoside analogues*, WO 0151490.

Jarvis, M. F., Yu, H., McGaraughty, S., Wismer, C. T., Mikusa, J., Zhu, C., Chu, K., Kohlhaas, K., Cowart, M., Lee, C.-H., Stewart, A. O., Cox, B. F., Polakowski, J., Kowaluk, E. A.: *Analgesic and anti-*

inflammatory effects of A-286501, a novel orally active adenosine kinase inhibitor, Pain **2002**, 96, 107-118.

Karlsten, R., Gordh, T., Post, C.: *Local antinociceptive and hyperalgesic effects in in the formalin test after peripheral administration of adenosine analogues in mice*, Pharmacol. Toxicol **1992**, 70, 434-438.

van der Klein, P. A. M., Kourounakis, A., Ijzerman, A.P.: *Allosteric modulation of the adenosine A1 receptor. Synthesis and biological evaluation of novel 2-amino-3-bentothiophenes as allosteric enhancers of agonist binding*, J. Med. Chem **1999**, 42, 3629-3635.

Lagerquist, B., Sylven, C., Beermann, B., Helmius, G., Waldenström, A.: *Intracoronary adenosine causes angina pectoris like pain – an inquiry into the nature of visceral pain*, Cardiovasc. Res. **1990**, 24, 609-613.

Li, X., Conklin, D., Ma, W., Zhu, X., Eisenach, J. C.: *Spinal noradrenergic activation mediates allodynia reduction from an allosteric adenosine modulator in a rat model of neuropathic pain*, Pain **2002**, 97, 117-125.

Linden, J., Sullivan, G., Sarembock, I. J., Scheld, M. W. (University of Virginia): *Methods and compositions for treating the inflammatory response*, WO 0072799.

Macdonald, R. L., Skerritt, J. H., Werz, M. A.: *Adenosine agonists reduce voltage-dependent calcium conductance of mouse sensory neurones in cell culture*, J. Physiol. **1986**, 370, 75-90.

Meert, T. F. and van Belle, H. (Janssen Pharmaceutica): *Use of draflazine-analogues for treating pain*, WO9857643.

Pastor-Anglada, M., Baldwin, S.A.: *Recent advanceses in the molecular biology and physiology of nucleoside and nucleobase transporters*, DDR **2001**, 52, 431-437.

Reddy, K.E. et al., 216th ACS National Meeting (Aug 23-27, Boston) **1998**.

Phillis, J.W.: *Adenosine as a neuroprotectant: therapeutic perspectives*, Exp. Rev. Neurother. **2002**, 2, 167-176.

Poon, A., Sawynok, J.: *Antinociceptive and anti-inflammatory properties of an adenosine kinase inhibitor and an adenosine deaminase inhibitor*, J. Eur. J. Pharmacol. **1999**, 384, 123-138.

Rivkees, S. A., Barbhaiya, H., IJzerman, A. P.: *Identification of the adenine binding site of the human A1 adenosine receptor*, J. Biol. Chem. **1999**, 274, 3617-3621.

Sauer, R., Maurinsh, J., Reith, U., Fülle, F., Klotz, K.-N., Müller, C. E.: *Water-soluble phosphate prodrugs of 1-propargyl-8-styrylxanthine derivatives, A_{2A}-selective adenosine receptor antagonists*, J. Med. Chem. **2000**, 43, 440-448.

Sen, R. P., Delicado, E. G., Miras-Portugal, M. T., Gualix, J.: *Nucleoside transporter and nucleotide vesicular transporter: two examples of mnemonic regulation*, DDR **2000**, 52, 11-21.

Tsuji, K., Terasaka, T., Nakamura, K. (Fujisawa Pharmaceuticals Corporation, Ltd.): *Imidazole compounds and their use as adenosine deaminase inhibitors*, WO 0153271.

11   P2 Receptors

Hagen-Heinrich Hennies,
Corinna Maul and Bernd
Sundermann

The physiological activity of adenine compounds has been under investigation for many years. Very early studies were published by Drury and Szent-Györgyi in 1929. Evidence first implicating ATP as an excitatory neurotransmitter in the somatosensory system came from studies by Holton and Holton who demonstrated that ATP is released from peripheral endings of primary sensory neurons (Holton and Holton, 1953; Holton, 1959). Then, in 1970, it was proposed that nonadrenergic, noncholinergic (NANC) nerves supplying the gut and bladder use ATP as a motor neurotransmitter (Burnstock et al., 1970; 1972a). In a pharmacological review, Burnstock introduced the term 'purinergic' and presented the first evidence for purinergic transmission in a wide variety of systems (Burnstock, 1972b).

The central release of ATP from dorsal horn synaptosomes was proven by White et al. (1985). Further studies (Sawynok et al., 1993) suggest that ATP can be released from central terminals of primary afferent neurons as well as from terminals of non-primary afferents within the dorsal horn and that ATP and GABA are co-transmitters at many synapses in the dorsal horn (Jo and Schlichter, 1999). After being released ATP acts on specific receptors, designated as P2 purinoreceptors, on the cell surface.

The release of ATP in the central nervous system

The P2 receptor nomenclature was prompted by evidence that extracellular ATP works through two different transduction mechanisms, namely intrinsic ion channels and G-protein coupled receptors (Benham and Tsien, 1987; Dubyak, 1991). In 1994 it was formally suggested that P2 receptors should be divided into two groups termed P2X and P2Y according to whether they are ligand-gated ion channels (Fig. 1) or are coupled to G-proteins - metabotropic receptors belonging to the heptahelical superfamily (Abbracchio and Burnstock, 1994; Barnard et al., 1994; Fredholm et al., 1994).

P2 nomenclature:

P2X   ligand-gated ion channels (ionotropic receptors)

P2Y   G-protein coupled receptors (metabotropic receptors)

As intensively reviewed by Ralevic and Burnstock (1998), studies on purinoceptors were accompanied by many pitfalls:

1. P2X receptors are multi-subunit receptors. They may exist as homomers or as heteromers; heteromers may have a different pharmacology in comparison with homomers

2. Cations can affect P2X channel activity very profoundly

3. Ligands previously regarded to be selective for P2Y receptors were found to be active at P2X channels also

4. Ecto-nucleotidases can alter agonist potencies (for review of extracellular metabolism of ATP see Zimmermann, 2000)

5. Antagonists used as P2 receptor blockers were found to be non-selective. In addition they are able to modulate ecto-nucleotidase activity also

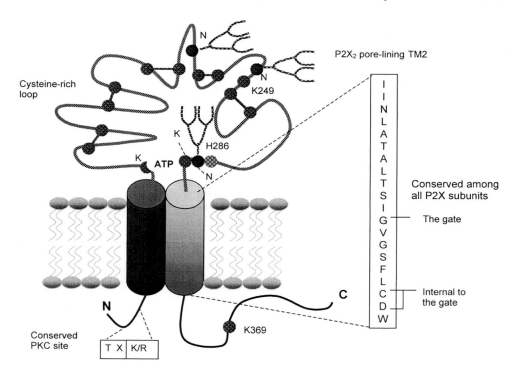

Figure 1: A representation of P2X subunit structure and function. P2X channels possess two transmembrane domains (TM); TM2 is believed to line the pore of the channel. The amino and carboxyl termini of the different P2X subunits are located intracellularly. The length of the amino termini is relatively constant among the different subunits and comprises about 20 - 30 residues. By contrast, the carboxy-terminal tails vary widely in length and range from 28 residues for $P2X_6$ to 242 for $P2X_7$. In the functional channel, the amino and carboxyl termini might be close to each other. P2X subunits have a conserved protein kinase C (PKC) site in the amino terminal tail, which is phosphorylated in $P2X_2$. Lysine residues extracellular to TM1 and TM2 contribute to the ATP-binding site, whereas K249 in $P2X_2$ forms a Schiff base with the antagonist PPADS. The extracellular loop of all P2X subunits contains 10 conserved cysteine residues. In addition, P2X subunits are glycosylated at three asparagine residues (N182, N239, N298). Finally, a histidine residue at 286 in human $P2X_4$ receptors contributes to H+ modulation, and the amino acids after splice site K369 determine desensitization in $P2X_2$ channels (adapted from Khakh, 2001).

The coexistence of different P2 receptors together with impure solutions caused by purine and pyrimidine degradation and interconversion as well as the lack of selective agonists and antagonists have led to some frustration in this field of research.

Recent reviews summarizing the functional properties of recombinant homomeric, recombinant heteromeric and native P2X receptors were published by Bianchi et al. (1999), Nörenberg and Illes (2000) and Khakh et al. (2001). In these publications the effects of the following agonists, antagonists (among others) as well as the ions Zn^{2+}, H^+ and Ca^{2+} on specified P2X-subtypes were described:

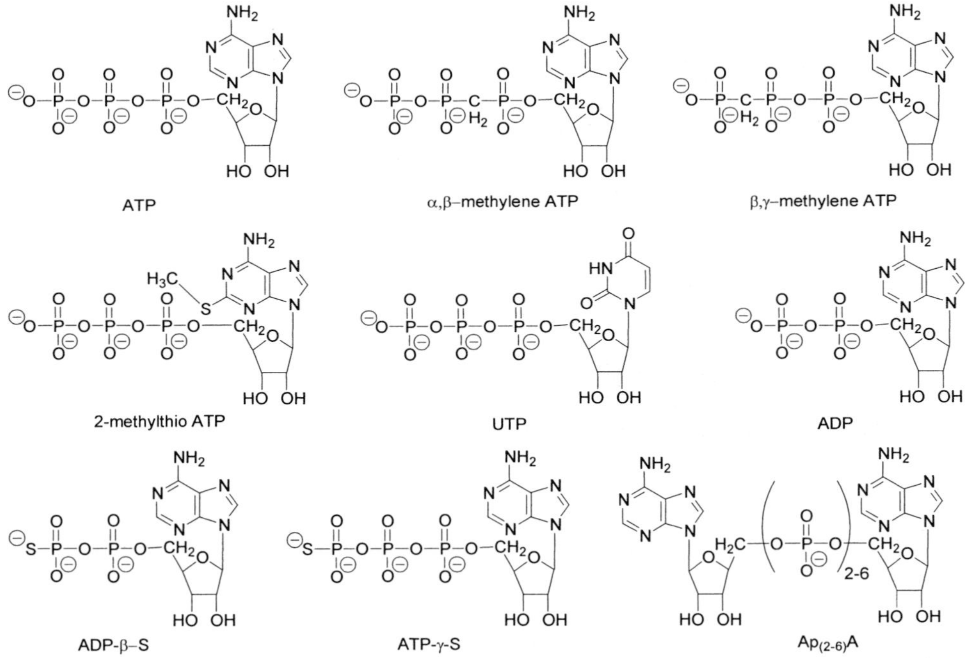

Scheme 1: P2X receptor agonists.

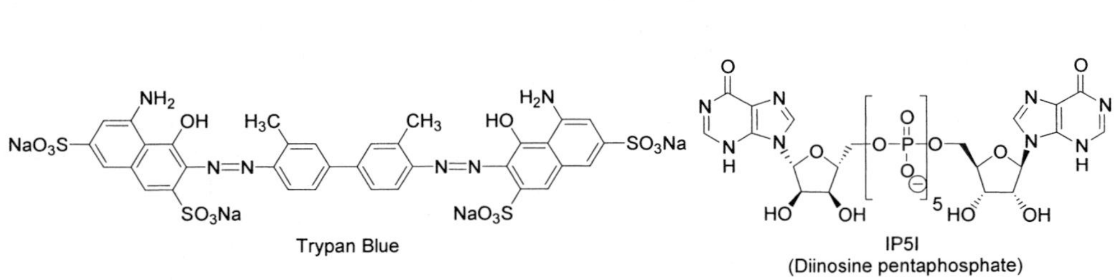

Scheme 2: P2X receptor antagonists.

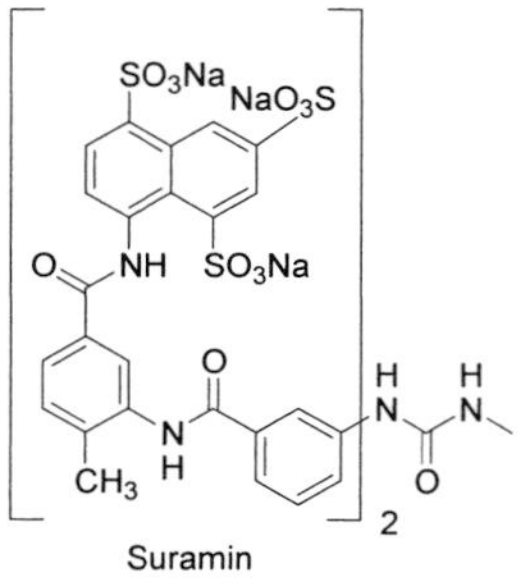

Suramin

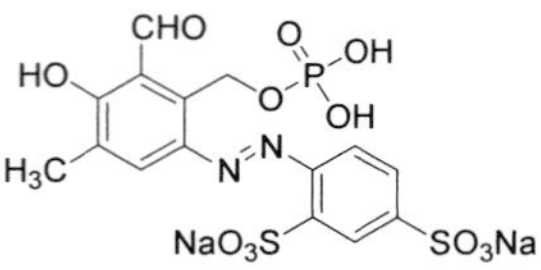

PPADS (pyridoxal phosphate-6-azophenyl -2'-4'-disulphonic acid)

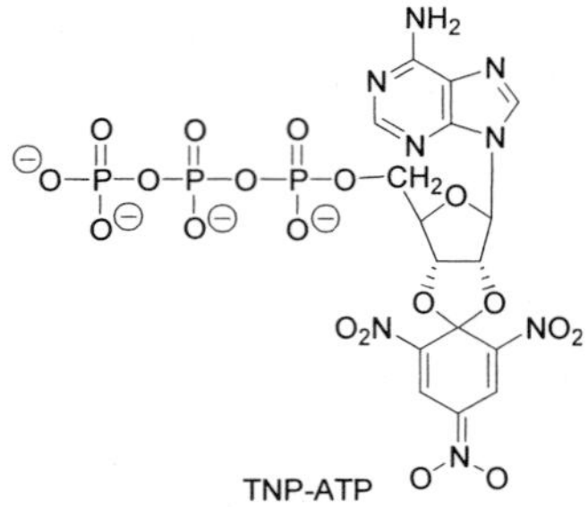

TNP-ATP (2',3'-(2,4,6-trinitrophenyl-ATP)

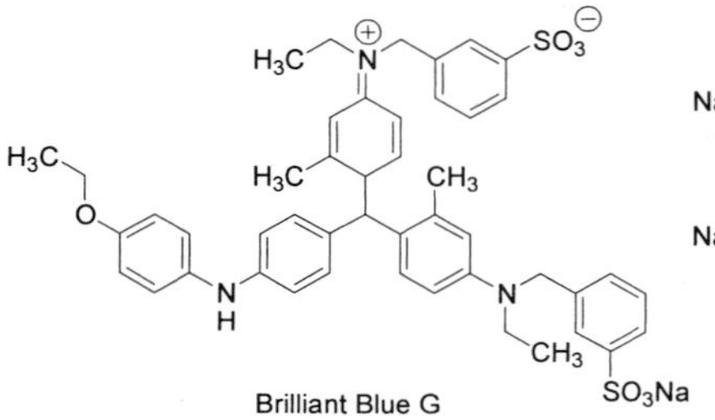

Brilliant Blue G

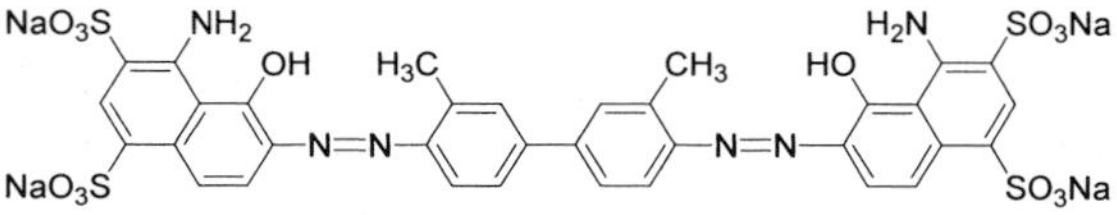

Evan's Blue

Scheme 2 continued.

Peripherally administered, ATP has pro-nociceptive effects

In behavioral tests, the actions of peripherally-administered ATP are pro-nociceptive. These nociceptive responses have been suggested to be due to direct activation of peripheral nerve terminals (Illes and Nörenberg, 1993). ATP produces depolarization when applied to the cell bodies of primary afferent neurons located within the dorsal root ganglia (DRG) (Jahr and Jessell, 1983). The depolarizing effect of ATP results from the activation of a non-selective cation channel (Bean, 1990) and is blocked by P2 purinoreceptor antagonists (Tsuda et al., 1999), indicating that excitation is mediated via ionotropic P2X purinoreceptors.

$P2X_{1-6}$ mRNA transcripts are expressed in sensory neurons of the dorsal root, nodose and trigeminal ganglia (Collo et al., 1996). Of these subunits one subtype, $P2X_3$, one of the seven P2X receptor subtypes known today (for overview see Alexander and Peters, 2000), has emerged as having a potentially important role in nociception because of its selective exprimation in cell populations enriched in nociceptors (Chen et al., 1995; Lewis et al. 1995, Tsuda et al., 1999, for minireview see Chizh et al., 2000). However, it is not clear if $P2X_3$ exists as a homomultimer or a heteromultimer with $P2X_2$ in sensory neurons *in vivo*. Evidence has been presented that capsaicin-sensitive, small DRG neurons may express

$P2X_3$ is expressed in cell populations enriched in nociceptors

mainly the homomultimeric $P2X_3$ subunit showing co-localization with vanilloid VR-1 receptors, while capsaicin-insensitive, medium-sized neurons express the heteromultimeric $P2X_{2/3}$ receptor. (Guo et al., 1999; Ueno et al., 1999).

As ATP seems to be involved in activating nociceptive sensory neurons through $P2X_3$-containing receptors, peripherally-acting antagonists selective for these receptors might be analgesics (Jarvis et al. (Abbott Laboratories), 2000). It is experimentally proven that pain induced by peripheral administration of ATP or the agonist α,β-methylene ATP is blocked by the non-selective P2 antagonists suramin and PPADS (Hamilton et al., 1999; Williams and Jarvis, 2000).

Pain induced by $P2X_3$ agonists is blocked by suramin and PPADS

Driessen et al. (1994) studied the effects of intrathecally applied P2 purinoceptor antagonists and agonists in the rat tail-flick test and rat formalin model. In the tail-flick test, the P2 antagonists suramin, Evans blue, Trypan blue and Reactive blue 2 (but not PPADS) caused moderate antinociception up to a doubling of the response latency. In contrast, the P2 agonists α,β-methylene ATP and 2-methylthio-ATP decreased the tail-flick latency up to 50%. In the formalin test, pretreatment with suramin 60 min prior to testing caused significant antinociception by decreasing the weighted pain intensity score up to 80 %.

Concerning human studies, only three reports have been reported (for review see Burnstock et al., 2000). Bleehen and Keele (1977) reported observations on the algogenic actions of adenosine compounds on blister base preparations. Coutts et al. (1981) injected ATP, ADP, AMP, adenosine, adenine and inosine intradermally. The area of erythema induced by the injection was delineated at 30 s. and again after a further 4.5 min when the size of the response was maximal. ATP, ADP and AMP evoked weal and flare responses in the skin in a dose-dependent manner. The rank order of potency was ATP > ADP > AMP; other metabolites were apparently inactive. Injections of ATP and high doses of ADP produced a sensation of persistent pain.

In 2000 Hamilton et al. reported that ATP in human skin elicits a dose-related pain response which is potentiated under conditions of hyperalgesia. The authors used iontophoresis to deliver ATP to the forearm skin of volunteers who rated the magnitude of the evoked pain on a visual analog scale. ATP consistently produced a modest burning pain, which began within 20 s. of starting iontophoresis and was maintained for several minutes. Persistent iontophoresis of ATP led to desensitization

Pain studies on humans with ATP

within 12 min but recovery from this was almost complete 1 h later. The pain produced by ATP was dependent on capsaicin-sensitive neurons, since in skin treated repeatedly with topical capsaicin pain was reduced to less than 25% of that elicited on normal skin. Moreover, ATP iontophoresed into skin 24 h after solar simulated radiation resulted in double the pain rating of normal skin. The pain response to saline was not altered after UV irradiation. The authors conclude that ATP produces pain by activating capsaicin-sensitive nociceptive afferents when applied to the skin.

Regulatory role of P2X$_3$ receptors

Experiments with P2X$_3$-knockout mice confirmed that P2X$_3$ receptors have a significant regulatory role in persistent inflammatory pain (Souslova et al., 2000), but ATP-evoked nociceptive behavior in mice is only partially reduced by disruption of the P2X$_3$ gene.

The role of P2Y$_1$ in pain sensation

In a recent paper Tominaga et al. (2001) present evidence that P2Y$_1$ receptors may also be involved in pain sensation. An accompanying commentary to this paper is given by Premkumar (2001) offering a scheme (see Fig. 2) of known second-messenger pathways that possibly modulate the vanilloid receptor (VR). Tominaga et al. (2001) show that in human embryonic kidney (HEK293) cells, stimulation of the endogenous metabotropic purinergic receptor P2Y$_1$ enhances the sensitivity of the heterologously expressed VR1 to capsaicin, protons, and temperature in a protein kinase C (PKC)-dependent manner. To further substantiate these findings, the authors co-expressed M1 muscarinic acetylcholine receptors and VR1 and demonstrated that, when pretreated with acetylcholine, the VR response induced by capsaicin or protons was potentiated. Finally, a similar potentiation of VR response by ATP could be observed in neurons from dorsal root ganglia. The authors conclude that ATP-induced nociception is partly caused by a potentiation of the VR response.Thus P2Y$_1$ receptors may represent a fruitful target for the development of drugs against pain. P2Y$_1$ knock-out mice were shown to have defective platelet aggregation and increased resistance to thromboembolism suggesting that potentially analgesic P2Y$_1$ antagonists may have antithrombotic side-effects (Boeynaems et al., 2001).

ATP-induced nociception is partly caused by a potentiation of the VR response

In view of the early results which indicated that mainly phosphorylated ATP derivatives had activity at P2 receptors, the identification of selective agents for one of the P2 receptors seemed to cause problems because of the difficulty in preventing such molecules from being rapidly broken down in the ordinary course of ATP metabolism (Jacobsen et al., 1995; Zimmermann, 2000).

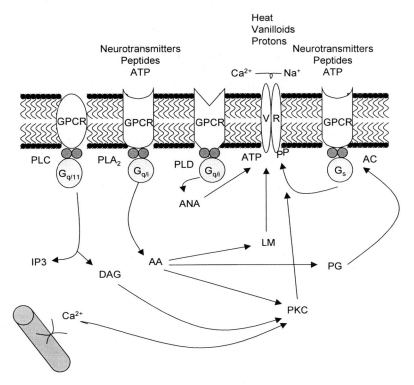

Figure 2: Known second-messenger pathways that modulate capsaicin or VRs. GPCR, G protein-coupled receptors; PLA$_2$, phospholipase A2; AC, adenylate cyclase; IP3, inositoltriphosphate; DAC diacylglycerol; LM, lipoxygenase metabolites; AA, arachidonic acid; ANA, anandamide; PG, prostaglandins; G$_{q/11}$, G$_{q/i}$, G$_s$, trimeric G-proteins (adapted from Premkumar, 2001)

Although a very reliable radioligand binding assay with use of a stable ATP analog (e.g. α, β-methylene ATP) and functional fluorescent assays suitable for a high throughput screening campaign are available, the search for a selective P2X$_3$ receptor antagonist has not been successful up to now. There are only few known compounds with agonistic or antagonistic activity (Lamprecht, 2000) for P2 receptors not selective for P2X$_3$ which can be used in assay characterization. Some ATP derivatives, e.g. 2', 3'-O-(2,4,6-trinitrophenyl)-ATP (TNP-ATP) and diinosine pentaphosphate (IP$_5$I) are rather potent and selective antagonists of P2X$_1$ and P2X$_3$ receptors (the former, but not the latter compound, also blocks the heteromeric P2X$_2$/P2X$_3$ receptor, see Dunn et al., 2000); however, their *in vivo* stability is limited.

The search for P2X receptor subtype selective ligands

In conclusion, activation of certain types of P2 receptors by ATP seems to be an important factor in several pain states. P2X$_3$ receptors, and P2Y$_1$ receptors represent an attractive target for the treatment of pain. Further progress in this area is hampered by the lack of potent and selective antagonists with sufficient *in vivo* stability.

Addendum

In addition to pain, experiments with P2X$_3$ knock-out mice (Cockayne et al., 2000; Souslova et al., 2000) have revealed surprising results. Cockayne et al. found, that P2X$_3$-null mice exhibit a marked urinary bladder hyporeflexia, characterized by decreased voiding frequency and increased bladder capacity, but normal bladder pressure. Antagonists to P2X$_3$ may therefore have therapeutic potential in the treatment of disorders of urine storage and voiding such as overactive bladder (Cook and McCleskey, 2000; Burnstock, 2001).

References

Abbracchio, M.P. and Burnstock, G.: *Purinoceptors: Are there families of P2X and P$_{2Y}$ purinoceptors?,* Pharmacol. Ther. **1994**, *64*, 445-475.

Alexander, S.P.H. and Peters, J.A.: *Receptor and ion channel nomenclature,* Trends Pharmacol. Sci. **2000**, Suppl., 72-75.

Barnard, E.A., Burnstock, G., Webb, T.E.: *G protein-coupled receptors for ATP and other nucleotides: A new receptor family,* Trends Pharmacol. Sci. **1994**, *15*, 67-70.

Bean, B.P.: *ATP-activated channels in rat and bullfrog sensory neurons: concentration dependence and kinetics,* J. Neurosci. **1990**, *10*, 1-10.

Benham, C.D. and Tsien, R.W.: *A novel receptor-operated Ca^{2+}-permeable channel activated by ATP in smooth muscle,* Nature (Lond) **1987**, *238*, 275-278.

Bianchi, B.R., Lynch, K.J., Touma, E., Niforatos, W., Burgard, E.C., Alexander, K.M., Park, H.S., Yu, H., Metzger, R., Kowaluk, E., Jarvis, M.F., Biesen, T. van: *Pharmacological characterization of recombinant human and rat P2X receptor subtypes,* Eur. J. Pharmacol. **1999**, *376*, 127-138.

Bleehen, T. and Keele, C.A.: *Observations on the algogenic actions of adenosine compounds on human blister base preparation,* Pain **1977**, *3*, 367-377.

Boeynaems, J.M., Robaye, B., Janssens, R., Suarez-Huerta, N., Communi, D.: *Overview of P2Y receptors as therapeutic targets,* Drug Dev. Res. **2001**, *52*, 187-189.

Burnstock, G., Campbell, G., Satchell, D., Smythe, A.: *Evidence that adenosine triphosphate or a related nucleotide is the transmitter substance released by non-adrenergic inhibitory nerves in the gut,* Br. J. Pharmacol. **1970**, *40*, 668-688.

Burnstock, G., Dumsday, B., Smythe, A.: *Atropine resistant excitation of the urinary bladder: the possibility of transmission via nerves releasing a purine nucleotide,* Br. J. Pharmacol. **1972a**, *44*, 451-461.

Burnstock, G.: *Purinergic nerves,* Pharmacol. Rev. **1972b**, *24*, 509-581.

Burnstock, G., McMahon, S.B., Humphrey, P.P.A., Hamilton S.G.: *ATP (P2X) Receptors and Pain,* Proceedings of the 9th World Congress on Pain. Progress in Pain Research and Management,

Vol. 16, **2000**, edited by M. Devor., M.C. Rowbotham, Z. Wiesenfeld-Hallin, 63-76. IASP Press, Seattle.

Burnstock, G.: *Purine-mediated signalling in pain and visceral perception,* Trends Pharmacol. Sci. **2001**, *22,* 182-188.

Chen, C. C., Akoplan, A. N., Sivilotti, N., Colquhoun, D., Burnstock, G., Wood, J. N.: *P2X purinoreceptor expressed by a subset of sensory neurons,* Nature **1995**, *377,* 428-431.

Chizh, B.A., Hennies, H., Wnendt S.: *P2X receptors as a target for the development of novel analgesics: where do we go from where we are?,* In 8th Mainzer Forum Medicinal Chemistry, 29 September **2000**, Institute of Pharmacy, Johannes Gutenberg-Universität, Mainz (Germany), Abstract pp. 64-66.

Cockayne, D.A., Hamilton, S.G., Zhu, Q.-M., Dunn, P.M., Zhong, Y., Novakovic, S., Malmberg, A.B., Cain, G., Berson, A., Kassotakis, L., Hedley, L., Lachnit, W.G., Burnstock, G., McMahon S.B., Ford A.P.D.W.: *Urinary bladder hyporeflexia and reduced pain-related behaviour in P2X$_3$-deficient mice,* Nature **2000**, *407,* 1011-1015.

Collo, G., North, R.A., Kawashima, E., Merlo-Pich, E., Neidhart, S., Surprenant, A., Buell, G.: *Cloning OF P2X5 and P2X6 receptors and the distribution and properties of an extended family of ATP-gated ion channels,* J. Neurosci. **1996**, *16,* 2495-2507.

Cook, S.P. and McCleskey E.W.: *ATP, pain and a full bladder,* Nature **2000**, *407,* 951-952.

Coutts, A.A., Jorizzo, J.L., Eady, R.A.J., Greaves, M.W., Burnstock G.: *Adenosine triphosphate-evoked vascular changes in human skin: mechanism of action,* Eur. J. Pharmacol. **1981**, *76,* 391-401.

Driessen, B., Reimann, W., Selve, N., Friderichs, E. and Bültmann, R.: *Antinociceptive effect of intrathecally administered P$_2$-purinoceptor antagonists in rats,* Brain Res. **1994**, *666,* 182-188.

Drury A.N. and Szent-Györgyi A.: *The physiological activity of adenine compounds with especial reference to their action upon the mammalian heart,* J. Physiol. (Lond) **1929**, *68,* 213-237.

Dubyak, G.R.: *Signal transduction by P$_2$-purinergic receptors for extracellular ATP,* Am. J. Respir. Cell Mol. Biol. **1991**, *4,* 295-300.

Dunn, P.M., Liu, M., Zhong, Y., King, B.F., Burnstock, G.: *Diinosine pentaphosphate: an antagonist which discriminates between recombinant P2X$_3$ and P2X$_{2/3}$ receptors and between two P2X receptors in rat sensory neurones,* Br. J. Pharmacol. **2000**, *130,* 1378-1384.

Fredholm, B.B., Abbracchio, M.P., Burnstock, G., Daly, J.W., Harden, K.T., Jacobson, K.A., Leff, P., Williams, M.: *Nomenclature and classification of purinoceptors,* Pharmacol. Rev. **1994**, *46,* 143-156.

Guo, A., Vulchanova, L., Wang, J., Li, X., Elde, R.: *Immunocytochemical localization of the vanilloid receptor 1 (VR1): relationship to neuropeptides, the P2X$_3$ purinoceptor and IB4 binding sites,* Eur. J. Neurosci. **1999**, *11,* 946-958.

Hamilton, S.G., Wade, A., McMahon, S.B.: *The effect of inflammatory mediators on nociceptive behaviour induces by ATP analogues in the rat,* Br. J. Pharmacol. **1999**, *126,* 326-332.

Hamilton, S.G., Warburton, J., Bhattachajee, A., Ward, J., McMahon S.B.: *ATP in human skin elicits a dose related pain response which is potentiated under conditions of hyperalgesia,* Brain **2000**, *123,* 1238-1246.

Holton, F.A, and Holton P.: *The possibility that ATP is a transmitter at sensory nerve endings,* J. Physiol. (Lond) **1953**, *119,* 50-51.

Holton, P.: *The liberation of ATP on antidromic stimulation of sensory nerves,* J. Physiol. (Lond) **1959**, *145,* 494-504.

Illes, P. and Nörenberg, W.: *Neuronal ATP receptors and their mechanism of action,* Trends Pharmacol. Sci. **1993**, *14,* 50-54.

Jacobsen, K.A., Fischer, B., Maillard, M.: *Biologically active ATP analogs,* US5620676 (**1995**).

Jahr, C.E. and Jessel, T.M.: *ATP excites a subpopulation of rat dorsal horn neurones,* Nature **1983**, *304,* 730-733.

Jarvis, M.F., Lynch, K.J., Burgard, E.C., Vanbiesen, T., Kowaluk, E.A., (Abbot Laboratories): *The P2X₃ receptor, methods of altering P2X₃ receptor activity and the use thereof*, WO0063379 (**2000**).

Jo, Y.H. and Schlichter, R.: *Synaptic corelease of ATP and GABA in cultured spinal neurons*, Nat. Neurosci. **1999**, *3*, 241-245.

Khakh, B.S., Burnstock, G., Kennedy, C., King, B.F., North, A., Séguéla, Ph., Voigt, M., Humphrey P.P.A.: *International Union of Pharmacology. XXIV. Current Status of the Nomenclature and Properties of P2X Receptors and Their Subunits,* Pharmacol. Rev. **2001**, *53*, 107-118.

Khakh, B.S.: *Molecular physiology of P2X receptors and ATP signalling at synapses,* Nature Rev. Neurosci. **2001**, *2*, 165-174.

von Kügelgen, I. and Wetter, A.: *Molecular pharmacology of P2Y-receptors,* Naunyn-Schmiedeberg's Arch. Pharmacol. **2000**, *362*, 310-323.

Lamprecht, G.: *Agonists and antagonists acting at P2X receptors: selectivity profiles and functional implications*, Naunyn-Schmiedeberg's Arch. Pharmacol. **2000**, *362*, 340-350.

Lewis, C., Neidhart, S., Holy, C., North, R. A., Buell, G., Suprenant, A.: *Coexpression of P2X2 and P2X3 receptor subunits can account for ATP-gated currents in sensory neurons*, Nature **1995**, *377*, 432-435.

Nörenberg, W. and Illes, P.: *Neuronal P2X receptors: localisation and functional properties,* Naunyn-Schmiedeberg's Arch. Pharmacol. **2000**, *362*, 324-339.

Premkumar, L.S.: *Commentary: Interaction between vanilloid receptors and purinergic metabotropic receptors: Pain perception and beyond,* Proc. Natl. Acad. Sci. USA **2001**, *98*, 6537-6539.

Ralevic, V. and Burnstock, G.: *Receptors for purines and pyrimidines,* Pharmacol. Rev. **1998**, 50, 413-492.

Sawynok, J., Downie, J. W., Reid, A. R., Cahill, C. M., White, T. D.: *ATP release from dorsal spinal cord synaptosomes: characterization and neuronal origin*, Brain Res. **1993**, *610*, 32-38.

Souslova, V., Cesare, P., Ding, Y., Akopian, A.N., Stanfa, L., Susuki, R., Carpenter, K., Dickinson, A., Boyce, S., Hill, R., Nebenius-Oosthuizen, D., Smith A.J.H., Kidd, E.J., Wood, J.N.: *Warm-coding deficits and aberrant inflammatory pain in mice lacking P2X3 receptors*, Nature **2000**, *407*, 1015-1017.

Tominaga, M., Wada, M., Masu, M.: *Potentiation of capsaicin receptor activity by metabotropic ATP receptors as a posible mechanism for ATP-evoked pain and hyperalgesia*, Proc. Natl. Acad. Sci. USA **2001**, *98*, 6951-6956.

Tsuda, M., Ueno, S., Inoue, K.: *Evidence for the involvement of spinal endogenous ATP and P2X receptors in nociceptive responses caused by formalin and capsaicin in mice*, Br. J. Pharmacol. **1999**, *128*, 1497-1504.

Ueno, S., Tsuda, M., Iwanga, T., Inoue, K.: *Cell-type specific ATP-activated responses in the rat dorsal root ganglion neurons*, Br. J. Pharmacol. **1999**, *126*, 429-436.

Williams, M. and Jarvis, M.F.: *Purinergic and pyrimidinergic receptors as potential drug targets*, Biochem. Pharmacol. **2000**, *59*, 1173-1185.

White, T.D., Downie, J. W., Leslie, R. A.: *Characteristics of K⁺- and veratridine-induced release of ATP from synaptosomes prepared from dorsal and ventral spinal cord*, Brain Res. **1985**, *334*, 372-374.

Zimmermann, H.: *Extracellular metabolism of ATP and other nucleotides,* Naunyn-Schmiedeberg's Arch. Pharmacol. **2000**, *362*, 299-309.

12   Natural and Synthetic Cannabinoids

Corinna Maul and Bernd Sundermann

For many thousand years *cannabis sativa* has been a valuable source of hemp fibre. The (ab)use of its psychoactive constituents has also been know in many cultures for a very long time. With the advent of superior alternative medications the medical use of cannabis extracts faded in the last century. Cannabis was removed from the US Pharmacopoeia in 1942 and from the British Pharmacopoeia in 1976 when it was classified as a drug with no therapeutic benefit.

Nevertheless and despite the widely illegal recreational use of cannabis the effects of cannabinoids on the brain still are under active investigation. The discovery of neuronal receptor proteins for cannabinoids and the existence of endogenous cannabinoid substances (Sullivan, 2000) are the most important milestones to date.

At least 60 bioactive compounds are contained in herbal cannabis. Δ^9-Tetrahydrocannabinol (Δ^9-THC) (Mechoulam and Gaoni, 1967), cannabidiol and cannabinol are the major psychoactive or adjuvant ingredients. Cannabinoids act through at least two different G-protein coupled receptors named CB_1 and CB_2 receptors.

Oral preparations of Δ^9-THC (dronabinol, marinol) and the synthetic structural analog nabilone are marketed as suppressants of nausea and vomiting provoked by antitumor agents. Furthermore Δ^9-THC is employed to stimulate the appetite of AIDS patients.

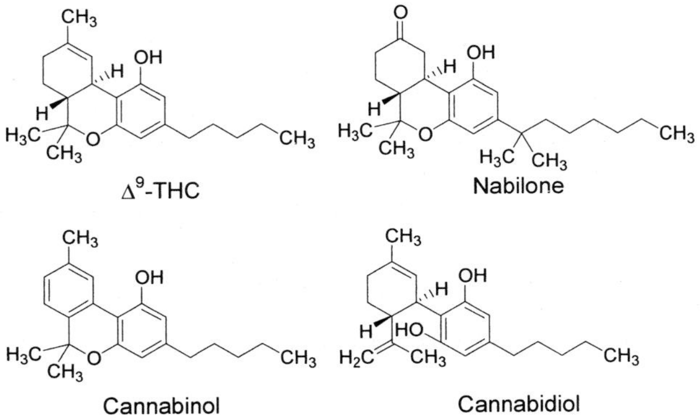

Figure 1: Structures of natural cannabinoids and nabilone.

In addition to these indications the pharmacology of cannabinoids promises a range of further potential applications. Cannabinoids have been shown to produce antinociception in animals and humans, so analgesia is

Synthetic tool compounds:

CP 55,940
(non-selective agonist)

WIN 55,212-2
(moderately CB$_2$-selective
agonist)

SR 141716A
(CB$_1$-selective antagonist)

SR 144528
(CB$_2$-selective antagonist)

Cannabinoid receptors

one of the important features of cannabinoids with therapeutic prospects (Segal, 1986; Fuentes et al., 1999).

One particular feature of plant-derived cannabinoids is their high lipid solubility, which indicates that limited gastrointestinal absorption and bioavailability are significant barriers to their development as therapeutics. For this reason cannabis is traditionally smoked, providing the most predictable and titratable route for administration. For therapeutic development pulmonary deliveries of cannabinoid aerosols are under investigation as an alternative.

Besides the classical cannabinoids there are other structural classes with cannabinoid activity: the *non-classical cannabinoids* typified by CP-55,940 and the *aminoalkylindols* exemplified with WIN 55,212-2. The 1H-pyrazole-3-carboxylic acid amide derivatives SR 141716A (Rinaldi-Carmona et al., 1994) and SR 144528 (Rinaldi-Carmona et al., 1998) were discovered to be moderately selective cannabinoid receptor antagonists.

The antinociceptive activity of cannabinoid receptor agonists has been widely investigated. Δ^9-THC has been most intensively studied. It exhibits antinociceptive activity in a wide range of animal models of acute pain (e.g. tail flick, hot plate) when administered orally, systemically or directly into brain or spinal cord. Δ^9-THC is also effective in models of inflammatory and neuropathic pain (overview: Pertwee, 2001). Other cannabinoids such as WIN 55,212 also show analgesic properties in acute and neuropathic pain models (Bridges et al. 2001). The antinociceptive effects could only be antagonized with the CB$_1$ selective antagonist SR 141716a and not with the CB$_2$ selective antagonist SR 144528. However, the motor effects of cannabinoids complicate interpretation of behavioral studies assessing motor reactions to noxious stimuli, but electrophysiological studies also support the behavioral findings. It was shown that cannabinoids selectively modulate the activity of nociceptive neurons in the spinal dorsal horn by actions at CB$_1$ receptors. This modulation represents a suppression of pain neurotransmission because the inhibitory effects are selective for pain-sensitive neurons and are observed with different modalities of noxious stimulation (Hohmann et al., 1999).

CB$_1$ receptors are found in particularly high concentrations within the central nervous system, but also on some peripheral neurons as well as in certain non-neuronal tissues (Herkenham et al., 1990). CB$_2$ receptors mainly occur in immune cells where they can mediate an immunosuppressant effect (Iwamura et al., 2001). Both

CB_1 and CB_2 seem to couple to inhibitory G_i and/or G_o proteins. CB_1 receptors are known to effect adenylate cyclase, a variety of potassium and calcium currents, and the mitogen-activated protein kinase pathway. CB_1 receptors have been shown to activate at least six subtypes of G_i and G_o proteins, supporting reports that they effect a wide variety of intracellular signaling systems. In contrast to CB_1 receptors, CB_2 receptors do not seem to effect ion currents directly (Breivogel et al., 2001).

It has been demonstrated that cannabinoids act to suppress action potential-evoked calcium rises in the presynaptic terminal, thereby decreasing transmitter release. The action potential-evoked rise in intraterminal calcium was decreased by postsynaptic depolarization. This postsynaptic depolarization induced reduction of presynaptic calcium was prevented by application of antagonists to the CB_1 receptor (Kreitzer and Regehr, 2001). Cannabinoid-induced decreases in synaptic transmission have been shown to result from an inhibition of N- and P/Q-type calcium channels, the subtypes through which calcium influx occurs during evoked transmitter release (Twitchell et al., 1997).

Influence of cannabinoids on Ca^{2+} currents

Several lines of investigation indicate an interaction between the opioid and cannabinoid system (Welch and Eads, 1999). There is also evidence that a physiological stimulation of metabotrobic glutamate and NMDA receptors is required for cannabinoid-induced analgesia (Palazzo et al., 2001).

Interactions with the opioid and glutamate systems

Investigations on CB_1 receptor knock-out mice have shown that the animals appear healthy and fertile, but with an increased mortality rate. They display reduced locomotor activity, increased ring catalepsy and hypoalgesia in the hot plate and formalin test. Interestingly in this study administration of Δ^9-THC still induced antinociception in the tail flick test, but not in the hot plate test, which indicates that not all CNS effects of Δ^9-THC are mediated by the CB_1 receptor. The molecular basis for the antinociceptive and other effects remains to be determined, but may involve an as yet unknown neuronal receptor (Zimmer et al., 1999). This hypothesis is supported by results from [^{35}S]GTPγS binding studies stimulated by anandamide and WIN 55,212-2 in brain membranes from both $CB_1^{+/+}$ and $CB_1^{-/-}$ mice. Both ligands were able to activate an unknown receptor which should be related to CB_1 and CB_2 because two chemically unrelated cannabinoid agonists produced pharmacological effects and activate this receptor. Interestingly the classical cannabinoids like THC do not activate G-proteins

Studies with CB_1 receptor knock-out mice suggest the existence of an as yet unknown neuronal cannabinoid receptor - potentially a new target for pain research

in brain membranes from $CB_1^{-/-}$ mice (Breivogel et al., 2001; Di Marzo et al., 2000a).

Δ^9-THC

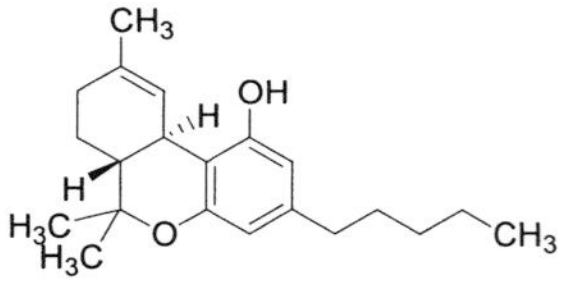

Δ^9-THC is marketed as marinol or dronabinol for the treatment of chemotherapy-induced nausea and vomiting in Australia, Canada, Israel, South Africa and the USA. It was granted orphan drug status in the US for the stimulation of appetite and prevention of weight loss in patients with a confirmed diagnosis of AIDS. Δ^9-THC is in phase I trials for spasticity, multiple sclerosis and post-operative pain. Several small clinical studies have confirmed the effectiveness of Δ^9-THC as an analgesic, with doses of 15 to 20 mg being comparable to 60 to 120 mg of codeine (Williamson and Evans, 2000).

In the 1970s the biosynthesis of cannabinoids was investigated with radiolabeling experiments. ^{14}C-labeled mevalonate and malonate were shown to be incorporated into tetrahydrocannabinolic acid and cannabichromenic acid at very low rates (< 0.02%). Until 1990 the precursors of all terpenoids, isopentenyl diphosphate and dimethyl-allyl diphosphate were believed to be biosynthesized via the mevalonate pathway. Subsequent studies, however, proved that many plant terpenoids are biosynthesized via the recently discovered deoxyxylulose phosphate pathway (Eisenreich et al., 1998; Rohmer, 1999). It was shown that the C_{10}-terpenoid moiety of cannabinoids is biosynthesized entirely or predominantly (>98%) via this pathway (Fellermeister et al., 2001). The phenolic moiety is generated by a polyketide-type reaction sequence.

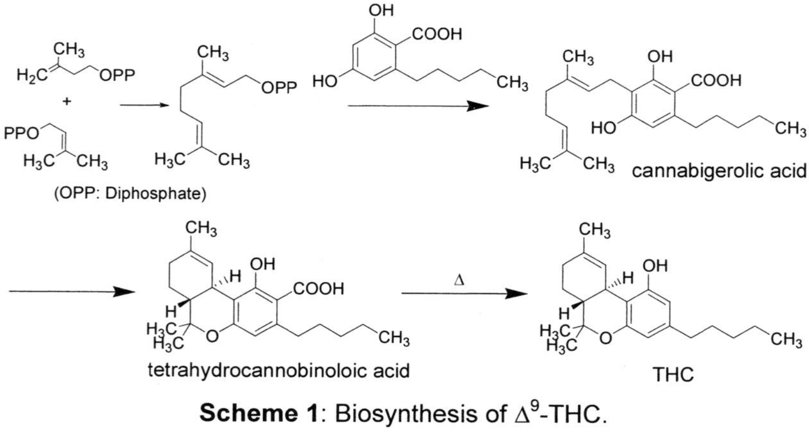

[1972-08-3], (-)-(Z)-(6aR,10aR)-6,6,9-Trimethyl-3-pentyl-6a,7,8,10a-tetra-hydro-6H-benzo[c]chromen-1-ol, "(-)-trans-Δ^9-tetrahydro-cannabinol" $C_{21}H_{30}O_2$

Trade names: Marinol, THC, Unimed, Compassia

Scheme 1: Biosynthesis of Δ^9-THC.

The oxidocyclization of cannabigerolic acid to tetrahydro-cannabinolic acid is catalyzed by tetrahydrocannabinolic acid synthase without any cofactors or coenzymes. This enzyme was recently identified together with two other specific enzymes, cannabidiolic acid and cannabi-chromenic acid synthase which transform cannabigerolic acid to cannabidiolic acid and cannabichromenic acid (Morimoto et al., 1999; Taura et al., 1996).

The psychoactive ingredients of *cannabis sativa* are finally formed when its leaves are dried at elevated temperature so that e.g. tetrahydrocannabinolic acid is decarboxylated to Δ^9-THC.

Nabilone

Nabilone, a synthetic cannabinoid, is marketed by Eli Lilly for the treatment of chemotherapy-induced nausea and vomiting in Canada and Great Britain.

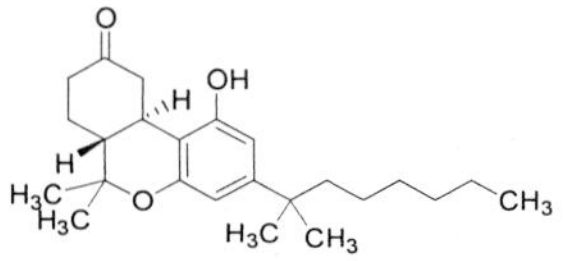

[51022-71-0], (6a*R*,10a*R*)-3-(1,1-Dimethyl-heptyl)-1-hydroxy-6,6-dimethyl-6,6a,7,8,10,10a-hexahydro-benzo[c]chromen-9-one, $C_{24}H_{36}O_3$

Trade name: Cesamet

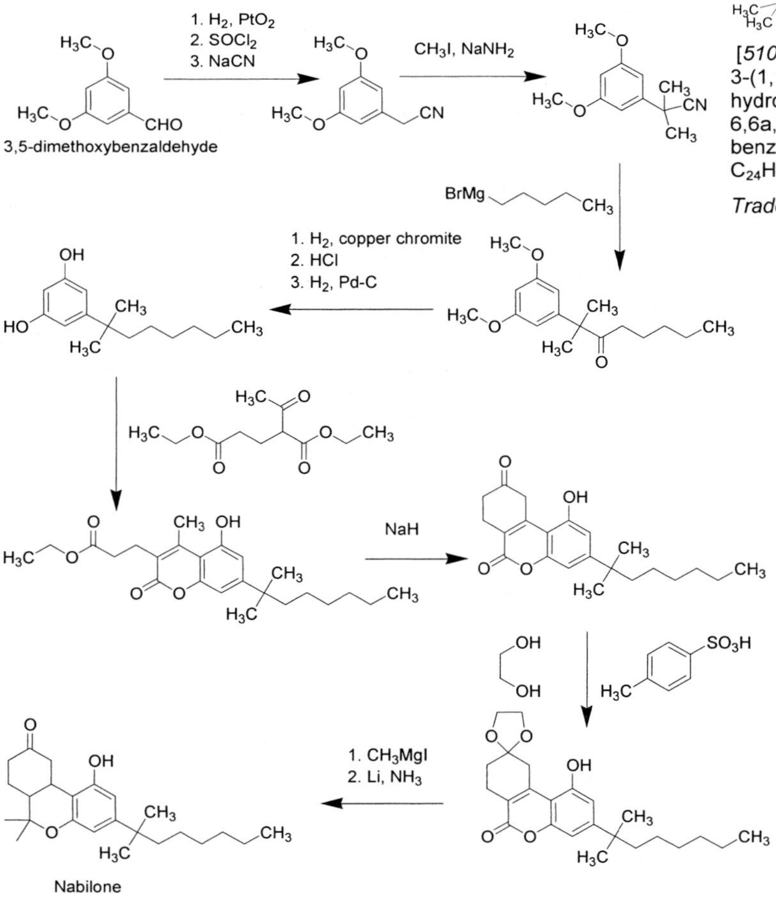

Scheme 2: Synthesis of nabilone.

Anandamide

[*94421-68-8*], all-(*Z*)-Eicosa-
5,8,11,14-tetraenoic acid (2-
hydroxy-ethyl)-amide,
$C_{22}H_{37}O_2$

2-Arachidonyl-glycerol

The finding that endogenous derivatives of the non-oxidative metabolism of polyunsaturated fatty acids could bind to and activate the cannabinoid receptors opened a new era in research on the possible therapeutic use of cannabinoids. Endogenous cannabinomimetic compounds have pharmacological properties similar to the exogenous compounds and thus offer new strategies for the pharmacological modulation of cannabinoid receptor activity. The endocannabinoids discovered so far are the anandamides which are ethanolamides of n-6 poly-unsaturated fatty acids with at least three double bonds and 20 carbon atoms of which the C20:4 anandamide is simply known as anandamide, and 2-arachidonoyl glycerol, a well known intermediate of phosphoglyceride and di- or tri-glyceride metabolism. The pharmacology, particularly of anandamide, has been extensively studied over recent years.

Anandamide was isolated from water-insoluble fractions of the porcine brain. It binds to CB_1 with rather moderate affinity (Ki 61 nM) and a low affinity for the CB_2 receptor (Ki 1930 nM). The name anandamide is based on its chemical nature (an amide) and the Sanskrit word ananda meaning bliss. The chemical structure of anandamide can be divided into two major molecular fragments: a polar ethanolamido head group and a hydrophobic arachidonyl chain. The polar head group comprises a secondary amide functionality with an N-hydroxyalkyl substituent while the lipophilic fragment is a non-conjugated *cis* tetraolefinic chain and an n-pentyl chain reminiscent of the lipophilic side chain found in the classical cannabinoids. A number of anandamide analogs have been synthesized and demonstrated to have considerable selectivity for the CB_1 receptor in comparison to the CB_2 receptor.

Anandamide was shown to alleviate nociception in several behavioral animal models, e.g. the hot plate and formalin test (Calignano et al., 2001). A most interesting aspect of anandamide with respect to pain research is that it seems to bind to the hypothetical third cannabinoid receptor (Di Marzo et al., 2000b): In the hot plate test anandamide is still antinociceptive in $CB_1^{-/-}$ mice, which is consistent with the observation that the selective CB_1 receptor antagonist SR 141716A does not block motor inhibitory and antinociceptive effects of anandamide in wild-type mice.

Like other arachidonate-derived endogenous compounds the endocannabinoids seem to be synthesized and released by cells on demand. The hydrolysis of phospholipid precursors, also probably embedded in the plasma membrane, seems to be necessary for the production of both anandamide and 2-arachidonyl-glycerol. The release of these compounds from cells does not appear to be vesicle mediated. However, unlike other eicosanoids no enzyme has been characterized so far as being uniquely responsible for anandamide or 2-achidonyl-glycerol formation. Anandamide is produced in neurons and leukocytes together with other N-acyl-ethanolamines from the hydrolysis of the corresponding N-acyl-phosphatidyl-ethanolamines. None of the enzymes responsible for the release of anandamide from membrane phospholipids appears to be used selectively for the formation of this endocannabinoid. The pathways leading to endocannabinoid biosynthesis seem to be part of more complex mechanisms regulating membrane phospholipid remodeling and intracellular second messenger levels, so the development of drugs selectively interfering with anandamide biosynthesis appears, at the moment, to be a difficult task.

The degradation of anandamide is catalyzed by fatty acid amide hydrolase (FAAH). Investigations on FAAH knock-out mice have shown that they cannot effectively degrade anandamide so they have 15-fold higher endogenous levels than wild-type mice. The mice seem normal until injected with anandamide, then they behave similar to wild-type mice treated with THC. The knock-out mice, even without anandamide treatment, have reduced pain sensitivity which can be reversed by a cannabinoid receptor antagonist, indicating that increased endogenous anandamide in FAAH knock-out mice affects their pain pathways. Therefore selective FAAH inhibitors might provide a selective method of using the cannabinoid signaling system for chronic pain relief.

Anandamide is approved by the FDA as an appetite enhancer. Its analgesic activity is under preclinical investigation by Yissum.

Inhibition of fatty acid hydrolase (FAAH) – a new target for pain research?

FAAH-inhibitor, 2 nM
(Boger et al., 2001)

Current Developments

Other developments in the area of cannabinoid analgesics include a marijuana patch being investigated by the American Cancer Society for the relief of chronic pain, nausea and vomiting associated with chemotherapy (Cancer Drug News, Feb. 2000, 30). Several cannabinoid agonists are reported by Pharmaprojects to be in the stage of preclinical evaluation. A range of recently published patent applications reveals that new compounds with cannabimimetic activity are being intensively investigated. A selection of these new compounds is given in Figure 2:

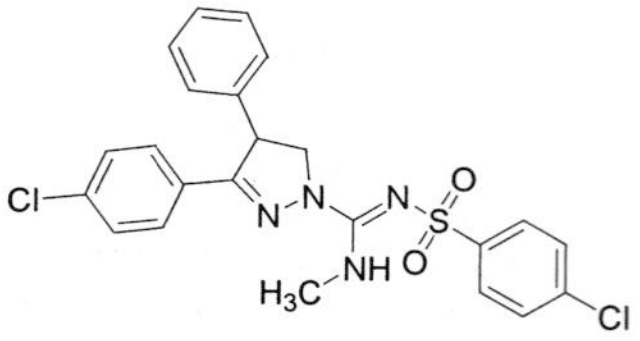

CB₁ receptor antagonist, claimed to be analgesic (Lange et al., Solvay, WO0170700)

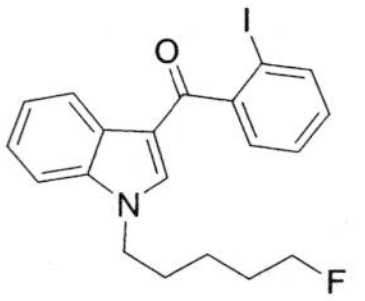

subnanomolar CB₁ receptor ligand (Makriannis and Deng, University of Conneticut, WO0128557)

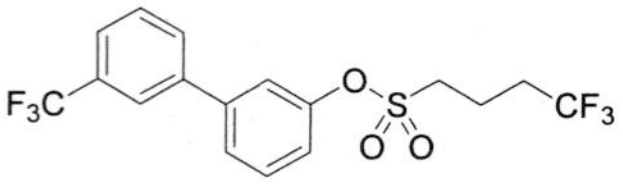

analgesic (Heil et al., Bayer, WO0174763)

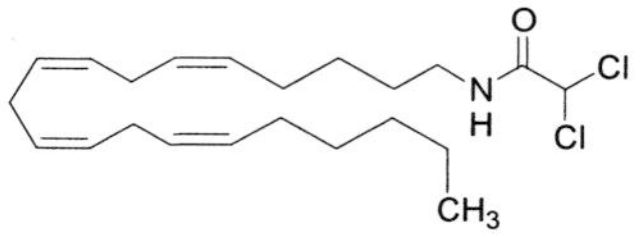

subnanomolar CB₁ receptor ligand (Makriannis and Deng, University of Conneticut, WO0128498)

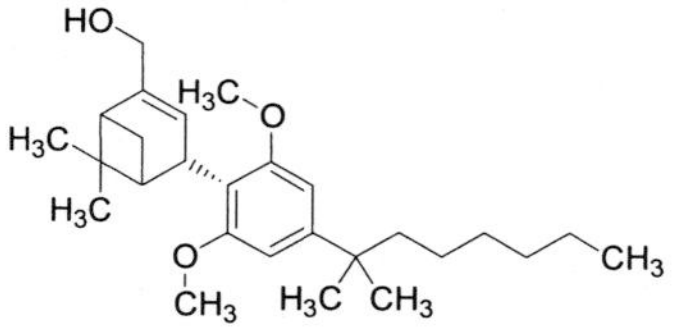

HU-308, analgesic (Fride et al., Yissum, WO0132169)

Figure 2: Compounds recently disclosed in patent applications.

References

Boger, D.L., Miyauchi, H., Hedrick, M.P.: *α-Keto Heterocycle Inhibitors of Fatty Acid Amide Hydrolase: Carbonyl Group Modification and α-Substitution*, Bioorg. Med. Chem. Lett. **2001**, *11*, 1517-1520.

Breivogel, C.S., Griffin, G., Di Marzo, V., Martin, B.R.: *Evidence for a new G protein-coupled cannabinoid receptor in mouse brain*, Mol. Pharmacol. **2001**, *60*, 155-163.

Bridges, D., Ahmad, K., Rice, A.S.: The synthetic cannabinoid WIN55,212-2 attenuates hyperalgesia and allodynia in a rat model of neuropathic pain, Br. J. Pharmacol. **2001**, *133*, 586-594.

Calignano, A., La Rana, G., Piomelli, D.: *Antinociceptive activity of the endogenous fatty acid amide, palmitylethanolamide*, Eur. J. Pharmacol. **2001**, *419*, 191-198.

Di Marzo, V., Breivogel, C.S., Tao, Q., Bridgen, D.T., Razdan, R.K., Zimmer, A.M., Zimmer, A., Martin, B.R.: *Levels, metabolism, and pharmacological activity of anandamide in CB1 cannabinoid receptor knockout mice*, J. Neurochem. **2000**a, *75*, 2434-2444.

Di Marzo, V., Bisogno, T., De Petrocellis, L.: *Endocannabinoids: New targets for drug development*, Cur. Pharmaceut. Design **2000**b, *6*, 1361-1380.

Eisenreich, W., Schwarz, M., Cartayrade, A., Arigoni, D., Zenk, M.H., Bacher, A.: *The deoxyxylulose phosphate pathway of terpenoid biosynthesis in plants and microorganisms*, Chem. Biol. **1998**, *5*, R221-233.

Fellermeister, M., Eisenreich, W., Bacher, A., Zenk, M.H.: *Biosynthesis of cannabinoids*, Eur. J. Biochem. **2001**, *268*, 1596-1604.

Fride, E., Breuer, A., Hanus, L., Tchilibon, S., Horowitz, M., Mechoulam, R., Garzon, A. (Yissum Research Development Company of the Hebrew University), *Agonist specific for the peripheral cannabinoid receptor*, WO 0132169.

Fuentes, J.A., Ruiz-Gayo, M., Manzanares, J., Vela, G., Reche, I., Corchero, J.: *Cannabinoids as potential new analgesics*, Life Sci. **1999**, *65*, 675-685.

Heil, M., Meier, H., Naab, P., Voerste, A., De Vry, J.-M.-V., Denzer, D., Mauler, F., Lustig, K., Hinz, V., Allerheiligen, S. (Bayer AG), *Aryl and Heteroaryl Sulfonates*, WO0174763 (**2001**).

Hohmann, A.G., Tsou, K., Walker, J.M.: *Cannabinoid suppression of noxious heat-evoked activity in wide dynamic range neurons in the lumbar dorsal horn of the rat*, J. Neurophysiol. **1999**, *81*, 575-583.

Herkenham, M., Lynn, A.B., Little, M.D., Johnson, M.R., Melvin, L.S., de Costa, B.R., Rice, K.C.: *Cannabinoid receptor localization in brain*, Proc. Natl. Acad. Sci. USA **1990**, *87*, 1932-6.

Iwamura, H., Suzuki, H., Ueda, Y., Kaya, T., Inaba T.: *In vitro and in vivo pharmacological characterization of JTE-907, a novel selective ligand for cannabinoid CB2 receptor*, J. Pharmacol. Exp. Ther. **2001**, *296*, 420-425.

Kreitzer, A.C., Regehr, W.G.: *Cerebellar depolarization-induced suppression of inhibition is mediated by endogenous cannabinoids*, J. Neurosci. **2001**, *21*, RC174.

Lange, J., Kruse, C., Tipker, J., Tulp, M., van Vliet, B. (Solvay Pharmaceuticals): *4,5-Dihydro-1H-pyrazole derivatives having CB_1-antagonistic activity*, WO0170700 (**2001**).

Makriannis, A., Deng, H. (University of Conneticut): *Cannabimimetic indole derivatives*, WO0128557 (**2001**).

Makriannis, A., Deng, H. (University of Conneticut): *Retro-anandamides, high affinity and stability cannabinoid receptor ligands*, WO0128498 (**2001**).

Mechoulam, R. and Gaoni, Y.: *Recent advances in the chemistry of hashish*, Fortschr. Chem. Org. Naturst. **1967**, *25*, 175-213.

Morimoto, S., Taura, F., Shoyama, Y.: *Biosynthesis of cannabinoids in* Cannabis sativa L., Phytochem. **1999**, *2*, 103-113.

Palazzo, E., Marabese, I., de Novellis, V., Oliva, P., Rossi, F., Berrino, L., Rossi, F., Maione, S.: *Metabotropic and NMDA glutamate receptors participate in the cannabinoid antinociception*, Neuropharmacology **2001**, *40*, 319-326.

Pertwee, R.G.: *Cannabinoid receptors and pain*, Prog. Neurobiol. **2001**, *63*, 569-611.

Rinaldi-Carmona, M., Le Duigou, A., Oustric, D., Barth, F., Bouaboula, M., Carayon, P., Casellas, P., Le Fur, G.: *Modulation of CB1 cannabinoid receptor functions after a long-term exposure to agonist or inverse agonist in the Chinese hamster ovary cell expression system*, J. Pharmacol. Exp. Ther. **1998**, *287*, 1038-1047.

Rinaldi-Carmona, M., Bart, F., Heaulme, M., Shire, D., Calandra, B., Congy, C., Martinez, S., Maruani, J., Neliat, G., Caput, D., et al.: *SR141716A, a potent and selective antagonist of the brain cannabinoid receptor*, FEBS Lett. **1994**, *350*, 240-244.

Rohmer, M.: *The discovery of a mevalonate-independent pathway for isoprenoid biosynthesis in bacteria, algae and higher plants*, Nat. Prod. Rep. **1999**,*16*, 565-574.

Segal, M.: *The therapeutic effects of cannabinoids*, In Cannabinoids as Therapeutic Agents, **1986**, edited by R. Mechoulam, 105-120, CRC Press, Boca Raton, USA.

Sullivan, J.M: *Cellular and molecular mechanisms underlying learning and memory impairments produced by cannabinoids*, Learn. Mem. **2000**, *7*, 132-139.

Taura, F., Morimoto, S., Shoyama, Y.: *Purification and characterization of cannabidiolic-acid synthase from* Cannabis sativa L., J. Biol. Chem. **1996**, *271*, 17411-17416.

Twitchell, W., Brown, S., Mackie, K.: *Cannabinoids inhibit N- and P/Q-type calcium channels in cultured rat hippocampal neurons*, J. Neurophysiol. **1997**, *78*, 43-50.

Welch, S.P. and Eads, M.: *Synergistic interactions of endogenous opioids and cannabinoid systems*, Brain Res. **1999**, *848*, 183-190.

Williamson, E.M. and Evans, F.J.: *Cannabinoids in clinical practice,* Drugs **2000**, *60*, 1303-1314.

Zimmer, A., Zimmer, A.M., Hohmann, A.G., Herkenham, M., Bonner, T.I.: *Increased mortality, hypoactivity, and hypoalgesia in cannabinoid CB1 receptor knockout mice*, Proc. Natl. Acad. Sci. USA **1999**, *96*, 5780-5785.

13   Vanilloids and the VR1 Receptor

Robert Frank

Introduction

Pain is initiated when the peripheral terminals of a subgroup of sensory neurons called nociceptors (Caterina and Julius, 1999) are activated. Nociceptor-specific cation channels, so-called vanilloid receptors, are the neuronal membrane recognition sites that serve as the molecular target for capsaicin, the main pungent ingredient in hot chilli peppers and related irritant compounds (Szallasi and Blumberg, 1990). A functional vanilloid receptor - called VR1 - activated not only by capsaicin but also by noxious heat (>43°C) and low pH (protons) has been cloned from rat (Caterina et al., 1997) and man (Hayes et al., 2000). So VR1 can be regarded as an integrator of chemical and physical stimuli that elicit pain.

Hot peppers and painful heat both activate sensory nerve fibers through an ion channel, known as vanilloid receptor subtype 1 (VR1). When activated, the channel opens, allowing an influx of calcium and sodium ions. The influx depolarizes neuronal pain fibers, initiating a nerve impulse through the dorsal root ganglion (DRG) to the brain. Noxious heat also activates VR1, explaining why our mouths feel hot when we eat chilli peppers.

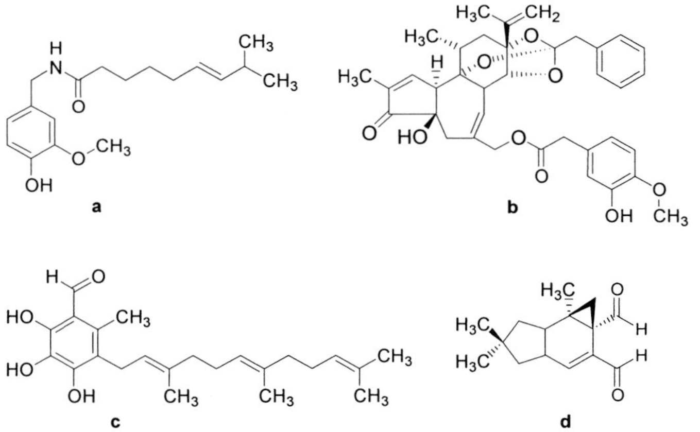

Scheme 1: Chemical structures of natural vanilloid receptor agonists: **a**, capsaicin, the irritant principle in hot peppers; **b**, resiniferatoxin (RTX), isolated from the cactus-like plant *Euphorbia resinifera*; **c**, the triprenyl phenol scutigeral, found in an edible, non-pungent mushroom; **d**, the sesquiterpenoid dialdehyde isovelleral, found in pungent mushrooms.

VR1 Receptor Structure, Localization and Signaling

VR1 is homologous to members of TRP (Harteneck et al., 2000), the transient receptor potential family of putative store-operated Ca^{2+} channels first identified in the *Drosophila* phototransduction pathway (Montell and Rubin, 1989; Caterina et al., 1997). These ion channels comprise six transmembrane domains with N-terminal anykrin

Frank

repeats (Clapham, 1996). The protein most likely exists in a multimeric form and forms a cation-selective ion channel with a preference for Ca^{2+} (Caterina et al., 1997). Although binding and Ca^{2+} uptake were initially believed to detect independent vanilloid receptor subtypes (Szallasi and Blumberg, 1996), VR1 can account for both the binding and functional activity of vanilloid ligands that show R- (resiniferatoxin-) and C- (capsaicin-) type structure-activity relations in rat dorsal root ganglion (DRG) neurons expressing native vanilloid receptors (Szallasi et al., 1999).

VR1 is a polytopic protein containing six trans-membrane segments with an additional short hydrophobic stretch between transmembrane regions 5 and 6, which is believed to be associated with the channel pore. There are three possible protein kinase A phosphorylation sites on the VR1 that might play a role in receptor desensitisation.

Vanilloid receptors are expressed by a subset of primary sensory neurons in dorsal root and trigeminal ganglia where their expression is regulated by nerve growth factor (Winter et al., 1993) and by a subpopulation of vagal (nodose ganglion) neurons sensitive to brain-derived neurotrophic factor (Helliwell et al., 1998). They have also been detected in several brain nuclei including the pre-optic area, locus coeruleus, medial hypothalamus, reticular formation and ventral thalamus (Acs et al., 1996; Sasamura et al., 1998). A more widespread distribution of VR1 within the CNS and on blood mononuclear cells has been reported recently (Mezey et al., 2000). Thus, VRs in the brain (and putative endogenous vanilloids) have been suggested to be involved in control of emotions, learning and satiety, to name just a few exciting possibilities (Mezey et al., 2000).

Binding to VR1 can be measured using [³H]RTX (Szallasi and Blumberg, 1990) or [¹²⁵I]RTX (Wahl et al., 2001). Furthermore, vanilloid receptor distribution can be visualized by [³H]RTX autoradiography (Szallasi, 1995) *in situ* hybridization (Caterina et al., 1997) or immunostaining (Tominaga et al., 1998). The heterogeneity of vanilloid-induced biological responses predicts the existence of vanilloid receptor subtypes. Vanilloids have been found to evoke several kinetically distinct currents in sensory neurons (Liu and Simon, 1996; Petersen et al., 1996).

Potential vanilloid receptor subtypes

Homologs of VR1 with a high threshold (> 52°C) for activation by noxious heat, or sensitivity to membrane stretch, provisionally termed vanilloid receptor-like protein (VRL-1) (Caterina et al., 1999) and stretch-inactivated channel (SIC) (Suzuki et al., 1999), respectively, have been identified. Neither channel is activated by vanilloid agonists (Caterina et al., 1999; Suzuki et al., 1999). A mouse ortholog of VRL-1 acts as a growth factor regulated channel (GRC) permeable to Ca^{2+} ions (Kanzaki et al., 1999). A splice variant of VR1 (VR.5'sv) that lacks the majority of the intracellular N-terminal domain is refractory to activation by vanilloid agonists, protons or noxious thermal stimuli (Schumacher et al., 2000). An additional homologue of VR1, variously termed OTRPC4 (Strotmann et al., 2000), VR-OAC (Liedtke et al., 2000), Trp12 (Wissenbach et al., 2000) or VRL-2 (Delany et al., 2000), is reported to be an osmotically regulated nonselective channel (Liedtke et al., 2000; Strotmann et al., 2000).

Treatment with vanilloid agonists leads to the activation of distinct subpopulations of primary sensory neurons (nociceptors), with somata in dorsal root, trigeminal as well as nodose ganglia (Holzer, 1991). These neurons transmit nociceptive information back to the central nervous system (afferent function), whereas their peripheral terminals are sites of release for a variety of pro-inflammatory neuropeptides (efferent function) such as calcitonin gene-related peptide (CGRP) or the tachykinin substance P (SP, NK1). Excitation of these neurons by vanilloids is followed by a long-lasting refractory state referred to as desensitization (Jancsó, 1968) or, under certain conditions such as neonatal treatment (Jancsó et al., 1977), may lead to gross neurotoxicity.

Effects of vanilloid agonists

Actual and Potential Applications of Natural and Synthetic Vanilloids

Human disorders which today are of interest in the context of vanilloid treatment can in general be divided into three categories (Winter et al., 1995):

(1) Disease states in which currently available capsaicin solutions or creams are clearly beneficial, such as non-allergic (vasomotor) rhinitis (Stjarne et al., 1989; Lacroix et al., 1991; Marabini et al., 1991; Filiaci et al., 1994), urinary bladder hyperreflexia (Fowler et al., 1992; Geirsson et al., 1995) and notalgia parestetica (Leibsohn, 1992).

(2) Pathological conditions in which capsaicin itself is not sufficiently active, but more potent vanilloids are expected to be of greater therapeutic value. For example: diabetic neuropathy (Ross and Varipapa, 1989), postherpetic neuralgia (Watson et al., 1988; Bernstein et al., 1989), chronic distal painful poly-neuropathy (Low et al., 1995), post-mastectomy pain syndrome (Watson et al., 1989), Guillain-Barré syndrome (Morgenlander et al., 1990), reflex sympathetic dystrophy (Cheshire and Snyder, 1990), vulvar vestibulitis (Friedrich, 1988).

(3) Innovative uses for novel, receptor subtype-selective vanilloids (see below), e.g. weight control.

Capsaicin

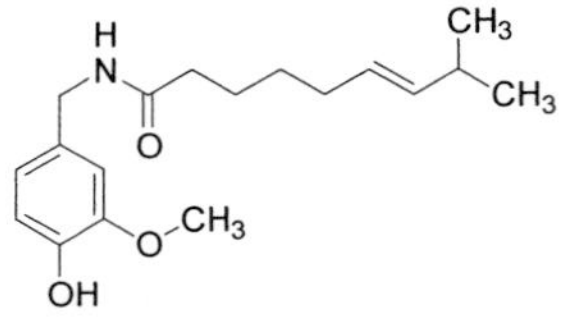

[404-86-4], trans-8-Methyl-N-vanillyl-6-nonenamide, $C_{18}H_{27}NO_3$, M_r 305.42, *mp* 62-65 °C

Trade names: Axsain (GB), Capsin, Capzasin, No pain (USA), Mioton (BG), Zacin (GB, IRL), Zostrix (AUS, CAN, USA), Capsacin (ES).

The vanilloid agonist capsaicin has been in use for decades as a pharmacological tool. In principle, all the three characteristic effects of capsaicin – excitation, desensitisation, neurotoxicity – can be used therapeutically, but desensitization to capsaicin is of particular interest as a novel approach to mitigate neuropathic pain insensitive to traditional pain-killers such as opiates (Szallasi and Blumberg, 1993; Winter et al., 1995). Capsaicin binding leads to Na^+ influx resulting in action potential generation (perceived as pain), and to Ca^{2+} accumulation (Wood, 1993). The increasing cytoplasmic Ca^{2+} concentration first impairs neuronal functions (desensitization) and may ultimately kill the affected neurons (Bleakman et al., 1990; Dray, 1992).

Synthesis: The synthesis of capsaicin is shown below (Gannett et al., 1988). For clinical use capsaicin is isolated from chilli pepper (*Capsicum annum*).

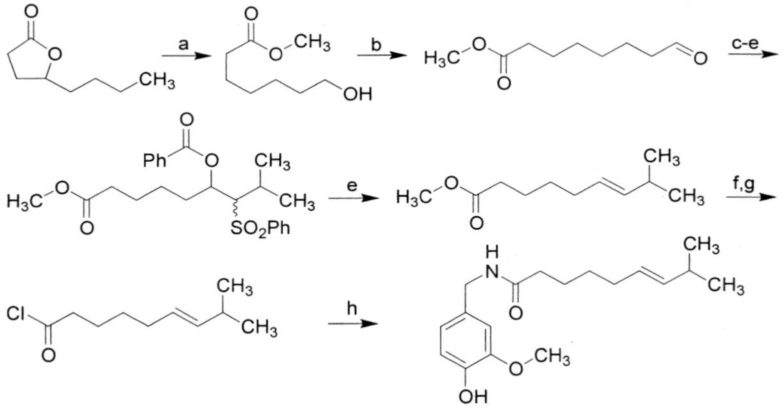

(a) MeOH, H^+; (b) PCC, NaOAc, CH_2Cl_2; (c) Butylphenylsulphone, -78°C, *n*-BuLi; (d) -78°C, then 0°C; (e) -78°C, C_6H_5COCl; (f) Na(Hg), MeOH, -20°C; (g) KOH, EtOH; (h) $SOCl_2$; (i) Vanillylamine, pyridine, rt, 3 days (Gannett et al., 1988).

Scheme 2: Synthesis of capsaicin.

Clinical use: Being a vanilloid agonist capsaicin is used based on counter irritation and desensitization. It is a standard ingredient in a variety of over-the-counter drugs used worldwide to relieve muscle ache. Through the existence of vanilloid-sensitive nerves in the human urinary bladder, capsaicin is beneficial in the treatment of urge incontinence (motor form bladder hypersensitivity and sensory form detrusor hyperflexia). Whereas toothache is a traditional indication, topical capsaicin has additional therapeutic value in atypical odontalgia, burning mouth syndrome and vasomotor rhinitis. Topical capsaicin has also been tried as an adjuvant analgesic in a variety of neuropathic pain conditions such as postherpetic neuralgia, painful diabetic neuropathy and postmastectomy pain syndrome, as well as in osteo- and rheumatoid arthritis (Winter et al. 1995; Sasamura et al., 1998; Szallasi and Blumberg, 1999).

The most important adverse effect of capsaicin is the initial burning sensation that it produces. Intravesical capsaicin induces intense suprapubic pain during intravesical instillation that may be made tolerable by lidocaine in some but not all patients. Capsaicin also frequently causes a transient worsening of the urinary conditions before improvement of symptoms due to desensitization of bladder afferents becoming evident. In patients with high spinal cord lesions capsaicin might provoke life-threatening autonomic dysreflexia.

Capsaicin is poorly absorbed through the human skin and is extensively metabolized (Szallasi and Blumberg, 1999), which explains why capsaicin creams are less active than expected on the basis of animal experimentation (Winter et al., 1995; Szallasi and Blumberg, 1999). When administered via a catheter into the human urinary bladder capsaicin is a powerful drug that relieves detrusor hyperreflexia (Winter et al., 1993; de Groat, 1997; Chancellor and de Groat, 1999). However, capsaicin administration is also very painful and might activate undesirable autonomic reflexes if absorbed into the circulation through the bladder mucosa (Cruz, 1998).

Adverse effects of capsaicin

Resiniferatoxin

Resiniferatoxin (RTX) is a daphnane diterpenoid contained in the irritant latex of some succulent African *Euphorbias*. Its total synthesis has been described as a 40 step asymmetric synthesis (Wender et al., 1997; see below), but for clinical use RTX isolated from *Euphorbia resinifera*.

Clinical use: Resiniferatoxin has been characterized as an ultrapotent sensory neuron desensitizing agent. It is 100 to 10,000 times more potent than capsaicin, has a longer duration of action, is much less irritating, and is substantially more effective in producing neural desensitization. Clinical studies have demonstrated the utility of RTX in humans for the treatment of urinary urge incontinence, also known as detrusor hyperactivity, detrusor instability, detrusor hyperreflexia, or uninhibited bladder. It can also be used against pain associated with diabetic neuropathy and in the treatment of migraine and rhinitis. RTX is at present undergoing clinical trials investigating its ability to suppress detrusor instability

[57444-62-9], 4-Hydroxy-3-methoxy-[(2S,3aR,3bS, 6aR,9aR,9bR,10R,11aR)-3a,3b,6,6a,9a,10,11,11a-octahydro-6a-hydroxy-8,10-dimethyl-11α-(1-methyl-ethenyl)-7-oxo-2-(phenyl-methyl)-7H-2,9β-epoxy-azuleno[5,4-e]-1,3-benzo-dioxol-5-yl]benzeneacetic acid, $C_{37}H_{40}O_9$, M_r 628.71.

Trade names: Afferon RTX (USA, CH).

(Cruz et al., 1997; Cruz, 1998; Lazzeri et al., 1998), an important cause of urinary incontinence.

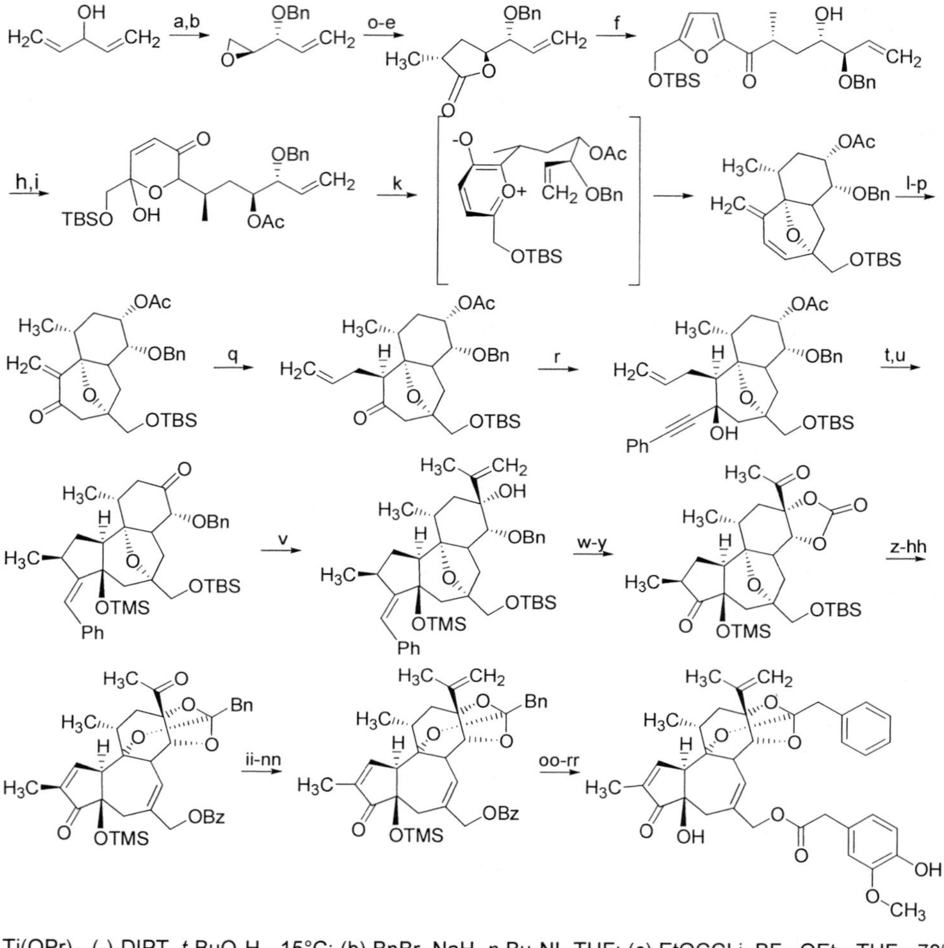

(a) Ti(OPr)₄, (-)-DIPT, t-BuO₂H, -15°C; (b) BnBr, NaH, n-Bu₄NI, THF; (c) EtOCCLi, BF₃•OEt₂, THF, -78°C; (d) TsOH, CH₂Cl₂; (e) LDA, -78°C, then MeI; (f) TBS-protected furfuryl alcohol, n-BuLi, THF, -78°C; (g) AcCl, pyridine, CH₂Cl₂, 0°C; (h) NaBH₄, MeOH, 0°C; (i) m-CPBA, THF, 0°C; (j) Ac₂O, DMAP, pyridine; (k) DBU, CH₃CN, 80°C; (l) H₂ (49 psi), 10% Pd/C, EtOAc; (m) Ph₃PCH₂, THF, reflux; (n) AcCl, DMAP, pyridine, 0°C; (o) SeO₂, t-BuO₂H, CH₂Cl₂; (p) MnO₂, CH₂Cl₂; (q) CH₂=CHLi, CuCN, Et₂O, -60°C; (r) PhCCLi, LiBr, THF, -78°C; MSTFA; (s) TMSCl, imidazole, CH₂Cl₂; (t) Cp₂ZrBu₂, THF, -78°C; HOAc; (u) TPAP, NMO, CH₂Cl₂; (v) CH₂=C(Me)MgBr, THF, 0°C; (w) O₃, CH₂Cl₂-MeOH, -78°C; (NH₂)₂CS, -78°C; (x) H₂ (45 psi), 20% Pd(OH)₂/C, EtOAc, MeOH; (y) triphosgene, pyridine, CH₂Cl₂, 0°C; (z) 49% HF, CH₃CN, 0°C; (aa) Tf₂O, pyridine, CH₂Cl₂, 0°C; n-Bu₄NI, CH₃CN; (bb) Rieke Zn, EtOH, reflux; (cc) SeO₂-t-BuO₂H, THF-HMPA (10:3), 80°C; (dd) SOCl₂, propylene oxide-Et₂O (1:2), 0°C; (ee) AgOBz-KOBz, 18-crown-6, CH₃CN; (ff) 0.5 M NaOH in aq. dioxane; (gg) DMAP, 2,4,6-Cl₃-PhC(O)C(O)CH₂Ph, toluene; (hh) 0.5% HClO₄ in MeOH; (ii) TMSCH₂Li, THF, -78°C; (jj) 49% HF, CH₃CN; (kk) BzCl, pyridine, DMAP, CH₂Cl₂; (ll) MSTFA, DMAP, DABCO, CH₃CN, 110°C; (mm) NBS, THF; (nn) Li₂CO₃, LiBr, DMF, 150°C; (oo) TBAF, THF, 0°C; (pp) Ba(OH)₂, MeOH; (qq) 2,4,6-Cl₃-PhC(O)OC(O)CH₂(4'-OAc)(3'-OMe)Ph, DMAP, toluene; (rr) pyrrolidine, CH₂Cl₂ (Wender et al., 1997).

Scheme 3: Synthesis of resiniferatoxin.

In comparison to capsaicin RTX has four major advantages:

(1) Because of its ultrapotency it may be used in much lower concentrations (Surh and Lee, 1995).

(2) Its use leads to desensitization (tachyphylaxis) rather than to irritation, which is the main factor limiting the therapeutic use of capsaicin.

(3) It has a much broader therapeutic window: full desensitization to pain or neurogenic inflammation may be achieved by means of a single RTX injection and without unacceptable toxicity.

(4) Unlike capsaicin it not only suppresses chemogenic pain, but is effective against noxious heat-evoked pain in normal rats as well as cold-evoked pain in animals with spinal cord injury.

RTX has its own shortcomings. Most importantly, RTX is expensive to isolate from natural sources and is difficult to synthesize. So there is a need for structurally simplified, orally active vanilloids. Whether either unsaturated dialdehydes or triprenyl phenols could serve as templates for the synthesis of such improved vanilloids remains to be explored.

Shortcomings of resiniferatoxin

Other Compounds

Other exogenous agonists at vanilloid receptors include novel capsaicin analogs that lack pungency or compounds that lack a vanilloid (o-hydroxymethoxy- or o-dimethoxyphenyl) moiety, for example unsaturated sesquiterpenoid dialdehydes or triprenyl phenols (see Introduction). Furthermore, the cannabinoid receptor agonist anandamide (see Chapter 11, *Cannabinoids*) and several eicosanoid products of lipoxgenases also activate vanilloid receptors (Hwang et al., 2000) and are putative endogenous agonists. Vanilloid receptor activity can also be induced by the activation of protein kinase C and the latter has been suggested to couple certain algesic stimuli, e.g. bradykinin, to signalling via vanilloid receptors (Cesare et al., 1999; Premkumar and Ahern, 2000).

Anandamide

DA-5018, NK1 antagonist, Phase II (Dong-A)

Olvanil, vanilloid agonist development ceased (Procter & Gamble)

Nonivamide, NK1 antagonist (Procter & Gamble)

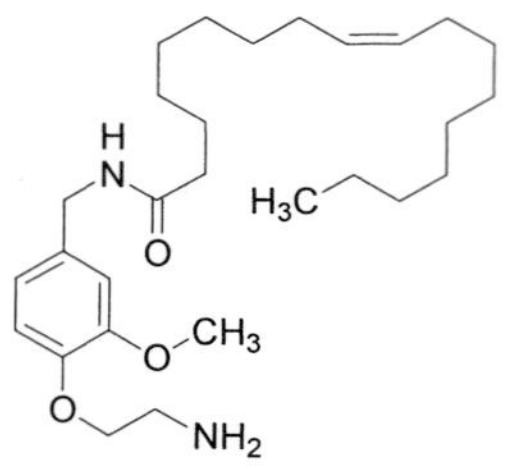

NE-21610,
vanilloid agonist
(Procter & Gamble)

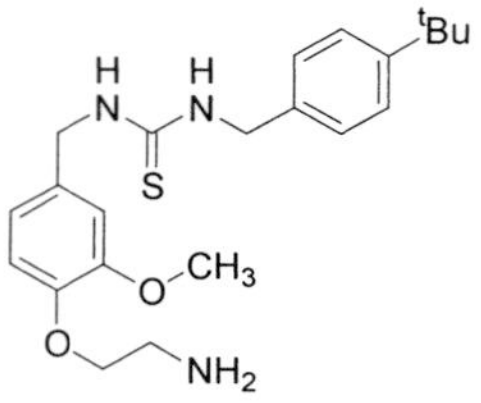

SDZ-249-482,
unspecified vanilloid agonist,
development ceased (Novartis)

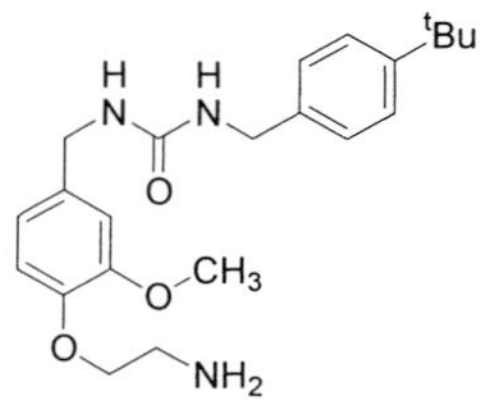

SDZ-249-665, unspecified
vanilloid agonist, preclinical studies
against neuropathic and
inflammatory pain (Novartis)

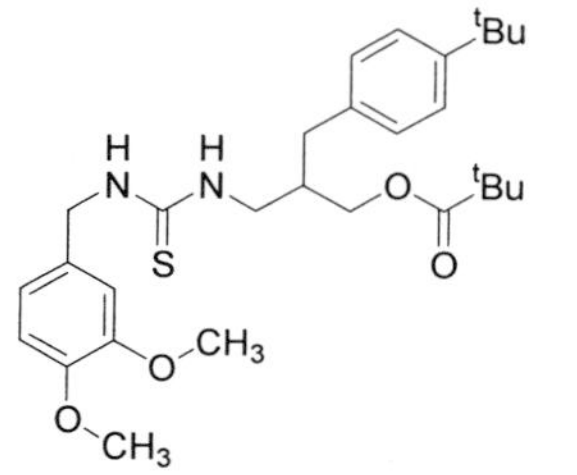

6d-I NIH, vanilloid antagonist,
preclinical analgesic,
(NIH)

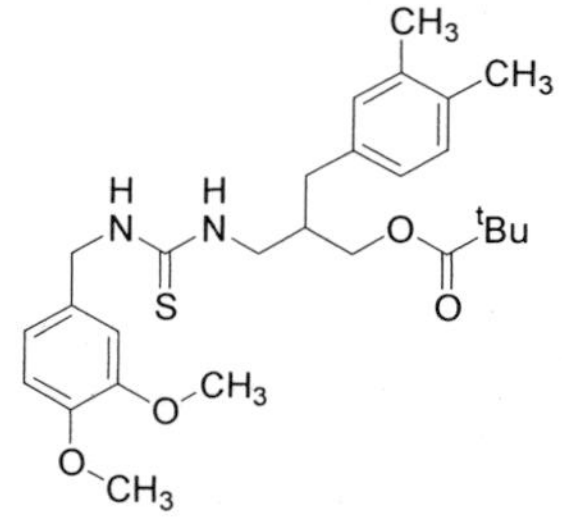

6b-I NIH, vanilloid antagonist,
preclinical analgesic,
(NIH)

Scheme 4: Structures of selected vanilloid like compounds.

The hot-tasting sesquiterpene dialdehyde polygodial was first isolated from water pepper (*Polygonum hydropiper*, Fukuyama et al., 1982).

The only current therapeutic use of an unsaturated 1,4-dialdehyde in the Western hemisphere is the use of polygodial (Kolorex® Capsules and Cream) to control localized candidiasis. According to the producer polygodial damages the cell wall of *Candida albicans* and other fungi (Sterner and Szallasi, 1999).

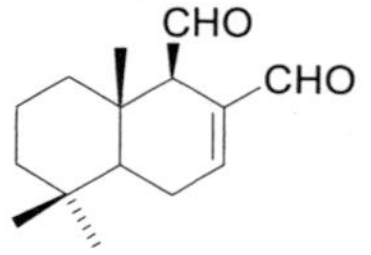

Polygodial [6754-20-7], 5,5,8a-Trimethyl-1,4,4a,5,6, 7,8,8a-octa-hydronaphthalene-1,2-dicarbaldehyde, $C_{15}H_{22}O_2$, M_r 234.33. *Trade name*: Kolorex® (NZ).

VR1 Antagonists

Known antagonists of vanilloid receptors include capsazepine, which acts competitively but with low potency at the capsaicin binding sites (Bevan et al., 1992), iodo-RTX, which binds with high affinity (Wahl et al., 2001), the unselective antagonist ruthenium red (Amann and Maggi, 1991) and synthetic arginine-rich hexapeptides (Planells-Cases et al., 2000), which are putative channel blockers.

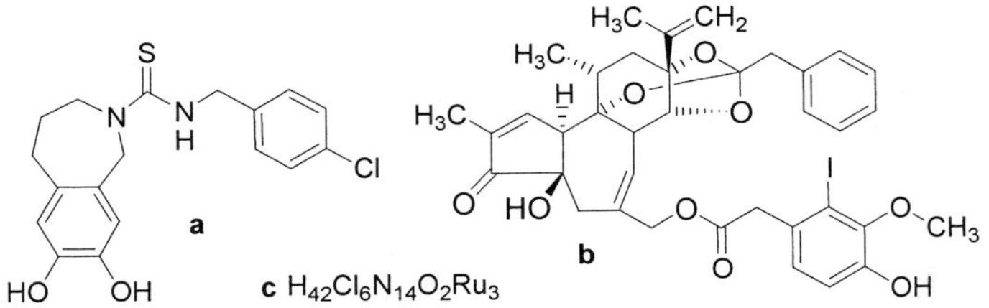

Scheme 5: Chemical structures of known vanilloid receptor antagonists: **a**, capsazepine, a weak but competitive synthetic compound from Novartis, **b**, iodo-resiniferatoxin, a potent and competitive synthetic compound from Novo Nordisk, **c**, ruthenium red, a weak, non-competitive and non-selective antagonists.

Contrary to the currently used (rapidly) desensitizing VR1 agonists capsaicin and RTX, selective VR1 antagonists are potentially useful for the treatment of pain and other pathological conditions without pronounced adverse effects (e.g. burning sensation). But whether the blockade of VR1 by potent and selective antagonists is as useful still remains to be proven. The one potent and selective VR1 antagonist known today - iodo-RTX - has received much attention but is a scarce and potentially chemically unstable compound needing further characterization.

Potential use for potent and selective VR1 antagonists

References

Acs, G., Palkovits, M., Blumberg, P.M.: *Specific binding of [3H]resiniferatoxin by human and rat preoptic area, locus ceruleus, medial hypothalamus, reticular formation and ventral thalamus membrane preparations*, Life Sci. **1996**, *59*, 1899-1908.

Amann, R. and Maggi, C.A.: *Ruthenium red as a capsaicin antagonist*, Life Sci. **1991**, *49*, 849-856.

Bernstein, J.E., Korman, N.J., Bickers, D.R., Dahl, M.V., Millikan, L.E.: *Topical capsaicin treatment of chronic postherpetic neuralgia*, J. Am. Acad. Dermatol. **1989**, *21*, 265-270.

Bevan, S., Hothi, S., Hughes, G., James, I.F., Rang, H.P., Shah, K., Walpole, C.S., Yeats, J.C.; *Capsazepine: a competitive antagonist of the sensory neurone excitant capsaicin*, Br. J. Pharmacol. **1992**, *107*, 544-552.

Bleakman, D., Brorson, J.R., Miller, R.J.: *The effect of capsaicin on voltage-gated calcium currents and calcium signals in cultured dorsal root ganglion cells*, Br. J. Pharmacol. **1990**, *101*, 423-431.

Caterina, M.J., Schumacher, M.A., Tominaga, M., Rosen, T.A., Levine, J.D., Julius, D.: *The capsaicin receptor: a heat-activated ion channel in the pain pathway*, Nature **1997**, *389*, 816-824.

Caterina, M.J. and Julius, D.: *Sense and specificity: a molecular identity for nociceptors*, Curr. Op. Neurobiol. **1999**, *9*, 525-530.

Caterina, M.J., Rosen, T.A., Tominaga, M., Brake, A.J., Julius, D.: *A capsaicin-receptor homologue with a high threshold for noxious heat*, Nature **1999**, *398*, 436-441.

Cesare, P., Dekker, L.V., Sardini, A., Parker, P.J., McNaughton, P.A.: *Specific involvement of PKC-epsilon in sensitization of the neuronal response to painful heat*, Neuron **1999**, *23*, 617-624.

Chancellor, M.B. and de Groat, W.C.: *Intravesical capsaicin and resiniferatoxin therapy: spicing up the ways to treat the overactive bladder*, J. Urology **1999**, *162*, 3-11.

Cheshire, W.P. and Snyder, C.R.: *Treatment of reflex sympathetic dystrophy with topical capsaicin. Case report*, Pain **1990**, 42, 307-311.

Clapham, D.E. : *TRP is cracked but is CRAC TRP?*, Neuron **1996**, *16,* 1069-1072.

Clapham, D.E.: *Some like it hot: spicing up ion channels.* Nature **1997**, *389,* 783-784.

Cruz, F.: *Desensitization of bladder sensory fibers by intravesical capsaicin of capsaicin analogs, a new strategy for treatment of urge incontinence in patients with spinal detrusor hyperreflexia or bladder hypersensitivity disorders.* Inter. Urogynecol. Journal **1998**, *9,* 214-220.

Cruz, F., Guimaraes, M., Silva, C., Reis M.: *Suppression of bladder hyperreflexia by intravesical resiniferatoxin*, Lancet **1997**, *350,* 640-641.

Delany, N.S., Hurle, M., Facer, P., Alnadaf, T., Plumpton, C., Kinghorn, I., See, C.G., Costigan, M., Anand, P., Woolf, C.J., Crowther, D., Sanseau, P., Tate, S.N.: *Identification and characterization of a novel human vanilloid receptor-like protein, VRL-2*, Physiological Genomics **2001**, *4,* 165-174.

Dray, A.: *Neuropharmacological mechanisms of capsaicin and related substances*, Biochem. Pharmacol. **1992**, *44,* 611-615.

Filiaci, F., Zambetti, G., Ciofalo, A., Luce, M., Masieri, S., Lovecchio, A.: *Local treatment of aspecific nasal hyperreactivity with capsaicin*, Allergo. Immunopatho. **1994**, *22,* 264-268.

Fowler, C.J., Jewkes, D., McDonald, W.I., Lynn, B., de Groat, W.C.: *Intravesical capsaicin for neurogenic bladder dysfunction*, Lancet **1992**, *339,* 1239.

Friedrich, E.G.: *Therapeutic studies on vulvar vestibulitis*, J. Reprod. Med. **1988**, *33,* 514-518.

Fukuyama, Y., Sato, T., Asakawa, Y., Takemoto, T.: *A potent warburganal and related drimane-type sesquiterpenoid from polygonum hydropiper*, Phytochemistry **1982**, *21,* 2895-2898.

Gannett, P.M., Nagel, D.L., Reilly, P.J., Lawson, T., Sharpe, J., Toth, B.: *The Capsaicinoids: Their separation, synthesis, and mutagenicity*, J. Org. Chem. **1988**, *53,* 1064-1071.

Geirsson, G., Fall, M., Sullivan, L.: *Clinical and urodynamic effects of intravesical capsaicin treatment in patients with chronic traumatic spinal detrusor hyperreflexia*, J. Urol. **1995**, *154,* 1825-1829.

de Groat, W.C.: *A neurologic basis for the overactive bladder*, Urology **1997**, *50,* 36-52.

Harteneck, C., Plant, T.D., Schultz, G.: *From worm to man: three subfamilies of TRP channels*, Trends Neurosci. **2000**, *23,*159-166.

Hayes, P., Meadows, H.J., Gunthorpe, M.J., Harries, M.H., Duckworth, D.M., Cairns, W., Harrison, D.C., Clarke, C.E., Ellington, K., Prinjha, R.K., Barton, A.J., Medhurst, A.D., Smith, G.D., Topp, S., Murdock, P., Sanger, G.J., Terrett, J., Jenkins, O., Benham, C.D., Randall, A.D., Gloger, I.S., Davis, J.B.: *Cloning and functional expression of a human orthologue of rat vanilloid receptor-1*, Pain **2000**, *88,* 205-215.

Helliwell, R.J., McLatchie, L.M., Clarke, M., Winter, J., Bevan, S., McIntyre, P.: *Capsaicin sensitivity is associated with the expression of the vanilloid (capsaicin) receptor (VR1) mRNA in adult rat sensory ganglia*, Neurosci. Lett. **1998**, *250,* 177-180.

Holzer, P.: *Capsaicin: cellular targets, mechanisms of action, and selectivity for thin sensory neurons*, Pharmacol. Rev. **1991**, *43,* 143-201.

Hwang, S.W., Cho, H., Kwak, J., Lee, S.Y., Kang, C.J., Jung, J., Cho, S., Min, K.H., Suh, Y.G., Kim, D., Oh, U.: *Direct activation of capsaicin receptors by products of lipoxygenases: endogenous capsaicin-like substances*, Proc. Natl. Acad. Sci. USA **2000**, *97,* 6155-6160.

Jancsó, N.: *Desensitization with capsaicin and related acylamides as a tool for studying the function of pain receptors*, edited by K. Lin, D. Armstrong, E.G. Prado, Pharmacology of Pain, **1968**, Pergamon Press, Oxford, 33-55.

Jancsó, G., Kiraly, E., Jancso-Gabor ,A.: *Pharmacologically induced selective degeneration of chemosensitive primary sensory neurones*, Nature **1977**, *270,* 741-743.

Kanzaki, M., Zhang, Y.Q., Mashima, H., Li, L., Shibata, H., Kojima, I.: *Translocation of a calcium-permeable cation channel induced by insulin-like growth factor-I*, Nature Cell Biology **1999**, *1*, 165-170.

Lacroix, J.S., Buvelot, J.M., Polla, B.S., Lundberg, J.M., *Improvement of symptoms of non-allergic chronic rhinitis by local treatment with capsaicin*, Clin. Exp. Allergy **1991**, *21*, 595-600.

Lazzeri, M., Spinelli, M., Beneforti, P., Zanollo, A., Turini, D.: *Intravesical resiniferatoxin for the treatment of detrusor hyperreflexia refractory to capsaicin in patients with chronic spinal cord diseases*, Scandinavian J. Urol. Nephrol. **1998**, *32*, 331-334.

Leibsohn, E.: *Treatment of notalgia paresthetica with capsaicin*, Cutis **1992**, *49*, 335-336.

Liedtke, W., Choe, Y., Marti-Renom, M.A., Bell, A.M., Denis, C.S., Sali, A., Hudspeth, A.J., Friedman, J.M., Heller, S.: *Vanilloid receptor-related osmotically activated channel (VR-OAC), a candidate vertebrate osmoreceptor*, Cell **2000**, *103*, 525-535.

Liu, L. and Simon, S.A.: *Capsaicin-induced currents with distinct desensitization and Ca2+ dependence in rat trigeminal ganglion cells*, J. Neurophysiol. **1996**, *75*, 1503-1514.

Low, P.A., Opfer-Gehrking, T.L., Dyck, P.J., Litchy, W.J., O'Brien, P.C.: *Double-blind, placebo-controlled study of the application of capsaicin cream in chronic distal painful polyneuropathy*. Pain **1995**, *62*, 163-168.

Marabini, S., Ciabatti, P.G., Polli, G., Fusco, B.M., Geppetti, P.: *Beneficial effects of intranasal applications of capsaicin in patients with vasomotor rhinitis*, Eur. Arch. of Oto-Rhino-Laryngol. **1991**, *248*, 191-194.

Mezey, E., Toth, Z.E., Cortright, D.N., Arzubi, M.K, Krause, J.E., Elde, R., Guo, A,. Blumberg, P.M., Szallasi, A.: *Distribution of mRNA for vanilloid receptor subtype 1 (VR1), and VR1-like immunoreactivity, in the central nervous system of the rat and human*, Proc. Natl. Acad. Sci. USA **2000**, *97*, 3655-3660.

Montell, C. and Rubin, G.M.: *Molecular characterization of the Drosophila trp locus: a putative integral membrane protein required for phototransduction*, Neuron **1989**, *2*,1313-1323.

Morgenlander, J.C., Hurwitz, B.J., Massey, E.W.: *Capsaicin for the treatment of pain in Guillain-Barre syndrome*, Ann. Neurol. **1990**, *28*, 199.

Petersen, M., Lamotte, R,H., Klusch, A., Kniffki, K.D.: *Multiple capsaicin-evoked currents in isolated rat sensory neurons*, Neuroscience **1996**, *75*, 495-505.

Planells-Cases, R., Aracil, A., Merino, J.M., Gallar, J., Perez-Paya, E., Belmonte, C., Gonzalez-Ros, J.M., Ferrer-Montiel, A.V.: *Arginine-rich peptides are blockers of VR-1 channels with analgesic activity*, FEBS Lett. **2000**, *481*, 131-136.

Premkumar, L.S. and Ahern, G.P.: *Induction of vanilloid receptor channel activity by protein kinase C*, Nature **2000**, *408*, 985-990.

Ross, D.R. and Varipapa, R.J.: *Treatment of painful diabetic neuropathy with topical capsaicin*, New Engl. J. Med. **1989**, *321*, 474-475.

Sasamura, T., Sasaki, M., Tohda, C., Kuraishi, Y.: *Existence of capsaicin-sensitive glutamatergic terminals in rat hypothalamus*, Neuroreport **1998**, *9*, 2045-1048.

Schumacher, M.A., Moff, I., Sudagunta, S.P., Levine, J.D.: *Molecular cloning of an N-terminal splice variant of the capsaicin receptor. Loss of N-terminal domain suggests functional divergence among capsaicin receptor subtypes*, J. Biol. Chem., **2000**, *275*, 2756-2762.

Singer, W., Opfer-Gehrking, T.L,. McPhee, B.R., Hilz, M.J., Low, P.A.: *Influence of posture on the Valsalva manoeuvre*, Clin. Sci. **2001**, *100*, 433-440.

Sterner, O. and Szallasi, A.: *Novel natural vanilloid receptor agonists: new therapeutic targets for drug development*, Trends Pharmacol. Sci. **1999**, *20*, 459-465.

Strotmann, R., Harteneck, C., Nunnenmacher, K., Schultz, G., Plant, T.D.: *OTRPC4, a nonselective cation channel that confers sensitivity to extracellular osmolarity*, Nature Cell Biol. **2000**, *2*, 695-702.

Stjarne, P., Lundblad, L., Lundberg, J.M., Anggard, A.: *Capsaicin and nicotine-sensitive afferent neurones and nasal secretion in healthy human volunteers and in patients with vasomotor rhinitis*, Br. J. Pharmacol. **1989**, *96*, 693-701.

Surh, Y.J. and Lee, S.S.: *Capsaicin, a double-edged sword: toxicity, metabolism, and chemopreventive potential*, Life Sci. **1995**, *56*, 1845-1855.

Suzuki, M., Sato, J., Kutsuwada, K., Ooki, G., Imai, M.: *Cloning of a stretch-inhibitable nonselective cation channel*, J, Biol. Chem., **1999**, *274*, 6330-6335.

Szallasi, A.: *Autoradiographic visualization and pharmacological characterization of vanilloid (capsaicin) receptors in several species, including man*, Acta Physiol. Scand. **1995** (Suppl.), *629*,1-68.

Szallasi, A. and Blumberg, P.M.: *Specific binding of resiniferatoxin, an ultrapotent capsaicin analog, by dorsal root ganglion membranes*, Brain Res. **1990**a, *524*, 106-111.

Szallasi, A. and Blumberg, P.M.: *Resiniferatoxin and its analogs provide novel insights into the pharmacology of the vanilloid (capsaicin) receptor*, Life Sci. **1990**b, *47*,1399-1408.

Szallasi, A. and Blumberg, P.M.: *Mechanisms and therapeutic potential of vanilloids (capsaicin-like molecules)*, Adv. Pharmacol. **1993**, *24*, 123-155.

Szallasi, A. and Blumberg, P.M.: *Vanilloid receptors: new insights enhance potential as a therapeutic target*, Pain **1996**, *68*, 195-208.

Szallasi, A,. Blumberg, P.M., Annicelli, L.L., Krause, J.E., Cortright, D.N.: *The cloned rat vanilloid receptor VR1 mediates both R-type binding and C-type calcium response in dorsal root ganglion neurons*, Mol. Pharmacol. **1999**, *56*, 581-587.

Szallasi, A. and Blumberg, P.M.: *Vanilloid (Capsaicin) receptors and mechanisms*, Pharmacol. Rev. **1999**, *51*, 159-212.

The Capsaicin Study Group: *Treatment of painful diabetic neuropathy with topical capsaicin: a multicenter, double-blind, vehicle-controlled study*, Arch. Intern. Med. **1991**, *151*, 2225-2229.

Tominaga, M., Caterina, M.J., Malmberg, A.B., Rosen, T.A., Gilbert, H., Skinner, K., Raumann, B.E., Basbaum, A.I., Julius, D.: *The cloned capsaicin receptor integrates multiple pain-producing stimuli*. Neuron **1998**, *21*, 531-543.

Wahl, P., Foged, C., Tullin, S., Thomsen, C.: *Iodo-resiniferatoxin, a new potent vanilloid receptor antagonist*, Mol. Pharmacol. **2001**, *59*, 9-15.

Watson, C.P., Evans, R.J., Watt, V.R.: *Post-herpetic neuralgia and topical capsaicin*, Pain **1988**, 33, 333-340.

Watson, C.P., Evans, R.J., Watt, V.R., *The post-mastectomy pain syndrome and the effect of topical capsaicin*, Pain **1989**, *38*, 177-186.

Wender, P,A., Jesudason, C.D., Nakahira, H., Tamura, N., Tebbe, A.L., Ueno, Y.: *The first synthesis of a daphnane diterpene – the enantiocontrolled total synthesis of (+)-resiniferatoxin*, J. Am. Chem. Soc. **1997**, *119*, 12976-12977.

Winter, J., Walpole, C.S., Bevan, S., James, I.F: *Characterization of resiniferatoxin binding sites on sensory neurons: co-regulation of resiniferatoxin binding and capsaicin sensitivity in adult rat dorsal root ganglia*, Neuroscience **1993**, *57*, 747-757.

Winter, J., Bevan, S., Campbell, E.A.: *Capsaicin and pain mechanisms*, Br. J. Anaesthesia **1995**, *75*, 157-168.

Wissenbach, U., Bodding, M., Freichel, M., Flockerzi, V.: *Trp12, a novel Trp related protein from kidney*, FEBS Letters **2000**, *485*, 127-134.

Wood, J.N. (Ed.): *Capsaicin in the Study of Pain*, Academic Press, New York, **1993**.

14   Substance P/NK₁ Receptors

Gregor Bahrenberg and
Corinna Maul

Introduction

In 1930, substance P (SP) was discovered by von Euler and Gaddum as an unidentified substance - referred to as P on tracings and protocols - present in alcoholic extracts of equine brain and intestine (von Euler and Gaddum, 1931). The early experiments were mostly concerned with its stimulating effect on smooth muscle and its vasodilator properties, later interest focussed on its role as a neurotransmitter or neuromodulator (von Euler, 1981). It took another 40 years to definitely establish the structure of hypothalamic SP (Chang et al., 1971). The development of SP receptor agonists and antagonists, and more recently the employment of transgenic mice, contributed to further elucidation of its sensory function (review: Harrison and Geppetti, 2001). This function and the anatomy of its expression (demyelinated sensory fibers, small and medium-sized neurons of spinal horn substantia gelatinosa) strongly suggest an important role as a mediator of pain and chronic inflammation (Otsuka and Yoshioka, 1993; Hill, 1994; Iversen, 1998; Zubrzycka and Janecka, 2000). Therefore, in the last 20 years, antagonists of SP and the SP-preferring receptor, called neurokinin-1 (NK₁) receptor, have been studied for their contribution in pain relief and a variety of conditions, including inflammation, asthma, emesis, anxiety and migraine (Wahlestedt, 1998). Herein, these efforts, especially with respect to pain, and their clinical rewards are critically reviewed.

Substance P and its Receptor

SP is an undecapeptide and the most abundant and best characterized of the neurokinin (tachykinin) group of peptides, which are defined by the common C-terminal amino acid sequence Phe-X-Gly-Leu-Met-NH₂. This group includes neurokinin A (NKA) and neurokinin B (NKB), but also neuropeptide K (NPK) and neuropeptide gamma (NPγ) (reviewed in: Saria, 1999; Hökfelt et al., 2001). The actions of SP, NKA and NKB are respectively mediated through G-protein linked receptors, designated NK₁, NK₂ and NK₃ and characterized by seven putative transmembrane helices (Maggio, 1988; Regoli et al., 1989; Nakanishi, 1991; Cascieri et al., 1992). The stimulation of tachykinin NK₁ receptors activates several second messenger systems that are stimulators of phosphatidyl inositol turnover via phospholipase C, arachidonic acid mobilization via phospholipase A₂ and cyclic adenosine

Substance P
Arg-Pro-Lys-Pro-Gln-Gln-
Phe-Phe-Gly-Leu-MetNH₂

Neurokinin A
Hys-Lys-Thr-Asp-Ser-Phe-
Val-Gly-Leu-MetNH₂

Neurokinin B
Asp-Met-His-Asp-Phe-Phe-
Val-Gly-Leu-MetNH₂

monophosphate accumulation via adenylyl cyclase (Mitsuhashi et al., 1992; Nakajima et al., 1992; Takeda et al., 1992; Seabrook and Fong, 1993; Garcia et al., 1994; Mochizuki et al., 1994; Saria, 1999). The rank order of potency of the neurokinin agonists for the neurokinin-1 (NK_1) receptor is SP>NKA>NKB, while the rank orders of potency for the other two subtypes (NK_2, NK_3) are NKA>NKB>SP and NKB>NKA>SP, respectively (Helke et al., 1990; Fong et al., 1992; Maggi and Schwartz, 1997). Substitutions of part of segments from NK_1 demonstrated that both the extracellular and transmembrane domains of the NK_1 receptor are involved in the binding of SP. The C-terminal sequence of SP is essential for activity at the NK_1 receptor, the minimum length of a fragment with reasonable affinity for the receptor is a C-terminal hexapeptide (Saria, 1999).

Evidence for a Role of SP in Nociception

Distribution of SP

Distribution of SP and its preferred receptor indicates a role in nociception. SP and NKA are suggested as primary afferent neurotransmitters because the gene precursor for these (preprotachykinin A) is found in unmyelinated primary sensory afferent neurons (Weihe, 1990; Duggan and Weihe, 1991; Rupniak and Hill, 1999). After synthesis in the cell bodies of sensory nerve fibers (located in spinal or cranial sensory ganglia), SP and NKA are released from terminals within the CNS and within peripheral tissues (Hill, 1986). In the CNS, SP neurons are present in the tegmental nuclei of the medulla, the central nucleus of amygdala and in the spiny neurons of the striatum that project into the medial segment of the globus pallidus and the substantia nigra pars reticulata. Fewer SP neurons are present in the dentate gyrus of the hippocampus. Some neurons are also present in layers V and VI of the cortex and project into the upper layers (Penney, 1996).

Distribution of NK1 receptors

The striatum, the nucleus accumbens, the hippocampus, the lateral nucleus of the hypothalamus, the habenula, the interpeduncular nucleus, the nucleus of the tractus solitarius, the raphe nuclei and the medulla oblongata are rich in tachykinin NK_1 receptors (Otsuka and Yoshioka, 1993). The predominant expression of NK_1 receptors within the spinal dorsal horn is consistent with the assumption that SP and NKA are important messengers here (Bleazard et al., 1994). The distribution of NK_1 receptors in the peripheral nervous system and in the gut are discussed elsewhere (McLean, 1996; Quartara and Maggi, 1997, 1998).

Surprisingly, the vanilloid receptor ligand capsaicin supplied the first experimental evidence for the association between SP and nociception (Gasparovic et al., 1964). Capsaicin depletes small primary afferents of at least SP, if not all of their peptide content, and this was accompanied by hypoalgesia. SP depolarizes the ventral root of an isolated rat spinal cord preparation (Konishi and Otsuka, 1974), and has also been shown to excite and/or depolarize neurons in the dorsal root (Urban et al., 1985). Furthermore, in studies on the larger laminae IV and V neurons, the selective NK$_1$ agonist, [Sar^9, Met(O$_2$)^{11}]substance P, was the most potent ligand tested (Morris et al., 1992). Fleetwood-Walker et al. (1987) reported that the NK$_1$ selective agonist [Met-O-Me^{11}]substance P excited neurons in laminae IV and V of cat spinal cord. Salter and Henry (1991), using iontophoretic application, demonstrated that presumed NK$_1$ receptor activation preferentially excited nociceptive neurons. Intrathecal administration of SP to a decerebrate, spinalized rat was found to facilitate the hamstring flexion reflex (Wiesenfeld-Hallin and Duranti, 1987), indicating that release of SP in the spinal cord may mediate hyperalgesia following tissue injury. Prolonged or intense noxious stimulation caused the release of SP in the vicinity of NK$_1$ receptors in the dorsal horn (Shults et al., 1984; Duggan et al., 1987). In addition, SP induces specific patterns of c-Fos expression in distinct regions (paraventricular, dorsomedial, parabrachial nuclei, medial thalamus) of the rat brain (Spitznagel et al., 2001). To sum up, one of the functions of SP is thought to be related to transmission of pain information into the central nervous system.

SP from primary afferents has a number of other effects on target cells besides pain transmission, e.g. vasodilatation, plasma protein extravasation, mast cell degranulation, recruitment of inflammatory cells, stimulation of secretion and muscle contraction (Maggi, 1997). The role of SP as an endogenous vasodilator in cerebral circulation and resulting effects on pain production have been discussed by Beattie et al. (1995a).

Quartara and Maggi (1998) summarize evidence for the involvement of NK$_1$ receptors in nociceptive transmission as follows: (1) NK$_1$ receptors are expressed at appropiate anatomical locations for noxious input in the spinal cord. (2) Spinal cord NK$_1$ receptor expression undergoes regulation after noxious manipulation. (3) The signal transmitted by activation of NK$_1$ receptors is a slowly-developing sustained depolarization, while the fast synaptic input to second order sensory neurons is

Sensory function of SP

Capsaicin

SP and nociception

Other effects of SP

Evidence for the involvement of NK$_1$ receptors in nociceptive transmission

mediated by excitatory amino acids. (4) Responses of second order sensory neurons to NK_1 receptor activation are enhanced by peripheral tissue injury or inflammation. (5) Tachykinin NK_1 receptor antagonists act synergistically to inhibit N-methyl-D-aspartate (NMDA)-mediated nociceptive transmission.

SP and NK_1 receptor knock-out mice

Further experimental evidence for the involvement of SP in pain perception came from knock-out animals. Mice, in which the preprotachykinin A gene was disrupted, showed significantly reduced responses in tests that involved more intense noxious stimuli (Cao et al., 1998). De Felipe et al. (1998) disrupted the NK_1 receptor, and found the characteristic amplification ('wind up') and intensity coding of nociceptive reflexes to be absent. NK_1 receptor knock-out mice show no changes in *acute* nociception tests. In contrast, SP and NK_1 receptor knock-out mice show reduction in responses to inflammatory stimuli. Nerve injury-induced mechanical but not thermal hyperalgesia is attenuated in NK_1 receptor knock-out mice, when inducing chronic neuropathic pain by unilateral ligation of the L5 spinal nerve (Mansikka et al., 2000).

SP and noradrenaline

Recently published work suggests that SP acting at the NK_1 receptor, when unopposed by tonic release of noradrenaline, causes chronic thermal hyperalgesia (Jasmin et al., 2002; reviewed in: Hill, 2002) The authors used mice lacking the gene coding for dopamine β-hydroxylase (DBH), the enzyme responsible for synthesis of noradrenaline from dopamine. The DBH knock-out resulted in a decreased nociceptive threshold to thermal, but not mechanical, stimuli and decreased efficacy of morphine. NK_1 receptor antagonists reversed the hyperalgesia in the DBH knock-out mice, confirming that the responses are operated through SP and NK_1 receptors. From these data, it is proposed that (at least in mice) SP and opioids have opposite effects on pain behavior with the pronociceptive effects of substance P being balanced by the antinociceptive effects of opioids.

In addition, several painful clinical conditions, including peripheral neuropathy, fibromyalgia and osteoarthritis, are associated with increased levels of SP in human cerebrospinal fluid (Rupniak and Kramer, 1999).

Peptidic SP antagonists

Following from the notion that an SP (or NK_1) antagonist might be useful for pain relief, several peptide and non-peptide antagonists have been discovered. The first peptide antagonists of SP were obtained in the early 1980s (review: Maggi et al., 1993). They have invariably been developed through the modification of one or more of the 11 amino acids that comprise substance P, mainly based on substitution with D-amino acids (Folkers et al., 1981).

The most potent of this first generation of tachykinin antagonists is [D-Arg^1,D-Trp^{7,9},Leu^{11}]SP, named spantide I (Folkers et al., 1984). An important advance was the discovery of SP analogs with N-terminal truncation of SP containing two or three D-Trp residues, such as in [D-Pro^4, D-Trp^{7,9,10}]SP (Regoli et al., 1984). For studies of the NK$_1$ receptor in the central and peripheral nervous system, [D-NicLys^1,3-Pal^3,D-Cl$_2$Phe^5,Asn^6,D-Trp^{7,9},Nle^{11}]SP,   also known as spantide II (Folkers et al., 1990), has been introduced (where D-NicLys^1 is N epsilon-nicotinoyllysine, Pal^3 is 3-(3-pyridyl)alanine, D- Cl$_2$Phe^5 is 3,4-dichloro-D-phenylalanine, and Nle is norleucine). Further examples of SP-derived antagonists are the peptidic antagonists [D-Pro^9,Pro^{10},Trp^{11}]-substance P,   [D-Pro^9,MeLeu^{10},Trp^{11}]-substance P, and the D-Pro^9-(S)-spirolactam derivatives GR82334 (see below) and GR72251 (Ward et al., 1990; Lavielle et al., 1994). Interestingly, these antagonists interact with different receptors in the guinea pig ileum bioassay, as they differ in their potencies to inhibit the spasmogenic activity evoked by the NK$_1$ receptor selective agonist [Pro^9]substance P or by septide, [pGlu^6,Pro^9]-substance P-(6-11) (Lavielle et al., 1994). Although peptidic antagonists proved useful as experimental tools to analyze SP or NK$_1$ receptor function (Hakanson and Sundler, 1985), they possess poor pharmacokinetic properties and relatively broad *in vivo* activities (residual agonist activity, degranulation of mast cells, local anesthetic properties, neurotoxic effects). It seemed likely that therapeutic effects would not be fully recognized until non-peptide, metabolically stable antagonists became available.

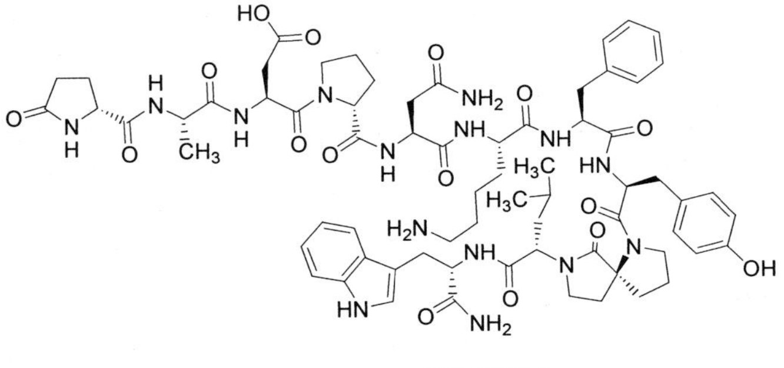

Spantide I & II

GR 82334

Non-Peptide Antagonists for NK₁ Receptors

Early attempts to synthesize non-peptide antagonists were hampered by the sequence diversity of the primary sequence of the NK₁ receptors from humans and rats, which influenced the potency of the compounds studied (Sachais et al., 1993; Saria, 1999). Appropriate models, with NK1 receptors closer to the human sequence, had to be established in gerbils, rabbits, and guinea pigs.

CP-96,345
[(2S,3S)-cis-2-(diphenyl methyl)-N-[(2-methoxyphenyl)-methyl]-1-aza-bi-cyclo[2.2.2] octan-3-amine]
$C_{28}H_{32}N_2O$, MW 412,57
[132746-60-2]

The first high-affinity, non-peptide antagonist of the tachykinin NK₁ receptor was discovered by researchers from Pfizer Central Research during a chemical file-screening approach and named CP-96,345 (Snider et al., 1991a; McLean et al., 1991; Watling, 1992; Ito et al., 1993). CP-96,345 displaced [³H]substance P binding to NK₁ sites with a K_i of 0.6 nM (equipotent with SP), and yielded a pA_2 of 8.7 in the relaxation assay of the dog carotid artery previously contracted with noradrenaline. These effects are specific for the 2S,3S configuration of CP-96,345 and for competitive antagonism at NK₁ sites. SP-induced salivation (10 nmol/kg i.v. SP), which is mediated by the NK₁ receptor, was inhibited by CP-96,345 (3.4 mg/kg i.v.), while the acetylcholine-evoked salivation response was not impaired (Snider et al., 1991b). CP-96,345 readily blocked the excitation produced by iontophoretic substance P or by nociceptive inputs to dorsal horn neurons in cats and rhesus monkeys (Radhakrishnan and Henry, 1991; Dougherty et al., 1993). In guinea pig brain, CP-96,345 inhibited 100 nM SP-induced increases in the firing rate of locus coeruleus neurons with an IC_{50} value of 90 nM (McLean et al., 1991). In rats it antagonized the flexor reflex facilitation produced by intrathecal application of SP in a dose-dependent manner (Xu et al., 1992). CP-96,345 has shown its antinociceptive activity in several mouse and rat pain models. Racemic CP-96,345 (30 mg/kg i.p.) induced a long-lasting increase in reaction time using the mouse hotplate test (Lecci et al. 1991). Moreover, inflammatory pain models in rat (intraplantar injection of 2% carrageenan or 5% formalin) revealed the antinociceptive activity of CP-96,345 (Birch et al., 1992). CP-96,345 has been reported to be a potent inhibitor of tachykinin-mediated neurogenic inflammation in the rat, blocking the SP-evoked fall in blood pressure and the mustard oil-induced plasma extravasation (Lembeck et al., 1992). Unfortunately, a major drawback of CP-96,345 is that it blocks sodium and calcium channels at high concentrations (Caesar et al., 1993), which itself caused analgesia not resulting from antagonism of the binding of SP to NK₁ receptors (Nagahisa et al., 1992).

Nevertheless, with the development of CP-96,345 the binding site for non-peptide antagonists and SP could be analyzed in parallel. It was found that SP binds at the extracellular ends of the transmembrane helices, whereas the small hydrophobic, non-peptide antagonists bind deeper in between the transmembrane segments (Hökfelt et al., 2001).

Pfizer's follow-up compound, CP-99,994 (Desai and Rosen, 1993), has a high affinity for NK_1 sites present on human IM-9 cells (K_i 0.17nM), but is essentially devoid of affinity at NK_2 and NK_3 sites and L-type Ca^{2+} channel sites (Watling and Krause, 1993). Peripherally administered CP-99,994 (0.1-10 mg/kg s.c.) antagonized the locomotor response induced in guinea pigs by intracerebroventricular injection of the selective NK_1 receptor agonist [Sar^9, $Met(O_2)^{11}$]SP. Previous studies suggest that CP-99,994 penetrates the blood brain barrier in rodents (McLean et al., 1993), and several arguments support a spinal action in the inhibition of prolonged chemical stimulation (Seguin et al., 1995).

The non-peptide NK_1 antagonist RP-67580 [((3aR,7aR)-7,7-diphenyl-2-(1-imino-2-(2-methoxyphenyl)ethyl)per-hydroisoindole)] can block the mechanical allodynia induced by the conditioning of C-fiber stimulation (Ma and Woolf, 1995), and attenuates progressive hypersensitivity of flexor reflex during experimental inflammation in rats (Ma and Woolf, 1997). Furthermore, RP-67580 in a range of 20-200 nmol antagonizes in a dose-dependent manner the sensitizing effect of SP in inflamed knee joints (Pawlak et al., 2001), and, when infused into the ventral tegmental area, prevents footshock stress-induced analgesia in the formalin test (Altier and Stewart, 1999). RP-67580 was as potent as morphine in various analgesic tests (Garret et al.,1991). RP-67580 displayed no activity at either NK_2 or NK_3 receptors in binding and *in vitro* functional assays (Betancur et al., 1997). However, at high concentrations, RP-67580 also exerts non-specific effects on Ca^{2+} channels.

For CP-96,345 and RP-67580, and also other NK_1 antagonists, marked species variants were observed in pharmacological studies. RP-67580 has a higher affinity for the rat and mouse NK_1 receptors, whereas CP-96,345 preferentially binds to human and guinea pig NK_1 receptors. CP-96,345 has a 90-fold selectivity for the human NK_1 receptor over the rat NK_1 receptor, while the agonist SP shows no such selectivity (Sachais et al., 1993).

Binding sites for substance P and the non-peptide antagonists

CP-99,994

RP-67580

SR140,333, WIN51,708,
WIN62,577

In mice, three further NK$_1$ antagonists - SR140,333, WIN51,708 and WIN62,577 - inhibited the late phase of formalin-induced licking, but failed to modify the tail-flick response at non-ataxic doses (Seguin et al., 1995). Examples of non-peptide antagonists for tachykinin receptors are listed in Table 1:

Table 1: Non-peptide antagonists for tachykinin receptors (adapted from Betancur et al.,1997).

Receptor subtypes	Endogenous ligands	Selective antagonists	
NK$_1$	SP>NKA>NKB	CP96349, SR140333, WIN51708, CGP49823, LY303870, L161664, L742694, CP122721, CAM4750, GR205171,	RP67580, CP99994, WIN62577, PD154075, LY306740, L733060, RPR100893, CAM4515, GR203040, MEN10930
NK$_2$	NKA>NKB»SP	SR48968,	GR159897
NK$_3$	NKB>NKA>SP	SR142801, SB223412	PD161182,

Mixed NK$_1$/NK$_2$ antagonist:
MDL105212A

NKA, neurokinin A; NKB, neurokinin B; SP, substance P.

SR140,333, Nolpitantium chloride

1-(2-{3-(3,4-Dichloro-phenyl)-1-[2-(3-isopropoxy-phenyl)-acetyl]-piperidin-3-yl}-ethyl)-4-phenyl-1-azonia-bicyclo[2.2.2]octane; chloride, C$_{37}$H$_{45}$Cl$_3$N$_2$O$_2$, MW 656,12, [153050-21-6]

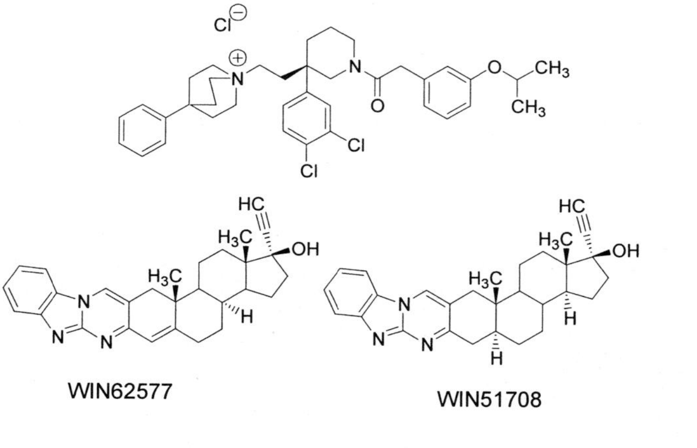

WIN62577

WIN51708

Scheme 1: Examples for non-peptide NK$_1$ antagonists.

Two further NK$_1$ receptor antagonists, described for the first time in the early 1990s, are FK888 and FK224. FK888 is a dipeptide derivative, synthesized by the Fujisawa group via a rational design strategy from the lead compound [D-Pro^4,D-Trp^{7,9,10},Phe^{11}]SP$_{4-11}$. FK888 is a compound with extremely high affinity for NK$_1$ receptors which inhibits [^{3}H]SP binding to guinea pig lung membranes with a K$_i$ of 0.69 nM and displays a pA$_2$ of 9.29 versus SP-induced contractions of the guinea pig ileum (Fujii et al., 1992; Watling and Krause, 1993). FK224 is a mixed NK$_1$/NK$_2$ antagonist (Morimoto et al., 1992), which passed first clinical evaluations in the treatment of obstructive airway disease (Soneoka et al., 1995). A 4-mg dose inhibited the bronchoconstrictor effect in 10 asthmatic patients when given by inhalation 20 min before challenge with bradykinin (Ichinose et al., 1992). In addition, FK224 may have therapeutic potential in the treatment of arthritis, as it blocks carragenenan- and SP-induced plasma leakage in the rat knee-joint in a dose-dependent manner.

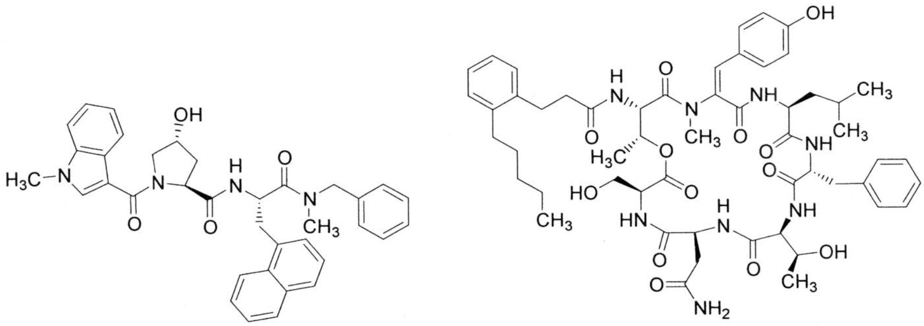

FK888   FK224

Scheme 2: Examples for synthetic peptide derivatives with NK$_1$ agonistic activity.

NK$_1$ receptor antagonists vary significantly in their abilities to penetrate the CNS following systemic administration. Poorly brain-penetrant compounds include SR140333, LY303870, RPR100893, and CGP 49823, whereas those with exceptionally good CNS penetration include the piperidines CP-99,994 and GR203040, the piperidine ether L-733,060, and morpholines such as L-742,694 (Rupniak and Hill, 1999). Putatively resulting from poor penetration of the blood brain barrier, LY303870 and RPR100893 are examples of NK$_1$ antagonists with poor efficacy and potency against inflammatory and neuropathic hyperalgesia in the guinea pig after oral administration. In contrast, the NK_1 receptor antagonist SDZ NKT343 (Ko and Walpole, 1996) produced 67% and 100% reversal of inflammatory and neuropathic hyperalgesia, respectively, at comparatively low oral doses (Urban and Fox, 2000). Therefore, SDZ NKT343 is clearly the most effective and potent NK_1 receptor antagonist in animal models. Unfortunately, clinical confirmation of the antihyperalgesic effects of SDZ NKT343 is not available.

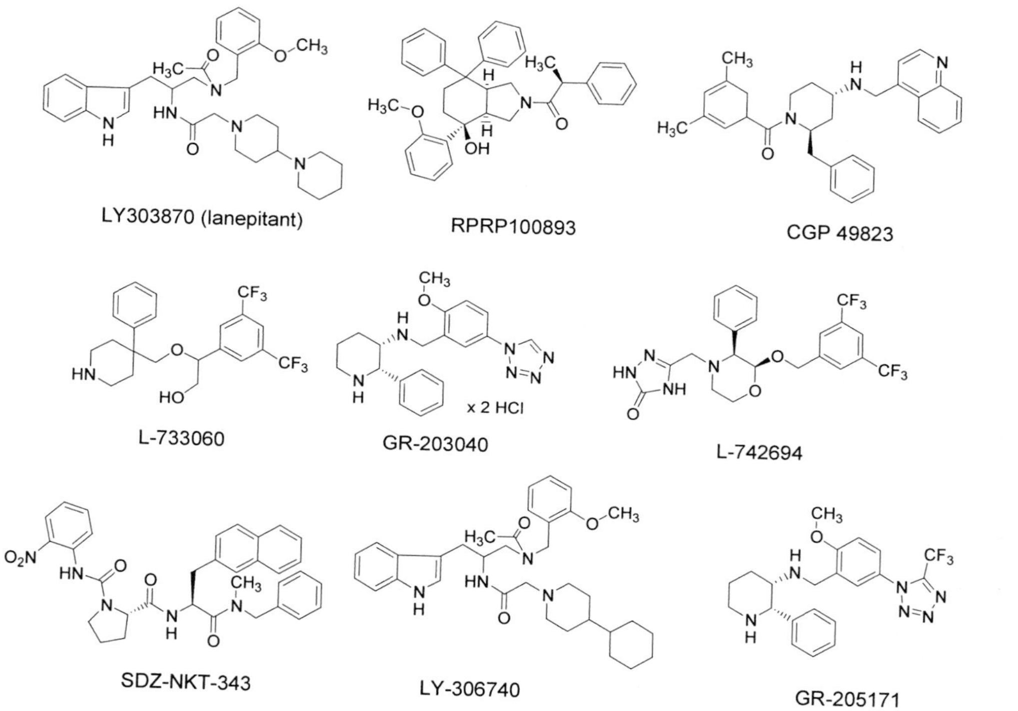

LY303870 (lanepitant)

RPRP100893

CGP 49823

L-733060

GR-203040

L-742694

SDZ-NKT-343

LY-306740

GR-205171

Scheme 3: Selection of non-peptide antagonists for NK_1 receptors.

Moreover, duration of central NK_1 receptor blockade is a critical point, as anesthetic-like nerve block caused by non-specific effects on ion channels in peripheral tissues could mask the selective antinociceptive effects of blocking NK_1 receptors in the spinal cord. The long-acting NK_1 antagonist L-733,060 maintained blockade of central NK_1 receptors at a time when peak plasma drug levels had subsided. Therefore, in paw licking experiments, the inhibitory effect of L-733,060 appeared to be due to central NK_1 receptor blockade (Rupniak et al., 1996).

NK$_1$ receptor antagonists exhibit weak potency in acute pain, whereas antinociceptive effects can only be observed after persistent peripheral inflammation, i.e. models of chronic pain (Radhakrishnan et al., 1998; Saria, 1999). This view has been confirmed with the discovery of the even more selective SDZ NKT343, mentioned above (Walpole et al., 1998a,b).

It should be mentioned here that discovery of the tachykinin receptor antagonists has not been limited to the NK$_1$ receptor, as non-peptide antagonists for the NK$_2$ receptor (e.g SR48,968) and NK$_3$ receptor (e.g. SR142,801) are known.

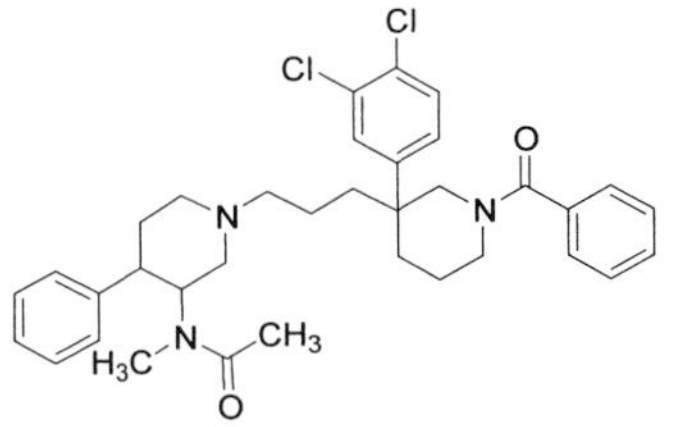

SR-142801 (Osanetant)
phase II clinical trials for
schizophrenia, depression,
and anxiety
(Sanofi-Synthelabo)

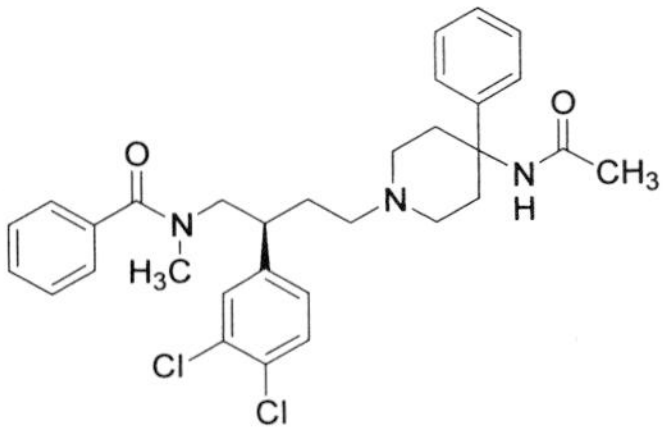

SR-48968 (Saredutant)
phase II clinical trials for asthma,
incontinence, and depression
(Sanofi-Synthelabo)

Scheme 4: NK$_2$ and NK$_3$ receptor antagonists in clinical trials.

Non-Peptide SP Antagonists

Non-peptide SP antagonists belong to a number of different structural classes: steroids, perhydroisoindolones, benzylamino and benzylether quinuclidine, benzylamino piperidines, benzylether piperidines, other piperidine-based structures and tryptophan-based antagonists (Quartara and Maggi, 1997; Argyropoulos and Nutt, 2000). From these, only two compounds progressed to Phase II trials in depression. The Novartis compound NKP608 is in Phase II trials for depression and social phobia, as well as chronic bronchitis (Argyropoulos and Nutt, 2000). MK869, also known as L754,030, from Merck was studied for depression. In clinical trials carried out at four sites, MK869 was found to be well tolerated, and its efficacy in major depressive disorder, was comparable to that of the serotonine uptake inhibitor paroxetine (20 mg daily, a moderate clinical dose; Kramer et al., 1998; Wahlestedt 1998). In addition, MK869 caused a lesser degree of sexual dysfunction. On the other hand, the high dose (300 mg) of MK869, producing micromolar plasma levels, and

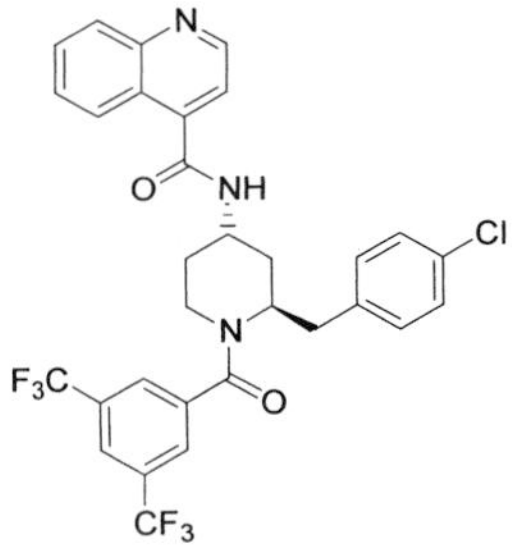

NKP608

MK869
(L-754,030)

Clinical pain studies

delayed onset of clinical efficacy (no effect before 2 to 3 weeks), presented no real progress compared to known monoamine uptake inhibitors. Trials with MK869 for treatment of depression were suspended in Phase II. Trials for anxiety disorders and schizophrenia continue. The compound has also been tested for emesis (Navari et al., 1999).

Clinical Use of SP or NK$_1$ Receptor Antagonists for the Treatment of Pain

Before the first clinical studies started, there was a strong expectation that NK$_1$ antagonists would be clinically efficacious analgesics. But the clinical trials have been very disappointing in terms of confirming the efficacy of NK$_1$ receptor antagonists in alleviating pain. NK$_1$ receptor antagonists fail to provide the level of sensory blockade required to produce clinical analgesia in humans (Rupniak and Kramer, 1999; Hill, 2000). However, the number of published clinical pain trials for NK$_1$ receptor antagonists remains limited, and many of the studies are only presented in abstract form. Results for clinical pain trials with different NK$_1$ antagonists have been summarized in Table 2 (according to Rupniak and Hill (1999)).

Table 2: Analgesic activity of NK$_1$ receptor antagonists (Rupniak and Hill 1999; with preliminary findings).

Clinical condition	Compound	Effect
dental pain	CP99994 (0.75 mg/kg, i.v.)	analgesia equivalent to ibuprofen
	CP122721 (200 mg, p. o.)	weak analgesia
	MK869 (300 mg, p. o.)	no analgesia
ostheoarthritis	LY303870 (600 mg, p.o., b.i.d.)	no analgesia
neuropathic pain	CP99994 (0.1 mg/kg, i.v.)	no analgesia
	LY303870 (200 mg, b.i.d.)	no analgesia
	MK869 (300 mg, p. o.)	no analgesia
migraine	RPR100893 (20 mg, p.o.)	no analgesia
	LY303870 (240 mg, p.o.)	no analgesia
	L758298 (60 mg, i.v.)	no analgesia
	GR205171 (25 mg, i.v.)	no analgesia

Assessment of dental pain following molar extraction represents one of the clinical evaluation methods for analgesic efficacy of NK₁ antagonists. During one study for postoperative dental pain, CP-99,994 (750 µg/kg i.v., over 5 h) was observed to be as effective as ibuprofen (Dionne et al., 1996). Findings with other NK₁ antagonists have been less encouraging. It is noteworthy that L-754,030 (300 mg p.o.) was reported to be ineffective as an analgesic for postoperative dental pain (Reinhardt et al., 1998), whereas it was clinically effective in antagonizing the effects of SP on forearm blood flow in humans (Newby et al., 1999). However, we should take into account that the dental pain model is considered to be a model of acute pain. Therefore, its use as a test setting for NK₁ receptor antagonism in humans is questionable, given that results from behavioral studies and knock-out mice suggest that a role for NK₁ receptor antagonists in acute pain is unlikely. For osteoarthritis with moderate joint pain, the effects of LY303870 (lanepitant) were compared against the reference analgesic, naproxen, in one clinical study (Goldstein, 1998). LY303870 was found to be ineffective when given as a twice daily treatment at doses up to 600 mg per-orally for 3 weeks.

In a study of painful peripheral neuropathy, CP99,994 (≤ 100 µg/kg i.v., over 2 h) had no analgesic effect (Suarez et al., 1994). Thus, to date clinical studies indicate that NK1 receptor antagonists are unlikely to be general analgesics (Rupniak and Kramer, 1999).

Clinical Use of NK₁ Receptor Antagonists for the Treatment of Migraine, Depression and Emesis

Clinical trials with NK₁ receptor antagonists for migraine, depression, and emesis were considerably more succesful than those for pain. These studies are excellently reviewed by May and Goadsby (2000, 2001).

Migraine headache is characterized by an intense unilateral throbbing pain, likely caused by diameter changes in extracranial, and most likely intracranial, arteries (Wolff, 1963). The source of the migraine headache is still not clear. The dura mater and its small vessels are suggested as an important parameter of headache pain. Mechanisms during initiation of migraine attacks may be explained by the model of neurogenic inflammation in the dura, characterized by plasma protein extravasation, vasodilatation, increased endothelial permeability and mast cell degranulation (Buzzi and Moskowitz, 1990; Moskowitz, 1992). In animal models of neurogenic inflammation, GR-203040 (Beattie et al. (Glaxo Wellcome), 1995b), lanepitant (LY-303870, Phebus et al. (EliLilly & Co), 1997), GR-82334 (O´Shaughnessy

Clinical studies for migraine

and Connor (Glaxo Wellcome), 1994), dapitant (RPR-100893, Lee et al. (Aventis Pharma AG), 1994), RP-67580 (Shepheard et al. (Aventis), 1993) and CP-99994 (Shepheard et al. (Pfizer), 1995) are all highly potent in blocking plasma protein extravasation. These results provide a substantial part of the preclinical rationale for the study of NK_1 antagonists in migraine. The first study employed RPR 100,893 at doses up to 20 mg (Diener, 1995), no headache relief was found. Similarly, in a double-blind, placebo-controlled, three-way crossover study, the NK_1 antagonist lanepitant (LY 303870), in doses up to 240 mg orally, was inactive in migraine (Goldstein et al., 1996).

Under the assumption that these compounds were not convincingly lipophilic, 25 mg GR205171 (Connor et al., 1998) and up to 60 mg L-758,298 (Norman et al., 1998) were administered intravenously. But again, these antagonists had no significant effect over placebo-controls in the double-blind studies. Most recent clinical evidence suggests, however, that perhaps vasoconstrictor properties are required to some degree to provide antimigraine effects, and this may be the reason why treatment with highly selective substance P receptor antagonists is insufficient (Cutler et al., 2000; May and Goadsby, 2001).

L-758298

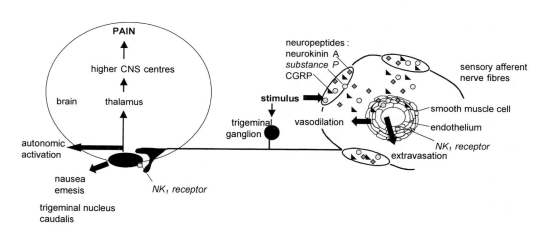

Figure 1: Diagrammatic representation of the putative pathophysiological mechanisms involved in the development of migraine headache and the potential sites of action of NK_1 receptor antagonists (adapted from Longmore et al., 1997).

Clinical studies for depression

The localization of SP in brain regions that coordinate stress responses, as well as behavioral studies with mice lacking the receptor for SP (De Felipe, 1998), suggest that NK₁ receptor antagonists might have psychotherapeutic properties. CGP49823 possesses significant anxiolytic properties (File, 1997). MK869 (non-peptide substance P antagonist) was tested in the treatment of moderate to severe depression, in a proof-of-concept study, as already described. The efficacy of MK869, as with other antidepressants, was expressed 2 to 3 weeks following the onset of treatment, suggesting the possibility of a common pathway for the action of antidepressants (Nutt, 1998; Wahlestedt, 1998). But the real progress was that co-morbid anxiety was treated very effectively with MK869 (Kramer et al., 1998; Nutt, 1998).

Several NK₁ receptor antagonists (including CP-99,994, GR203040, GR205171 and CP-122,721), due to their anti-emetic activity, offer the prospect of a novel approach for the control of emesis associated with, for instance, cancer chemotherapy. L754,030 has been shown to prevent emesis after treatment with cisplatin (Navari et al., 1999). Oral CP-122,721 200 mg decreased emetic episodes compared with ondansetron (4 mg i.v.) during the first 24 h after gynecologic surgery (Gesztesi et al., 2000). The NK₁ antagonists appear to be no more effective than $5HT_3$ receptor antagonists in preventing acute emesis. But they are well tolerated, and could prove useful, in combination with other compounds, as an alternative for delayed emesis (Hesketh, 2001). Effects of SP/NK₁ receptor antagonists on schizophrenia and affective disorders are reviewed by Rupniak and Kramer (1999).

Clinical studies for emesis

CP-122721

GR-205171

Conclusions and Implications for Future Studies

The trials described so far have commonly shown a lack of usefulness of NK₁ receptor antagonists in the treatment of pain. But we do not know whether the failure of the selected compounds is a matter of pharmacodynamics (e.g. poor penetration of the blood brain barrier) or a genuine discrepancy between animal and human pain pathophysiology (Urban and Fox, 2000). Hence, animal tests should carefully be chosen whether they are predictive or not, and it would be helpful if a wider range of conditions could be examined (Hill, 2000a). Therefore, new preclinical analysis methods should be developed for a more effective judgement of likely clinical outcomes.

Furthermore, the discovery of novel compounds with higher therapeutic potential can be foreseen. A selection of compounds which were filed recently for the treatment of pain and migraine is given below. As all of the non-peptide tachykinin receptor antagonists arose from targeted screening of large substance libraries using a robust radioligand binding assay, future high throughput techniques will provide further compounds with better pharmacological properties. Combination of such substances with existing analgesics could prove to be beneficial. Such co-medications will prove helpful in patients affected not only by chronic pain but also depression. As a result, we should not give up the studies with NK$_1$ receptor antagonists with respect to analgesis!

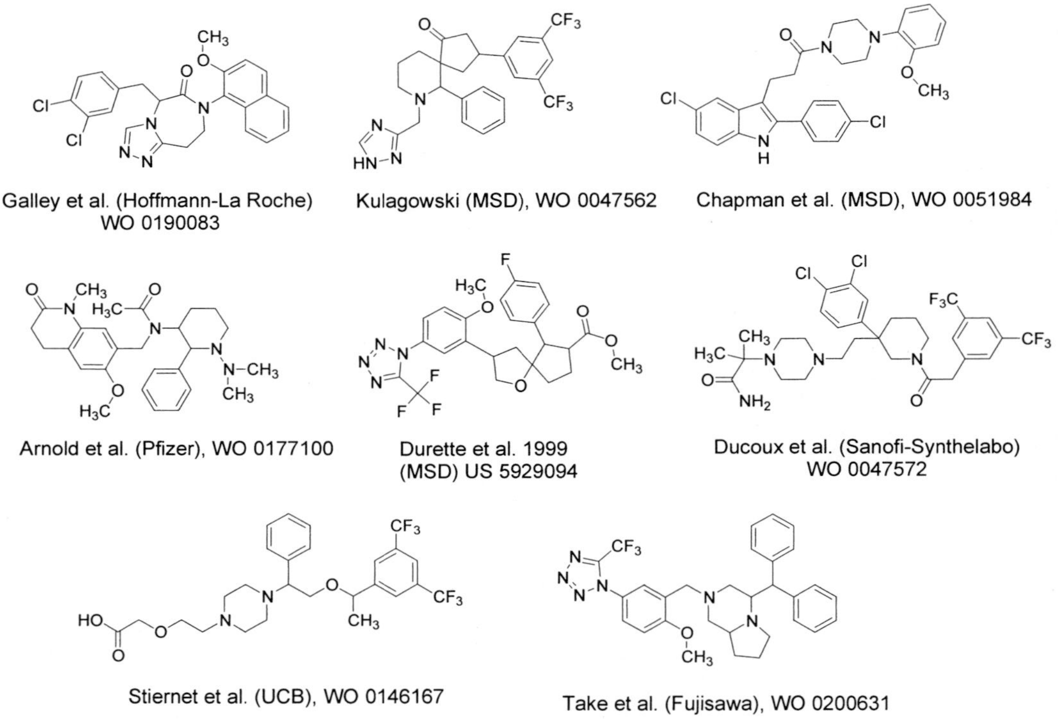

Galley et al. (Hoffmann-La Roche) WO 0190083	Kulagowski (MSD), WO 0047562	Chapman et al. (MSD), WO 0051984
Arnold et al. (Pfizer), WO 0177100	Durette et al. 1999 (MSD) US 5929094	Ducoux et al. (Sanofi-Synthelabo) WO 0047572
Stiernet et al. (UCB), WO 0146167		Take et al. (Fujisawa), WO 0200631

Scheme 5: Selection of substanceP/NK1-antagonists filed for the treatment of pain and migraine.

References

Altier, N. and Stewart, J.: *The tachykinin NK-1 receptor antagonist, RP-67580, infused into the ventral tegmental area prevents stress-induced analgesia in the formalin test*, Physiol. Behav. **1999**, *66*, 717-721.

Argyropoulos, S. V. and Nutt, D. J.: *Substance P antagonists: novel agents in the treatment of depression,* Exp. Opin. Invest. Drugs **2000**, *9*, 1871-1875.

Arnold, E. P., Chappie, T. A., Huang, J., Humphrey, J. M., Nagel, A. A., O'Neill, B. T., Sobolov-Jaynes, S. B., Vincent, L. A. (Pfizer): *Benzoamide piperidine containing compounds and related compounds,* **WO 0177100**.

Beattie, D. T., Connor, H. E., Hagan, R. M.: *Recent developments in tachykinin NK₁ receptor antagonists: prospects for the treatment of migraine headache*, Can. J. Physiol. Pharmacol. **1995a**, *73*, 871-877.

Beattie, D. T., Beresford, I. J., Connor, H. E., Marshall, F. H., Hawcock, A. B., Hagan, R. M., Bowers, J., Birch, P.J., Ward, P.: *The pharmacology of GR203040, a novel potent and selective non-peptide tachykinin NK1 receptor antagonist*, Br. J. Pharmacol.**1995b**, *116*, 3149-3157.

Betancur, C., Azzi, M., Rostene, W.: *Nonpeptide antagonists of neuropeptide receptors: tools for research and therapy*, Trends Pharmacol. Sci. **1997**, *18*, 372-383.

Birch, P. J., Harrison, S. M., Hayes, A. G., Rogers, H., Tyers, M. B.: *The non-peptide NK1 receptor antagonist, (+/-)-CP-96,345, produces antinociceptive and anti-oedema effects in the rat,* Br. J. Pharmacol. **1992**, *105*, 508-510.

Bleazard, L., Hill, R. G., Morris, R.: *The correlation between the distribution of the NK₁ receptor and the actions of tachykinin agonists in the dorsal horn of the rat indicates that substance P does not have a functional role on substantia gelatinosa (lamina II) neurons*, J. Neurosci. **1994**, *14*, 7655-7664.

Buzzi, M. G. and Moskowitz, M. A.: *The anti-migraine drug sumatriptan (GR 43175), selectively blocks neurogenic plasma extravasation from blood vessels in dura mater*, Br. J. Pharmacol. **1990**, *99*, 202-206.

Caesar, M., Seabrook, G. R., Kemp, J. A.: *Block of voltage-dependent sodium currents by the substance P receptor antagonist CP96,345 in neurones cultured from rat cortex*, Br. J. Pharmacol. **1993**, *109*, 918-924.

Cao, Y. Q., Mantyh, P. W., Carlson, E. J., Gillespie, A.-M., Epstein, C. J., Basbaum, A. I.: *Primary afferent tachykinins are required to experience moderate to intense pain*, Nature **1998**, *392*, 390-394.

Cascieri, M. A., Huang, R.-R. C., Fong, T. M., Cheung, A. H., Sadowski, S., Ber, E., Strader, C. D.: *Determination of the amino acid residues in substance P conferring selectivity and specificity for the art neurokinin receptors*, Mol. Pharmacol. **1992**, *41*, 1096-1099.

Chang, M. M., Leeman, S. E., Niall, H. D.: *Amino-acid sequence of substance P*, Nat. New Biol. **1971**, *232*, 86-87.

Chapman, K. T., Dinnell, K., Elliott, J., Hollingworth, G. J., Hutchins, S. M., Shaw, D. E., Willoughby, C. A. (Merck, Sharp & Dohme): *2-Aryl indole derivatives as antagonists of tachykinin*, WO 0051984.

Connor, H., Bertin, L., Gillies, S., Beattie, D., Ward, P.: *Clinical evaluation of a novel, potent, CNS penetrating NK1 receptor antagonist in the acute treatment of migraine*, Cephalalgia **1998**, *18*, 392.

Cutler, N., Gomez-Mancilla, B., Leibowitz, M., Fleishaker, J.: *A study of safety and efficacy in patients with acute migraine, using PNU-142633, a selective 5-HT1D agonist*, Cephalalgia **2000**, *20*, 268.

De Felipe, C., Herrero, J. F., O´Brien, J. A., Palmer, J. A., Doyle, C. A., Smith, A. J. H., Laird, J. M. A., Belmonte, C., Cervero, F., Hunt, S. P.: *Altered nociception, analgesia and aggression in mice lacking the receptor for substance P*, Nature **1998**, *392*, 394-397.

Desai, M. C. and Rosen, T. J. (Pfizer, Inc., U.S.A.): *Preparation of 3-aminopiperidine derivatives and related nitrogen-containing heterocycles*, WO9301170.

Diener, H. C. (RPR100893-201 migraine study group): *Substance P antagonist RPR100893-201 is not effective in human migraine attacks.* 6th Int. Headache Res. Sem. Nov.17-19 Copenhagen, Denmark **1995**.

Dionne, R. A., Max, M. B., Parada, S., Gordon, S. M., McLean, D. B.: *Evaluation of a neurokinin₁ antagonist, CP-99,994, in comparison to ibuprofen and placebo in the oral surgery model*, Clin. Pharmacol. Therap. **1996**, *59*, 216.

Dougherty, P. M., Palecek, M., Paleckova, V., Sorkin, L. S., Willis, W. D.: *The role of NMDA, non-NMDA, and NK1 receptors in the excitation of spinothalamic tract neurons in anaestetized monkeys*, J. Physiol. **1993**, *459*, 209P.

Ducoux, J. P., Emonds-Alt, X., Gueule, P., Proietto, V. (Sanofi-Synthelabo): *(1-Phenacy-3-phenyl-3-piperidylethyl)piperidine derivatives, method for the production thereof and pharmaceutical compositions containing the same*, WO 0047572.

Duggan, A. W. and Weihe, E.: *Central transmission of impulses in nociceptors: events in the superficial dorsal horn*, in Towards a new pharmacology of pain, **1991**, edited by A. Basbaum and J. M. Besson, 35-67, Wiley & Sons, Chichester.

Duggan, A. W., Morton, C. R., Zhao, Z. Q., Hendry, I. A.: *Noxious heating of the skin releases immunoreactive substance P in the substantia gelatinosa of the cat: a study with antibody microprobes*, Brain Res. **1987**, *403*, 345-349.

Durette, P., Kopka, I., MacCoss, M., Mills, S., (Merck & Co.): *Heteroaryl spiroethercycloalkyl tachykinin receptor antagonists*, EP 5929094 (**1999**).

File, S. E.: *Anxiolytic action of a neurokinin 1 receptor antagonist in the social interaction test*, Pharmacol. Biochem. Behav. **1997**, *58*, 747-752.

Fleetwood-Walker, S. M., Mitchell, R., Hope, P. J., El-Yassir, N., Molony, V.: *The roles of tachykinin and opioid receptor types in nociceptive and non-nociceptive processing in superficial dorsal horn*. In Fine afferent nerve fibers and pain, **1987**, edited by R. F. Schmidt, H. G. Schaible, C. Vahle-Hinz, 239-247, VCH, Weinheim.

Folkers, K., Feng, D. M., Asano, N., Hakanson, R., Wiesenfeld-Hallin, Z., Leander, S.: *Spantide II, an effective tachykinin antagonist having high potency and negligible neurotoxicity*, Proc. Natl. Acad. Sci. U.S.A. **1990**, *87*, 4833-4835.

Folkers, K., Hakanson, R., Horig, J., Jie-Cheng, X., Leander, S.: *Biological evaluation of substance P antagonists*, Br. J. Pharmacol. **1984**, *83*, 449-456.

Folkers, K., Hörig, J., Rosell, S., Björkroth, U.: *Chemical design of antagonists of substance P*, Acta Physiol. Scand. **1981**, *111*, 505-506.

Fong, T. M., Huang, R.-R. C., Strader, C. D.: *Localization of agonist and antagonist binding domains of the human neurokinin-1 receptor*, J. Biol. Chem. **1992**, *267*, 25664-25667.

Fujii, T., Murai, M., Morimoto, H., Maeda, Y., Yamaoka, M., Hagiwara, D., Miyake, H., Ikari, N., Matsuo, M.: *Pharmacological profile of a high affinity dipeptide NK1 receptor antagonist, FK888*, Br. J. Pharmacol. **1992**, *107*, 785-789.

Galley, G., Goergler, A., Godel, T., Heck, R. (Hoffmann-La Roche): *1,4-Diazepan-2,5-dione derivatives and their use as NK-1 receptor antagonists*, WO 0190083.

Garcia, M., Sakamoto, K., Shigekawa, M., Nakanishi, S., Ito, S.: *Multiple mechanisms of arachidonic acid release in Chinese hamster ovary cells transfected with cDNA of substance P receptor*, Biochem. Pharmacol. **1994**, *48*, 1735-1741.

Garret, C., Carruette, A., Fardin, V., Moussaoui, S., Peyronnel, J.-F., Blanchard, J.-C., Laduron, P. M.: *Pharmacological properties of a potent and selective nonpeptide substance P antagonist*, Proc. Natl. Acad. Sci. U.S.A. **1991**, *88*, 10208-10212.

Gasparovic, K., Hadzovik, S., Stern, P.: *Contribution of the theory that substance P has a transmitter role in sensory pathways*, Med. Exp. **1964**, *10*, 303-306.

Gesztesi, Z., Scuderi, P. E., White, P. F., Wright, W., Wender, R. H., D'Angelo, R., Black, L. S., Dalby, P. L., MacLean, D.: *Substance P (neurokinin-1) antagonist prevents postoperative vomiting after abdominal hysterectomy procedures*, Anesthesiology **2000**, *93*, 931-937.

Goldstein, D.: *Lanipetant in osteoarthritic pain*, Clin. Pharmacol. Therap. **1998**, *63*, PI 24.

Goldstein, D., Wang, O., Saper, J., Stoltz, R., Silberstein, S., Mathew, N.: *Ineffectiveness of neurokinin-1 antagonist in acute migraine: a crossover study*, Cephalalgia **1996**, *17*, 785-790.

Hakanson, R. and Sundler, F.: *Tachykinin Antagonists*, Fernström Foundation Series. (Elsevier, Amsterdam, NL **1985**).

Harrison, S. and Geppetti, P.: *Substance P*, Int. J. Biochem. Cell Biol. **2001**, *33*, 555-576.

Helke, C. J., Krause J. E., Mantyh, P. W., Couture, R., Bannon, M. J.: *Diversity in mammalian tachykinin peptidergic neurons: multiple peptides, receptors, and regulatory mechanisms*, FASEB J. **1990**, *4*, 1606-1615.

Hesketh, P. J.: *Potential role of the NK1 receptor antagonists in chemotherapy-induced nausea and vomiting*, Support. Care Cancer **2001**, *9*, 350-354.

Hill, R.G.: *Current perspectives on pain*, Sci. Prog. Oxf. **1986**, *70*, 95-107.

Hill, R. G.: In *The Tachykinin Receptors* (ed. Buck, S.H.) 471-498 (Humana, Totowa, NJ, **1994**).

Hill, R. G.: *NK1 (substance P) receptor antagonists— why are they not analgesic in humans?* Trends. Pharmacol. Sci. **2000**, *21*, 244-246.

Hill, R. G.: *Reply: will changing the testing paradigms show that NK1 receptor antagonists are analgesic in humans?* Trends Pharmacol. Sci. **2000**, *21*, 465.

Hill, R. G.: *Substance P, opioid, and catecholamine systems in the mouse central nervous system (CNS)*, Proc. Natl. Acad. Sci. U.S.A. **2002**, *99*, 549-551.

Hökfelt, T., Pernow, B., Wahren, J.: *Substance P: a pioneer amongst neuropeptides*, J. Internal Med. **2001**, *249*, 27-40.

Ichinose, M., Nakajima, N., Takahashi, T., Yamauchi, H., Inoue, H., Takishima, T.: *Protection against bradykinin-induced bronchoconstriction in asthmatic patients by neurokinin receptor antagonist*, Lancet **1992**, *340*, 1248-1251.

Ito, F., Kondo, H., Shimada, K., Nakane, M., Lowe, J., A. III, Rosen, T. J., Yang, B. V. (Pfizer Inc., U.S.A.): *Preparation of 2-diphenylmethyl-3-benzylaminoquinuclidines as substance P antagonists*, WO9221677.

Iversen, L.: *Substance P equals pain substance?* Nature **1998**, *392*, 334-335.

Jasmin, L., Tien, D., Weinshenker, D., Palmiter, R. D., Green, P. G., Janni, G., Ohara, P. T.: *The NK$_1$ receptor mediates both the hyperalgesia and the resistance to morphine in mice lacking noradrenaline*, Proc. Natl. Acad. Sci. U.S.A. **2002**, *99*, 1029-1034.

Ko, S.Y. and Walpole, C. (Sandoz Ltd., Switz.): *Preparation of carbamoylprolylnaphthylalanineamides and related compounds as tachykinin antagonists*, WO9618643.

Konishi, S. and Otsuka, M.: *Excitatory action of hypothalamic substance P on spinal motoneurons of newborn rats*, Nature **1974**, *252*, 734-735.

Kramer, M. S., Cutler, N., Feighner, J., Shrivastava, R., Carman, J., Sramek, J. J., Reines, S. A., Liu, G., Snavely, D., Wyatt-Knowles, E., Hale, J. J. et al.: *Distinct mechanism for antidepressant activity by blockade of central substance P receptors*, Science **1998**, *281*, 1640-1645.

Kulagowski, J. J. (Merck, Sharp & Dohme): *Spirocyclic ketones and their use as tachykinin antagonists*, WO 0047562.

Lavielle, S., Brunissen, A., Carruette, A., Garret, C., Chassaing, G.: *Highly potent substance P antagonists substituted with beta-phenyl- or beta-benzyl-proline at position 10*, Eur. J. Pharmacol. **1994**, *258*, 273-276.

Lembeck, F.: *The 1988 Ulf von Euler Lecture*, Acta Physiol. Scand. **1988**, *133*, 435-454.

Lembeck, F., Donnerer, J., Tsuchiya, M., Nagahisa, A.: *The non-peptide tachykinin antagonist, CP-96,345, is a potent inhibitor of neurogenic inflammation*, Br. J. Pharmacol. **1992**, *105*, 527-530.

Lecci, A., Giuliani, S., Patacchini, R., Viti, G, Maggi, C. A.: *Role of NK1 tachykinin receptors in thermonociception: effect of (+/-)-CP96,345, a non-peptide substance P antagonist, on the hot plate test in mice*, Neurosci, Lett. **1991**, *129,* 299-302.

Lee, W. S., Moussaoui, S. M., Moskowitz, M. A.: *Blockade by oral or parenteral RPR100893 (a non-peptide NK1 receptor antagonist) of neurogenic plasma protein extravasation within guinea pig dura mater and conjunctiva*, Br. J. Pharmacol. **1994**, *112*, 920-924.

Longmore, J., Hill, R. G., Hargreaves, R. J.: *Neurokinin-receptor antagonists: pharmacological tools and therapeutic drugs*, Can. J. Physiol. Pharmacol. **1997**, *75*, 612-621.

Ma, Q.-P. and Woolf, C. J.: *Involvement of neurokinin receptors in the induction but not the maintenance of mechanical allodynia in rat flexor motoneurones*, J. Physiol. **1995**, *486*, 769-777.

Ma, Q.-P. and Woolf, C. J.: *Tachykinin NK_1 receptor antagonist RP67580 attenuates progressive hypersensitivity of flexor reflex during experimental inflammation in rats,* Eur. J. Pharmacol. **1997**, *322*, 165-171.

Maggi, C. A., Patacchini, R., Rovero, P., Giachetti, A.: *Tachykinin receptors and tachykinin receptor antagonists*, J. Auton. Pharmacol. **1993**, *13*, 23-93.

Maggi, C. A.: *Tachykinins as peripheral modulators of primary afferent nerves and visceral sensitivity*, Pharmacol. Res. **1997**, *36*, 153-169.

Maggi, C. A. and Schwartz, T. W.: *The dual nature of the tachykinin NK_1 receptor*, Trends Pharmacol. Sci. **1997**, *18*, 351-355.

Maggio, J.E.: *Tachykinins*, Annu. Rev. Neurosci. **1988**, *11*, 13-28.

Mansikka, H., Sheth, R. N., DeVries, C., Lee, H., Winchurch, R., Raja, S. N.: *Nerve injury-induced mechanical but not thermal hyperalgesia is attenuated in neurokinin-1 receptor knockout mice*, Exp. Neurol. **2000**, *162*, 343-349.

May, A. and Goadsby, P. J.: *Substance P receptor antagonists in the therapy of migraine*, Exp. Opin. Invest. Drugs **2001**, *10*, 673-678.

May, A. and Goadsby, P. J.: *NK_1 receptor antagonists and migraine,* Current Opin. In CPNS Invest. Drugs **2000**, *2*, 167-170.

McLean, S.: *Nonpeptide antagonists of the NK1 tachykinin receptor,* Med. Res. Rev. **1996**, *16*, 297-317.

McLean, S., Ganong, A., Seymour, P. A., Snider, R. M., Desai, M. C., Rosen, T., Bryce, D. K., Longo, K. P., Reynolds, L. S., Robinson, G., Schmidt, A. W., Siok, C., Heym, J.: *Pharmacology of CP-99,994; a nonpeptide antagonist of the tachykinin neurokinin-1 receptor*, J. Pharmacol. Exp. Ther. **1993**, *267*, 472-479.

McLean, S., Ganong, A. H., Seeger, T. F., Bryce, D. K., Pratt, K. G., Reynolds, L. S., Siok, C. J., Lowe, J. A.III, Heym, J.: *Activity and distribution of binding sites in brain of a nonpeptide substance P (NK1) receptor antagonist*, Science **1991**, *251*, 437-439.

Mitsuhashi, M., Ohashi, Y., Shichijo, S., Christian, C., Sudduth, K. J., Harrowe, G., Payan, D. G.: *Multiple intracellular signaling pathways of the neuropeptide substance P receptor*, J. Neurosci. Res. **1992**, *32*, 437-443.

Mochizuki, O. N., Nakajima, Y., Nakanishi, S., Ito, S.: *Characterization of the substance P receptor-mediated calcium influx in cDNA transfected Chinese hamster ovary cells. A possible role of inositol1,4,5-triphosphate in calcium influx*, J. Biol. Chem. **1994**, *269*, 9651-9658.

Morimoto, H., Murai, M., Maeda, Y., Yamaoka, M., Nishikawa, M., Kiyotoh, S., Fujii, T.: *FK 224, a novel cyclopeptide substance P antagonist with NK_1 and NK_2 receptor selectivity,* J. Pharmacol. Exp. Ther. **1992**, *262*, 398-402.

Morris, R., Bleazard, L., Hill, R. G.:*The responses of neurons, in the deep dorsal horn of rat spinal cord slices in vitro, to the application of neurokinin agonists are correlated with their responses to peripheral nerve stimulation*, J. Physiol. **1992**, *452*, 252P.

Moskowitz, M. A.: *Neurogenic vs. vascular mechanisms of sumatriptan and ergot alkaloids in migraine*, Trends Pharmacol. Sci. **1992**, *13*, 307-311.

Nagahisa, A., Asai, R., Kanai, Y., Murase, A., Tsuchiya-Nakagaki, M., Nakagaki, T., Shieh, T. C., Taniguchi, K.: *Non-specific activity of CP96,345 in models of pain and inflammation*, Br. J. Pharmacol. **1992**, *107*, 273-275.

Nakajima, Y., Tsuchida, K., Negishi, M., Ito, S., Nakanishi, S.: *Direct linkage of three tachykinin receptors to stimulation of both phosphatidylinositol hydrolysis and cyclic AMP cascades in transfected Chinese hamster ovary cells*, J. Biol. Chem. **1992**, *267*, 2437-2442.

Nakanishi, S.: *Mammalian tachykinin receptors*, Annu. Rev. Neurosci. **1991**, *14*, 123-136.

Navari, R. M., Reinhardt, R. R., Gralla, R. J., Kris, M. G., Hesketh, P. J., Khojasteh, A., Kindler, H., Grote, T. H., Pendergrass, K., Grunberg, S. M., Carides, A. D., Gertz, B. J.: *Reduction of cisplatin-*

induced emesis by a selective neurokinin-1-receptor antagonist. L-754,030 Antiemetic Trials Group, N. Engl. J. Med. **1999**, *340*, 190-195.

Newby, D. E., Sciberras, D. G., Ferro, C. J., Gertz, B. J., Sommerville, D., Majumdar, A., Lowry, R. C., Webb, D. J.: *Substance P-induced vasodilatation is mediated by the neurokinin type 1 receptor but does not contribute to basal vascular tone in man*, Br. J. Clin. Pharmacol. **1999**, *48*, 336-344.

Norman, B., Panebianco, D., Block, G.: *A placebo-controlled, in-clinic study to explore the preliminary safety and efficacy of intravenous L-758,298 (a prodrug of the NK1 receptor antagonist L-754,030) in the acute treatment of migraine*, Cephalalgia **1998**, *18*, 407.

Nutt, D. J.: *Substance P antagonists: a new treatment for depression?* Lancet **1998**, *352*, 1644-1646.

O´Shaughnessy, C. T. and Connor, H. E.: *Investigation of the role of tachykinin Nk1, NK2 receptors and CGRP receptors in neurogenic plasma protein extravasation in dura mater*, Eur. J. Pharmacol. **1994**, *263*, 193-198.

Otsuka, M. and Yoshioka, K.: *Neurotransmitter functions of mammalian tachykinins*, Physiol. Rev. **1993**, *73*, 229-308.

Pawlak, M., Schmidt, R. F., Heppelmann, B., Hanesch U.: *The neurokinin-1 receptor antagonist RP67580 reduces the sensitization of primary afferents by substance P in the rat*, Eur. J. Pain **2001**, *5*, 69-79.

Penney, J. B., Jr.: *Neurochemical neuroanatomy*. In Neuropsychiatry **1996**, edited by B. S. Fogel, R. B. Schiffer, S. M. Rao, 145-171, Williams and Wilkins, Baltimore, MD.

Phebus, L. A., Johnson, K. W., Stengel, P. W., Lobb, K. L., Nixon, J. A., Hipskind, P. A.: *The non-peptide NK-1 receptor antagonist LY303870 inhibits neurogenic dural inflammation in guinea pigs*, Life Sci. **1997**, *60*, 1553-1561.

Quartara, L. and Maggi, C. A.: *The tachykinin NK₁ receptor: Part I. ligands and mechanisms of cellular activation*, Neuropeptides **1997**, *31*, 537-563.

Quartara, L. and Maggi, C.A.: *The tachykinin NK₁ receptor: Part II. Distribution and pathophysiological roles*, Neuropeptides **1998**, *32*, 1-49.

Radhakrishnan, V., Iyengar, S., Henry, J.L.: *The nonpeptide NK1 receptor antagonists LY303870 and LY306740 block the responses of spinal dorsal horn neurons to substance P and to peripheral noxious stimuli*, Neuroscience **1998**, *83*, 1251-1260.

Radhakrishnan, V. and Henry, J. L.: *Novel substance P antagonist, CP-96345, blocks responses of cat spinal dorsal horn neurons to noxious cutaneous stimulation and to substance P,* Neurosci. Lett. **1991**, *132*, 39-43.

Regoli, D., Escher, E., Drapeau, G., D´Orleans-Juste, P., Mizrahi, J.: *Receptors for substance P. III. Classification by competitive antagonists.*, Eur. J. Pharmacol. **1984**, *97*, 179-189.

Regoli, D., Drapeau, G., Dion, S., D´Orleans-Juste, P.: *Receptors for substance P and related neurokinins*, Pharmacology **1989**, *38*, 1-15.

Reinhardt, R. B., Laub, J. B., Fricke, J. R., Polis, A. B., Gertz, B. J.: *Comparison of a neurokinin₁ antagonist, L-754,030, to placebo, acetaminophen and ibuprofen in the dental pain model,* Clin. Pharmacol. Therap. **1998**, *63*, PI 124.

Rupniak, N. M. J. and Kramer, M.S.: *Discovery of the anti-depressant and anti-emetic efficacy of substance P receptor (NK₁) antagonists,* Trends Pharmacol. Sci. **1999**, *20*, 485-490.

Rupniak, N. M. J.and Hill, R. G.: *Neurokinin antagonists*. In Novel aspects in pain management: opioids and beyond, **1999**, edited by J. Sawynok and A. Cowan, 135-155, Wiley-Liss, New York.

Rupniak, N.M.J., Carlson, E.J., Boyce, S., Webb, J.K., Hill, R.G.: *Enantio-selective inhibition of the formalin paw late phase by the NK₁ receptor antagonist L-733,060 in gerbils,* Pain **1996**, *67*, 189-195.

Sachais, B. S., Snider, R. M., Lowe, J. A. III, Krause, J. E.: *Molecular basis for the species selectivity of the substance P antagonist CP-96,345,* J. Biol. Chem. **1993**, *268*, 2319-2323.

Salter, M. W. and Henry, J. L.: *Responses of functionally identified neurons in the dorsal horn of the cat spinal cord to substance P, neurokinin A and physalaemin*, Neuroscience **1991**, *43*, 601-610.

Saria, A.: *The tachykinin NK1 receptor in the brain: pharmacology and putative functions*, Eur. J. Pharmacol. **1999**, *375*, 51-60.

Seabrook, G. R. and Fong, T. M.: *Thapsigargin blocks the mobilisation of intracellular calcium caused by activation of human NK_1 (long) receptors expressed in Chinese hamster ovary cells,* Neurosci. Lett. **1993**, *152*, 9-12.

Seguin, L., Le Marouille-Girardon, S., Millan, M.J.: *Antinociceptive profiles of non-peptidergic neurokinin$_1$ and neurokinin$_2$ receptor antagonists: a comparison to other classes of antinociceptive agent*, Pain **1995**, *61*, 325-343.

Shepheard, S. L., Williamson, D. J., Hill, R. G., Hargreaves, R. J.: *The non-peptide neurokinin-1 receptor antagonist, RP 67580, blocks neurogenic plasma extravasation in the dura mater of rats*, Br. J. Pharmacol. **1993**, *108*, 11-12.

Shepheard, S. L., Williamson, D. J., Williams, J., Hill, R. G., Hargreaves, R. J.: *Comparison of the effects of sumatriptan and the NK-1 antagonist CP-99,004 on plasma extravasation in dura mater and c-fos RNA expression in trigeminal nucleus caudalis of rats*, Neuropharmacology **1995**, *34*, 255-261.

Shults, C. W., Quirion, R., Chronwall, B., Chase, T. N., O'Donohue, T. L.: *A comparison of the anatomical distribution of substance P and substance P receptors in the rat central nervous system* Peptides **1984**, *5*, 1097-1128.

Snider, R. M., Constantine, J. W., Lowe, J. A. III, Longo, K. P., Lebel, W. S., Woody, H. A., Drozda, S. E., Desai, M. C., Vinick, F. J., Spencer, R. W.: *A potent nonpeptide antagonist of the substance P (NK1) receptor*, Science **1991a**, *251*, 435-437.

Snider, R. M., Longo, K. P., Drozda, S. E., Lowe, J. A. III., Leeman, S. E.: *Effect of CP-96,345, a nonpeptide substance P receptor antagonist, on salivation in rats*, Proc. Natl. Acad. Sci. U.S.A. **1991b**, *88*, 10042-10044.

Soneoka, K., Shuto, H., Fujii, T. (Fujisawa Pharmaceutical Co., Ltd., Japan): *Use of peptides for the manufacture of a medicament for treatment of chronic obstructive pulmonary disease, mental disease, ond other diseases*, WO9420126.

Spitznagel, H., Baulmann, J., Blume, A., Unger, T., Culman, J.: *C-FOS expression in the rat brain in response to substance P and neurokinin B*, Brain Res. **2001**, *916*, 11-21.

Stiernet, F., Genicot, C., Soie, M.-A., Moureau, F., Ryckmans, T., Taverne, T., Henichart, J.-P., Neuwels, M., Goldstein, S.: *α-Arylethylpiperazine derivatives as neurokinin antagonists*, WO 0146167.

Suarez, G. A., Opfer-Gehrking, T. L., McLean, D. B., Low, P. A.: *Double-blind, placebo-controlled study of the efficacy of substance P (NK1) receptor antagonist in painful peripheral neuropathy*, Neurology **1994**, *44*, 373P.

Takeda, Y., Blount, P., Sachais, B. S., Hershey, A. D., Raddatz, R., Krause, J. E.: *Ligand binding kinetics of substance P and neurokinin A receptors stably expressed in Chinese hamster ovary cells and evidence for differential stimulation of inositol 1,4,5-trisphosphate and cyclic AMP second messenger responses*, J. Neurochem. **1992**, *59*, 740-745.

Take, K., Kasahara, C., Shigenaga, S., Azami, H., Eikyu, Y., Nakai, K., Morita, M. (Fujisawa Pharmaceutical Co.): *Benzhydryl derivatives*, WO 0200631.

Urban, L.A. and Fox, A.J.: *NK_1 receptor antagonists-are they really without effect in the pain clinic?* Trends Pharmacol. Sci. **2000**, *21*, 462-464.

Urban, L., Willets, J., Randic, M., Papka, R. E.: *The acute and chronic effects of capsaicin on slow excitatory transmission in rat dorsal horn,* Brain Res. **1985**, *330*, 390-396.

Von Euler, U. S. and Gaddum, J. H.: *An unidentified depressor substance in certain tissue extracts*, J. Physiol. (London) **1931**, *72*, 74-87.

Von Euler, U. S.: *The history of substance P*, Trends Neurosci. **1981**, *V4 (N10)*, 4.

Wahlestedt, C.: *Reward for persistence in substance P research*, Science **1998**, *281*, 1624-1625.

Walpole, C. S. J., Brown, M. C. S., James, I. F., Campbell, E. A., Mcintyre, P., Docherty, R., Ko, S., Hedley, L., Ewan, S., Buchheit, K.-H., Urban, L. A.: *Comparative, general pharmacology of SDZ NKT 343, a novel, selective NK1 receptor antagonist*, Br. J. Pharmacol. **1998a**, *124*, 83-92.

Walpole, C., Ko, S. Y., Brown, M., Beattie, D., Campbell, E., Dickenson, F., Ewan, S., Hughes, G. A., Lemaire, M., Lerpiniere, J., Patel, S., Urban, L.: *2-Nitrophenylcarbamoyl-(S)-prolyl-(S)-3-(2-naphthyl)alanyl-N-benzyl-N-methylamide (SDZ NKT 343), a potent human NK1 tachykinin receptor antagonist with good oral analgesic activity in chronic pain models*, J. Med. Chem. **1998b**, *41*, 3159-3173.

Ward, P., Ewan, G. B., Jordan, C. C., Ireland, S. J., Hagan, R. M., Brown, J. R.: *Potent and highly selective neurokinin antagonists*, J. Med. Chem. **1990**, *33*, 1848-1851.

Watling, K. J.: *Nonpeptide antagonists herald new era in tachykinin research*, Trends Pharmacol. Sci. **1992**, *13*, 266-269.

Watling, K. J. and Krause, J. E.: *The rising sun shines on substance P and related peptides*, Trends Pharmacol. Sci. **1993**, *14*, 81-84.

Weihe, E.: *Neuropeptides in primary afferent neurons*. In Primary afferent neurons, **1990**, edited by W. Zenker, and W. Neuhuber, 127-159, Plenum Press, New York.

Wiesenfeld-Hallin, Z. and Duranti, R.: *D-Arg¹, D-Try⁷,⁹, Leu¹¹-substance P (spantide) does not antagonise substance P-induced hyperexcitability of the nociceptive flexion withdrawal reflex in the rat*, Acta Physiol. Scand. **1987**, *129*, 55-59.

Wolff, H. G.: In Headache and other head pain **1963**, edited by H. G. Wolff, Oxford University Press, New York, MD.

Xu, X. J., Dalsgaard, C. J., Wiesenfeld-Hallin, Z.: *Intrathecal CP-96,345 blocks reflex facilitation induced in rats by substance P and C-fiber-conditioning stimulation*, Eur. J. Pharmacol. **1992**, *216*, 337-344.

Zubrzycka, M. and Janecka, A.: *Substance P: transmitter of nociception*, Endocrine Reg. **2000**, *34*, 195-201.

15   CGRP₁-Receptor Antagonists

Clemens Gillen

Introduction

Calcitonin gene-related peptide αCGRP is a 37-amino acid neuropeptide that was first identified in 1982 as an extremely potent vasodilator (Amara et al., 1982). It is generated by alternative splicing from the calcitonin gene and has a characteristic 7-amino acid ring formed by a disulfide bridge between position 2 and 7 and an amidated N-terminus. A second CGRP homolog, βCGRP, with high sequence homology was subsequently isolated and is derived from a different gene. Both peptides display rather similar biological effects that include vasodilatation, increased regional blood flow, hypotension and tachycardia.

The high expression in pain-relevant areas of the nervous system together with its dual role as potent vasodilator and excitatory neuromodulator suggested a role for CGRP in pain or migraine and led to intense research on this topic.

First identification of CGRP as an extremely potent vasodilator

CGRP Family of Peptides

The CGRP family of peptides includes the 37-amino acid neurotransmitter CGRP, the 52-amino acid adreno-medullin, found predominantly in vascular cells and adrenal tissue and the 37-amino acid amylin found in pancreatic islet β-cells. These peptides share a 6-amino acid ring structure, formed by an intramolecular disulfide bridge.

```
human_CGRPα          ACDTATCVTHRLAGLLSRSGGVVKNNFVPTN-VGSKAF-NH₂ 37
human_CGRPβ          ACNTATCVTHRLAGLLSRSGGMVKSNFVPTN-VGSKAF-NH₂ 37
rat_CGRPα            SCNTATCVTHRLAGLLSRSGGVVKDNFVPTN-VGSEAF-NH₂ 37
rat_CGRPβ            SCNTATCVTHRLAGLLSRSGGVVKDNFVPTN-VGSKAF-NH₂ 37
rat_amylin           KCNTATCATQRLANFLVHSSNNFGAILSSTN-VGSNTY-NH₂ 37
rat_adrenomedullin YRQSMNQGSRSTGCRFGTCTMQKLAHQIYQFTDKDKDGMAPRNKISPQGY-NH₂ 50
                     *  .**. ::**  : :   .        : . * :..: :
```

Figure 1: Comparison of the CGRP family peptides. The amino acids are annotated in the following way: small and hydrophobic in plain text, acidic in bold, basic in bold italics and hydroxyl or amine in italics. "*" Indicates identical or conserved residues in all peptides; ":" indicates conserved substitutions and "." indicates semi-conserved substitutions.

Receptor Pharmacology

CGRP₁ and CGRP₂ receptor
subtypes

The first pharmacological tools available for studying the CGRP receptor were derivatives of CGRP. The N-terminally truncated fragment CGRP(8-37) is antagonistic, whereas a linear peptide like ([Acetamidomethyl-cysteine^{2,7}]CGRP (Cys(ACM^{2,7})CGRP)) behaves as an agonist. The analysis of these CGRP peptide analogs *in vitro* and *in vivo* allowed the subdivision into a CGRP₁ and a CGRP₂ receptor subtype, a nomenclature initially proposed by Dennies et al. (1989). The CGRP₁ receptor subtype is antagonized by CGRP(8-37) (pA₂ = 7.7) and Cys(ACM^{2,7})CGRP is weak or inactive as an agonist. As a functional example for the CGRP₁ receptor the guinea pig atrium is used.

Evidence for further CGRP
receptor subtypes

The CRGP₂ receptor subtype is selectively activated by Cys(ACM^{2,7})CGRP, but only weakly antagonized by CGRP(8-37) (pA₂ = 6.5). A prototypical *in vitro* bioassay to study the CGRP₂ receptor is the rat vas deferens. The above-mentioned nomenclature is under discussion, because it is based on poorly selective and weak agonists and antagonists but the CGRP₁/CGRP₂ subdivision is still generally used. Evidence for further CGRP receptor subtypes comes from studies demonstrating CGRP(8-37)-insensitive βCGRP-activated receptors. More recently, the use of the non-peptide antagonist BIBN-4096BS suggests a further subtype expressed in rat vas deferens. Although CGRP was one of first neuropeptides to be identified, the molecular basis of the two CGRP receptors is still under debate.

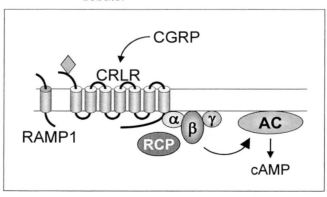

Figure 2: Model of the CGRP₁ receptor complex. The CGRP₁ receptor is a heteromer of CRLR and RAMP1 that couples predominantly via G$_S$ proteins to adenylate cyclase (AC). The receptor component protein (RCP) is essential for G protein activation.

Molecular characterization
of CGRP₁

The reason for these difficulties became apparent after successful molecular characterization of the CGRP₁ receptor. The $CGRP_1$ receptor has a unique phenotype since it is a receptor complex built up by a classical heptahelical G protein-coupled receptor, the so called calcitonin receptor-like receptor (CRLR) and the receptor-associated modifying protein 1 (RAMP-1). In addition another protein, the receptor component protein (RCP) binds intracellularly to the CRLR/RAMP-1 complex and is essential for the efficient activation of G_S proteins (Juaneda et al., 2000; see Fig. 2). The molecular basis of the $CGRP_2$ receptor and the additional subtypes is currently unknown.

Signaling

Activation of the CGRP receptor is linked to several intracellular pathways. The CRLR/RAMP1 heteromer can couple to pertussis toxin- (PTX-) insensitive G proteins, leading to production of cAMP (Main et al., 1998). The same authors also found coupling through PTX-sensitive G proteins, suggesting that the recombinant $CGRP_1$ receptor may signal through G_i and G_o proteins. Using primary cultures of rat neonatal spinal cord an increase in cGMP could be observed, suggesting that the CGRP receptor also couples to the guanylcyclase (Parsons and Seybold, 1997) although this effect only became apparent at high CGRP concentrations. In non-neuronal cells a coupling of the native CGRP receptor to the MAP kinase signaling pathway (Kawase et al., 1999) and to phospholipase C leading to increased intracellular Ca^{2+} concentrations was found (Drissi et al., 1998). In conclusion, the most important signaling mechanism is undoubtedly the G_s protein-mediated increase in cAMP concentrations.

Evidence for a Role of CGRP in Migraine

The pathophysiology of migraine is still under debate. The predominant current opinion is that migraine is a neurovascular disorder with the primary trigger potentially occurring in the CNS. This trigger ultimately leads to vasodilatation with a subsequent activation of trigeminal afferent sensory neurons activating central `nociceptive´ neurons projecting to higher pain centers (see Fig. 3; for review see: Hargreaves and Shepheard, 1999).

Several lines of investigation have provided evidence to support the theory that CGRP plays a role in migraine. CGRP is the most abundant primary afferent peptide in trigeminal sensory nerves. Since CGRP is one of the most potent vasodilators known and the $CGRP_1$ receptor is

Animal studies supporting a role for CGRP in migraine

expressed on the endothelial cells of the meningeal arteries CGRP is presumed to be a key mediator of meningeal vasodilatation. In addition to these physiological considerations several animal studies support the proposal that $CGRP_1$ receptors play a role in migraine. Stimulation of the trigeminal ganglion in anesthetized rats leads to meningeal vasodilatation, which could be inhibited by the CGRP1 antagonist CGRP(8-37) (Kurosawa et al., 1995). This experiment implied that CGRP were elevated after trigeminal stimulation, an observation that had been reported by Goadsby and Edvinsson (1993). Interestingly, these elevated CGRP levels could be reduced by treatment with migraine drugs like sumatriptan or dihydroergotamine (Goadsby and Edvinsson, 1993).

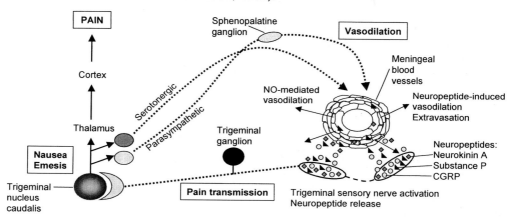

Figure 3: Integrated hypothesis of pathogenesis of migraine headache and associated symptoms, and role of trigeminovascular system (adapted from P.J. Goadsby and R.J. Hargreaves). Intense neurometabolic cortical activity such as cortical spreading depression (CSD) is a trigger for migraine. The release of potassium ions and protons, neurotransmitters and metabolites into the extracellular space causes transient hyperemia and vasodilation in cortex, pia vessels and dura mater. This sensitizes and ultimately activates perivascular trigeminal afferents which transmit impulses to the trigeminal ganglia and the trigeminal nucleus caudalis (TNC). Impulses from the TNC are carried rostrally to brain structures involved in pain processing and perception. Depolarization of the trigeminal afferents leads to the retrograde perivascular release of vasoactive neuropeptides such as neurokinin A, substance P and CGRP. Activation of the ipsilateral TNC leads to stimulation of the superior salivatory nucleus (SSN) and parasympathetic efferents via the spenopalatine ganglion. Postganglionic parasympathetics promote vasodilation and augment flow releasing vasoactive intestinal peptide, nitric oxide and acetylcholine into the dura mater.

Another study described the CGRP-induced histamine release from dural mast cells that could be blocked by CGRP(8-37) (Ottoson and Edvinsson, 1997). Therefore

CGRP together with substance P may also play a role in migraine-associated neurogenic inflammation.

The analysis of CGRP plasma levels in human volonteers was found to be a important diagnostic parameter, since elevated plasma levels were found in patients with acute migraine and in patients with cluster headache (Edvinsson and Goadsby, 1994) as well as in humans after trigeminovascular stimulation. In accordance with the above-mentioned animal studies the elevated CGRP levels in migraineurs were reported to be reduced by sumatriptan or dihydroergotamine (Goadsby and Edvinsson, 1993). A mechanistic explanation was given by Durham and Rosso (1999) who found that sumatriptan can directly repress CGRP secretion from cultured trigeminal neurons. Here the activation of $5HT_1$ receptors inhibits the release via an increase in phosphorylase activity that is likely mediated by a sustained elevated level of intracellular calcium. In conclusion, there is strong evidence that a $CGRP_1$ antagonist should provide effective treatment for migraine and cluster headache.

Elevated CGRP levels in patients with migraine or cluster headache

In Vivo Evidence for a Role in Pain

CGRP is highly abundant in somatic sensory nerves. Here CGRP often coexists with other neuropeptides such as substance P. Immunocytochemical studies have shown that substance P is nearly always associated with CGRP in small type DRG neurons, whereas CGRP can be localized without substance P (Wiesenfeld-Hallin et al., 1984). In the periphery the CGRP released by sensory neurons leads to vasodilatation and together with neuropeptides like substance P mediates neurogenic inflammation. CGRP is also released in the dorsal horn following peripheral noxious stimulation. Like SP, it also produces slow depolarization of spinal dorsal horn neurons and can potentiate the depolarizing effect of SP. Three different strategies were used to clarify the role of the CGRP receptors in pain. The $CGRP_1$ antagonist CGRP(8-37) was tested in pain models. In order to antagonize endogenous CGRP an anti-CGRP antiserum was given intrathecally in several pain models. The generation and behavioral analysis of αCGRP-deficient mice completes the picture.

The antinociceptive effect of CGRP(8-37) was observed in different pain types of such as abdominal pain (p-phenylquinone induced writhing, Saxen et al., 1994; acetic acid-induced writhing, Friese et al., 1997), visceral pain (colorectal distension model, Plourde et al., 1997), burn pain (heat-induced hyperalgesia; Lofgren et al., 1997), and

Antinociceptive effect of the CGRP antagonist CGRP(8-37) in several pain models central neuropathic pain (spinal hemisection; Bennett et al., 2000). No effect was observed in mouse tail-flick as a model of acute pain (Saxen et al., 1994).

In order to block the effects of spinally released CGRP, an antiserum against CGRP was tested in several models of chronic pain and was found to be antinociceptive in models of chronic inflammatory pain such as adjuvant-arthritis (Kuraishi et al., 1988) or carrageenan-induced hyperalgesia (Kawamura et al., 1989). In addition this antiserum inhibited the repeated cold stress-induced hyperalgesia in rats (Satoh et al., 1992).

CGRP$^{-/-}$ mice show reduced hyperalgesia

The antinociceptive effects seen with CGRP(8-37) or anti-CGRP antiserum are in line with the hyperalgesia found in αCGRP-deficient mice produced by Salmon et al. (1999). The CGRP$^{-/-}$ mice showed in comparison with CGRP$^{+/+}$ mice a reduced hyperalgesia during chronic inflammatory pain, elicited by injection of formalin or capsaicin into the hindpaw (Salmon et al., 2001). The authors also described reduction in abdominal pain, since the intraperitoneal injection of acetic acid yielded fewer writhing reactions. The injection of carrageenan into the hind paw of CGRP$^{-/-}$ mice showed reduced edema formation and indicates a role for CGRP in neurogenic inflammation.

A second αCGRP-deficient mouse was produced by Hoff et al. (1998) in order to study the role of calcitonin. CGRP$^{-/-}$ mice are born normally, are fertile and live a normal life span. These mice were tested in a model of chronic arthritis, where a mixture of kaolin/carrageenan was injected into the knee joint and in comparison to wild type mice failed to develop secondary hyperalgesia (Zhang et al., 2001).

Assuming that we can apply these results to the human situation, CGRP$_1$ antagonists may also be effective for treatment of chronic inflammatory and visceral pain but not for acute pain. A thorough evaluation of this receptor in neuropathic pain is still missing.

Nonpeptidic Antagonists and their Current Status

In 1997 scientists from SmithKline Beecham published a series of quinine analogs as CGRP antagonists (Daines et al.1997, WO9709046). These compounds displayed only weak affinities for the human CGRP receptor in the micromolar range and were therefore not of great importance (Daines et al., 1997).

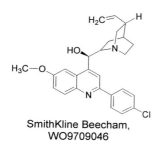

SmithKline Beecham, WO9709046

A major breakthrough in the field was the development of the first highly potent non-peptide CGRP receptor antagonist BIBN-4096BS (Eberlein et al. (Boehringer

Ingelheim) DE19911039, 2000; for a review see: Doods et al., 2001). This compound, a Tyr-Lys dipeptide derivative, is a pure antagonist with high affinity towards the human CGRP₁ receptor (K_i = 14.4 pM).

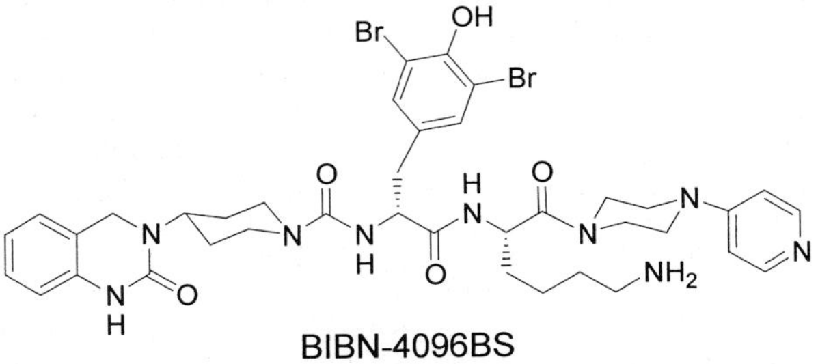

BIBN-4096BS

In studies using human cerebral vessels BIBN-4096BS was able to reverse CGRP-mediated vasodilatation (Doods et al., 2000). Stimulation of the marmoset trigeminal ganglion leads to an increase in facial blood flow. In this model of neurogenic inflammation, BIBN-4096BS showed a rapid and dose-dependent inhibition of the increased blood flow (Doods et al., 2000). Furthermore, in anesthetized marmosets BIBN-4096BS inhibited CGRP-mediated neurogenic vasodilatation in doses from 0.001 to 0.03 mg/kg, whereas concentrations up to 1 mg/kg BIBN-4096BS did not affect cardiovascular parameters (Doods et al., 2000). This may be explained by low basal CGRP levels. Although high doses of CGRP are cardioprotective, the CGRP₁ antagonist BIBN-4096BS had no negative effect on myocardial infarct size or release of creatine phosphate kinase. In conclusion BIBN-4096BS may provide a therapeutic migraine intervention without cardiovascular side-effects (Wu et al., 2001). In a recent publication it was shown that the CGRP-induced relaxation of human coronary arteries was blocked by BIBN-4096BS with a pA2 value of 10.4 compared to an pA2 value of 10.2 in human cerebral arteries. In contrast to the results in marmosets described above, this study assumes cardiovascular side-effects for this compound (Edvinsson et al., 2002). BIBN-496BS is currently in phase II clinical studies for the treatment of migraine.

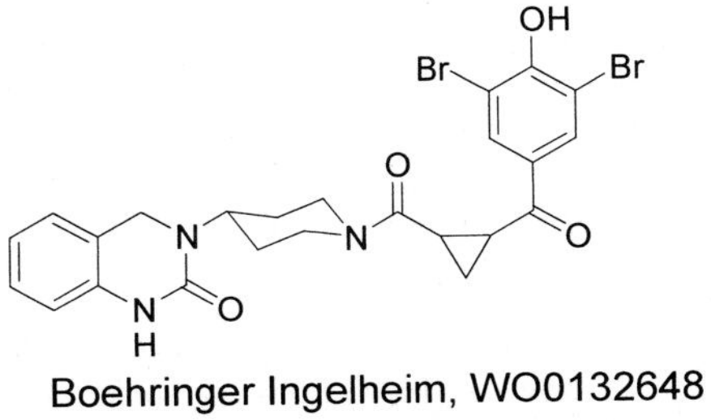

Boehringer Ingelheim, WO0132648 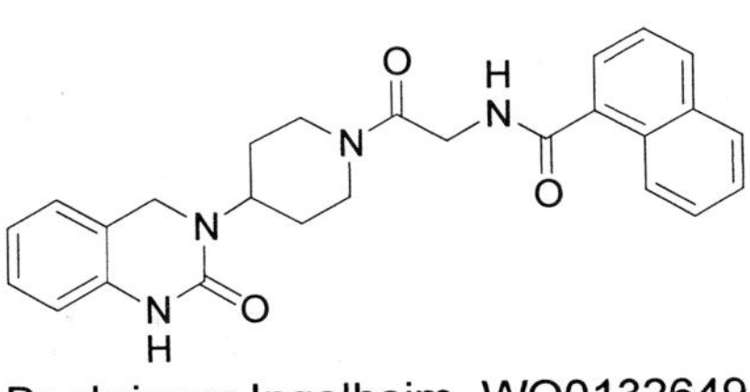   Boehringer Ingelheim, WO0132649

Based on this structure Boehringer Ingelheim synthesised and filed patents on compounds where the dipeptide core of BIBN-496BS is replaced by a cyclopropyl ring (Eberlein et al., WO0132648). In a recent patent application Boehringer Ingelheim also claimed naphtalenes, piperidines, imidazoles, and quinazolines as CGRP receptor antagonists without disclosing any functional properties of the molecules (Rudolf et al., WO0132649). In addition piperidine-substituted amino acids have been filed by Boehringer Ingelheim (Rudolf et al., WO0149676).

Interestingly Boehringer Ingelheim has also filed a patent application on a structure that is derived directly from BIBN-4096BS and can be described as a De-Lys-BIBN-4096BS-derivative (Rudolf et al., WO9811128). This so called 'compound 1' (WO9811128) was resynthesized by scientists from Merck, Sharp and Dohme and presented as a functional CGRP receptor blocker in human SK-N-MC cells with a pK_i value of 7.8 and in human cerebral arteries with a pK_i value of 7.7 (Edvinsson et al., 2001). In porcine coronary arteries 'compound1' demonstrated no antagonistic effect (Hasback et al., 2001) that may be explained by a species-specific binding profile.

SmithKline Beecham is another company with interests in CGRP receptor antagonists and has filed patent applications for two structural classes, the 3,4-dinitrobenzamides (Daines et al., WO9809630) and 4-sulfinyl benzanilides (Daines et al., WO9856779).

Boehringer Ingelheim, WO9811128

CGRP antagonists from SmithKline Beecham:
a) SB-(+)-273779, b) WO9809630, c) WO9856779.

One of these 4-sulfinyl benzanilides, SB-(+)-273779 inhibited ^{125}I-labeled CGRP binding to SK-N-MC cells and human cloned $CGRP_1$ receptor with K_i values of 310 nM and 250 nM, respectively (Aiyar et al., 2001). Detailed binding analysis suggests that this compound has irreversible binding characteristics. The authors demonstrated that SB-(+)-273779 inhibits several CGRP-mediated effects such as vasodilation of the pulmonary artery, [14C]deoxyglucose uptake in L6 cells or decrease in blood pressure in anesthetized rats (Aiyar et al., 2001). Unfortunately SB-(+)-273779 exhibits several limitations including poor solubility, poor oral availability and a short half life of ~10 min that precluded an extensive *in vivo* characterization (Aiyar et al., 2001).

The activities of Merck, Sharp and Dohme have also led to a patent application disclosing benzamidoyl-piperidine derivatives to be CGRP antagonists (Hill et al., WO0018764). The compounds are claimed to inhibit [^{125}I]CGRP binding to SK-N-MC cell membranes with K_i values below 10 µM.

It is interesting to note that although several major pharmaceutical companies have tried to develop CGRP antagonists, only few compounds have been published. Together with the fact that most of them are bulky structures - like BIBN-4096BS or 'compound 1' (WO9811128) - this may indicate a general structural hindrance in the development of small molecule CGRP antagonists. At the moment BIBN-4096BS remains to be the only compound that is suitable for studying the role of CGRP in clinical trials.

Merck, Sharp and Dohme, WO0018764

Perspectives

There are several lines of evidence that propose a key role for CGRP in the pathophysiology of migraine. In current practice, the first line treatment for migraine are NSAIDS but the triptans as mixed 5HT1b/D agonists are the gold standard. Several triptans are on the market now that differ mainly in onset of action and oral availability. However there is a high percentage of non-responders (up to 30%) and a high recurrency rate (25-35%) with all these compounds. For this reason new and effective drugs are needed. After the failure of several new approaches such as NK1 antagonists, endothelin antagonists and inhibitors of protein plasma extravasation, potential migraine treatment is based on targets like CGRP or NO (for review see: Doods et al., 2001). Therefore the results of the clinical trials with BIBN-4096BS for acute migraine attacks are awaited with great interest. The evidence for the role of CGRP antagonists in chronic pain is quite convincing, since an antinociceptive/hypoalgesic effect has been shown with the peptidic antagonist CGP(8-37), an anti-CGRP antiserum and αCGRP-deficient mice. However, a thorough evaluation of the non-peptidic tools in different animal models of pain is essential but hampered by the fact that a central acting analgesic is needed here. On the molecular level the nature of the different CGRP receptor subtypes has to be elucidated. For this purpose the non-peptidic antagonists are also useful. Current clinical studies using BIBN-4096BS will show if CGRP antagonists provide effective treatment for migriane with fewer side effects. If these studies have a positive outcome, this class of drugs may be of use in further indications like chronic pain or inflammation.

References

Amara, G.S., Jonas, V., Rosenfeld, M.G., Ong, E.S., Evans, R.M.: *Alternative RNA processing in calcitonin gene expression generates mRNAs encoding different polypeptide products*, Nature **1982**, *298*, 240-244.

Aiyar, N., Daines, D.R., Disa, J., Chambers, P.A., Sauermelch, C.F., Quiniou, M., Khandoudi, N., Gout, B., Douglas, S.A., Wilette, R.N.: *Pharmacology of SB-273779, a nonpeptide calcitonin gene-related peptide 1 receptor antagonist*, J. Pharmacol. Exp. Ther. **2001**, *296*, 768-775.

Bennett, A.D., Chastain, K.M., Hulsebosch, C.E.: *Alleviation of mechanical and thermal allodynia by CGRP(8-37) in a rodent model of chronic central pain*, Pain **2000**, *86*, 163-175.

Boyer, J.-C., Christen, M.-O., Balmes, J.-L., Bali, J.-P., Bianchi, B.: *Calcitonin gene-related peptide-induced relaxation of isolated human colonic smooth muscle cells through different intracellular pathways*, Biochem. Pharmacol. **1998**, *56*, 1097-1104.

Daines, R.A., Sham, K.K.C., Taggert, J.J., Kingsbury, W.D., Chan, J., Breen, A., Disa, J., Aiyar, N.: *Quinine analogs as non-peptide calcitonin gene-related peptide (CGRP) receptor antagonists*, Bioorg. Med. Chem. Lett. **1997**, *7*, 2673-2676.

Daines, R.A. (SmithKline Beecham Corporation, USA*)*: *Preparation of 3,4-dinitrobenzamides as calcitonin gene-related peptide receptor ligands*, WO9809630 (**1998**).

Daines, R.A. (SmithKline Beecham Corporation, USA): *Preparation of quinine and quinidine compounds as antagonists of the Calcitonin gene-related Peptide (CGRP) receptor*, WO9709046 (**1997**).

Daines, R.A, Chambers, P.A. (SmithKline Beecham Corporation, USA): *Preparation of 4-sulfinyl benzamides as calcitonin gene-related peptide antagonists*, WO9856779 (**1998**).

Dennies, T.B., Fournier, A., St. Pierre, S., Quirion, R: *Structure activity profile of calcitonin gene-related peptide in peripheral and brain tissues. Evidence for receptor multiplicity*, J. Pharmacol. Exp. Ther. **1989**, *251*, 718-725.

Doods, H., Hallermayer, G., Wu, D., Entzeroth, M., Rudolf, K., Engel, W., Eberlein, W.: *Pharmacological profile of BIBN-4096BS, the first selective small molecule CGRP antagonist*, Br. J. Pharmacol. **2000**, *129*, 420-423.

Doods, H.: *Development of CGRP antagonists for the treatment of migraine*, Curr. Opin. Invest. Drugs **2001**, *2*, 1261-1268.

Drissi, H., Lasmoles, F., Le Mellay, V., Marie, P.J., Lieberherr, M.: *Activation of phospholipase C-beta1 via Galphaq/11 during calcium mobilization by calcitonin gene-related peptide*, J. Biol. Chem. **1998**, *273*, 20168-20174.

Durham, P.L., and Russo, A.F.: *Regulation of calcitonin gene-related peptide secretion by a serotonergic antimigraine drug*, J. Neurosci. **1999**, *19*, 3423-3429.

Eberlein, W., Engel, W., Rudolf, K., Doods, H., Hallermeyer, G., Bauer, E. (Boehringer Ingelheim): *Preparation of 3-(1-cyclopropylcarbonyl-4-piperidinyl)-3,4-dihydro-2(1H)-quinazolines as calcitonin gene-related peptide antagonists*, WO0132648 (**2001**).

Eberlein, W., Rudolf, K., Dreyer, A., Müller, S.G., Doods, H., Bauer, E. (Boehringer Ingelheim): *Preparation of amino-acid derivatives for use as calcitonin gene-related peptide antagonists*, DE19911039 (**2000**).

Edvinsson, L. and Goadsby, P.: *Neuropeptides in migraine and cluster headache*, Cephalalgia **1994**, *14*, 320-327.

Edvinsson, L., Sams, A., Jansen-Olesen, I., Tajti, J., Kane, S.A., Rutledge, R.Z., Koblan, K.S., Hill, R.G., Longmore, J.: *Characterization of the effects of a non-peptide CGRP receptor antagonist in SK-N-MC cells and isolated human cerebral arteries*, Eur. J. Pharmacol. **2001a**, *415*, 39-44.

Edvinsson, L., Alm, R., Shaw, D., Rutledge, R.Z., Koblan, K.S., Longmore, J., Kane, S.A.: *Effect of the CGRP receptor antagonist BIBN4096BS in human cerebral, coronary and omental arteries and in SK-N-MC cells*, Eur. J. Pharmacol. **2001b**, *415*, 39-44.

Friese, N., Diop, L., Chevalier, E., Angel, F., Riviere, P.J.M., Dahl, S.G.: *Involvement of prostaglandins and CGRP-dependent sensory afferents in peritoneal irritation-induced visceral pain*, Reg. peptides **1997**, *70*, 1-7.

Goadsby, P.J. and Edvinsson, L.: *The trigeminovascular system and migraine: Studies characterizing cerebrovascular and neuropeptide change seen in human and cats*, Ann. Neurol. **1993**, *33*, 48-56.

Hargreaves, R.J. and Shepheard, S.L.: *Pathophysiology of migraine. New insights*, Can. J. Neurol. Sci. **1999**, *26*, 512-519.

Hasback, P., Sams, A., Schifter, S., Longmore, J., Edvinsson, L.: *CGRP receptor mediating CGRP-, adrenomedullin- and amylin-induced relaxation in porcine coronary arteries. Characterization with ´Compound1´ (WO9811128), a non-peptide antagonist*, Br. J. Pharmacol. **2001**, *133*, 1405-1413.

Hill, R.G., Patchett, A.A., Yang, L. (Merck Sharp and Dohme Limited, USA): *Preparation of N-4-(oxobenzimidazolyl)piperidinocarbonyl]arylglycinamides as CGRP antagonists*, WO0018764 (**2000**).

Juaneda, C., Dumont, Y., Quirion, R.: *The molecular pharmacology of CGRP and related peptide receptor subtypes*, Trends Pharmacol. Sci. **2000**, *21*, 432-438.

Kawamura, M., Kuraishi, Y., Minami, M., Satoh, M.: *Antinociceptive effect of intrathecally administered antiserum against calcitonin gene-related peptide on thermal and mechanical noxious stimuli in experimental hyperalgesic rats*, Brain Res. **1989**, *497*, 199-203.

Kawase, T., Okuda, K., Wu, C.H., Yoshie, H., Hara, K., Burns, D.M.: *Calcitonin gene-related peptide acts as a mitogen for human Gin-1 gingival fibroblasts by activating the MAP kinase signalling pathway*, J. Periodontal Res. **1999**, *34*, 160-168.

Kuraishi, Y., Nanayama, T., Ohno, H., Minami M., Satoh M.: *Antinociception induced in rats by intrathecal administration of antiserum against calcitonin gene-related peptide*, Neurosci. Lett. **1988**, *92*, 325-329.

Kurosawa, M., Messlinger, K., Pawlak, M., Schmidt, R.F.: *Increase of meningeal blood flow after electrical stimulation of rat dura mater encephali: mediation by calcitonin gene-related peptide*, Br. J. Pharmacol. **1995**, *114*, 1397-1402.

Lofgren, O., Yu, L.C., Theodorsson, E., Hansson, P., Lundeberg T.: *Intrathecal CGRP(8-37) results in a bialteral increase in hindpaw withdrawal latency in rats with a unilateral thermal injury*, Neuropeptides **1997**, *31*, 601-607.

Main, M., Brown, J., Brown, S., Fraser, N.J., Foord, S.M.: *The CGRP receptor can couple via pertussis toxin sensitive and insensitive G proteins*, FEBS Letters **1998**, *441*, 6-10.

Ottoson, A. and Edvinsson, L.: *Release of histamine from dural mast cells by substance P and calcitonin gene-related peptide*, Cephalalgia **1997**, *17*, 166-74.

Parsons, A.M. and Seybold, V.S.: *Calcitonin gene-related peptide induces the formation of second messengers in primary cultures of neonatal rat spinal cord*, Synapse **1997**, *26*, 235-242.

Plourde, V., St-Pierre, S., Quirion, R.: *Calcitonin gene-related peptide in viscerosensitive response to colorectal distension in rats*, Am. J. Physiol. **1997**, *36*, G191-G196.

Rudolf, K., Eberlein, W., Dreyer, A., Müller, S.G., Doods, H., Bauer, E. (Boehringer Ingelheim*)*: *Preparation of piperidine-substituted amino-acids for use in treatment of CGRP-mediated disorders*, WO1049676 (**2001**).

Rudolf, K., Eberlein, W., Engel, W., Doods, H., Hallermeyer, G., Bauer, E. (Boehringer Ingelheim): *Preparation of naphtalenes, piperidines, imidazoles, and quinazolines as calcitonin gene-related peptide antagonists*, WO0132649 (**2001**).

Rudolf, K., Eberlein, W., Engel, W., Pieper, H., Doods, H., Hallermeyer, G., Entzeroth, M., Wienen, W. (Karl Thomae GmbH, Germany): *Preparation of modified amino acids and their use as calcitonin gene-related peptide antagonists in pharmaceutical compositions*, WO9811128 (**1998**).

Salmon, A.-M., Damaj, M.I., Sekine, S., Picciotto, M.R., Marubio, L., Changeux, J.-P.: *Modulation of morphine analgesia in αCGRP mutant mice*, Neuroreport **1999**, *10*, 849-854.

Salmon, A.-M., Damaj, M.I., Marubio, L.M., Epping-Jordan, M.P., Merlo-Pich, E., Changeux, J.-P.: *Altered neuroadaption in opiate dependence and neurogenic inflammatory nociception in αCGRP deficient mice*, Nature **2001**, *56*, 357-358.

Satoh, M., Kuraishi, Y., Kawamura, M.: *Effects of intrathecal antibodies to substance P, calcitonin gene-related peptide and galanin on repeated cold stress-induced hyperalgesia: comparison with carrageenan-induced hyperalgesia*, Pain **1992**, *49*, 273-278.

Saxen, M.A., Smith, F.L., Dunlow, L.D., Dombrowski, D.S., Welch, S.P.: *The hypothermic and antinociceptive effects of intrathecal injection of CGRP(8-37) in mice*, Life Sci. **1994**, *55*, 1665-1674.

Wiesenfeld-Hallin, Z., Hökfelt, T., Lundberg, J.M., Forssmann, W.G., Reinecke, M., Tschopp, F.A., Fischer, J.A.: *Immunoreactive calcitonin gene-related peptide and substance P coexist in sensory neurons to the spinal cord and interact in spinal behavioural responses to the rat*, Neurosci. Lett. **1984**, *52*, 199-203.

Wu, D., Van Zwieten, P.A., Doods, H.N.: *Effects of calcitonin gene-related peptide (CGRP) and BIBN-4096BS on myocardial ischemia in anesthetized rats*, Acta Pharm. Sin. **2001** in press.

Zhang, L., Hoff, A.O., Wimalawansa, S.J., Cote, G.J., Gagel., R.F., Westlund, K.F.: *Arthritic calcitonin/α calcitonin gene-related peptide knockout mice have reduced nociceptive hypersensitivity*, Pain **2001**, *89*, 265-273.

16   Nitric oxide :
Potential of NO Donors and NO Synthase Inhibitors for the Treatment of Pain

Corinna Maul, Hagen-Heinrich Hennies and Bernd Sundermann

In recent years, nitric oxide (NO) has emerged as one of the most interesting mediators of normal and patho physiological processes. NO is a highly reactive free radical, a lipophilic gas with a very short half-life in the range of 5 - 30 s under bioassay conditions (Palmer et al., 1987). NO is rapidly converted to nitrogen dioxide (NO_2), which again rapidly forms the more stable metabolites nitrite (NO_2^-) and nitrate (NO_3^-).

Direct vascular effects of NO

As Furchgott, Ignarro and Murad have shown, NO is essential for keeping blood vessels wide open to maintain blood flow and pressure. In atherosclerosis, in which plaques occlude the coronary arteries, the cells lining the blood vessels produce less NO. The work that led to the Nobel prize in 1998 explains why patients with chest pain (angina pectoris) caused by atherosclerosis get relief from pills containing nitroglycerine, which, once it has entered the smooth muscle cells, releases NO (Ignarro, 1999; Furchgott, 1999; Murad, 1999).

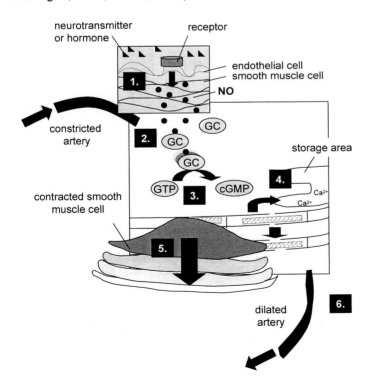

Figure 1: Mechanism of action of NO.
1. Neurotransmitter or hormone bind to receptors on endothelial cells lining the artery, which in response releases nitric oxide (NO). 2. NO molecules from the endothelium travel into smooth muscle cells, where they activate the enzyme, guanylyl cyclase (GC). 3. GC converts guanosine triphosphate (GTP) to cyclic guanosine monophosphate (cGMP). 4. cGMP causes calcium ions to enter storage areas of the cell. The lowered concentrations of calcium ions (Ca^{++}) set off a cascade of cellular reactions that cause the cell's contractile filaments (myosin and actin) to slide apart. 5. Smooth muscle cells relax. 6. Blood vessel dilates.

Arginine: source of
endogenous NO

In mammalian cells NO is produced by the oxidation of the terminal guanidino nitrogen of L-arginine (L-arg) by nitric oxide synthase (NOS). According to patent literature, NOS inhibitors have been one of the most intensively investigated research areas in industry of the last couple of years.

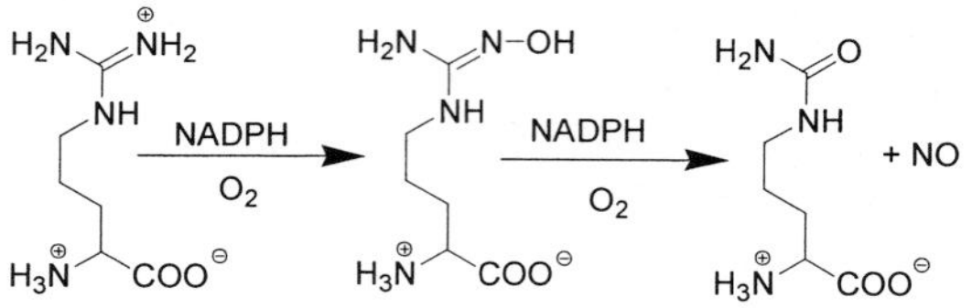

Scheme 1: NO formation from L-arg catalyzed by NOS.

Identification of three
isoforms: nNOS, eNOS,
iNOS

nNOS and the NMDA
receptor are closely
coupled: in nNOS-deficient
mice, effects induced by
PCP, an NMDA receptor
antagonist, were not
obtained (Bird et al. 2001)

Three distinct isoforms of NOS have been identified (Knowles and Moncada, 1994). Molecular cloning has shown these to share 50 - 60% homology. There is a constitutive form (neuronal NOS, nNOS), whose activity is regulated by Ca^{2+} and calmodulin, and which is found in neuronal tissue, both centrally and peripherally. nNOS is believed to play a role in the production of NO as a neurotransmitter. NO production in the brain is initiated by glutamate binding to the NMDA receptor, which is closely coupled to nNOS. A second, Ca^{2+}/calmodulin-requiring, constitutive enzyme (endothelial cell NOS, eNOS) is present in vascular endothelium where it regulates blood pressure and vascular tone. A third, Ca^{2+}-independent isoform (inducable NOS, iNOS) is induced in activated macrophages and other cell types by numerous inflammatory stimuli including lipopolysaccharide (LPS) and cytokines (e.g. IL-1) (Hobbs et al., 1999). Once induced, iNOS manufactures large amounts of NO over many hours and can have either a beneficial effect (e.g. host defense response) or a harmful effective induction is uncontrolled. iNOS has been implicated in the pathology of a large number of inflammatory conditions.

Localization of constitutive
NOS isoforms

The constitutive isoforms of NOS are mainly, but not only, localized in the tissues where they were originally identified. In some brain regions, eNOS and nNOS occur in the same cell populations (Dinerman et al., 1994). In mice it was shown that hippocampal neurons express eNOS, and nNOS was found in human bronchi as well as in human skeletal muscle (Hobbs et al., 1999). In coronary arteries of eNOS knock-out mice, nNOS-derived NO, via activation of cGMP, takes over the role of eNOS and maintains blood flow-induced vessel dilation (Huang et al., 2002).

All NOS proteins possess a bi-domain structure, and dimerization to homodimers (≥ 260 kDa each), is required for enzyme activity (see Table1).

Activation of NOS through dimerization

Table 1: Characteristics of human NOS isoforms.
(Adapted from Wattanapitayakul, Young et al., 2000).

Isoform	MW (kDA)	Chromosome localization (Gene structure)	Gene size (kb)	Expressional regulation	Calcium dependence
NOS1 (nNOS)	160	12q24.2 (29 exons, 28 introns)	> 200	constitutive but highly regulated	yes
NOS2 (iNOS)	130	17q11.2-q12 (26 exons, 25 introns)	37	inducible by cytokines	no
NOS3 (ecNOS)	135	7q35-q36 (26 exons, 25 introns)	21	constitutive but highly regulated	yes

Known Features of NOS Protein Structure

The C-terminal portion of the NOS protein closely resembles to cytochrome P-450 reductase, possesses many of the same cofactor binding sites, and basically performs the same functions. Consequently, this portion is often referred to as the reductase domain. At the extreme C-terminus is an NADPH binding region, which is conserved in all NOS and aligns perfectly with that of cytochrome P-450 reductase. The NADPH binding site is followed, in turn, by flavin adenine dinucleotide (FAD) and flavin mononucleotide (FMN) consensus sequences.

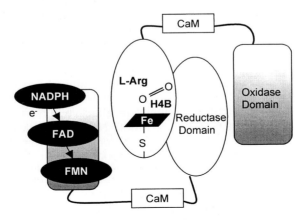

Figure 2: Hypothetical structure of NOS.

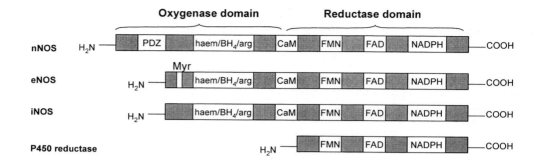

Figure 3: Schematic representation of nitric oxide synthase isoforms and cytochrome P450 reductase. Haem, heme; PDZ, PDZ domain (GLGF repeats); CaM, calmodulin; FMN, flavin mononucleotide; FAD, flavin adenine dinucleotide (adapted from Hobbs et al., 1999).

Unlike cytochrome P-450 reductase, NOS is a self-sufficient enzyme in that the oxygenation of its substrate, L-arginine, occurs at the heme-site in the N-terminal portion, termed the oxygenase domain, of the protein. Stoichiometric amounts of heme are present in NOS and are required for catalytic activity.

Nitroglycerine – an NO Donor Causing Severe Headache

The analgesic activity of NO synthase inhibitors has not been known for a long time, although a connection was suggested. The discoverer of nitroglycerine, Ascanio Sobrero, had noted that exposure to this chemical can cause severe headaches. Alfred Nobel, who spent much of his time experimenting with this substance, must have had experienced this effect and later on, when nitroglycerine was produced on an industrial scale, it is reasonable to assume that it posed a serious medical and environmental problem, especially for his collaborators (Ringertz, 2000). On the other hand, Lauder Brunton, a distinguished British physician, had found in 1867 that organic nitrates were effective in relieving angina pectoris pain. When in 1890 Nobel´s physicians recommended nitroglycerine as a remedy for his heart disease he declined it because he knew about the headaches caused by this compound.

NOS Inhibitors as Potential Analgesics

The analgesic effect of 2-amino-4-methylpyridine was reported in 1958 (Fastier and McDowall). In 1980 the compound was described as a "morphine-like analgesic" (Bergman and Elam). A recent study published by Pfizer suggests that 2-amino-4-methylpyrdine acts by inhibiting neuronal NO synthesis (Pettipher et al. 1997).

The analgesic effect of NOS inhibitors refers to the inhibition of nNOS and, in the case of inflammation, iNOS. Knock-out experiments support this thesis: mice lacking iNOS have a delay in the expression of neuropathic pain following a chronic constriction injury of nerves associated with neuropathic pain (Levy et al., 2001). For physiological changes observed in nNOS-, iNOS- and eNOS-knock-out mice, see Table 2.

2-Amino-4-methyl-pyridine, NOS inhibitor with analgesic activity [695-34-1]

Table 2: Physiological changes observed in nNOS-, iNOS- and eNOS-knock-out mice (adapted from Wattanapitayakul, Young and Bauer 2000).

Knock-out-mice	Physiological changes and responses to diseases	References
NOS1 (nNOS)	Resistance to cerebral ischemia	Huang et al. (1994)
	Reduction in dendrite numbers	Inglis et al. (1998)
	Resistance to NMDA-induced neurotoxicity *in vitro* and *in vivo*	Ayata et al. (1997); Dawson et al. (1996)
	Resistance to MPTP-induced neurotoxicity in the brain	Przedborski et al. (1996)
	Enhanced aggression in male mice	Nelson and Young (1998)
	Reduced aggression in female mice	Gammie and Nelson (1999)
	Deficiency in nocturnal motor coordination	Kreigfeld et al. (1999)
	Altered urinary bladder structure	Burnett et al. (1997)
	Pyloric sphincter hypertrophy, enlarged stomach	Huang et al. (1993)
NOS2 (iNOS)	Increased susceptibility to bacterial infection	Shiloh et al. (1999)
	Increased susceptibility to tuberculosis	MacMicking et al. (1997)
	Susceptible to experimental autoimmune encephalitis	Fenyk-Melody et al. (1998)
	Ssceptible to endotoxin-induced uveitis	Smith et al. (1998)
	Neuroprotective after endogenous traumatic brain injury	Sinz et al. (1999)
NOS3 (eNOS)	Hypertension and decreased heart rate Increased plasma renin activity Lack of response to ACh and calcium ionophore Increased sensivity to phenylephrine, serotonin, and nitroglycerine	Shesely et al. (1996); Kojda et al. (1999)
	Impaired ovulation and oocyte meiotic maturation	Jablonka-Shariff and Olson (1998)

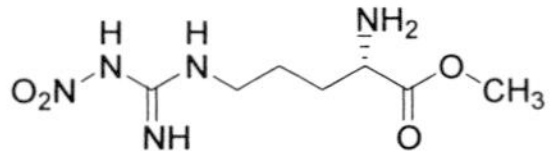

L-NAME (N-Nitro-L-arginine-methylester), [50903-99-6]

Antinociceptive properties of NO

dual effect of nitric oxide donors in nociception

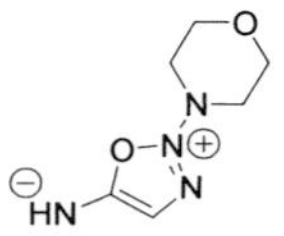

SIN-1 (NO-donor)
[26687-79-6]

Studies to elucidate the functional role of NO have used inhibitors of NO synthase such as L-NAME and L-NMMA (see below). Systemic and intrathecal injections of NO synthase inhibitors have been shown to reduce noxious responses to formalin and carrageenan-induced hyperalgesia (Sakurada et al., 2001). Furthermore, NO-induced mechanical hyperalgesia has been reported to be mediated by supraspinal centers and does not occur in *in vitro* preparations of the spinal cord.

On the other hand, NO can also be antinociceptive in that it exerts a tonically inhibitory action on the background activity of dorsal horn neurons. The increase in background activity occurs almost exclusively in nociceptive neurons (Trudrung et al., 2000).

This may explain the conflicting effects observed with NO or NO donors on laboratory animals or on humans. Transdermal nitroglycerine was used successfully in the management of shoulder pain syndrome due to supraspinatus tendinitis, and as a co-adjuvant in opiate therapy for the control of cancer pain. NSAIDs releasing NO, e.g. nitroparacetamol, are described to exhibit greater antinociceptive activities than their parent compounds (al-Sawayeh et al., 2000). In a study investigating the antinociceptive effect of the NO donor SIN-1 it was shown that SIN-1 has an antinociceptive effect at low doses but a pronociceptive effect at higher doses (Sousa and Prado, 2001).

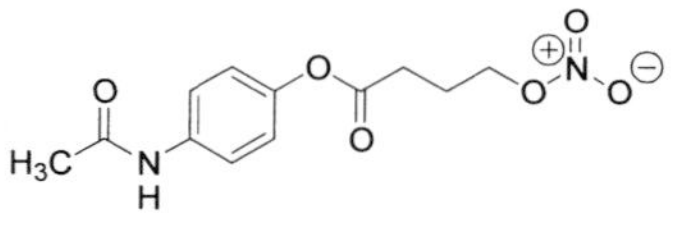

Nitroparacetamol, phase I clinical trials
(NicOx 2001)

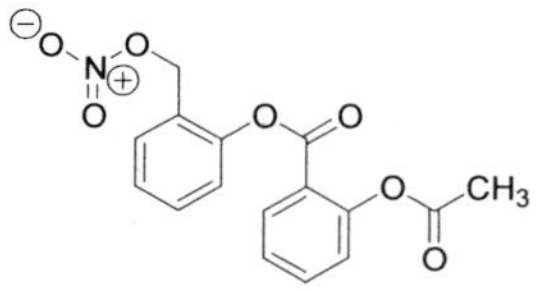

NO-ASA, has been in phase I clinical trials for pain, and is now developed for cardiovascular indications (phase II, NicOx) [175033-36-0]

Scheme 2: NO donors in clinical trials.

Nitric Oxide Inhibitors and Migraine

Nitric oxide inhibition has an analgesic effect in patients with chronic tension-type headache, probably due to a reduction in central sensitization at the level of the spinal dorsal horn, trigeminal nucleus or both (Ashina, 2002).

Increasing scientific evidence suggests a key role for NO in migraine. This evidence is mainly based on experimental studies using two different human headache models (Olesen and Jansen-Olesen, 2000).

Clinical studies have suggested that migraine patients more often experience a migraine-like headache in association with nitroglycerine administration than do non-migraineurs. In controlled double-blind trials it has been shown that migraine-sufferers develop a genuine migraine attack following nitroglycerine infusion after a time lapse of several hours. This induced migraine headache is preceded by an immediate headache response during the infusion (Olesen et al. 1993).

Moreover, migraine sufferers have been found to be hypersensitive to histamine in controlled trials. The activation of endothelial H1-receptors induces the formation of NO (Jansen-Olesen et al., 1997). Thus, the increased sensitivity to histamine in migraine sufferers may also been explained by hypersensitivity to activation of the NO pathway.

Targinine (L-NMMA)

The L-arginine derivative targinine was investigated by GlaxoWellcome for the treatment of severe hypotension resulting from septic shock. Phase III clinical trials were discontinued due to concerns from an interim analysis which showed a higher mortality rate among patients treated with targinine compared to the placebo group. Targinine had previously been in development for migraine. In 15 migraine patients (phase II, 6 mg/kg i.v. infusion, 15 min), targinine significantly reduced migraine pain, phonophobia and photophobia, and although it increased mean arterial pressure by 17% and decreased the heart rate by 21%, patients were unaffected by these changes (Lassen et al., 1997).

Targinine (L-NMMA)

5-Guanidino-2-methylamino-pentanoic acid, $C_7H_{16}N_4O_2$, MW 188,23

TRIM

TRIM is an extremely weak NOS inhibitor. The compound was reported to be 40-fold more selective for nNOS and eNOS over iNOS (Moore, King's College London). Potential for the treatment of chronic pain was suggested, but, as far as we know, no development has been reported since 1997.

TRIM, 1-(2-Trifluoromethyl-phenyl)-1H-imidazole, $C_{10}H_7F_3N_2$, MW 212,17

ONO-1714

ONO-1714 has reached phase II clinical trials for the treatment of hypotension and septic shock. The compound is a very potent and competitive inhibitor of the human iNOS with no selectivity over the neuronal form and 10-fold selectivity over eNOS. The compound is very active *in vivo*, reducing LPS-stimulated NO production in a mouse model with an ID_{50} value of 0.1 mg/kg s.c.. In 2000, the analgesic activity of ONO-1714 was filed by Ono Pharmaceuticals (Naka and Kobayashi).

ONO-1714, 7-Chloro-5-methyl-2-aza-bi-cyclo[4.1.0]hept-3-ylidene-amine, $C_7H_{11}ClN_2$, MW 158,63, [214479-33-1]

A wide variety of new NOS inhibitors have been reported over the last couple of years, but clinical data have not been available up to now. A selection of NOS inhibitors patented recently is shown in the following scheme :

The NOS enzyme activities can be determined by different test systems cited in the literature (e.g. Green et al. 1982; Feelisch and Noak, 1987; Mayer et al., 1989; Bredt and Snyder 1990; Archer, 1993; etc.).

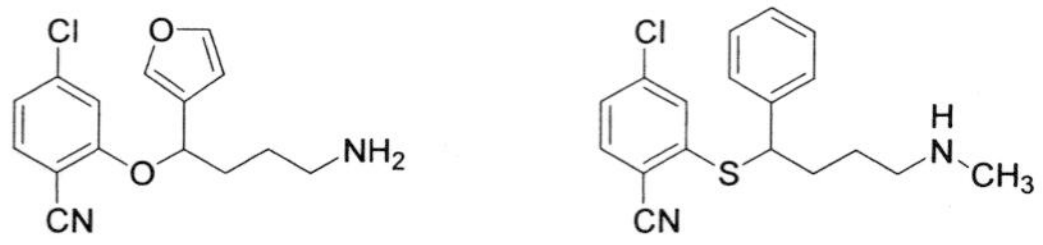

Cheshire et al., AstraZeneca, WO 0162713; WO 0162714;
WO 0162721; WO 0162704

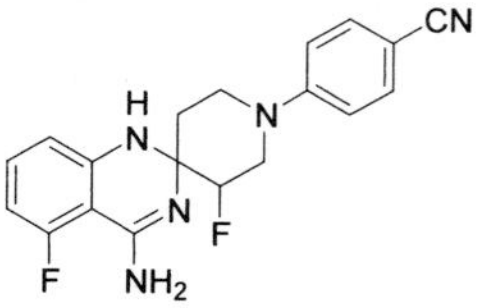

Walpole et al., AstraZeneca, WO 0158867

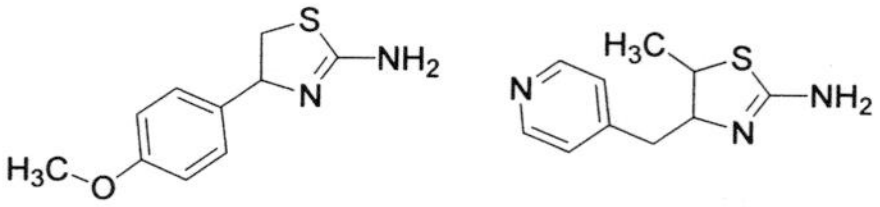

Carry et al., Aventis Pharma, WO 0193867; WO 0194325

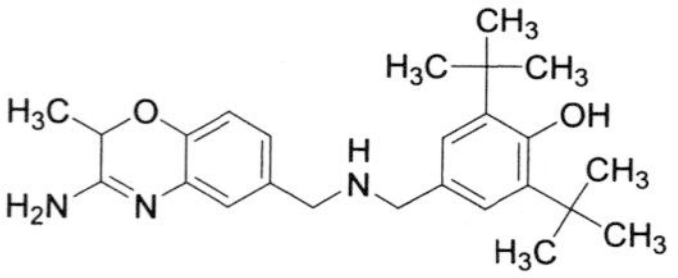

Hölscher et al., Schering, WO 0181324

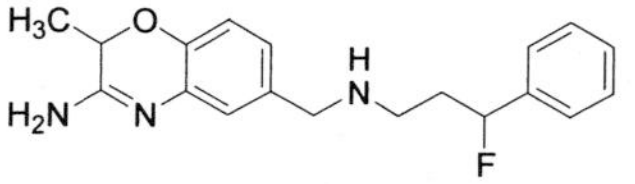

Rehwinkel et al., Schering, WO 0181323

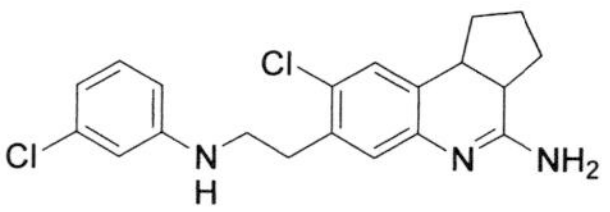

Jaroch et al., Schering, WO 0017167

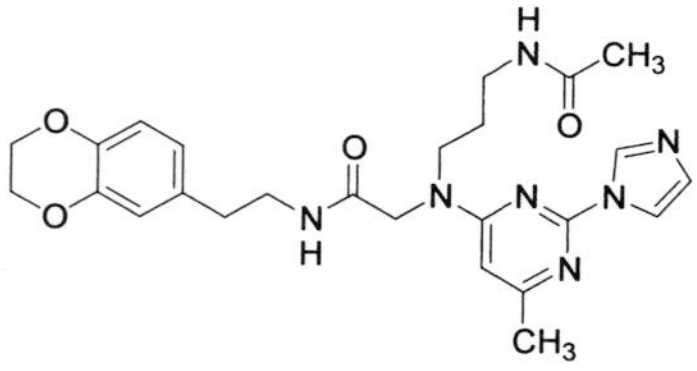

Arnaiz et al., Berlex, WO 0114371

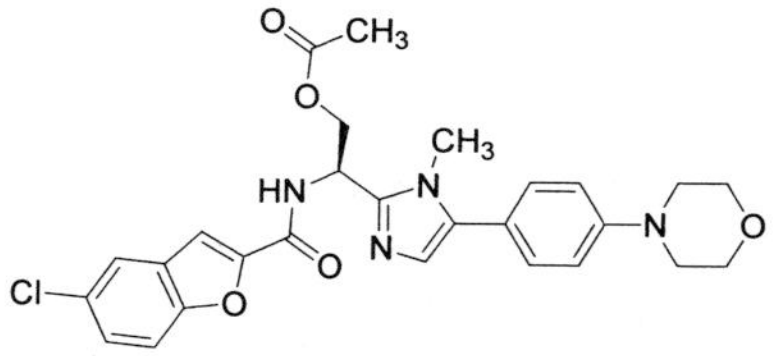

Sakai et al., Fujisawa, WO 0102387

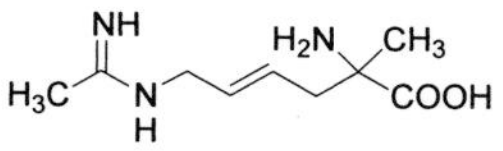

Durley et al., Pharmacia, WO 0222559

Scheme 3: NOS-inhibitors patented recently.

There is no doubt that NO plays a key role in pain sensation and migraine, which makes NO synthase an interesting target for pain research. Recent overviews have been published by Lowe (2000) and Cheshire (2001).

References

al-Sawayeh, O. A., Futter, L. E., Clifford, R. H., Moore, P. K.: *Nitroparacetamol exhibits anti-inflammatory and anti-nociceptive activity,* Br. J. Pharmacol. **2000**, *130*, 1453-1456.

Archer, S., (Review): *Measurement of nitric oxide in biological models,* FASEB Journal **1993**, 7, 349-360.

Arnaiz, D. O., Baldwin, J. J., Davey, D. D., Devlin, J. J., Dolle, R. E., Erickson, S. D., Mcmillan, K., Morrissey, M. M., Ohlmeyer, M. H. J., Pan, G., Paradkar, V. M., Parkinson, J., Philips, G. B., Ye, B., Zhao, Z. (Berlex Laboratories): *N-heterocyclic derivatives as NOS-inhibitors,* WO 0114371.

Ashina, M.: Nitric oxide synthase inhibitors for the treatment of chronic tension-type headache, Exp. Op. Pharm. **2002**, *3*, 395-399.

Ayata, C., Ayata, G., Hara, H., Matthews, R.T., Beal, M.F., Ferrante, R.J., Endres, M., Kim, A., Christie, R.H., Waeber, C., Huang, P.L., Hyman, B.T., Moskowitz, M.A.: *Mechanisms of Reduced Striatal NMDA Excitotoxicity in Type I Nitric Oxide Synthase Knock-Out Mice,* J. Neurosci. **1997**, *17*, 6908-6917.

Babu, B. R. and Griffith, O. W.: *Design of isoform-selective inhibitors of nitric oxide synthase,* Curr. Opin. Chem. Biol. **1998**, *2*, 491-500.

Bergman, F. and Elam, R.: *On the mechanism of action of 2-amino-4-methylpyridine, a morphine-like analgesic,* Arch. Int. Pharmacodyn. **1980**, *247*, 275-282.

Bird, D. C., Bujas-Bobanovic, M., Robertson, H. A., Dursun, S. M.: *Lack of phencyclidine-induced effects in mice with reduced neuronal nitric oxide synthase,* Psychopharmacology **2001**, *155*, 299-309.

Birkinshaw, T., Cheshire, D., Mete, A. (AstraZeneca): *Novel phenylheteroalkylamine derivatives,* WO 0162713.

Boer R., Ulrich, W.-R., Klein, T., Mirau, B., Haas, S., Baur, I.: *The Inhibitory potency and selectivity of arginine substrate site nitric-oxide synthase inhibitors is solely determined by their affinity toward the different isoenzymes,* Mol. Pharmacol. **2000**, *58*, 1026-1034.

Bredt, D.S. and Snyder, S.H.: *Isolation of nitric oxide synthetase, a calmodulin-requiring enzyme,* Proc. Natl. Acad. Sci. USA **1990**, *87*, 682-685.

Burnett, A.L., Calvin, D.C., Chamness, S.L., Liu, J.X., Nelson, R.J., Klein, S.L., Dawson, V.L., Dawson, T.M., Snyder, S.H.: *Urinary bladder-urethral sphincter dysfunction in mice with targeted disruption of neuronal nitric oxide synthase models idiopathic voiding disorders in humans,* Nat. Med. **1997**, 3, 571-574.

Carry, J.-C., Damour, D., Guyon, C., Mignani, S., Bacque, E., Bigot, A (Aventis Pharma): *2-Aminothiazoline derivatives and their use as NO-synthase inhibitors,* WO 0194325.

Carry, J.-C., Damour, D., Guyon, C., Mignani, S., Bigot, A, Bacque, E., Tabart, M. (Aventis Pharma): *4,5-Dihydro-thiazo-2-ylaminederivatives and their use as NO-synthase inhibitors,* WO 0193867.

Cheshire, D. R.: *Use of nitric oxide synthase inhibitors for the treatment of inflammatory disease and pain,* IDrugs **2001**, *4*, 795-803.

Cheshire, D., Connolly, S., Cox, D., Mete, A. (AstraZeneca): *Novel phenylheteroalkylamine derivatives,* WO 0162714.

Cheshire, D., Connolly, S., Cox, D., Millichip, I. (AstraZeneca): *Novel use of phenylheteroalkylamine derivatives,* WO 0162721.

Cheshire, D., Connolly, S., Cox, D.,Hamley, P., Mete, A., Pimm, A. (AstraZeneca): *Novel use of phenylheteroalkylamine derivatives,* WO 0162704.

Dawson, V.L., Kizushi, V.M., Huang, P.L., Snyder S.H., Dawson, T.M.: *Resistance to neurotoxicity in cortical cultures from neuronal nitric oxide synthase-deficient mice,* J. Neurosci **1996**, *16*, 2479-2487.

Dinerman, J. L., Dawson, T. M., Schell, M. J., Snowman, A., Snyder, S. H.: *Endothelial nitric oxide synthase localized to hippocampal pyramidal cells: implications for synaptic plasticity*, Proc. Natl. Acad. Sci. **1994**, *91*, 4214-4218.

Durley, R., Sikorski, J., Hansen, D., Promo, M. A., Webber, R. K., Pitzele, B. S., Awasthi, A. K., Moorman, A. E. (Pharmacia Corporation): *2-Amino-2-alkyl-4-hexenoic and hexynoic acid derivatives useful as nitric oxide synthase inhibitors*, WO 0222559.

Fastier, F. N. and McDowall, M. A.: *Analgesic activity of 4-methyl-2-aminopyridine and some related compounds*, Aust. J. Exp. Biol. **1958**, *36*, 491-498.

Feelisch M. and Noack, E.A.: *Correlation between nitric oxide formation during degradation of organic nitrates and activation of guanylate cyclase,* Eur. J. Pharmacol. **1987**, *139*, 19-30.

Fenyk-Melody, J.E., Garrison, A.E., Brunnert, S.R., Weidner, J.R., Shen, F., Shelton, B.A., Mudgett, J.S.: *Experimental autoimmune encephalomyelitis is exacerbated in mice lacking the NOS2 gene,* J. Immunol. **1998**, *160*, 2940-2946.

Furchgott, R. F.: *Endothelium-derived relaxing factor: discovery, early studies and identification as nitric oxide (Nobel lecture)*, Angew. Chem. Int. Ed. **1999**, *38*, 1870-1880.

Gammie, S.C. and Nelson, R.J., *Maternal aggression is reduced in neuronal nitric oxide synthase-deficient mice,* J. Neurosci. **1999**, *19*, 8027-8035.

Green, L.C., Wagner, D.A., Glogowski, J., Skipper, P.L., Wishnok, J.S., Tannenbaum,S.R.: *Analysis of nitrate, nitrite, and [15N]nitrate in biological fluids,* Anal. Biochem. **1982**, *126*, 131-138.

Hobbs, A. J., Higgs, A., Moncada, S.: *Inhibition of nitric oxide synthase as potential therapeutic target*, Annu. Rev. Pharmacol. Toxicol. **1999**, *39*, 191-220.

Hölscher, P., Jautelat, R., Rehwinkel, H., Jaroch, S., Sülzle, D., Hillmann, M., Burton, G. A., McDonald, F. M. (Schering AG): WO 0181324.

Huang, A., Sun, D., Shesely, E. G., Levee, E. M., Koller, A., Kaley, G.: *Neuronal NOS-dependant dilation to flow in coronary arteries of male eNOS-KO mice,* Am. J. Physiol. Heart Circ. Physiol. **2002**, *282*, H429-H436.

Huang, P.L., Dawson, T.M., Bredt, D.S., Snyder, S.H., Fishman, M.C.: *Targeted disruption of the neuronal nitric oxide synthase gene,* Cell **1993**, *75*, 1273-1286.

Huang, Z., Huang, P.L., Panahian, N., Dalkara, T., Fishman, M.C., Moskowitz, M.A.: *Effects of cerebral ischemia in mice deficient in neuronal nitric oxide synthase,* Science **1994**, *265*, 1883-1885.

Ignarro, I. J.: *Nitric oxide: a unique endogenous signalling molecule in vascular biology* (Nobel lecture) Angew. Chem. Int. Ed. **1999**, *38*, 1882-1892.

Inglis, F.M., Furia, F., Zuckerman, K.E., Strittmatter, S.M., Kalb, R.G.: *The role of nitric oxide and NMDA receptors in the development of motor neuron dendrites,* J. Neurosci. **1998**, *18*, 10493-10501.

Jablonka-Shariff, A. and Olson, L.M.,*The role of nitric oxide in oocyte meiotic maturation and ovulation: meiotic abnormalities of endothelial nitric oxide synthase knock-out mouse oocytes,* Endocrinology **1998**, *139*, 2944-2954.

Jansen-Olesen, I., Ottosson, A., Cantera, L., et al.: *Role of endothelium and nitric oxide in histamine-induced responses in human cranial arteries and detection of mRNA encoding H1 and H2 receptors by RT-PCR,* Br. J. Pharmacol. **1997**, *121*, 41-48.

Jaroch, S., Rehwinkel, H., Hölscher, P., Sülzle, D., Hillmann, M., Burton, G. A., McDonald, F. M.: *Aminoalkyl-3,4-dihydroquinoline derivatives as NO synthase inhibitors*, WO 0017167.

Knowles, R. G. and Moncada, S.: *Nitric oxide synthases in mammals*, Biochem. J. **1994**, *298*, 249-258.

Kojda, G., Laursen, J.B., Ramasamy, S., Kent, J.D., Kurz, S., Burchfield, J., Shesely, E.G., Harrison, D.G.: *Protein expression, vascular reactivity and soluble guanylate cyclase activity in mice lacking the endothelial cell nitric oxide synthase: contributions of NOS isoforms to blood pressure and heart rate control,* Cardiovasc. Res. **1999**, *42*, 206-213.

Kriegsfeld, L.J., Eliasson, M.J., Demas, G.E., Blackshaw, S., Dawson, T.M., Nelson, R.J., Snyder, S.H.: *Nocturnal motor coordination deficits in neuronal nitric synthase knock-out-mice,* Neuroscience **1999**, *89*, 311-315.

Levy, D., Kubes, P., Zochodne, D.W.: *Delayed peripheral nerve degeneration, regeneration, and pain in mice lacking inducible nitric oxide synthase,* J. Neuropathol. Exp. Neurol. **2001**, *60*, 411-421.

Lassen, L. H., Ashina, M., Christiansen, I., Olesen, J.: *Nitric oxide synthase inhibition in migraine,* The Lancet **1997**, *349*, 401-402.

Lowe, J. A.: *Nitric oxide synthase inhibitors: Recent patent activity,* IDrugs **2000**, *3*, 63-72.

MacMicking, J.D., North, R.J., LaCourse, R., Mudgett, J.S., Shah, S.K., Nathan, C.F.: *Identification of nitric oxide synthase as a protective locus against tuberculosis,* Proc. Natl. Acad. Sci. USA **1997**, *94*, 5243-5248.

Mayer, B., Schmidt, K., Humbert, P. and Böhme, E.: *Biosynthesis of endothelium-derived relaxing factor: a cytosolic enzyme in porcine aortic endothelial cells Ca^{2+}-dependently converts L-arginine into an activator of soluble guanylyl cyclase,* Biochem. Biophys. Research Commun. **1989**, *164*, 678-685.

Murad, F.: *Discovery of some of the biological effects of nitric oxide and its role in cell signalling* (Nobel lecture), Angew. Chem. Int. Ed. **1999**, *38*, 1856-1868.

Naka, M., Kobayashi, K.: *Analgesics,* WO 0074678.

Nelson, R.J., and Young, K.A.: *Behavior in mice with targeted disruption of single genes,* Neurosci. Biobehav. **1998**, *22*, 453-462.

Olesen, J., Iversen, H. K., Thomsen, L. L.: *Nitric oxide supersensitivity. A possible mechanism of migraine pain,* Neuroreport **1993**, *4*, 1027-1030.

Olesen, J. and Jansen-Olesen, I.: *Nitric oxide mechanisms in migraine,* Pathol. Biol. **2000**, *48*, 648-657.

Palmer, R. M. J., Ferrige, A. G., Moncada, S.: *Nitric oxide release accounts for the biological activity of endothelium-derived relaxing factor,* Nature **1987**, *327*, 524-526.

Pettipher, E. R., Hibbs, T. A., Smith, M. A., Griffiths, R. J.: *Analgesic activity of 2-amino-4-methylpyridine, a novel NO synthase inhibitor,* Inflamm. Res. **1997**, *46*, S135-S136.

Przedborski, S., Jackson-Lewis, V., Yokoyama, R., Shibata, T., Dawson, V.L., Dawson, T. M.: *Role of neuronal nitric oxide in 1-methyl-4-phenyl-1, 2, 3, 6-tetrahydropyridine (MPTP)-induced dopaminergic neurotoxicity,* Proc. Natl. Acad. Sci. USA **1996**, *93*, 4565-4571.

Rehwinkel, H., Hölscher, P., Jaroch, S., Sülzle, D., Hillmann, M., Burton, G. A., McDonald, F. M. (Schering AG): *Benzoxazine and benzothiazinederivatives and the use thereof in medicaments,* WO 0181323.

Ringertz, N.: *Alfred Nobel's health and his interest in medicine,* The official web side of the Nobel foundation [**2000**].

Sakurada, C., Sugiyama, A., Nakayama, M., Yonezawa, A., Sakurada, S., Tan-No, K., Kisara, K., Sakurada, T.: *Antinociceptive effect of spinally injected L-NAME on the acute nociceptive response induced by low concentrations of formalin,* Neurochem. Int. **2001**, *38*, 417-423.

Shesely, E.G., Maeda, N., Kim, H.S., Desai, K.M., Krege, J.H., Laubach, V.E., Sherman, P.A., Sessa, W.C., Smithies, O.: *Elevated blood pressures in mice lacking endothelial nitric oxide synthase,* Proc. Natl. Acad. Sci. USA **1996**, *93*, 13176-13181.

Shiloh, M.U., MacMicking, J.D., Nicholson, S., Brause, J.E., Potter, S., Marino, M., Fang, F., Dinauer, M., Nathan, C.: *Phenotype of mice and macrophages deficient in both phagocyte oxidase and inducible nitric oxide synthase,* Immunity **1999**, *10*, 29-38.

Sinz, E.H., Kochanek, P.M., Dixon, C.E., Clark, R.S., Carcillo, J.A., Schiding, J.K., Chen, M., Wisniewski, S.R., Carlos, T.M., Williams, D., DeKosky, S.T., Watkins, S.C., Marion, D.W., Billiar, T.R.: *Inducible nitric oxide synthase is an endogenous neuroprotectant after traumatic brain injury in rats and mice,* J. Clin. Invest. **1999**, *104*, 647-656.

Smith, J.R., Hart, P.H., Coster, D.J., Williams, K.A.: *Mice deficient in tumor necrosis factor receptors p55 and p75, interleukin-4, or inducible nitric oxide synthase are susceptible to endotoxin-induced uveitis,* Invest. Ophthalmol. Vis. Sci. **1998**, *39*, 658-661.

Sousa, A. M. and Prado, W. A.: *The dual effect of a nitric oxide donor in nociception,* Brain Res. **2001**, *897*, 9-19.

Thomsen, L. L. and Olesen, J.: *Nitric oxide theory of migraine,* Clin. Neurosci. **1998**, *5*, 28-33.

Trudrung, P., Wirth, U., Mense, S.: *Changes in the number of nitric oxide-synthesizing neurones on both sides of a chronic transection of the rat spinal cord,* Neurosci. Lett. **2000**, *287*, 125-128.

Walpole, C., Yang, H. (AstraZeneca): *Novel compounds,* WO 0158867.

Wattanapitayakul, S.K., Young, A.P., Bauer, J.A.: *Genetic variations in nitric oxide synthase isoforms,* Pharmaceut. News **2000**, *7*, 14-20.

Part IV

Outlook

Part IV

Outlook

17 The Future of Pain Management

Ulrich Jahnel and Clemens Gillen

Introduction

The current pharmacotherapy of pain is based mainly on two well established principles: non-steroidal anti-inflammatory drugs (NSAIDS) and opioids. Both of these classes suffer from drawbacks in clinical use. For some types of pain, where the efficacy of existing pain therapies is relatively high (e.g. opioids for perioperative pain or NSAIDS for inflammatory pain) , the need for new drugs is dictated by side-effect liabilities. Some of the NSAIDS are associated with gastric damage as well as kidney and liver toxicity, while the opioids can produce addiction, tolerance and dependence along with constipation, nausea, respiratory depression and sedation. Furthermore, for some indications such as neuropathic pain these classical strategies appear to be ineffective in a substantial number of patients. The urgent medical need for novel and safe analgesics with high efficacy has led to intense research for new targets, and those with the greatest potential are reviewed in this book.

In addition to the target- and substance-orientated chapters, this chapter presents additional strategies for pain relief along with the classification of different strategies within a hypothetical time schedule.

Near-term Improvements of Pain Therapy

An optimization of the two classical principles mentioned above was achieved by the generation of more selective compounds. For example, the cyclooxygenase-2- (COX-2) selective NSAIDS (Celecoxib, Rofecoxib) with improved gastric tolerance have entered the market with tremendous success (see Chapter 2). In addition, research in the opioid field has been directed towards the identification of selective ligands for the individual opioid receptor subtypes. At present a number of κ- and δ-receptor agonists are being analyzed in clinical trials (see Chapters 3, 9.1).

An alternative strategy uses the combination of known drugs such as tramadol and acetaminophen, thereby targeting multiple components of the pain pathway (Silverfield et al., 2002). This combination of opioids with NSAIDs is a well-established strategy that is part of the WHO scale for treatment of chronic pain.

Another strategy which exploits already established drugs is the development of new drug delivery systems. The transdermal delivery of opioids such as fentanyl (Durogesic®) or buprenorphine (Transtec®) using patch formulations has proven to be very successful. The continuous, long-lasting delivery of a strong opioid is especially suited to the treatment of severe chronic pain in elderly patients.

The intense research for additional pain targets resulted in the identification of several compounds which have entered the clinic, including glutamate receptor antagonists (see Chapter 7), nicotinic receptor agonists (see Chapter 8.1), muscarinic receptor agonists (see Chapter 8.2), sodium channel modulators (see Chapter 6.1), excitability blockers such as gabapentin (see Chapter 5) and adenosine receptor modulators (see Chapter 10). At present there are approximately 70 new analgesic compounds in clinical studies which will surely lead to substantial improvements within the next few years.

Midterm Improvements: The Visible Horizon

In order to gain more insight into the mechanisms underlying pain perception and in order to identify new targets for pain treatment, several strategies are currently used.

Genomics

The search for genes that are differentially expressed in certain pain-relevant tissues, e.g. dorsal root ganglia, versus other tissues or in pain-suffering animals versus control animals led to the identification of several pain-relevant target genes. For example the search for nociceptor-specific genes led to the identification of the TTX-resistant sodium channel SNS/$Na_{v1.8}$ (Akopian et al., 1996) and the purinergic receptor P2X3 (Chen et al., 1995). A different molecular procedure includes the use of degenerate primers and low-stringency homology screening using PCR to clone novel members of particular protein families. Using primers for G protein-coupled receptors and DRG-cDNA as a template, a new class of sensory neuron-specific receptors was recently identified (Lembo et al., 2002).

After completion of the human genome sequence with the reduced estimation of the number of human genes the focus has now switched to proteomic strategies. Future studies will focus on the pain-associated modification or translocation of pain-relevant proteins, and will elucidate signaling mechanisms by identifying protein-protein interactions.

Proteomics

These strategies led to the identification of several receptors for which the endogenous ligands were not known. The subsequent screening of peptidic compound libraries using functional receptor assays was successfully used for deorphanizing. Following this strategy the heptadecapetide nociceptin/orphanin FQ could be identified as the endogenous ligand for the orphan receptor ORL1 (see Chapter 9.2). A further pain-relevant example is the receptor for the neuropeptide FF (NPFF) that was deorphanized simultaneously by Bonini et al. and Elshourbagy et al. (2000).

Deorphanizing of G protein-coupled receptors

In a strategy complementary to that mentioned above, several compounds with well-known analgesic activity were used to identify their molecular targets. Successful examples include the isolation of the GABA$_B$ receptor using baclofen (Kaupmann et al., 1997) and the vanilloid receptor 1 using capsaicin (Caterina et al., 1997). In both cases an expression-cloning strategy was used that will be described briefly for the capsaicin receptor. Based on the fact that capsaicin causes a large influx of calcium into cells which contain its receptor, a DRG cDNA library was expressed in HEK293 cells which were subsequently screened for calcium influx after capsaicin treatment using the flurorescent calcium-sensitive dye Fura-2. The positive cells were shown to contain a novel cation-channel called vanilloid receptor subtype 1 (VR1, see Chapter 13).

Identification of targets for known analgesics

In order to validate this increasing number of potential pain targets, several strategies have been pursued by the pharmaceutical industry. An HTS screening of compound libraries is carried out in order to identify low molecular weight compounds that are subsequently tested in animal models of nociception. In the last few years, molecular genetic approaches have become more significant. In the knock-out approach, the specific deletion of the target gene leads to so-called knock-out mice which can be tested in models of nociception. Although this approach has its limitations due to developmental changes and

Strategies for target validation

compensatory alterations, it allows significant insights into the functional role of several pain targets such as VR1, adenosine receptors, or muscarinic receptors (see corresponding chapters). In the knock-down approach the target protein levels are reduced *in vivo* by the administration of antisense oligonucleotides into certain CNS regions. Pain targets analyzed with this strategy include the δ-opioid receptor (Wahlestedt et al., 2000), the TTX-R sodium channel $Na_{v1.8}$ (Lai et al., 2002) and the cannabinoid-receptor CB1 (Edsall et al., 1996).

As a result of the strategies described above for target identification and target validation, several new pain targets are in preclinical research with promising compounds like the ORL1 receptor antagonists (see Chapter 9.2), capsaicin receptor antagonists (see Chapter 13) or metabotropic glutamate receptor modulators (see Chapter 7.1). For these targets their relevance to the treatment of pain in man is still unknown and has to be proven by the forthcoming clinical studies. Nevertheless it is to be expected that some of these compounds will be successful and reach the market within the next 5 to 10 years.

Molecular Aspects of the Future

Given the intense research carried out in this field by several pharmaceutical companies and numerous academic groups it is to be expected that the list of new pain targets will increase further and will result in new pharmacological interventions.

There are several molecular approaches that are currently used with great success for target validation in animals and might also be used in humans. Three of these approaches will be discussed below.

Selective ablation of spinal pain-relevant neurons

This method which was developed by Mantyh et al. (1997) uses a conjugate of substance P and the ribosome-inactivating protein saporin for selective ablation of neurons in the dorsal spinal cord. After intrathecal administration of SP-SAP in adult rats, it is internalized and cytotoxic to the lamina I spinal cord neurons which express the substance P receptor. Histochemical analysis showed a reduction of NK1-positive lamina I neurons of approx. 85%. The animals showed normal behaviour, but a strongly reduced thermal and mechanical hyperalgesia after an intraplantar injection of capsaicin. In a second publication (Nichols et al., 1999) the authors demonstrated that this effect was dose-dependent, long-lasting (up to 200 days) and affected mechanical and thermal hyperalgesia during inflammatory as well as neuropathic pain. This method can be regarded as pain-reducing molecular surgery that may also be used for the treatment of incurable severe chronic pain in humans.

As described earlier, the antisense strategy was used successfully in animals for the validation of pain-associated target genes. This knock-down strategy could be directed against pronociceptive gene products, such as the NMDA receptor subunits, the NK1 receptors or the sodium channel $Na_{v1.8}$. However, it must be taken into account that the antisense oligonucleotides need to be injected directly into the CNS (e.g. intrathecally). It is still questionable whether antisense constructs will find a place in pharmacotherapy, given the fact that only one antisense ODN is currently on the market (Formivirsen® for treatment of cytomegalovirus-induced retinitis). The substantial improvements in nucleotide chemistry leading to ODNs of increased stability and reduced toxicity could open the way for a broader application of antisense-ODNs and may include their use as analgesics.

Antisense approaches for knock-down of pain relevant genes

The current report of the U.S. recombinant DNA advisory committee lists 509 approved human gene therapy protocols. Most of these protocols are for cancer followed by infectious diseases and virus infections. At the moment there is no human gene therapy protocol which targets chronic pain. In contrast to the antisense strategy, this molecular approach should lead to the overexpression of antinociceptive gene products, such as endogenous opioids. Indeed, overproduction of opioid peptides in primary sensory neurons or spinal cord-induced antihyperalgesic effects in various animal models of persistent pain (Finegold et al., 1999; Wilson et al., 1999; Braz et al., 2001; Goss et al., 2001). The recent significant and constant advances in vector system design suggest that these techniques will be available in the future for safe application in humans.

Gene transfer approaches to control pain

Mechanism-Based Diagnosis and Therapy of Pain

The pursuit of the pharmaceutical industry for a powerful wide-spectrum analgesic mechanism may find its limitations in the complexity of the mechanisms underlying chronic pain. In recent years the increasing availability of information regarding the molecular basis of pain perception and transmission has led to the proposal of a mechanism-based diagnosis and therapy for pain (Woolf and Decosterd, 1999; Dallel and Voisin, 2001; Woolf and Max, 2001). The induction of pain encompasses multiple components acting on different levels of the neuraxis and are inherently dynamic. A certain syndrome such as neuropathic pain may be accompanied by several symptoms such as spontaneous chronic or paroxysmal pain or allodynia. For instance, allodynia, which includes all situations in which the threshold of pain is lowered, may be due to one or several of the following mechanisms: nociceptor sensitization, central sensitization or regenerative sprouting of Aβ fibers. Therefore it is of great importance to identify in individual patients which mechanisms are responsible for their pain and to target treatment specifically at those mechanisms. This mechanism-based pain assessment can only be established by the concerted efforts of physicians, academic pain researchers, industry and government research funders. Together with the discovery of targets specific to particular pain mechanisms, a bridge between molecular neurobiology and the patient arriving at a clinic seems possible.

References

Akopian, A.N., Sivilotti, L., Wood, J.N.: *A tetrodotoxin-resistant sodium channel expressed by C-fibre associated sensory neurons,* Nature **1996**, *379*, 257-262.

Bonini, J.A., Jones, K.A., Adham, N., Forray, C., Artymyshyn, R., Durkin, M.M., Smith, K.E., Tamm, J.A., Boteju, L.W., Lakhlani, P.P., Raddatz, R., Yao, W.J., Ogozalek, K.L., Boyle, N., Kouranova, E.V., Quan, Y., Vaysse, P.J., Wetzel, J.M., Branchek, T.A., Gerald, C., Borowsky, B.: *Identification and characterization of two G protein-coupled receptors for neuropeptide FF,* J. Biol. Chem. **2000**, *15*, 39324-39231.

Braz, J., Beaufour, C., Coutaux, A., Epstein, A.L., Cesselin, F., Hamon, M., Pohl, M.: *Therapeutic efficacy in experimental polyarthritis of viral-driven enkephalin overproduction in sensory neurons,* J. Neurosci. **2001**, *21*, 7881-7888.

Caterina, M.J., Schumacher, M.A., Tominaga, M., Rosen, T.A., Levine, J.D., Julius, D.: *The capsaicin-receptor: a heat-activated ion channel in the pain-pathway,* Nature **1997**, *389*, 816-24.

Chen, C.-C., Akopian, A.N., Sivilotti, L., Colquhoun, D., Burnstock, G., Wood, J.N.: *A P2X purinoceptor expressed by a subset of sensory neurons,* Nature **1995**, *377*, 428-431.

Dallel, R. and Voisin, D.: *Towards pain treatment based on the classification of pain-generating mechanisms?*, Eur. Neurol. **2001**, *45*, 126-132.

Edsall, S.A., Knapp, R.J., Vanderah, T.W., Roeske, W.R., Consroe, P., Yamamura, H.I.: *Antisense oligonucleotide treatment to the brain cannabinoid receptor inhibits antinociception,* Neuroreport **1996**, *31*, 593-596.

Elshourbagy, N.A., Ames, R.S., Fitzgerald, L.R., Foley, J.J., Chambers, J.K., Szekeres, P.G., Evans, N. A., Schmidt, D.B., Buckley, P.T., Dytko, G.M., Murdock, P.R., Milligan, G., Groarke, D.A., Tan, K.B., Shabon, U., Nuthulaganti, P., Wang, D.Y., Wilson, S., Bergsma, D.J., Sarau, H.M.: *Receptor for the pain modulatory neuropeptides FF and AF is an orphan G protein-coupled receptor,* J. Biol. Chem. **2000**, *275*, 25965-25971.

Finegold, A.A., Mannes, A.J., Iadarola, M.J.: *A paracrine paradigm for in vivo gene therapy in the central nervous system: treatment of chronic pain,* Hum. Gene Ther. **1999**, *10*, 1251-1257.

Goss, J.R., Mata, M., Goins, W.F., Wu, H.H., Glorioso, J.C., Fink, D.J.: *Antinociceptive effect of a genomic herpes simplex virus-based vector expressing human proenkephalin in rat dorsal root ganglion,* Gene Ther. **2001**, *8*, 551-556.

Kaupmann, K., Huggel, K., Heid, J., Flor, P.J., Bischoff, S., Mickel, S.J., McMaster, G., Angst, C., Bittiger, H., Froestl, W., Bettler, B.: *Expression cloning of GABA(B) receptors uncovers similarity to metabotropic glutamate receptors,* Nature **1997**, *386*, 223-224.

Lai, J., Gold, M.S., Kim, C.S., Bian, D., Ossipov, M.H., Hunter, J.C., Porreca, F.: *Inhibition of neuropathic pain by decreased expression of the tetrodotoxin-resistant sodium channel, NaV1.8.,* Pain **2002**, *95*,143-152.

Lembo, P.M., Grazzini, E., Groblewski, T., O'Donnell, D., Roy, M.O., Zhang, J., Hoffert, C., Cao, J., Schmidt, R., Pelletier, M., Labarre, M., Gosselin, M., Fortin, Y., Banville, D., Shen, S.H., Strom, P., Payza, K., Dray, A., Walker, P., Ahmad, S.: *Proenkephalin A gene products activate a new family of sensory neuron-specific GPCRs,* Nature Neurosci. **2002**, *5*, 201-209.

Mantyh, P.W., Rogers, S.D., Honore, P., Allen, B.J., Ghilardi, J.R., Li, J., Daughters, R.S., Lappi, D.A., Wiley, R.G., Simone, D.A.: *Inhibition of hyperalgesia by ablation of lamina I spinal neurons expressing the substance P receptor,* Science **1997,** *278*, 275-279.

Nichols, M.L., Allen, B.J., Rogers, S.D., Ghilardi, J.R., Honore, P., Luger, N.M., Finke, M.P., Li, J., Lappi, D.A., Simone, D.A., Mantyh, P.W.: *Transmission of chronic nociception by spinal neurons expressing the substance P receptor,* Science **1999** *286*,1558-1561.

Silverfield, J.C., Kamin, M., Wu, S.C., Rosenthal, N.: *Tramadol/acetaminophen comination tablets for the reatment of osteoarthritis flare pain: a multicenter, outpatient, randomized, double-blind, placebo-controlled, parallel-group, ad-on study,* Clin. Ther. **2002**, *24*, 282-297.

Wahlestedt, C., Salmi, P., Good, L., Kela, J., Johnsson, T., Hokfelt, T., Broberger, C., Porreca, F., Lai, J., Ren, K., Ossipov, M., Koshkin, A., Jakobsen, N., Skouv, J., Oerum, H., Jacobsen, M.H., Wengel, J.: *Potent and nontoxic antisense oligonucleotides containing locked nucleic acids,* Proc. Natl. Acad. Sci. USA **2000**, *97*, 5633-5638.

Wilson, S.P., Yeomans, D.C., Bender, M.A., Lu, Y., Goins, W.F., Glorioso, J.C.: *Antihyperalgesic effects of infection with a preproenkephalin-encoding herpes virus,* Proc. Natl. Acad. Sci. USA **1999**, *96*, 3211-3216.

Woolf, C.J. and Decosterd, I.: *Implications of recent advances in the understanding of pain pathophysiology for the assessment of pain in patients,* Pain Suppl. **1999**, *6*, S141-S147.

Woolf, C.J. and Max, M.: *Mechanism-based pain diagnosis,* Anesthesiol. **2001**, *95*, 241-249.

Glossary

Helmut Buschmann,
Thomas Christoph and
Elmar Friderichs

Absorption

Process of taking in. Chemicals can be absorbed into the bloodstream after breathing or swallowing.

Active transport

Active transport is the carriage of a solute across a biological membrane from low to high concentration that requires the expenditure of (metabolic) energy.

Acute pain

A normal biological response to help protect the body against potentially harmful environmental stimuli. Typically acute pain is caused by identifiable stimuli, is short-lived and stops when the tissue injury that caused it has healed.

Addiction

The compulsive use of drugs for non-medical purpose. It is characterised by a craving for mood-altering drug effects, not painrelief. Addiction refers to a dysfunctional behaviour as opposed to the improved function and quality of life that result from pain relief. In cancer patients who use opioids for long-term pain relief addiction is extremely rare.

Adjuvants

Agents used as adjuncts or adjunctive therapies to opioid analgesics in total management of moderate-to-severe pain. They can directly diminish pain, counteract opioid side effects, or help manage concurrent psychiatric symptoms.

Address-message concept

Address-message concept refers to compounds in which part of the molecule is required for binding, (address) and part for the biological action (message) (IUPAC).

ADME

Absorption, Distribution, Metabolism, Excretion. See Pharmacokinetics.

Adverse effect

Undesirable and unintended, although not necessarily unexpected, result of therapy or other treatment.

A-fibres

A specific type of nerve fibre involved in the conduction of nociceptive impulses.

Affinity

Affinity is the tendency of a substance to associate with another. The affinity of a drug is its abillty to bind to its biological target (receptor, enzyme, transport system, etc. For pharmacological receptors it can be thought of as the frequency with which the drug, when brought into the proximity of a receptor by diffusion, will reside at a position of minimum free energy within the force, field of that receptor. For an agonist (or for an antagonist) the numerical representation of affinity is the reciprocal of the equilibrium dissociation constant of the ligand-receptor complex denoted KA, calculated as the rate constant for offset (k_{-1}) divided by the rate constant for onset (k_1).

Agonist

A substance that can stimulate a receptor type to transmit an intracellular message and thus initiate a cellular biochemical change. An agonist is an endogenous substance or a drug that can interact with receptors and initiate a physiological or a pharmacological response (contraction, relaxation, secretion, enzyme activation, etc). An agonist is a Drug that binds cellular receptors which are ordinarily stimulated by naturally occurring substances, triggering a response.

Allodynia

Pain due to a stimulus that does not usually provoke pain.

Alzheimer's disease

Progressive, neurodegenerative disease characterized (AD) by loss of function and death of nerve cells in several areas of the brain leading to loss of cognitive function such as memory and language.

Anaesthesia

Absence of all sensory modalities.

Anaesthetic

A compound that reversibly depresses nerve function, producing loss of ability to perceive pain or other sensations.

Analgesia

Absence of pain in response to a stimulation that would normally be painful.

Analgesic

A drug used primarily for relieving pain.

Analogue

An analogue is a drug whose structure is inspired by that of another drug but whose chemical and biological properties may be quite different (IUPAC). See Congener.

Animal Models of Pain

Animal models of nociception can be divided according to the therapeutic indication: Acute Pain, Migraine Pain, Inflammatory Pain, Visceral Pain, Neuropathic Pain. Different degrees of chronification (up to weeks in neuropathic pain models) and different stimuli (mechanical, thermal, chemical, electrical) are used depending on the experimental question. In most cases a nociceptive threshold (e.g. withdrawal latency of a paw) is determined. Sometimes, nociceptive intensities are determined e.g. in order to quantify hyperalgesia.

Antagonist

A substance that binds to a receptor type without activating it but which blocks the attachment of agonists to the receptor. An antagonist is according to this definition a drug-or a chemical entity that opposes the physiological effects of another. At the receptor level, it is a chemical entity that opposes the receptor associated responses normally induced by another agent. An antagonist is a Drug that binds a receptor without triggering a response.

Anticonvulsant

A compound commonly used for treating epilepsy but also has applications in treating pain (e.g. phenytoin, carbamezapine, gabapentin and sodium valproate).

Antisense molecule

An antisense molecule is an oligonucleotide or analogue thereof that is complementary to a segment of RNA or DNA and that binds to it and inhibits its normal function. (IUPAC).

Assay

Any combination of targets and compounds which is exposed to a detection device to measure chemical or biological activity.

Backache

Probably the second most common and probably the most expensive form of chronic pain in industrialised societies behind headache. It can be acute or chronic and has many causes. It is sometimes treated with epidural injections or injections into joints.

Bennet model of neuropathic pain

Nerve injury, followed by pain related behaviour, is induced by loose ligation of the ischiatic nerve of one hind paw of the rat. 3-4 weeks after ligation, neuropathic pain-like behaviour is seen as increased sensitivity towards heat and pressure stimuli (hyperalgesia). Also pain reactions toward non-noxious tactile (mechanical allodynia) or cold stimuli (cold allodynia) can be observed. Mechanical allodynia is tested with von Frey hairs and cold allodynia by putting the animals on metal plate cooled to 4 °C. The number of paw liftings is counted (Bennett and Xie, Pain **1988**, *33*, 87-107).

Bioinformatics

the use of search programmes (public domain, proprietary or in-house programmes) to analyse DNA and protein sequences to predict the function of a gene sequence.

Bioisostere

A bioisostere is a compound resulting from the exchange of an atom or of a group of atoms with another, broadly similar, atom or group of atoms. The objective of a bioisosteric replacement is to create a new compound presenting similar biological properties to the parent compound. The biolsosteric replacement may be physicochemically or topologically based (IUPAC).

Biotransformation

Biotransformation is the chemical conversion of substances by living, organisms or enzyme preparations derived therefrom (IUPAC).

Bone pain   Pain experienced in the bones either caused by osteoporosis or bone metastases in cancer patients.

Cell   Smallest membrane-bound biological unit capable of replication.

Cell membrane   The phospholipid bilayer that surrounds a cell, forming a selectively-permeable barrier.

Cellular assay   Assay run on whole living cells.

Central pain   Pain associated with a lesion of the central nervous system.

C-fibres   Afferent (inward) nerve fibres; most C-fibres are nociceptive, carrying pain impulses to the central nervous system.

Chemoinformatics   A generic term that encompasses the design, creation, organisation, storage, management, retrieval, analysis, dissemination, visualisation and use of chemical information, not only in its own right, but as a surrogate or index for other data, information and knowledge.

Chronic pain   Pain which lasts more than 6 months and which may continue in the absence of any identifiable tissue injury. Typically this type of pain can severely affect the patient's quality of life by causing intensive physical suffering. Chronic pain can also be divided into chronic cancer-related pain and chronic non-cancer pain, which have different methods of management.

Chung model of neuropathic pain Nerve injury in rats is induced by a tight ligation of the root of the spinal nerve at L5-L6. Animals show hyperalgesia and allodynia similar to the Bennet model. Tactile allodynia, measured with von Frey hairs, is the most reliable parameter of pain intensity in this model (Kim and Chung, Pain **1992**, *50*, 355-363).

Clinical Candidate   A compound (small molecule) that has achieved the first ever dose administered to the first human (including patients if they are the first humans to receive the compound).

Clinical trials   Research studies that involve patients.

Clone   Group of identical genes, cells, or organisms derived from a single ancestor.

Cloned DNA   Any DNA fragment that passively replicates in the host organism after it has been joined to a cloning vector.

Cloning   Process of making genetically identical copies.

Coenzyme   A coenzyme is a dissociable, low-molecular weight, non-proteinaceous organic compound (often nucleotide) participating in enzymatic reactions as acceptor or donor of chemical groups or electrons.

Rational drug design - use of high resolution molecular imaging techniques (NMR, x-ray crystallography) to identify the active site of the target molecule and construct an new active substance which binds to this active site.

Computer-aided/structural drug design

A congener is a substance literally con- (with) *generated* or synthesized by essentially the same synthetic chemical reactions and the same procedures. Analogues are substances that are analogous in some respect to the prototype and in chemical structure. Clearly congeners may be analogues or vice versa but not necessarily. The term congener, while most often a synonym for homologue, has become somewhat more diffuse in meaning so that the terms congener and analogue are frequently used interchangeably in the literature.

Congener

Inability to do without, in this context, a drug; a problem which can occur in particular with the long-term use of opioids.

Dependence

A complication of diabetes where painful nerve damage can affect the limbs (especially causing ulcers in the feet if the patient has poor blood circulation), intestinal and cardiovascular system.

Diabetic neuropathy

Docking studies are molecular modeling studies aiming at finding a proper fit between a ligand and its binding site (IUPAC).

Docking studies

A double-blind study is a clinical study of potential and marketed drugs, where neither the investigators nor the subjects know which subjects will be treated with the active principle and which ones will receive a placebo (IUPAC).

Double-blind study

Any chemical compound that may be used on humans to help in diagnosis, treatment, cure, mitigation, or prevention of disease or other abnormal conditions.

Drug

Drug targeting is a strategy aiming at the delivery of a compound to a particular tissue of the body (IUPAC).

Drug targeting

A dual action drug is a compound which combines two desired different, pharmacological actions at a similarly efficacious dose (IUPAC).

Dual action drug

Efficacy is the property that enables drugs to produce responses. It is convenient to differentiate the properties of drugs into two groups; those which cause them to associate with the receptors (affinity) and those that produce stimulus (efficacy). This term is

Efficacy

often used to characterize the level of maximal responses induced by agonists. In fact, not all agonists of a receptor- are capable of inducing identical levels of maximal responses. It depends on the efficiency of receptor coupling, i.e., from the cascade of events, which, from the binding- of the drug to the receptor, leads to the observed biological effect. Efficacy describes the relative intensity with which agonists vary in the response they produce even when they occupy the same number of receptors and with the same affinity. Efficacy is *not* synonymous to intrinsic activity (IUPAC).

Enzyme

Protein that acts as a catalyst, affecting the rate at which chemical reactions occur in cells. An enzyme is any molecular structure that catalyses a physiological chemical reaction.

Epidural

A form of intraspinal analgesia where the agent is injected into the epidural space that surrounds the dura mater, which is the membrane that contains the cerebo-spinal fluid directly outside the spinal cord.

Fibromyalgia

A disease characteristically affecting depressed, middle-aged women complaining of diffuse, symmetrical and persistent musculoskeletal pain/tenderness and sleep disturbance with no organic basis, or a real pathological entity. It requires more than a psychological/psychatric approach to treat effectively.

Formalin test

A small amount of formalin solution is injected into the hind paw of mice or rats. This induces a bi-phasic pain reaction and a specific pain-related behaviour. The first phase represents acute nociceptive pain, whereas the second phase indicates more persistent pain associated with inflammation and tissue damage. Pain behaviour is observed in both phases and measured by means of a scoring system. Besides opioids, compounds active against inflammatory and neuropathic pain can be detected (Dubuisson and Dennis, Pain **1977**, *4*, 161-174).

Gene

Unit of inheritance; a working subunit of DNA containing the code for a specific product, typically, a protein such as an enzyme.

Gene expression

Process by which a gene's coded information is translated into the structures present and operating in the cell (either proteins or RNAs).

Genetics

Scientific study of heredity how particular qualities or traits are transmitted from parents to offspring.

All the genetic material in the chromosomes of a particular organism; its size is generally given as its total number of base pairs.

Genome

Research and technology development efforts aimed at mapping and sequencing some or all of the genorne of human beings and other organisms.

Genome projects

Identification and functional characterization of genes; Genomics is the identification of previously unknown human DNA sequences encoding natural human proteins with previously unknown medical use that can be used as targets in Drug Discovery to discover novel therapeutic agents or administered for therapeutic benefit.

Genomics

Genetic constitution of an organism.

Genotype

An anaesthetising compound which results in a loss of consciousness; usually a gas or intravenously injected liquid. Often used together with a neuromuscular blocker.

General anaesthetic

any cellular macromolecule to which a ligand binds initiating an effect via a G-protein mechanism (Note that it will include only binding activity through binding domain and will not account for any further event that the protein may perform through its effector domain).

G-protein coupled receptor (GPCR)

A heteroreceptor is a receptor regulating the synthesis and/or the release of mediators other than its own ligand (IUPAC).

Heteroreceptor

Technique of rapidly searching for molecules with desired biological effects from very large compound libraries.

High-throughput-screening (HTS)

Compound found by screening to have a desired biological effect.

Hit (compound)

The term homologue is used to describe a compound belonging to a series of compounds differing from each other by a repeating unit, usually a methylene group (IUPAC).

Homologue

A model of thermal pain. Mice or rats are placed on a heated metal plate of variable temperature. Depending on the temperature (48-58 °C), a weak or strong pain stimulus is induced. Animals respond either by licking their paws or by jumping. Analgesics increase the latency for this pain reaction. The low temperature hot plate detects a broader spectrum of less efficacious analgesics in comparison to its high temperature modification or the tail flick test (Eddy and Leimbach; J. Pharmacol. **1953**, *107*, 385).

Hot plate test

Human Genome Project	International research effort aimed at mapping and sequencing all of the genome of the human beings and other organisms.
Hydrophilicity	Hydrophilicity is the tendency of a molecule to be solvated by water (IUPAC).
Hydrophobicity	Hydrophobicity is the association of non polar groups or molecules in an aqueous environment which arises from the tendency of water to exclude non polar molecules (IUPAC). See Lipophilicity.
Hyperalgesia	An increased response to a stimulus that is normally painful. Many cases of hyperalgesia have features of allodynia, however, the term hyperalgesia is used specifically when there is a response of increased pain to a stimulus that normally is painful.
Hyperesthesia	Increased sensitivity to stimulation, excluding special senses.
Hypoalgesia	Diminished sensitivity to a noxious stimulation.
ICH (International Conference on Harmonization)	The International Conference on Harmonisation of Technical Requirements for Registration of Pharmaceuticals for Human Use (ICH) brings together the regulatory authorities of Europe, Japan and the United States and experts from the pharmaceutical industry in the three regions to harmonise scientific and technical aspects of product registration. They make recommendations which will be adopted by the national / EU authorities after an approval process.
Intrathecal	A form of intraspinal anaesthesia or analgesia in which the agent is injected through the dura mater and arachnoid membrane into the cerebro-spinal fluid which surrounds the spinal cord.
IND	Investigational New Drug. Application must be approved by the Food and Drug Administration (FDA) before a drug can be tested in humans in clinical trials.
Intrinsic activity	Intrinsic activity is the maximal stimulatory response induced by a compound in relation to that of a criven reference compound. This term has evolved with common use. It was introduced by Ariens as a proportionality factor between tissue response and receptor occupancy. The numerical value of intrinsic activity (alpha) could ran from unity (for full agonists, i.e., agonist inducing the tissue maximal response) to zero (for antacyonists). The fractional values within this ran denoting partial agonists. Arien-8 original definition equates the molecular nature of alpha to maximal response only when response is a linear function of receptor occupancy. This function has

been verified. Thus, intrinsic activity, which is a drug and tissue parameter, cannot be used as a characteristic drug parameter for classification of drugs or drug receptors. For this purpose, a proportionality factor derived by null methods, namely, relative efficacy, should be used. Finally, "intrinsic activity" should not be used instead of "intrinsic efficacy". A "parcial agonist" should be termed "agonist with intermediate intrinsic efficacy" in a given tissue (IUPAC).

Inverse agonist

An inverse agonist is a drug which acts at the same receptor as that of an agonist, yet produces an opposite effect. Also called negative antagonists.

In vitro

In a test tube.

In vivo

In the living cell or organism as opposed to in vitro.

Ion channel

Receptor or carrier proteins which, when activated, allows the passage of ions across cell membranes.

Lead / Lead compound

As a result of the screening process used during drug discovery, active substances will be identified. Of these active substances, the compound that best fits the desired characteristics profile (pharmacological activity, lack of early toxicity, patentability, etc) will be declared a lead compound. Development activities will then begin to shift from a broad discovery program to a more focused development program centred around the lead compound.

Lead Candidate

A chemical entity (small molecule) or series (a set of structural analogues) that has shown sufficient activity and selectivity for the target, to form the basis for focused medicinal chemistry and optimisation of pharmacological properties.

Lead discovery

Lead discovery is the process of identifying active new chemical entities, which by subsequent modification may be transformed into a clinically useful drug (IUPAC). This phase begins at the initiation of target screening "start of target screening" milestone and concludes with the identification of the first chemical lead compound (or lead series) selected for optimisation - "lead series selected" milestone. It involves the testing of compounds, either *in vitro* or *in vivo*, to determine their target effect (e.g. molecular interaction or biological effects).

Lead generation

Lead generation is the term applied to strategies developed to identify compounds which possess a desired but non-optimized biological (IUPAC).

Lead optimization	Lead optimisation is the synthetic modification of a biologically active compound, to fulfill all stereoelectronic, physicochemical, pharmacokinetic and toxicologic required for clinical usefulness (IUPAC). This phase begins with the first chemical lead or lead series selected for optimisation (i.e. the "lead series selected" milestone) and concludes with a decision for an optimized compound to enter preclinical development (i.e. the "pre-clinical candidate selected" milestone). This phase consists of testing of a compound to determine the chemical structure that has the optimum potency and selectivity for the target in question. The phase includes the search for back-up compounds and may also include early ADME and toxicity evaluation.
Ligand	Chemical messenger, usually released by one cell to communicate with a different cell by binding to specific receptors on the receiving cell's surface.
Lipophilicity	Lipophilicity represents the affinity of a molecule for a lipophilic environment. It is commonly measured by its distribution behaviour in a biphasic system, either liquid-liquid (e.a. partition coefficient in 1-octanol / water) or solid-liquid (retention on reversed-phase high performance liquid chromatography *(RP-HPLC)* or thin-layer chromatography *(TLQ System)* (IUPAC). See Hydrophobicity.
Metabolism	The term metabolism comprises the entire physical and chemical processes involved in the maintenance and reproduction of life in which nutrients are broken down to generate energy and to give simpler molecules (catabolism) which by themselves may be used to form more complex molecules (anabolism). In case of heterotrophic organisms, the energy evolving from catabolic processes is made available for use by the organism (IUPAC).
Me-too drug	A me-too drug is a compound that is structurally very similar to already known drugs, with only minor pharmacological differences (IUPAC).
Molecular modeling	Molecular modeling is a technique for the investigation of molecular structures and properties using computational chemistry and graphical visualization techniques in order to provide a plausible three-dimensional representation under a given set of circumstances (IUPAC).
Ligand	Any atom or molecule attached to a central atom, usually a metallic element, in a co-ordination or complex compound.

Anaethestising compound that only acts on the area in which it is applied; usually in the form of a spray, gel cream, local injection into the skin or adjacent nerves where they function to block nerve impulses.

Local anaesthetic

A vascular disease causing an intensely painful unilateral headache that can last from a few hours to 72 hours or longer.

Migraine

Opioid is the preferred medical and pharmacological term for opium derivatives and analogues, narcotic having legal and other non medical connotations

Narcotic

New chemical entity. A new chemical entity is a compound not previously described in the literature.

NCE

New drug application. A document that combines all relevant data (with attachments) to allow the US FDA (or an other drug regulatory agency) to review and decide whether to approve marketing of a new drug. Detailed reports of chemistry; pharmacology, toxicology, metabolism, manufacturing, quality controls and clinical data along with proposed labelling are included.

NDA

Pain occurring in the area served by a sensory nerve, either because of compression or disease of that nerve, or else occurring without any apparent organic cause.

Neuralgia

Pain resulting from non-inflammatory dysfunction of the peripheral or central nervous system without nociceptor stimulation or trauma. Examples include post-herpetic neuralgia, complex regional pain syndromes, phantom pain and trigeminal neuralgia.

Neurogenic pain

Pain caused by functional abnormalities or structural lesions in the peripheral or central nervous system frequently arising from injury (e.g. surgery, accident or amputation), diseases (e.g. diabetes, herpes zoster or cancer), infarction or dysfunction of the nervous system. A damaged nerve may initiate signals in other nerves not associated with the injured area. It may either have a burning sensation or an aching sensation.

Neuropathic pain

The response to excitation of nociceptors. Although nociception may give rise to the experience of pain, pain may arise in the absence of nociception. Conversely, nociception may also occur in the absence of pain.

Nociception

Pain which occurs when intact peripheral nerve endings (nociceptors) are stimulated by noxious

Nociceptive pain

	mechanical, thermal or chemical stimuli (e.g. inflammatory pain).
Nociceptor	Peripheral nerve ending.
Noxious stimulus	A stimulus which is potentially or actually damaging to body tissue, however it does include instances where there is no lasting tissue damage, such as that which occurs as muscle pain due to excessive exercise.
nuclear receptor	Receptors which are associated to a cell nucleus.
Opiate	Refers to the drug whose origin is the opium poppy, including codeine and morphine.
Opioid	Any substance having activity at the opioid receptor. Opioids can also be grouped according to pharmacological activity: pure, partial agonists, antagonists or mixed agonist-antagonists.
Opioid receptors	The different types and subtypes of opioid receptors in the nervous system. The mu (μ), kappa (κ) and delta (δ) subtype are designated by corresponding Greek letters.
Orphan drug	An orphan drug is a drug for the treatment of a rare disease for which reasonable recovery of the sponsoring firm's research and development expenditure is not expected within a reasonable time. The term is also used to describe substances intended for such uses (IUPAC).
Orphan receptor	Receptor with unknown function binding known ligands.
Pain threshold	The least experience of pain that a person can recognise. It is the level at which 50% of stimuli are recognised as painful; it must be understood that pain is the experience of the patient, which is difficult to measure, whereas the stimulus intensity can be measured by the psychophysicist as an external event.
Pain tolerance level	The greatest level of pain that a person is prepared to tolerate. It should be understood that this a subjective experience and so its clinical value is limited.
Palliative care	A form of care which attempts to provide at least superficial or temporary relief of pain and suffering such as that which is provided for cancer and/or terminally-ill patients.
Partial agonist	A substance which partially (in comparison to an agonist) activates a receptor type to transmit an intracellular message. A partial agonist is an agonist which is unable to induce maximal activation of a

receptor population, regardless of the amount of drug applied.

Peptidomimetics are compounds containing non-peptidic structural elements that are capable of mimicking or antagonizing the biological action(s) of a natural parent peptide (IUPAC).

Peptidomimetic

Pain which occurs after a limb has been amputated or lost as if it were still there.

Phantom pain

Pharmacokinetics refers to the study of absorption, distribution, metabolism and excretion (ADME) of bioactive compounds in a higher organism (IUPAC).

Pharmacokinetics

A pharmacophore is the ensemble of steric and electronic features that are necessary to ensure the optimal supramolecular interactions with a specific biological taraget structure and to trigger (or to block) its biological response. A pharmacophore does not represent a real molecule or a real association of functional groups, but a purely abstract concept that accounts for the common molecular interaction capacities of a group of compounds towards their target structure. The pharmacophore can be considered as the largest common denominator shared by a set of active molecules. This definition discards a misuse often found in the medicinal chemistry literature which consists of naming as a pharmacophore simple chemical functionalities such as guanidines, sulfamides or imidazolines, or typical structural skeletons such as flavones, phenothiazines, prostaglandins or steroids (IUPAC).

Pharmacophore (pharmacophorie patterrn)

The first trials in humans that test a compound for safety, tolerance, and pharmacokinetics. The Phase I trials usually employ healthy volunteers and may expose up to about 50 individuals to the drug. For therapeutic biologics and known toxic compounds, e.g. anticancer agents, only patients with the targeted illness would be used. A Phase I study is a closely monitored clinical trial of a drug or vaccine conducted in a small number of healthy volunteers; used to determine toxicity, pharmacokinetics, preferred route of administration, and safe dosage range of a drug.

Phase I (clinical trial)

The first studies to define efficacy in patients. In general, 100-300 patients would be entered into. Various closely monitored clinical trials during this phase. Dose and dosing regimens are assessed for magnitude and duration of effect during this phase. Some companies further differentiate this phase into Phase 2A and 2B (proof of efficacy and dose finding). A phase II study is a controled clinical study of a drug

Phase II (clinical trial)

	or vaccine to identify common short-term side-effects and risks associated with the drug or vaccine, to collect information on its immunogenicity and to demonstrate its efficacy conducted on a limited number of patients with disease.
Phase III (clinical trial)	Expanded controlled and uncontrolled clinical trials intended to gather additional evidence of effectiveness for specific indications and to better understand safety and drug-related adverse effects. Phase III trials are usually large multicenter trials which collect substantial safety experience and may also include specialized studies needed for labelling (e.g. paediatric or elderly, comparative agents). Thousands of patients may be included in the Phase III trials.
Placebo	A placebo is an inert substance or dosage form which is identical in appearance, flavor and odour to the active substance or dosage form. It is used as a active control in a bioassay or in a clinical study (IUPAC).
Physical dependence	Involves the development of a withdrawal syndrome following abrupt discontinuation of treatment or a substantial reduction in dose. It is a normal expected response to continuous opioid therapy and does not mean that the patient is addicted.
Potency	Potency is the dose of drug required to produce a specific effect of given intensity as compared to a standard reference. Potency is a comparative rather than an absolute expression of drug activity. Drug potency depends on both affinity and efficacy. Thus, two agonists can be equipotent, but have different intrinsic efficacies with compensating differences in affinity (IUPAC).
Pre-clinical Candidate	An optimised (having sufficient potential as a therapeutic candidate to be tested in humans) compound (small molecule) selected to enter pre-clinical development.
Prodrug	A prodrug is any compound that undergoes biotransformation before exhibiting its pharmacological effects. Prodrugs can thus be viewed as drugs containing specialized non-toxic protective groups used in a transient manner to alter or to eliminate undesirable properties in the parent molecule (IUPAC).
Protease	Any enzyme that catalyzes the cleavage of a peptide or protein.
Protease inhibitors	Class of drugs designed to inhibit the enzyme protease.

Large, complex molecule composed of amino-acids. Proteins are essential to the structure, function, and regulation of the body. Examples are hormones, enzymes, and antibodies.

Protein

Complete profile of all expressed (produced) proteins within a cell, a tissue, or an entire organism at a given time.

Proteome

Analysis of the functions and interactions of proteins in healthy tissue compared to tissue affected by a disease. Proteomics includes the the separation, identification & characterisation of proteins present in a biological sample and comparison of disease and control samples to identify "disease specific proteins". These proteins may have potential as targets for drugs or as molecular markers of disease.

Proteomics

This test, performed in rats, is the classical model of inflammatory pain. Intraplantar injection of inflammatory stimuli such as carrageenan, kaolin, or complete Freund adjuvants (CFA) induces paw swelling and increased pain sensitivity. As pain stimulus pressure is applied on the inflammed paw and gradually increased until the animal responds by vocalisation or withdrawal of the paw. Analgesics increase the pressure threshold (Randall and Selitto, Arch. Int. Pharmacodyn. **1957**, *111*, 409-419).

Randall-Selitto test

Protein in a cell or on its surface that selectively binds a specific substance (ligand). Upon binding its ligand, the receptor triggers a specific response in the cell.

Receptor

Decreased breathing rate as brought on by analgesia/anaesthesia.

Respiratory depression

Any painful state of the supporting structures of the body such as bones, ligaments, joints, tendons or muscles. Arthritis is a form of rheumatism in which the joints have become inflamed.

Rheumatism

Structure-activity relationship is the relationship between chemical structure and pharmacological activity for a series of compounds (IUPAC).

Structure-activity relationship

Refers to a substance related to, or sharing the action of opium which has a strong action such as morphine (as opposed to weak action provided by codeine) and is used for treating chronic and moderate-to-severe pain only.

Strong opioid

This model represents intense nociceptive pain induced by heat. A hot lightbeam is focussed on the tail of a mouse or rat and the latency for the withdrawal of the tail, a brisk movement called 'tail

Tail flick test

flick', is determined. Only very potent analgesics such as opioids (e.g. morphine), α_2 adrenergic agonists (e.g. clonidine) and cholinomimetics (e.g. arecoline, epibatidine) dose-dependently increase tail flick latency up to a voluntarily fixed cut off time (D'Amour and Smith; J. Pharm. Exp. Ther. **1941**, 72, 74-79).

Target

Specific biological molecule, such as an enzyme, receptor or ion channel, assumed to be relevant to a certain disease. Most drugs work by binding to a target, thereby affecting its biological function.

Target identification

Identifying a molecule (often a protein) that is instrumental to a disease process (though not necessarily directly involved), with the intention of finding a way to regulate that molecule's activity for therapeutic purposes.

Target validation

Crucial step in the drug discovery process. Following the identification of a potential disease target, target validation verifies that a drug that specifically acts on the target can have a significant therapeutic benefit in the treatment of a given disease.

Teratogen

A teratogen is a substance that produces a malformation in a foetus.

Tolerance

Associated with drug dependence, this phenomenona may occur with chronic administration of a drug. It is characterised by the necessity to progressively increase the dose of the drug to produce its original effect. Tolerance is mainly caused by neuroadaptive changes in the brain.

Transporters

Carrier proteins which transport molecules across a cell membrane.

Trigeminal neuralgia

Pain characterised by an agonising shooting pain that starts at one side of the face for no apparent reason and can last from a few seconds to a few minutes. May be associated with multiple sclerosis.

Weak opioid

Refers to a substance related to, or sharing the action of opium. They have a weak action, such as codeine (as opposed to the strong action provided by morphine), and are used for treating mild-to-moderate pain (some are available as over-the-counter products).

WHO analgesic ladder

Developed by the World Health Organization and widely regarded as the best approach to the management of acute pain, chronic non cancer pain and chronic cancer pain. The analgesic ladder ascends from non-opioids through weak opioids to strong opioids according to the severity of the pain.

A pain reaction is induced in mice or rats by intraperitoneal injection of an irritant (e.g. acetic acid, phenylquinone, acetylcholine). This induces stretching movements called 'writhings'. The number of writhings, counted during time intervals of 20-30 min, represents pain intensity and is dose-dependently reduced by analgesics. This test detects almost all types of analgesics but is sensitive to unspecific effects such as sedation (Hendershot and Forsaith, J. Pharmacol. Exp. Ther. **1959**, *125*, 237-240).

Writhing test

Index